WORK

Promoting Participation and Productivity
Through Occupational Therapy

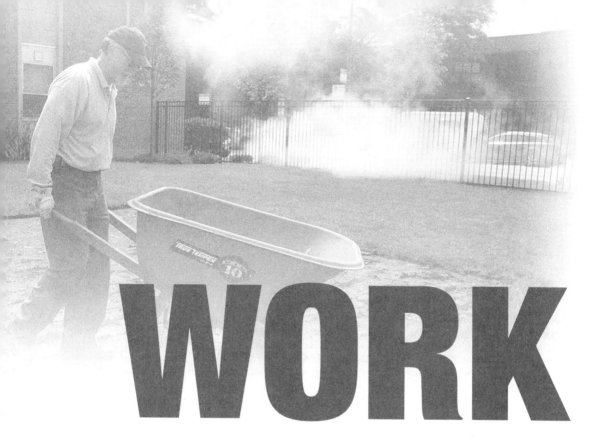

WORK

Promoting Participation and Productivity
Through Occupational Therapy

Brent Braveman, Ph.D, OTR/L, FAOTA
Director, Department of Rehabilitation Services
University of Texas MD Anderson Cancer Center
Houston, Texas

Jill J. Page, OTR/L
Page Consulting, LLC
Birmingham, Alabama

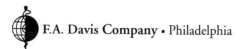 F.A. Davis Company • Philadelphia

F. A. Davis Company
1915 Arch Street
Philadelphia, PA 19103
www.fadavis.com

Copyright © 2012 by F. A. Davis Company

Printed in the United States of America

Last digit indicates print number: 10 9 8 7 6 5 4 3 2 1

Acquisitions Editor: Christa Fratantoro
Manager of Content Development: George W. Lang
Developmental Editor: Yvonne Gillam
Art and Design Manager: Carolyn O'Brien

As new scientific information becomes available through basic and clinical research, recommended treatments and drug therapies undergo changes. The author(s) and publisher have done everything possible to make this book accurate, up to date, and in accord with accepted standards at the time of publication. The author(s), editors, and publisher are not responsible for errors or omissions or for consequences from application of the book, and make no warranty, expressed or implied, in regard to the contents of the book. Any practice described in this book should be applied by the reader in accordance with professional standards of care used in regard to the unique circumstances that may apply in each situation. The reader is advised always to check product information (package inserts) for changes and new information regarding dose and contraindications before administering any drug. Caution is especially urged when using new or infrequently ordered drugs.

Library of Congress Cataloging-in-Publication Data

Work : promoting participation and productivity through occupational therapy / [edited by] Brent M. Braveman, Jill J. Page.
    p. ; cm.
Includes bibliographical references and index.
ISBN-13: 978-0-8036-0016-4
ISBN-10: 0-8036-0016-X
1. Occupational therapy. I. Braveman, Brent. II. Page, Jill J.
[DNLM: 1. Occupational Therapy—methods. 2. Occupational Therapy—psychology. 3. Employment—psychology. 4. Work—psychology. WB 555]
RM735.W578 2012
616.89'165—dc23

2011025293

Dedications

For my "Pumpkins" Ava and Alana because they make me smile.
Many thanks to my family, my dear friends who support
and guide me through life. And thank you to all of my
patients and colleagues who have taught me what occupational therapy,
work, and life is really all about.

Brent Braveman, PhD, OTR/L, FAOTA

For those who encouraged me when I thought my options were limited.
You will probably never know the impact you have had on my life.
Thank you.
Thanks and unending gratitude to my family
and my friends. Without you, the ride would be bumpy and boring.
To my professors, patients and peers who exposed me to the best
a profession can offer (you know who you are). I wake up every day
glad to be an occupational therapist because of people like you.

Jill J. Page, OTR/L

Contributors

Edna Alon, OT, MSc
Head of Occupational Therapy Department
Vocational Rehabilitation Center for the Youth
Tel Aviv-Jaffa

Paula Jo Belice, MS, OTR/L
Rush University Medical Center
Chicago, Illinois

Brent Braveman, PhD, OTR/L, FAOTA
Director of Rehabilitation Services
University of Texas MD Anderson Cancer Center
Houston, Texas

Betsy B. Burgos, EdS, MA, OTR/L, ATP
Independent Consultant/Provider
Adjunct Professor, Florida Gulf Coast University
Fort Myers, Florida

Susan M. Cahill, MAEA, OTR/L
Clinical Assistant Professor
Department of Occupational Therapy
University of Illinois at Chicago
Chicago, Illinois

Ricardo C. Carrasco, PhD, OTR/L, FAOTA
Chair, Department of Occupational Therapy
Nova Southeastern University
Tampa, Florida

Matthew B. Dodson, OTD, OTR/L
Supervisor, Outpatient Traumatic Brain Injury
Department of Occupational Therapy
Walter Reed Army Medical Center
Washington, D.C.

Rachel M. Eisfelder, MOT, OTR/L
Occupational Therapy–Rehabilitation Services
Truman Medical Center Behavioral Health
Kansas City, Missouri

Thomas F. Fisher, PhD, OTR, CCM, FAOTA
Professor and Chair
Department of Occupational Therapy
IU School of Health and Rehabilitation Sciences
Indiana University–Purdue University at Indianapolis
    Campus
Indianapolis, Indiana

Kirsty Forsyth, PhD, FCOT, OTR
Professor and Director of Firefly Research
Queen Margaret University
Edinburgh, Scotland

Rebecca Gewurtz, PhD, OT Reg (Ont.)
Assistant Professor, Occupational Therapy
School of Rehabilitation Science
McMaster University
Hamilton, Ontario

Jyothi Gupta, PhD, OT(C), OTR/L
Associate Professor
Doctor of Physical Therapy Program and
    Occupational Science and Occupational Therapy
    Program
St. Catherine University
Minneapolis, Minnesota

Susan Skees Hermes, MS, OTR/L, BCP
Level III Occupational Therapist
Children's Hospital Boston
Brookline, Massachusetts

Ev Innes, PhD MHPEd BAppSc(OT), AccOT
Associate Professor, Occupational Therapy
School of Health and Human Sciences
Southern Cross University
Coolangatta, Queensland, Australia

Vicki Kaskutas, MHS, OTD, OT/L
Assistant Professor in Occupational Therapy and
    Medicine
Washington University School of Medicine
St. Louis, Missouri

Arlene V. Kinney MEd OTR/L
Keiser University
University Department Chair, OTA Program
Fort Lauderdale, Florida

Jenica Lee, OTD, OTR/L
Chicago, Illinois

Kathryn Maltchev, OTR/L
Advisor, Health and Productivity
Health Fitness
McKinney, Texas

Debora Oliveira, Ed.S., M.S., OTR/L
Florida Agricultural and Mechanical University
Tallahassee, Florida

Jill J. Page, OTR/L
Owner, Page Consulting, LLC
Birmingham, Alabama

Susan Prior, BSc
Lead Research Practitioner
ACTIVATE Collaboration, Firefly Research
Queen Margaret University
Edinburgh, Scotland

Navah Z. Ratzon, OT, PhD
Department of Occupational Therapy
Steyer School of Health Professions
Sackler Faculty of Medicine
Tel Aviv, Israel

Dory Sabata, OTD, OTR/L, SCEM
Clinical Assistant Professor
KUMC Occupational Therapy Education
Kansas City, Kansas

T. Schejter-Margalit, OT, MSc
Research Assistant
Department of Occupational Therapy
Steyer School of Health Professions
Sackler Faculty of Medicine
Tel Aviv University
Tel Aviv, Israel

Supriya Sen, MS, OTR/L
Specialist in Occupational Therapy/Clinical Instructor
Department of Occupational Therapy
University of Illinois at Chicago
Chicago, Illinois

Shoshana Shamberg, OTR/L, MS, FAOTA
President, Abilities OT Services and Seminars
    (AOTSS), Inc.
Irlen Visual Learning Center of Maryland
Baltimore, Maryland

Annick Thibodeau, OTR/L
Return-to-Work Specialist
Georgetown, Texas

Timothy J. Wolf, OTD, MSCI, OTR/L
Assistant Professor of Occupational Therapy and
    Neurology
Washington University School of Medicine
Program in Occupational Therapy
St. Louis, Missouri

Reviewers

Susan E. Baptiste, MHSc, OTReg(Ont), FCAOT
Professor
Rehabilitation Science Department
McMaster University
Ontario, Canada

Kay Blose, MOT, OTR/L
Program Director
Occupational Therapist Assistant Program
Mountain State University
Beckley, West Virginia

Karen Cameron, PhD, OTD, MEd, OTR/L
Program Director and Associate Professor
Occupational Therapy Department
Alvernia University
Reading, Pennsylvania

Nancy E. Carson, MHS, OTR/L
Assistant Professor
Occupational Therapy Program
Medical University of South Carolina
Charleston, South Carolina

Patricia A. Crist, PfD, OTR, FAOTA
Chairperson and Professor
Occupational Therapy Program
Duquesne University
Pittsburgh, Pennsylvania

Kathleen T. Foley, PhD, OTR/L
Assistant Professor
Occupational Therapy Department
University of Alabama at Birmingham
Birmingham, Alabama

Ruth Ford, EdD, MSBS, OTR/L
Associate Dean and Program Director
Occupational Therapy Department
Belmont University
Nashville, Tennessee

Margaret Friesen, PhD, MEd, BOT, DipOT, OTReg(MB)
Assistant Professor
Occupational Therapy Department
University of Manitoba
Manitoba, Canada

Karen P. Funk, OTD, OTR, CEAS
Clinical Associate Professor
Rehabilitation Sciences, Occupational Therapy
    Department
University of Texas at El Paso
El Paso, Texas

Anita Hamilton, MOT, PhD
Assistant Professor
Occupational Therapy Department
University of Alberta
Alberta, Canada

Kimberly Hartmann, PhD, OTR/L, FAOTA
Associate Professor and Chair
Occupational Therapy Department
Quinnipiac University
Guilford, Connecticut

Liane Hewitt, DrPH, OTR/L
Associate Professor
Occupational Therapy Department
Loma Linda University
Loma Linda, California

Heather Javaherian, OTD, OTR/L
Associate Professor and Program Director
Occupational Therapy Department
Loma Linda University
Loma Linda, California

Leslie Johnson, BHSc OT
Instructor
School of Medical Rehabilitation
University of Manitoba
Manitoba, Canada

Nancy M. Klein, MS, OTR/L
Program Director
Occupational Therapist Assistant Department
St. Louis Community College
St. Louis, Missouri

Paula Kramer, PhD, OTR
Professor and Chair
Occupational Therapy Department
University of the Sciences in Philadelphia
Philadelphia, Pennsylvania

Linda M. Martin, PhD, OTR/L, FAOTA
Professor and Chair
Occupational Therapy and Community Department
Florida Gulf Coast University
Fort Myers, Florida

Christine Merchant, PhD, OTR/L
Associate Program Director
Occupational Therapy Department
Midwestern University
Glendale, Arizona

Jane O'Brien, PhD, OTR
Associate Professor
Occupational Therapy Department
University of New England
North Waterboro, Maine

Colleen Schneck, ScD, OTR/L, FAOTA
Professor and Chair
Occupational Therapy Department
Eastern Kentucky University
Richmond, Kentucky

Caroline Storr, BSc(OT), OT(C), MBA
Academic Coordinator of Clinical Education
Occupational Therapy Department
McGill University
Quebec, Canada

Acknowledgments

We would like to acknowledge the following people for their assistance in preparing this textbook and thank them for their thoughtful feedback, guidance, and support.

Marcia Finlayson, PhD, OT(C), OTR/L
University of Illinois at Chicago

Kathleen T. Foley, PhD, OTR/L
University of Alabama at Birmingham

Joy Hammel, PhD, OTR/L, FAOTA
University of Illinois at Chicago

Gary Kielhofner, DrPh, OTR/L, FAOTA
University of Illinois at Chicago

Deborah B. Pitts, Ph.D. (cand.), MBA, OTR/L, BCMH, CPRP
University of Southern California

Renee Taylor, PhD
University of Illinois at Chicago

Contents in Brief

Contents

SECTION II:
An Overview of Occupational Therapy Work-Related Service Settings and Populations 117

CHAPTER 8: **Older Workers: Maintaining a Worker Role and Returning
to the Workplace 172**

Jyothi Gupta and Dory Sabata

CHAPTER 9: **Mental Health and Work 198**

Rachel Eisfelder and Rebecca Gewurtz

CHAPTER 10: **Volunteerism and Play: Alternative Paths to Work Participation 221**

Brent Braveman

Purpose and Focus of the Book

Work is an area of occupation identified in the Occupational Therapy Practice Framework and is a major focus of time and energy for a majority of adults in modern society. Work can take the form of paid competitive employment, supported employment, or volunteer efforts, and the nature of work can vary tremendously in focus and in its requirements of workers. Work can require a complex mix of physical, social, cognitive, and perceptual skills, and occupational performance within the worker role is heavily influenced by interaction with the social and physical environments.

Our preparation for and involvement in work spans most of our lifetimes, starting in childhood as we learn habits that support the adoption of productive roles later in life. Occupational therapy practitioners provide transitional services to adolescents and young adults under the Individuals with Disabilities Education Act (IDEA) and through work-related services to develop skills or respond to challenges and support for continuing productive roles as we age. As the dream for a funded retirement beginning at the age of 65 has become more difficult to achieve, and as the life span has increased and some workers are choosing to remain in the workforce until late in their lives, the needs for work-related occupational therapy services with older adults has increased.

"Work and Industry" was named as one of six of the American Occupational Therapy Association's Centennial Vision priority areas. In the process of developing the Centennial Vision, drivers of change for occupational therapy services were identified, among them (a) aging and longevity, (b) the Internet and the Information Age, (c) diversity of the population, (d) stress and depression, and (e) changes in lifestyle choices and values. Each of these drivers influences the environment in which modern workers function and has implications for the level of need for occupational therapy services.

Occupational therapy practitioners are uniquely prepared to assess the influence of these drivers of change on work occupational performance and to help workers adapt to challenges to performance. Occupational therapy practitioners address work-related practice in a range of settings, including school systems, medical model settings, private practices, and the workplace itself. The assessment and intervention strategies utilized also include a wide variety of approaches, and practitioners must remain abreast of current practice trends and developments in theory and evidence. Practitioners must also continually scan the environment for changes in the many policies and laws at the local, state, national, and even international levels for their impact on the delivery of work related services.

Topics and Organization

This textbook provides a broad overview of work and work-related occupational therapy services. Because occupational therapy practitioners provide work-related services to a diverse group of consumers and clients and in a wide variety of settings, it is not practical to provide in-depth information on specific assessment and intervention strategies in every area. As a result, the authors of each chapter were asked to provide an introduction and overview of the topics at hand that can be supplemented with more specific information from other sources.

This text is divided into four general sections, although, as with any complex topic, it is important to recognize the interconnection of the chapters and not rigidly separate them. There are many ways that we must "connect the dots" as we consider how to comprehensively evaluate and intervene with any client.

An Introduction to Work and Occupational Therapy Work-Related Services

Chapters 1, 2, and 3 provide an introduction and overview of work in today's world, including cultural perspectives. The critically important development of the worker role across the life span and an occupational therapy perspective on work is discussed. Chapter 4 introduces the most commonly used occupational therapy conceptual practice models and related knowledge used in work-related practice. These models are discussed in more depth in later chapters in the book, and examples of specific applications are provided. Chapter 5 reviews the roles of the occupational therapist and the occupational therapy assistant in work-related occupational therapy and describes the opportunities for teamwork, partnerships, and autonomy.

1

Work in the Modern World
The History and Current Trends in Workers, the Workplace, and Working

Brent Braveman

Key Concepts

The following are key concepts addressed in this chapter:

- Work has played a major societal role throughout the world's history, and changes in the organization of work, its meaning, and the nature of work performed influence how we view working today.
- The occupational therapy profession has a long history of involvement in work-related practice grounded in the moral treatment of the mentally ill and the rehabilitation of wounded soldiers as a result of two world wars. Today, occupational therapy personnel provide a wide range of work-related interventions in a variety of settings and with a variety of populations across the life span.
- Occupational therapy work-related practice and vocational rehabilitation in general have been greatly influenced in the last century by legislation that protects the worker and persons with disabilities and provides resources to foster their participation in the workplace and in society.
- There have been dramatic shifts in the nature of work in modern society, and it is critical that occupational therapy personnel in the area of work-related practice are aware of trends taking place in work, the workplace, and the workforce.

Case Introduction—Opportunities in Work-Related Practice

When Hannah began her occupational therapy education, she assumed she was headed for practice in a traditional setting. She had volunteered in the occupational therapy department at a rehabilitation hospital prior to applying to graduate school and had a cousin who was an occupational therapy practitioner in a school system. However, as Hannah progressed through her program, she became aware of the full range of opportunities for occupational therapy practitioners and the increasingly varied settings in which they work. One of these areas is work-related practice.

At her state occupational therapy association conference, Hannah attended a presentation on Becoming an Entrepreneur, given by an occupational therapy practitioner who owned her own company that provided worksite injury prevention and rehabilitation services. Upon returning to school, she spent some time exploring the American Occupational Therapy Association's (AOTA's) website and learned that work and industry is one of its six focus areas for 2017, the year the occupational therapy profession will celebrate its 100th anniversary. Realizing that she would soon have to begin the process of choosing sites for her level I and level II fieldwork experiences, Hannah decided to learn more about occupational therapy's involvement in work-related practice and the seemingly growing career opportunities in this area.

Introduction

In today's world, one thing is sure: in one form or another, most of us will spend much of our adult lives working. In 2007, the average American who was employed full time spent 7.6 hours per day working (U.S. Bureau of Labor Statistics, 2008a). That means that the adult who begins working at age 22 and retires at age 65 and who receives 3 weeks of vacation each year will work over 80,000 hours in his or her adult life! Yet retiring at age 65 is becoming less common, and in difficult and turbulent economic times, a growing number of Americans have to work far beyond the average number of hours. Many Americans work at jobs at which they do not receive benefits such as paid time off. Others, particularly white-collar workers, often work hours that far exceed a typical 40-hour workweek. Elsewhere in the world, it is a slightly different story. In France, the average workweek is 35 hours. By law, French citizens are guaranteed 5 weeks of vacation and 12 holidays per year. By October 24 each year, the average American has worked as many hours as the average European will for the entire year (Tracy, 2007). In turbulent global economic times such as those experienced in 2009 and 2010, the work patterns of men and women around the world may be reexamined. However, regardless of cultural influences, most adults in modern society will spend the majority of their lives working.

The forms of work we perform have almost infinite variations and combinations of physical labor, cognitive and perceptual processing and problem solving, creative expression, and environmental demands and supports. However, whether an individual spends his or her day pounding a hammer, typing at a computer, bringing meals to patrons in a restaurant, or driving a tractor and feeding animals, all forms of work have some things in common. *Work* is a means of providing a financial or other source of reward to support our daily existence and help us to meet our need for food and shelter. And whether or not a person's work is highly valued by the individual or by society as a whole, working holds some meaning for the individual and is tied in some way to his or her identity as a worker and a person. Occupational therapy practitioners analyze the characteristics and demands of work as well as the capacities, interests, and characteristics of workers to understand how work fits in each client's life and to facilitate improved occupational performance.

Chapter 1 reviews how work has evolved and introduces you to work in modern society, particularly from the perspective of occupational therapy. The chapter considers the various functions of work and the different roles that working plays in people's lives as well as the varied meanings attached to work and the worker role. Important trends in the workplace and their possible implications on workers, particularly those with disabilities, are considered. Key *drivers of change,* such as the aging of the population, evolving technologies, and increasing racial diversity and immigration, and the implications of these drivers, are described. Finally, the potential impact that injury or disability can have on an individual's capacity for work is introduced here and explored throughout the text.

A Short History of Work

From a historical perspective, modern views of work as a positive and important activity that provides a significant contribution to individual meaning and life satisfaction are a recent development. The idea that work has intrinsic value for its own sake has not always been part of the human consciousness. Throughout much of our world's history, work was viewed as difficult and degrading. Working hard was not the expectation for everyone in early classical or medieval cultures. Work was seen as necessary to satisfy material needs, but philosophers such as Plato and Aristotle made it clear that most men labored "in order that the minority, the élite, might engage in pure exercises of the mind—art, philosophy, and politics" (Hill, 2005).

The period between roughly 476 AD and 1400 AD is usually called the *Middle Ages* or the *medieval period*. During this era, war was almost a constant in what is now Western Europe, and most workers were focused on daily life and survival. Religious and other leaders began to have an influence on how work was perceived and emphasized the positive outcomes of work, including self-sufficiency, decreased reliance on the church and society for survival, and improved quality of life. The nobles who resided in rural areas provided kings and rulers with protection in exchange for land. Working days were extremely long, and peasants worked the land in what was largely an agricultural economy (Fig. 1.1); in return they received protection and ownership rights for small plots of land (Davenport, 2007). Some trades and industries began to prosper in cities where work life was somewhat easier.

The population decrease caused by the plague during the late medieval period (1347–1352) led to a serious economic depression. Nearly 50 percent of the population in

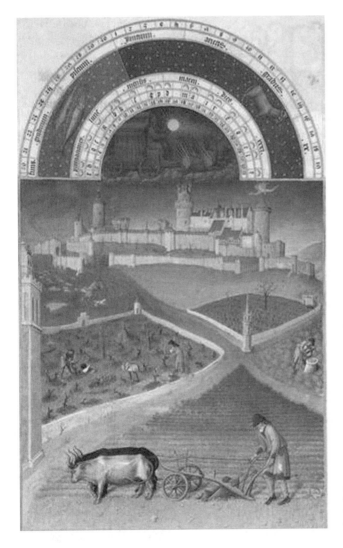

Figure 1.1 During the medieval period, workdays were long. Many workers lived on land owned by nobles and were involved primarily in agriculture.

Europe died. Merchants and trades people had fewer customers to whom they could sell their goods, and economic hardship increased. Because the plague was spread through close contact with others, those who could afford to do so abandoned the cities. As incidence of the plague decreased in the late 15th century, populations began to increase again, resulting in new demand for goods and services. A new middle class began to emerge as bankers, merchants, and tradespeople once again had a market for their goods and services. The types of work that people performed began to increase in variety, and the notion that a person would devote his life to the development and honing of skills in a particular type of work or craft became more common.

The *Renaissance* (meaning rebirth) was a cultural movement that began in Italy and spread throughout the rest of Europe, spanning roughly the 14th to the 17th century. During this time, knowledge from Greek, Arabic, and other cultures had a growing influence, especially in the areas of mathematics and science. The Renaissance reached its peak at different times in different cultures, beginning in Italy with the visual arts, and worked its way as far as England, where its achievements are most recognized in drama, theater, and literature (W.W. Norton and Company, 2008). The Renaissance saw the rise of strong central governments and an increasingly urban economy based on commerce and exchange of services rather than relying primarily on agriculture. Trade increased greatly during the Renaissance, and the exchange of metals, spices, and other materials had a dramatic impact on working life, resulting in further development of varied forms of work.

From 1500 to 1600 AD, populations in Europe grew dramatically, especially in cities. Work became central to survival, and new values arose regarding the place of work in society. German social scientist Max Weber described a set of values associated with the rise of industrial society, commonly called the *protestant work ethic* in writings first published in 1930. In brief, the protestant work ethic holds that we fulfill our duty to God by diligence and hard work with the resulting accumulation of goods acting as a reassuring sign of our eventual salvation (Weber, 2002).

The *Modern Era* generally refers to the period from the beginning of the *Industrial Revolution* in the 18th century and continuing to today. During the Industrial Revolution (approximately 1760–1830), major changes took place in agriculture, manufacturing, and transportation that spread throughout Europe and the world (Inikori, 2002). The mechanization of processes in the textile and iron-making industries and the refined use of coal resulted in a shift from a primarily manual labor market to an industry- and service-based economy that has continued until current times. The development of factories was a major draw to urban areas and fostered the development of cities. In turn, workers looked more to others to produce goods that they purchased to survive rather than growing or making their own goods, and this further fostered the initial development of a service economy. Women and children made up a large percentage of the workforce in some industries, such as the textile industry, while men were often involved in industries such as metalwork, building, and coal (Ross, 2007). The idea of work as a *calling* had been replaced by the concept of public usefulness. Workweeks were long: workers commonly worked more than 60 hours per week, and work conditions were often poor with many threats to workers' health (Hill, 2005). The values of self-sufficiency and hard work exuded during this time continue to influence current views of those who work and provide for themselves and those who do not but rely instead on social assistance.

During the 19th century, manufacturing became one of the dominant features of the U.S. economic system, particularly in the Northeast. By the early 20th century, the majority of Americans lived in towns or cities so they could work in factories (Mick and Wolff, 2008). The time between World War I and World War II is sometimes called the *Machine Age*. It was marked by the mass production of high-volume goods, including the automobile, on moving assembly lines; advances in architecture, including skyscrapers; gigantic production machinery, especially for producing and working metal; and vastly improved transportation services, including shipping, rail, and air travel. These advances had dramatic impacts on daily life. Some of these influences included mass marketing and consumerism, replacement of skilled crafts with low-skill laborers, growth of large corporations, and growth of strong labor unions in response. These changes continued to influence how we conceptualize work as a place we go to outside of the home and resulted in organizations (e.g., companies or corporations) assuming a central and lasting role as employers. Changes in work occurred, including a reduction of the typical workweek to 48 hours, and paid holidays were introduced by many employers (Ross, 2007).

> *These advances had dramatic impacts on daily life. Some of these influences included mass marketing and consumerism, replacement of skilled crafts with low-skill laborers, growth of large corporations, and growth of strong labor unions in response. These changes continued to influence how we conceptualize work as a place we go to outside of the home and resulted in organizations (e.g., companies or corporations) assuming a central and lasting role as employers.*

More efficient assembly-line techniques introduced in the early 20th century meant fewer workers could produce more goods at a lower cost. During the latter part of the century, productivity increases as a result of improvements in communication and other technologies caused a similar result. At the end of the 20th century, manufacturing accounted for approximately 30 percent of total gross domestic product in the United States (U.S. Department of Labor, 2000). Since 1970, the largest growth in jobs has been in the service sector (e.g., wholesale and retail trade, finance, real estate, transportation) with an increase of over 19 million jobs in the 10-year period between 1998 and 2008.

The information age (1970 to present) arose with the use of computer-based information systems to convert, store, protect, process, transmit, and retrieve information. Technological advances in this field have changed lifestyles around the world, and new industries focusing on the exchange of information and communication have flourished. As a result, there has been a shift from blue-collar jobs in manufacturing and industry to white-collar jobs in technical, managerial, and clerical positions. Some jobs in manufacturing and industry have also become more technical and necessitated a higher level of thinking on the job as machines were interfaced with computers and control systems became more complex (Hill, 2005). While Industrial Age blue-collar jobs often required low discretion, limited decision making, and limited judgment on the part of workers, information age jobs are characterized as the opposite. The term *knowledge worker* was coined by Peter Drucker to describe a new type of worker in today's society. A knowledge worker works with and produces *information* as a product (Drucker, 1957).

Today, work, workers, working, and the workplace continue to change. The service sector continues to grow, while there has been a decrease in agricultural and manufacturing jobs. Professional and business services and health care and social assistance, the industry sectors with the largest projected employment growth, will add 8.1 million jobs by 2016, more than half of the projected increase in total employment (U.S. Department of Labor, 2007). Entrepreneurism has become a major driving force in the United States and abroad. Small firms are responsible for one-half of the output of the private sector in the United States. Small companies comprise 96 percent of all exporters of U.S. goods, and 53 percent of the time these businesses are operated from home (U.S. Department of Labor, 2008). Options for working from home by *telecommuting* have increased, and in an effort to attract and retain workers, many employers offer flexibility in work hours and settings (Fig. 1.2).

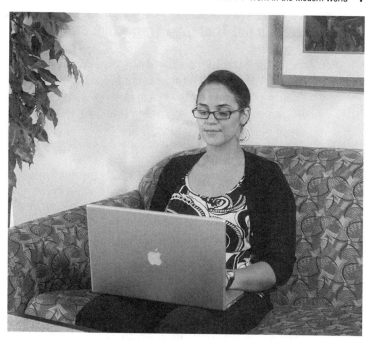

Figure 1.2 Workers today have many options that promote flexibility, including working from home or from remote locations, even while traveling.

The worker of today and tomorrow is also changing. It is projected that the percentage of those aged 55 and older in the U.S. workforce will grow by 46.7 percent, or nearly 5.5 times the growth rate for the labor force overall. Increases in the labor force will vary by race. Whites will remain the largest race group of workers, composing 79.6 percent of the labor force by 2016. The number of blacks will grow by 16.2 percent and will constitute 12.3 percent of the labor force. Asians will continue to be the fastest-growing race group, increasing by 29.9 percent, and will make up 5.3 percent of the labor force by 2016. Thirty-four percent of all businesses are owned by women, and the number of minority-owned businesses has increased by 168 percent. Unfortunately, the employment picture is not as positive for persons with disabilities. Only 52.3 percent of people with disabilities are employed compared to an employment rate of 82.1 percent for persons without disabilities. This picture has remained fairly stable despite that 72 percent of working-age people with disabilities indicate that they want to work (U.S. Department of Labor, 2008).

While much is often made of concerns over the effects of the aging workforce on the U.S. workplace, the fact is that the U.S. population is growing, and a growing population means a larger labor force, higher levels of production, more services, more creativity, more consumption, and a larger potential tax base. Over the last 25 years, Europe's young population (aged 14 and under) has decreased by 21 percent, and currently more elderly than children live in the European Union. In terms of workers and the workforce, much of Europe faces the opposite problem of the United States (European Union Center of North Carolina, 2008).

Many of these trends are explored in more depth throughout this text. They all have implications for work-related occupational therapy practice. To be most effective, we need to understand how the world of work is changing, how those changes impact the worker of today, and the opportunities they provide to assist our clients to pursue work as an important area of occupational performance.

An Occupational Therapy Perspective on Work

Occupational therapy practitioners help people *live life to its fullest* by engaging them in daily life activities that they find meaningful and purposeful. The profession's interest in human beings' ability to engage in everyday life activities characterizes the *domain* of occupational therapy. A profession's domain is those areas of human experience in which members of the profession offer assistance to others. The broad term that occupational therapy practitioners use to capture the breadth and meaning of "everyday life activity" is *occupation* (AOTA, 2008b).

Figure 1.3 and Table 1.1 represent the domain of occupational therapy. Occupational therapy practitioners consider all of the many types of occupations in which any individual, group, or population might engage within their domain of practice. *Work* is one of seven *areas of occupation* identified in the *Occupational Therapy Practice Framework: Domain and Process (OTPF)*. The other six areas of occupation include activities of daily living, instrumental activities of daily living, education, play, leisure, and social participation. No one area of occupation is more important than another, and the meaning and value of any occupation is always considered from the point of view of the person, group, organization, or community with which you are working. Table 1.2 summarizes examples of areas related to work that occupational therapy practitioners might address that are included in the OTPF. Included are activities needed for engaging in paid employment as well as in volunteer activities that might also be considered as work.

The definition of *occupation* varies in nuanced ways from source to source. In the OTPF, occupations are defined as "activities of everyday life, named, organized, and given value and meaning by individuals and a culture. Occupation is everything people do to occupy themselves including looking after themselves . . . enjoying life . . . and contributing to the social and economic fabric of their communities" (AOTA, 2008b). In the model of human occupation, a widely used occupational therapy conceptual practice model, an occupation is defined as "the doing of work, play or activities of daily living within a temporal, physical, and socio-cultural context that characterizes much of human life" (Kielhofner, 2008). Similar definitions are offered within other conceptual practice models.

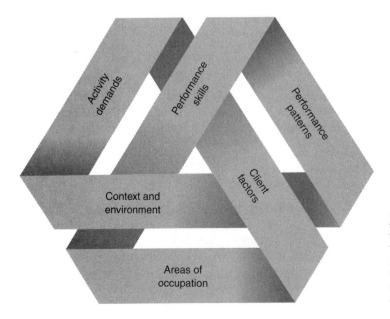

Figure 1.3 A representation of the Domain of Occupational Therapy from the Occupational Therapy Practice Framework: Domain and Process. Reprinted with permission from AOTA (American Occupational Therapy Association, 2008b).

Table 1.1 Domain of Occupational Therapy

Areas of Occupation	Client Factors	Performance Skills	Performance Patterns	Context and Environment	Activity Demands
• Activities of daily living (ADL) • Instrumental activities of daily living (IADL) • Rest and sleep • Education • Work • Play • Leisure • Social participation	• Values • Beliefs and spirituality • Body functions • Body structures	• Sensory perceptual • Motor and praxis • Emotional regulation • Cognitive • Communication • Social	• Habits • Routines • Roles • Rituals	• Cultural • Physical • Social • Personal • Spiritual • Temporal • Virtual	• Objects used and their properties • Space demands • Social demands • Sequencing and timing • Required actions • Required body functions • Required body structures

Reprinted with permission from AOTA (American Occupational Therapy Association, 2008a).

Table 1.2 Work as an Area of Occupation

Areas of Work-Related Occupation	Brief Description
Employment interests and pursuits	Identifying and selecting work opportunities based on assets, limitations, likes, and dislikes relative to work
Employment seeking and acquisition	Identifying and recruiting for job opportunities; completing, submitting, and reviewing appropriate application materials; preparing for interviews; participating in interviews and following up afterward; discussing job benefits; and finalizing negotiations
Job performance	Job performance including work skills and patterns; time management; relationships with coworkers, managers, and customers; creation, production, and distribution of products and services; initiation, sustainment and completion of work; and compliance with work norms and procedures
Retirement preparation and adjustment	Determining aptitudes, developing interests and skills, and selecting appropriate avocational pursuits
Volunteer exploration	Determining community causes, organizations, or opportunities for unpaid "work" in relationship to personal skills, interests, location, and time available
Volunteer participation	Performing unpaid "work" activities for the benefit of identified selected causes, organizations, or facilities

Reprinted with permission (American Occupational Therapy Association, 2008b).

The construct of an occupation is beautiful in its simplicity in that we are all familiar with occupations as they exist in our everyday experience. The use of the term in practice with individuals outside of the profession has proven to be problematic at times, however, because of confusion over its meaning and the use of *occupation* by other disciplines and laypersons when referring to a particular *job* or *profession*. This can be particularly true in work-related practice. As noted earlier, *work* is an area of occupation encompassing an enormous number and wide variety of individual occupations. Because the focus of this text is on the *area of occupation* called *work* and work-related occupational therapy intervention focuses on facilitating occupational performance (working), *work* and *working* are used for the most part throughout the text. This should not be misunderstood to lessen the importance and centrality of the term *occupation* in work-related practice. Work-related practice can and should be both *occupation based* and *evidence based*.

Occupational therapy's involvement in work-related practice can be traced back to the roots of the profession. As noted in the previous section, social and economic events have influenced views of work and the role work has played in society throughout our history. In the late 1700s, a new political agenda and social movement emerged in Western Europe that included a shift in attitudes toward the treatment of mentally ill persons. These persons had previously been subjected to harsh treatments such as regular *bleeding* and were chained up in prisonlike institutions (Ross, 2007). The focus of the new *moral treatment* was to replace brutality with kindness and idleness with occupation. Various forms of manual labor, including agriculture, tailoring, shoemaking, and sewing were some of the occupations used in the moral treatment of the insane (Gordon, 2009). Work activities were "often in keeping with gender and class norms of the time and women often were occupied with domestic work, knitting or sewing and men were occupied with manual labor such as horticulture, bricklaying, basket making or tailoring" (Ross, 2007).

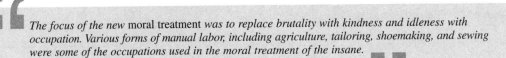

The focus of the new moral treatment *was to replace brutality with kindness and idleness with occupation. Various forms of manual labor, including agriculture, tailoring, shoemaking, and sewing were some of the occupations used in the moral treatment of the insane.*

This more compassionate approach also took hold in the United States in the mid-1800s. King and Olson (2009) note that soon after this movement began in the United States, "Work-related therapy was also used for people with physical disabilities to promote good health." From the first meeting of the *National Society for the Promotion of Occupational Therapy* (NSPOT; later renamed the American Occupational Therapy Association) in 1917, work-related practice was included within the scope of occupational therapy intervention. The titles "work cure" and "ergotherapy" were considered as possible titles for the profession before "occupational therapy" was adopted. Early founders of the profession, including T. B. Kidner and George Barton, advocated for the use of occupation as preliminary to and highly valued in vocational rehabilitation (Jacobs and Baker, 2000). The production of handcrafts and other goods was predominantly used in the therapeutic interventions of early occupational therapy. However, because the sale of these items provided financial assistance to the institutions that housed the clients and the clients received some profits from their sale, these interventions were in essence "work" related.

Until World War I (1914–1918), the occupational therapy profession was concerned primarily with working with persons with mental illness. However, as the United States became involved in the war, concern increased over rising numbers of returning soldiers with physical impairments. NSPOT collaborated with the military to recruit and train "reconstruction aides" to meet the needs of the injured. World War II presented a similar demand for those with skills to work with returning injured and disabled soldiers, and significant growth occurred in the profession of occupational therapy (Gordon, 2009). Federal legislation, including the Vocational Education Act of 1917, the Soldiers Rehabilitation Act of 1918, and the Civilian Vocational Rehabilitation Act of 1920, supported the training of reconstruction aides and provided formal support for the provision of work-related services for returning solders and to the general public (Jacobs and Baker, 2000). Table 1.3 briefly summarizes these acts and other key federal legislation related to vocational rehabilitation and work-related practice over the last century. Some of this legislation is addressed in more depth in later chapters.

Between World War I and World War II, a number of key events and movements laid the groundwork for occupational therapy to continue to develop its involvement in work-related practice. Theoretical developments in the field of psychology, including the psychodynamic paradigm (which emphasizes inner drives and past experiences in helping to explain current behavior) and behaviorism (which proposes that all actions of

Table 1.3 Key Legislation Relevant to Vocational Rehabilitation and Work-Related Occupational Therapy

Year and Name of Act	Focus of the Legislation
1917 Smith-Hughes Act	Federal funding for state vocational educational programs
1935 Social Security Act (Pub.L. 74-271)	Emphasized that vocational rehabilitation of persons with disabilities is a social responsibility and provided permanent authorization of the federal Vocational Rehabilitation Program
1943 Barden-LaFollette Act	Expanded the VR program, including emotionally disturbed and mentally retarded; began physical restoration services; authorized separate blind agencies to administer the VR program; and required states to submit a written state plan to the federal government
1954 Social Security Amendments (Pub.L. 83-761)	Established the Social Security disability program under Title II provisions for Social Security Disability Insurance (SSDI) to provide monthly disability insurance payments to workers with disabilities and their eligible dependents
1956 Social Security Amendments (Pub.L. 84-880)	Created the Social Security Disability Insurance (SSDI) program for disabled workers aged 50–64
1960 Social Security Amendments (Pub.L. 86-778)	Eliminated the restriction that disabled workers receiving SSDI benefits had to be aged 50 or older
1965 Vocational Rehabilitation Act Amendments (Pub.L. 89-333)	Expanded services to a broader population of rehabilitation clients and provided federal funds to help construct new rehabilitation centers and workshops
1973 Rehabilitation Act (Pub.L. 93-112)	Established the priority to serve persons with severe disabilities. Changed Vocational Rehabilitation Act to Rehabilitation Act. Established Title VI civil rights protection for people with disabilities, including Section 504, which prohibits discrimination against otherwise qualified persons with disabilities in any program or activity receiving federal funds
1980 Social Security Act Amendments (Pub.L. 96-265) and the related Omnibus Reconciliation Act (Pub.L. 96-499)	Authorized special cash payments (Section 1619[a]) and continued Medicaid eligibility (Section 1619[b]) for individuals who receive Supplemental Security Income (SSI) benefits but nonetheless engage in substantial gainful activity
1986 Rehabilitation Act Amendments (Pub.L. 99-506)	Broadened the Act's purposes, including rehabilitation engineering and supported employment services, and emphasizing services for persons with severe disabilities and individualized service planning. Specified that states must plan for individuals making the transition from school to work
1990 Americans with Disabilities Act (ADA; Pub.L. 101-336)	Provided a clear and comprehensive national mandate for the elimination of discrimination against individuals with disabilities, including titles on employment, public services (general and transportation), public accommodations and services operated by private entities, telecommunications, and miscellaneous provisions

(table continues on page 12)

Table 1.3 Key Legislation Relevant to Vocational Rehabilitation and Work-Related Occupational Therapy—cont'd

Year and Name of Act	Focus of the Legislation
1990 Individuals with Disabilities Education Act Amendments (IDEA; Pub.L. 101-476)	Renamed the Education of the Handicapped Act and reauthorized programs under the Act to improve support services to students with disabilities, especially in the areas of transition and assistive technology. Placement in the least restrictive environment was emphasized
1991 Civil Rights Act (Pub.L. 102-166)	Reversed numerous U.S. Supreme Court decisions that restricted the protections in employment discrimination cases and authorized compensatory and punitive damages under Title V of the Rehabilitation Act and Title I of the ADA
1994 School-to-Work Opportunities Act (Pub.L. 103-239)	Authorized funds for programs to assist students, including students with disabilities, in the transition from school to work
1996 Health Insurance Portability and Accountability Act (Pub.L. 104-191)	Improved access to health care for millions of Americans by guaranteeing that private health insurance is available, portable, and renewable and limiting preexisting condition exclusions
1998 Workforce Investment Act (WIA; Pub.L. 105-220)	Consolidated several employment and training programs including the Rehabilitation Act into statewide systems of workforce development partnerships. Required cooperative partnerships to create the statewide workforce development systems. Within the Rehabilitation Act, consumer choice is enhanced and the State Rehabilitation Advisory Council is renamed the State Rehabilitation Council and given expanded responsibilities to work with the state agency to jointly develop, agree to, and review state goals and priorities
1999 Ticket to Work and Work Incentives Improvement Act (TWIIA; Pub.L. 106-170)	Established the Ticket to Work and Self-Sufficiency Program to provide SSDI and SSI beneficiaries with a ticket they can use to obtain vocational rehabilitation services, employment services, and other support services from an employment network of their choice. It includes an array of provisions to eliminate Social Security and Medicaid disincentives to employment and to promote the development of supports and incentives for persons with disabilities to work
2008 Americans with Disabilities Amendments Act (ADAAA; Pub.L. 110-325)	Rejected strict interpretation of the definition of disability; prohibited the consideration of mitigating measures such as medication, prosthetics, and assistive technology in determining whether an individual has a disability; and clarified who qualifies for receipt of reasonable accommodations in the workplace

Reprinted with permission (Haworth, 2008).

an organism—including acting, thinking, and feeling—can and should be regarded as behaviors) were influential, as were the dramatic advances in science and medicine. World War II (1939–1945) resulted in greatly increased demand for rehabilitation services to treat injured soldiers. While the military reconditioning programs addressed the stated objective of assisting soldiers to return to civilian life and responsibilities, including vocational pursuits, vocational readiness was not the main focus of occupational therapy at this time; it tended to focus instead on reducing disability and improving activities of daily living (Gordon, 2009; Jacobs and Baker, 2000).

In the post–World War II era, continuing advances in medicine and rehabilitation and further federal legislation, including the Vocational Rehabilitation Act Amendments (Hill-Burton Act, Pub.L. 83-565) in 1954, fostered increased attention to vocational rehabilitation. This act included extensive revision to the original act: financing improvements and funding for research and demonstration projects, counselor education, and construction of rehabilitation facilities (Haworth, 2008). Changes in social security, including the creation of Social Security Disability Insurance (SSDI) in 1956 and expansion of covered persons in 1960, provided public funds for disabled workers. Occupational therapy practitioners in mental health played a central role in assessing work skills and work placement, and concurrent improvements in pharmacological treatment of mental illness supported the development of industrial rehabilitation programs in psychiatric institutions. Despite these improvements, little progress was made during the 1960s in occupational therapy's involvement in vocational rehabilitation outside of mental health settings, and the profession paid increased attention to physical rehabilitation.

The 1960s and 1970s was a time of questioning and reflection for the occupational therapy profession as it examined its focus in the midst of quickly evolving medical science. Effective treatments for tuberculosis and poliomyelitis (two major client groups for occupational therapy) had been introduced in the 1950s with great success. There had been a shift toward specialization in the profession, and practitioners began addressing particular aspects of the person rather than the holistic needs of the person (Ross, 2007). Increasingly, occupational therapy scholars raised concern about the trend for the profession to drift toward more technical application of skills and more reliance on *mechanistic* or *reductionistic* paradigms to guide the profession. Educational programs for occupational therapy practitioners had increasingly emphasized content related to neurology, biomechanics, and other knowledge related to physical rehabilitation. While this helped to advance practice specifically related to physical aspects of occupational performance, less attention was paid to psychosocial elements of occupational performance. However, Mary Reilly and others began to call for a return to the most important elements of the field's first paradigm, and Reilly led the development of a renewed focus on occupation. The resulting concepts, *occupational behavior*, introduced themes such as the motivation for occupation, the organization of occupation in time through habits and roles, and the importance of the environment in supporting or impeding adaptation (Kielhofner, 2009).

At the same time, legislation during the 1960s, 1970s, and 1980s provided increased incentives for the professions of occupational therapy to become more involved in work-related practice and vocational rehabilitation (see Table 1.3). Employers and health insurers also developed a deeper interest in preventing injury in the workplace and aiding injured workers to return more quickly to the workplace. As a result, programs and interventions designed to assess a worker's capacity to work, to improve this capacity (e.g., improve capacity for occupational performance), and to prevent or minimize long-term impairment and disability were increasingly developed. Occupational therapy practitioners became involved in *industrial rehabilitation* and *work hardening* programs. The AOTA produced several official documents describing the role of occupational therapy in work-related practice. These included a position paper named "The Role of the Occupational Therapist in the Vocational Rehabilitation Process" (1980) and "Work Hardening Guidelines" (1986). These programs of the 1980s were well received, and in 1988, the Commission on Accreditation of Rehabilitation Facilities (CARF) developed accreditation standards to help standardize the content and quality of these programs. Jacobs and Baker (2000) noted that "this document primarily ensured uniformity and quality within work rehabilitation and stressed a comprehensive approach to work therapy involving a coordinated interdisciplinary team of occupational therapy practitioners, physical therapists, psychologists, and vocational specialists. The programs addressed both biomechanical and psychosocial work injury management problems."

Over the last two decades, considerable advances have been made in the profession's involvement in work-related practice concurrently with additional public support and concern for helping people, including those with disabilities, to enter and remain in the workforce. As a result of the efforts of many leaders in the field, occupational therapy has regained its focus on occupation as a profession, and this focus includes trends in work-related practice such as the development of *onsite work programs*. The focus of these programs is to return an injured worker to work as quickly as possible and to provide intervention at the worksite by involving the worker in real-life, real-job work occupations. This transformation has required the field to recapture its original orientation and retain important technology accumulated during the mechanistic paradigm. It also has required that the field correct some of the problems that surfaced during the mechanistic paradigm (Kielhofner, 2009). There has been steady focus on developing the science of the occupational therapy profession, including development and validation of conceptual models of practice upon which work-related practice can be based. Among other models, advances in knowledge have been gained in the biomechanical, cognitive, motor-control, and model of human occupation conceptual practice models. These efforts have included the development of tools for application of theory in practice, such as assessments based on occupational therapy conceptual practice models, including "The Worker Role Interview" and "The Work Environment Impact Scale" (Braveman, et al., 2005; Fenger, Braveman, and Kielhofner, 2008; Moore-Corner, Kielhofner, and Olson, 1998). There has been renewed focus on returning to practice based not only on the use of occupation but also on evidence (Finlayson and Braveman, 2005).

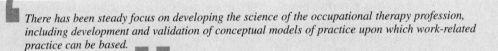

There has been steady focus on developing the science of the occupational therapy profession, including development and validation of conceptual models of practice upon which work-related practice can be based.

Several key pieces of legislation were passed in the 1990s: the Americans with Disabilities Act of 1990 (ADA; Pub.L. 101-336), the Health Insurance Portability and Accountability Act of 1996 (HIPAA; Pub.L. 104-191), and the Ticket to Work and Work Incentives Improvement Act of 1999 (TWWIIA; Pub.L. 106-170). The ADA provided a clear national mandate to eliminate discrimination against individuals with disabilities. The act includes five titles: (1) employment, (2) public services (general and transportation), (3), public accommodations and services operated by private entities, (4) telecommunications, and (5) miscellaneous provisions. Chapter 16 provides an in-depth discussion of the ADA and its relationship to work-related practice. The HIPAA improved access to health care for millions of Americans by guaranteeing that private health insurance is available, portable, and renewable and by limiting preexisting condition exclusions (Haworth, 2008). The TWWIIA has assisted those attempting to enter or return to work in two ways. The Work Incentives Improvement Act portion of the legislation allowed individuals receiving SSI and SSDI recipients to maintain premium-free Medicare Part A coverage for approximately 6 years after they return to work, creating a health insurance safety net if they could not find employment. The Ticket to Work and Self-Sufficiency Program (TWSSP) segments of the legislation gave SSI and SSDI recipients a "ticket" in the form of a paper document to obtain employment services, support services, and vocational rehabilitation from an employment network of their choice: the intent of the TWSSP was to enable individuals with disabilities to exert greater choice, control, and self-direction of the employment services they receive and to promote competition among agencies providing employment services for individuals with disabilities, leading to improved services.

A recent piece of key legislation is the *Americans with Disabilities Amendments Act of 2008*. This act was drafted in response to decisions by the U.S. Supreme Court that "narrowed the definition of disability so much that people with serious conditions such as epilepsy, muscular dystrophy, cancer, diabetes, and cerebral palsy have been determined to not meet the definition of disability under the ADA." The act "effectively rejects strict interpretation of the definition of disability, strikes more of a balance between employer and employee interests, prohibits the consideration of medications, prosthetics, and assistive technology in determining whether an individual has a disability, and provides that reasonable accommodations are only required for individuals who can demonstrate they have an impairment that substantially limits a major life activity, or a record of such impairment. Accommodations need not be provided to an individual who is only 'regarded as' having an impairment" (Committee on Education and Labor, 2008).

Occupational Therapy Work-Related Practice Today

Today occupational therapy practitioners provide work-related interventions in a wide range of settings and with many different populations across much of the life span. Table 1.4 provides a brief description of some of these settings and the focus of occupational therapy intervention. It is not a complete list, but provides an overview of some work-related practice opportunities for occupational therapy practitioners.

Table 1.4 Examples of Work-Related Occupational Therapy Practice

Area of Practice	Brief Description
Injury prevention	Providing individual intervention and indirect consultation to prevent injuries at the workplace through job analysis, workplace redesign, and employee education in proper body mechanics and safety
Preemployment screening	Assessment of a potential employee's capacities to determine if the individual is capable of performing essential job duties
Sheltered workshops	Protective settings that provide employment opportunities for people with disabilities and/or those from disadvantaged backgrounds, such as ethnic minority groups, the long-term unemployed, and those returning to the workforce after a period of rehabilitation
Supported employment	Provision of job coaching, employment counseling, skills training, and other supportive services to a worker who is employed in a competitive paid position
Ergonomic assessment and intervention	Designing work systems and environments by applying the theory, principles, data, and methods in order to optimize human well-being and overall system performance
Transition planning in school settings	Preparing students to leave the school setting and enter employment and community living as part of services mandated under the Individuals with Disabilities Education Act (IDEA).
Wellness and health promotion	Wellness programs promote a healthy balance of the mind, body, and spirit to result in an overall feeling of well-being; health promotion is focused on enabling people to increase control over and to improve their health
Work hardening and work conditioning	Intervention, including exercise and work simulation, focused on increasing an individual's biomechanical, neuromuscular, cardiovascular, behavioral, and vocational functioning

(table continues on page 16)

Table 1.4 Examples of Work-Related Occupational Therapy Practice—cont'd

Area of Practice	Brief Description
Case management	The process of assessing, planning, facilitating, and advocating for options and services to meet an individual's health needs through communication and available resources to promote quality cost-effective outcomes
Community-based organizations	Services provided at a variety of community and nonprofit organizations, including prevocational training, skills training, development of work habits, resume and interview preparation, etc.

Work can be an area of concern for persons across most of the life span. Children and adolescents develop the habits and skills that prepare them to assume a worker role through participation in household chores and other occupations within the home and in schools. Part-time employment such as babysitting, mowing lawns, shoveling snow, completing odd jobs, or working for a formal organization in a paid position allows teenagers to further develop work habits and skills to prepare them for working as adults.

For adults, work serves a number of functions. Beyond providing a source of income and sustenance, work provides structure and a daily routine around which we organize our lives. Working provides an opportunity for interacting and socializing with others through the performance of work occupations as well as formal and informal social functions associated with workplaces. Many adults find great personal meaning in their work and experience it as a source of fulfillment, gaining a sense of mastery and strong identity from their work. Persons can spend their entire adult lives working at and developing a career in order to leave some form of legacy as a result of their efforts. While this is not true for all workers, and we all know people who work at jobs they dislike, work serves functions far beyond being a means to earn a living and to obtain food and shelter.

Today, working remains an issue for many older adults. As America's large and influential baby boom generation approaches and passes the traditional retirement age of 65, the vision of a traditional retirement is changing for many to include a new vision of a work-filled retirement. A report published by Rutgers University in 2005 noted that while more than a quarter of American workers still expect their 60s and 70s to be devoted to leisure or community service, the majority of workers say that full-time or part-time work will be either necessary or desirable (Reynolds, Ridley, and Van Horn, 2005a). Nearly 7 in 10 workers expect to continue to work full time or part time following retirement from their main job, including 15 percent who expect to start their own business. Only 13 percent expect to stop working entirely. Some older adults would like to retire and leave work but are financially unable to do so. For 20 percent of seniors over 65 years old, Social Security is their only source of income, and for two-thirds it is the major source of income (U.S. Senate Special Committee on Aging, 2008). This fixed income may not be sufficient to pay for the high cost of living and often requires supplemental income. Many workers want to continue to work on at least a part-time basis because of rewards other than financial. Some even want to begin new careers or open their own businesses. Older adult workers have some special needs because of age-related neurological, cognitive, sensorimotor, and psychological changes, and growing attention is being paid in work-related practice to helping the older worker continue to work successfully. Chapter 8 explores the needs of older workers in more depth.

In addition to intervening across the age span, work-related occupational therapy practice can involve direct intervention, consultation, and educational services in a variety of settings and with varied populations. You were briefly introduced to some of these settings, populations, and types of intervention in Table 1.4. Later chapters focus on some of these intervention areas more specifically. Occupational therapy practice has broadened since its inception to include interventions focused on prevention of work-related illnesses and promotion of health and wellness, and it has moved beyond intervening with individuals to working with groups of employees, companies, other types of organizations, and communities. In the next section, we explore some of the trends occurring in the workplace and with today's workers.

Trends in the Workplace and the Worker

As illustrated so far, the evolution of work and working in society can be characterized by constant change in the types of work performed, the characteristics of workers, and the workplace. Over the past two centuries, developments in technology have reshaped the world we live in, solved untold numbers of challenges to our health and well-being, and created new threats.

As we move toward the 100th anniversary of the occupational therapy profession in 2017 and beyond, we can be sure that change in society and in work will continue at an epic pace. The AOTA identified work and industry as one of six centennial vision practice areas, noting that there will be great opportunities for occupational therapy practitioners in work-related practice (AOTA, 2008a; 2007). In addition to the continued need for occupational therapy practitioners in traditional areas of work-related practice, such as injury management, occupational therapists are starting their own businesses and providing consulting services to companies on topics such as injury prevention, reasonable accommodations for workers with special needs, and ergonomic evaluations (Brachtesende, 2005). To capitalize on these opportunities, we must anticipate, identify, and understand work-related trends as much as possible.

Researchers with the Rand Corporation identified three trends likely to shape the future of work in this century: (1) shifting demographic patterns, (2) the pace of technological change, and (3) the path of economic globalization (Rand Corporation, 2007). Some of the implications of these trends include the following:

- More employees working in decentralized firms with more individualized relationships with their employers, including telecommuting and working from home.
- Slower labor-force growth with increased reliance on women, older workers, and people with disabilities to replace the fewer numbers of younger workers entering the workforce.
- More emphasis on retraining and lifelong learning to increase competitiveness in the global economy and to help shift workers from unskilled low-technology work to higher-skilled and more technologically demanding work.
- While wages may rise, there will be less of a tie between employment and access to fringe benefits, placing a higher financial burden on employees to be totally self-sufficient (Rand Corporation, 2007).

Many trends and influences in the workplace are interrelated and combine in their effects on work and the worker. For example, technological change is closely influenced by the trend toward globalization of industry and production, and vice versa. The technologies underlying the Internet and telecommunications have increased information flow among countries, speeding the rate of globalization. At the same time, according to the

U.S. Department of Labor, "The spread of free markets and free trade has promoted greater competition worldwide, creating strong incentives for domestic producers to adopt new technologies and requiring workers to become more technologically savvy" (2000). The Society for Human Resource Management identified eight themes in workplace trends that also reflect those found by the Rand Corporation (see Box 1.1).

In addition to the larger societal and global trends affecting the workplace, other trends affect the experience of the worker on a day-to-day basis. While some trends, such as increased flexibility in work schedules, have been beneficial for workers, there are also disadvantages associated with some trends (Fig. 1.4). For example, workers who rely heavily on new wireless technologies say these technologies make their jobs easier (80%), make it easier to share ideas (73%), and give them flexibility in the hours they work (58%). On the minus side, communications technology increases demands that they work more hours (46%), increases job-related stress (49%), and makes it harder to disconnect from work at home and on weekends (49%) (Claburn, 2008). Table 1.5 presents some of the most commonly identified trends and changes in the workplace and some of their advantages and disadvantages.

Box 1.1 Themes in Workplace Trends

- The importance of globalization and integrating markets.
- Demographic change and its impact on diversity and labor availability.
- The implications of increased health-care costs.
- Immigration and global labor mobility.
- Skills shortages and a greater emphasis on talent management.
- The growing importance of demonstrating ethics and corporate social responsibility.
- The influence of new technologies, especially social networking and human resources technologies.
- A greater reliance on metrics.

(Society for Human Resource Management, 2007)

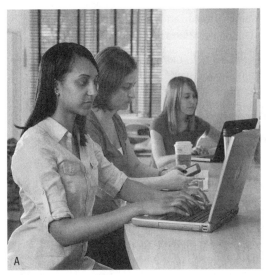 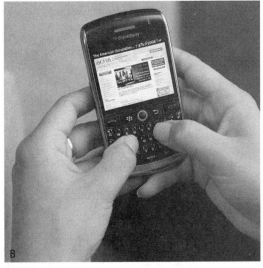

Figure 1.4 Evolving wireless technologies are both an advantage and a possible strain on today's workers, allowing them to access e-mail and the Internet almost anywhere.

Table 1.5 Examples of Trends in the Workplace and Their Advantages and Disadvantages

Workplace Trend	Advantages	Disadvantages
Electronic communication • Cellular phones • E-mail • Personal digital assistants	• Easier to share ideas • Increased flexibility • Increased access to information while traveling and commuting	• Added stress • Increased work hours • Harder to disconnect from work in the evening or on weekends • Increased interruptions and more difficulty concentrating on tasks
Telecommuting and working from home	• Less time commuting • Lowered stress • More flexibility in addressing varied work hours in a national and global economy	• More threats of distraction • Less consistent social interaction with coworkers • More feeling of disconnection
Flextime	• Increased convenience to manage personal commitments such as children • Increased sense of empowerment	• Connecting with peers and being an effective team member more difficult • Potential for more workplace conflict
Job sharing and contingent workers	• Increased flexibility • Increased mobility • More cross training and likelihood of support from others	• Less access to traditional benefits such as health insurance and paid time off • Potential for more workplace conflict
Part-time work	• More opportunity for parents and older workers • Increased flexibility	• Less access to traditional benefits such as health insurance and paid time off
Increased attention to health and fitness, including increased regulation of behavior (e.g., smoking)	• Improved health and sense of well-being • Improved productivity	• Less personal choice • More sense of intrusion of work into personal life

The rate of change in today's world has grown exponentially. Cellular phones and personal computers have been commercially available only for approximately 30 years and have infiltrated every aspect of our lives and changed the ways many of us perform our jobs. While they now are commonplace and we rely on them and take them for granted, they have only gained wide acceptance and accessibility during the work life of today's middle-aged workers. We might wonder what sorts of changes in technology and the workplace might happen in the next three decades and how we will experience work and working in 2040 and beyond.

Trends in Worker Demographics

There have been major shifts in the last century in the type of work that people perform and in where they work. For example, over the past decade, the service sector has overtaken agriculture as the prime employer of women around the globe. In 2007, 36.1 percent of employed women worked in agriculture and 46.3 percent in services. In comparison, male sectoral shares were 34.0 percent in agriculture and 40.4 percent in services (International Labour Organization, 2008). The U.S. Department of Labor (2000) noted that three out of four U.S. workers were in occupations that did not require a bachelor's degree and predicted that distribution to remain stable for at least the next two decades with workers in occupations requiring short-term and on-the-job training composing nearly 40 percent of the workforce.

More women are working than ever before, but globally they also have been more likely than men to get low-productivity, low-paid, and vulnerable jobs with no social protection or basic rights and no voice at work (International Labour Organization, 2008). However, we are seeing changes in the educational level of women, and women are now entering many fields and professions once dominated by men. Beginning in 1991, more women were enrolled at colleges and universities in the United States than men, and this trend has continued with the percentage of women increasing. In 2005, about 43 percent of women ages 18 to 24 were enrolled in college, compared with 35 percent of young men. Between 1970 and 2005, the gender composition has shifted so that women now make up the majority—54 percent—of the over 10 million young adults enrolled in college (Mather and Adams, 2007).

Older workers are one of the fastest growing components of the U.S. workforce. The U.S. Bureau of Labor Statistics estimated that between 2002 and 2012, the number of workers 55 years and older is expected to grow by nearly 50 percent, far outpacing increases in the number of workers aged 16 to 54. By 2012, workers 55 and older will make up about 20 percent of the labor force (Toossi, 2004). A worker who will be 65 in the year 2015 was born in 1950 in the post–World War II era. While these baby boomers grew up expecting to enjoy a traditional retirement, they may now be faced with the need or desire to continue to work. In general, this cohort of adults has lived through prosperous economic times. They are better educated than previous generations and have more disposable income than any generation before. They have witnessed dramatic changes in technology, although there may be a wide range of skill and capacity for its use within the workers who make up this cohort. The personal computer was introduced to homes in the 1980s when these workers were already in their 30s. Although the number of computers is now estimated at 1 billion worldwide with another billion projected by 2014, not all adults are computer literate. According to a study by the Pew Charitable Trusts in 2006 of 17,766 people in 17 countries, 76 percent of U.S. respondents said they used a computer at least occasionally at home or at work, and 70 percent used the Internet (O'Brien, 2006). While some aging workers are completely technologically savvy and are familiar with the latest wireless communication and other technologies, others might still be considered *computer illiterate.*

Authors of a report based on a national survey on the changing views of workers toward retirement noted, "The traditional notion of retirement—where one stops working completely and enjoys leisure time with friends and family—is obsolete." They found that about two-thirds of respondents viewed retirement from full-time work as an opportunity for continued productive employment. Seven of 10 workers expected to continue to work full time or part time following retirement from their main job, including 15 percent who planned to start their own business (Reynolds, Ridley, and Van Horn, 2005b). Workers may continue to work beyond traditional retirement age for many reasons, among them the following:

- Changing jobs more frequently. The average person born in the later years of the baby boom held 10.8 jobs from age 18 to age 42. Nearly two-thirds of these jobs were held from ages 18 to 27 (U.S. Bureau of Labor Statistics, 2008b).
- Fewer companies offering fully funded pension plans and a shift to requiring employees to fund their own retirement.

- Extended life expectancy with a new record high reported in 2006 of 78.1 years (National Center for Health Statistics, 2008).
- Working for enjoyment and satisfaction (as evidenced by workers starting second careers and opening their own businesses).

There also have been changes and trends related to men in the workplace. The following statistics were cited in a 2005 report by the National Bureau of Economic Research related to trends in hours worked by men in the United States (Kuhn and Lozano, 2005):

- Between the 1980 Census and 2005 American Community survey, the share of employed-for-pay U.S. men who worked more than 48 hours per week rose from 16.6 to 24.3 percent.
- Salaried men are much more likely to work long hours than are hourly paid men, with an increase from 24.4 to 30.1 percent.
- While older men were less likely to work long hours in 1979, this reversed by 2006, with older men becoming more likely to work longer hours.
- Longer hours are much more common among college graduates than among workers with less education.

Based on these statistics, contrary to what one might guess, the primary reason for men working longer hours is *not* solely economic need, since those with more education and who are salaried and more likely to have benefits such as health care and paid leave are *more* likely to work long hours.

The dichotomy between time spent at work and time spent in leisure and self-development occupations found in the United States and other industrialized countries is relatively new. As recently as the mid-20th century, workdays were very long (typically over 12 hours) and many persons worked seven days a week. Paid time off, vacations, and other benefits were not provided in many forms of labor. As we move to make the profession of occupational therapy more *globally connected*, we must recognize that more than 80 percent of the world's population still lives this way! To the majority of people in developing countries, work was and is the primary focus of life. Many persons around the world would perceive the contrast between "work" and "personal life" to be both artificial and perplexing. While time may be dedicated to families and communities, little leisure time is available to pursue hobbies, self-interests, or self-improvement (Vaknin, 2007).

> *Many persons around the world would perceive the contrast between "work" and "personal life" to be both artificial and perplexing. While time may be dedicated to families and communities, little leisure time is available to pursue hobbies, self-interests, or self-improvement.*

In fact, most of the world's workers live in developing countries. Of 3.1 billion workers, 73 percent live in developing countries, while only 14 percent live in advanced industrial countries. Some 46 million new workers join the world's labor force each year, mostly in developing countries. While the world's labor force is concentrated in developing countries, its capital and skills are concentrated much more heavily in advanced industrial countries (Ghose, Majid, and Ernst, 2008).

A growing challenge facing the workforce in industrialized countries like the United States is the mismatch between the number of low-skilled workers and the demand created by high-skilled jobs. This mismatch has arisen as a result of deindustrialization, skill-biased technological change, and growing specialization in skill-intensive products induced by globalization. These factors have been steadily reducing the demand for low-skilled labor despite the dwindling number of low-skilled workers and increasing the demand for high-skilled labor despite the rapidly increasing number of high-skilled workers (Ghose, et al., 2008). Although, according to projections by the U.S. Department of Labor, the 10 occupations with the fastest employment growth between now and 2016 represent employment areas calling for a variety of education and skill levels. These 10 occupations are listed in Box 1.2.

Trends in People With Disabilities and Work

So far you have read about many shifts and trends in the workplace and in workers in general in the United States and around the globe. But how do these employment trends relate to persons living with a disability? And do all clients in work-related practice have a disability? Let's start with the second question first.

In work-related practice, occupational therapy practitioners may provide intervention to prevent an impairment, injury, or disability from ever happening; they may work with an injured worker to prevent the onset of a disabling condition and to return the injured worker to the workplace; or they may work with a person who has a disability to help him or her gain employment or return to work. The term *disability* can be defined in different ways. According to the ADA, an individual is considered to have a disability if he or she has a physical or mental impairment that substantially limits one or more major life activities, has a record of such an impairment, or is regarded as having such an impairment (U.S. Department of Justice Civil Rights Division, 2006). Current disability scholars, as part of a *social model of disability* or the *disability model*, emphasize that "the problem (of disability) is defined as a dominating attitude by professionals and others, inadequate support services when compared with society generally, as well as attitudinal, architectural, sensory, cognitive, and economic barriers, and the strong tendency for people to generalize about all persons with disabilities, overlooking the large variations within the disability community" (Kaplan, 2008). Under this model, disability occurs only in the context of inadequate environmental supports to allow a person with physical, cognitive, or other challenges to fully participate in society. Disability therefore is defined by the mismatch between an individual and environmental demands.

There are some noticeable differences between employment for persons with disabilities and employment for those in society in general. Based on the 2000 census, about 49.7 million Americans (including all age groups) have a disability, and about two-thirds

---

Box 1.2   The 10 Occupations With the Largest Projected Employment Growth, 2006–2016

1. Registered nurses
2. Retail salespersons
3. Customer service representatives
4. Food preparation and food service workers
5. Personal and home care aides
6. Postsecondary teachers
7. Janitors and cleaners
8. Nursing aides, orderlies, and attendants
9. Bookkeeping, accounting, and auditing
10. Waiters and waitresses

(U.S. Department of Labor, 2007)

of these individuals have a severe disability. Fifty-six percent of those between the ages of 16 and 64 who have a disability (18.6 million people) were employed. Of those, 60.1 percent of men and 51.4 percent of women with disabilities are employed (Waldrop and Stern, 2003). The overall employment rate for persons with disabilities hovers around 35 percent compared to 75 percent of the general population, and this statistic has not changed significantly since World War II (National Organization on Disability, 2007).

Trends in labor-force participation by persons with disabilities have been the focus of several studies. For example, women with disabilities, in particular younger women with disabilities, experienced a larger increase in labor-force participation rates than did women without disabilities (Trupin and Yelin, 2003). However, men with disabilities, especially older men, experienced a larger decrease in labor-force participation rates than did men without disabilities. This relationship was stronger among minority groups with disabilities: nonwhite women have not experienced gains proportional to white women with disabilities, while nonwhite men with disabilities fared even worse than did white men with disabilities (Boni-Saenz, Heinemann, Crown, and Emanuel, 2005). Data from the U.S. Census Bureau's 2001 current population survey indicated that while the majority (82%) of working-age Americans is in the labor force, and 65 percent are working full time, less than one-third of people with disabilities are in the labor force (29%), and only 18 percent are working full time. During difficult economic times, people with disabilities who want to work often face additional barriers to entering the workforce. These barriers include lack of physical access to the workplace, employers reluctant to hire people with disabilities, lack of transportation, potential loss of Social Security income or federally funded health insurance, lack of experience, and insufficient access to employment services (Dixon, Kruse, and Van Horn, 2003).

It is also important to consider the variations in working hours, whether persons are working part time or full time, and whether they can find employment for as many hours as they would like or if they are *underemployed*. From 1984 to 2000, the percentage of nondisabled workers aged 18 to 64 who were employed part time decreased slightly, but the percentage of disabled workers of the same ages employed part time increased. Most of this gain occurred between the passage of the ADA in 1990 and its full implementation in 1994 (Hotchkiss, 2004). Two factors may be behind this trend. Employers may see offering part-time employment as a low-cost method to accommodate a worker's disability, and more disabled workers receiving SSI or SSDI may be working under the new work incentives under social security that allow a recipient with a disability to work part time while maintaining his or her benefits.

The pattern of part-time employment for persons with disabilities exists in other countries as well. For example, in a national interview survey of 2,000 disabled people of working age (men aged 16 to 64, women aged 16 to 59) in the United Kingdom, the following results were found in regard to employment and persons with disabilities (Meager, Bates, Dench, Honey, and Williams, 1998):

- Disabled people are more likely than nondisabled people to work in manual and low-skilled occupations and less likely to work in managerial, professional, and high-skilled occupations (11% of disabled people are in managerial occupations, compared with 15% of nondisabled people).
- Nearly three-quarters of disabled people work full time, a similar proportion to nondisabled people. Only 25 percent of disabled people working part time say that they do so because of their disability, although people with more severe disabilities are slightly more likely to work part time (19% of disabled part-timers have a "severity core" of 4 or more, compared with 14% of full-timers).
- There is a strong increase with age in the rate of self-employment among disabled people (corresponding to the pattern among the nondisabled population).

- Nearly two-thirds (64%) of disabled people in work have no special working arrangements, and of those who do, the commonest is flextime (15%). Most of those with flexible working arrangements (94%) say that the arrangements are not associated with their disability.

It is important to remember when considering the topic of disability and work that many disabilities are not related to physical challenges or impairments but may be cognitive in nature or related to mental health. According to the World Health Organization (2004), mental disorders are the leading cause of disability in the United States for individuals between the ages of 15 and 44 years. Four nationally representative surveys conducted between 1989 and 1998 found that people who had any mental illness (but who were not necessarily disabled by these disorders) had lower employment rates (48%–73%) than people who did not report mental illness (76%–87%). Employment rates for people who met criteria for disabling mental illness were even lower, ranging from 32 to 61 percent, and lower still—22 to 40 percent—among those with diagnoses associated with high levels of disability such as schizophrenia and related disorders (Cook, 2006). Barriers to employment have been identified as (1) low educational attainment, (2) lowered productivity and higher absenteeism, (3) unfavorable labor market conditions that impact persons with disabilities more than the nondisabled, (4) lack of effective vocational and clinical services, (5) labor force discrimination, (6) lack of legislative protection, (7) poverty level income, (8) linkage of health care to disability beneficiary status, (8) employment disincentives in social security work benefits, and (9) ineffective work incentive legislation.

Chapter Summary

Chapter 1 reviewed the changing role that work has played in society throughout the world's history. There have been dramatic changes over the centuries in the nature of work performed as we have moved from a primarily agricultural-based economy to an emphasis on industry and manufacturing to today's economy that is significantly driven by the service industries. Just as dramatic have been shifts in where we work and in trends taking place in the workplace and the workforce. Technology has reshaped the workforce, and the advent of personal computers and wireless communication has created tremendous flexibility and other advantages for the worker, although the disadvantages that these technologies can create must be recognized as well. Demographic changes in race, gender, and age are increasingly influencing the workplace, and projections are that this will continue for the coming decades.

This chapter also reviewed the history of the involvement of the occupational therapy profession in work-related practice since its early grounding in the moral treatment of the mentally ill and the rehabilitation of wounded soldiers in the two world wars. Today, occupational therapy practitioners provide a wide range of work-related interventions in a variety of settings and with a variety of populations across much of the life span. The influences on occupational therapy work-related practice by legislation that protects the worker and persons with disabilities and provides resources to foster their participation were also explored.

Coming chapters explore in more depth some of these concepts as well as specific aspects of work-related assessment and intervention. Related concepts, such as how we develop an identity as a worker, the influence of culture and the need to become culturally competent practitioners, and the roles of the occupational therapist and the occupational therapy assistant, are also discussed in depth.

Case Resolution

As Hannah explored options for completing one of her fieldwork experiences in the area of work-related practice, she was astounded by the possibilities. While she had learned about the roots of the occupational therapy profession and the historical ties between work and the occupational therapy profession in one of her foundational courses, she had not realized that occupational therapy practitioners provided such a wide range of interventions in the area of work-related practice today. As she explored AOTA's website and began reading the literature written by occupational therapy scholars and scientists, she learned that occupational therapy practitioners provide prevention services in private clinics and at job sites, provide a wide range of services to persons across the life span to help them enter the workplace and succeed, and work in traditional settings such as hospitals and mental health services. However, she also became aware that emerging areas of practice included ergonomics and workplace consultation on areas such as the Americans with Disabilities Act.

As she considered choosing sites for her fieldwork experiences, Hannah decided she would pursue an experience in one of the many work-related practice settings near her university. She realized she could use much of the knowledge and skills that she was gaining in her education related to physical, cognitive, and psychosocial functioning in her practice. She also learned that there would be many career opportunities for her after she graduated.

References

American Occupational Therapy Association (AOTA). (1980). The role of the occupational therapist in the vocational rehabilitation process. *American Journal of Occupational Therapy, 34,* 881–883.

American Occupational Therapy Association (AOTA). (1986). Work hardening guidelines. *American Journal of Occupational Therapy, 40,* 841–843.

American Occupational Therapy Association (AOTA). (2007). Ad hoc reports examine vision-related practice areas. Retrieved from www.aota.org/News/Centennial/Background/AdHoc/ 39452.aspx.

American Occupational Therapy Association (AOTA). (2008a). AOTA's centennial vision. Retrieved from www.aota .org/News/Centennial/Background/36516.aspx?FT=.pdf.

American Occupational Therapy Association (AOTA). (2008b). Occupational therapy practice framework: Domain and process, 2nd ed. *American Journal of Occupational Therapy, 62,* 625–683.

Boni-Saenz, A. A., Heinemann, A. W., Crown, D. S., & Emanuel, L. L. (2005). The business of employing people with disabilities: Four case studies—Multi-case study report. University of Illinois at Urbana–Champaign: Disability Research Institute.

Brachtesende, A. (2005). New markets emerge from society's needs. *OT Practice.* Retrieved from www.aota.org/Educate/EdRes/StuRecruit/Working/38380.aspx.

Braveman, B., Robson, M., Velozo, C., Kielhofner, G., Fisher, G. S., Forsyth, K., et al. (2005). *The Worker Role Interview (Version 10).* Chicago: Model of Human Occupation Clearinghouse, Department of Occupational Therapy.

Claburn, T. (2008). Networked workers: Connected, distracted, stressed. *InformationWeek.* Retrieved from www.informationweek.com.

Committee on Education and Labor: U.S. House of Representatives. (2008). ADA Amendments Act of 2008.

Cook, J. A. (2006). Employment barriers for persons with psychiatric disabilities: Update of a report for the President's Commission. *Psychiatric Services, 57,* 1391–1405.

Davenport, J. (2007). *The Age of Feudalism.* Detroit: Lucent Books.

Dixon, K. A., Kruse, D., & Van Horn, C. E. (2003). Restricted access: A survey of employers about people with disabilities and lowering barriers to return to work. New Brunswick, NJ: Rutgers University, John J. Heldrich Center for Workforce Development.

Drucker, P. F. (1957). *Landmarks of Tomorrow: A Report on the New Post-Modern World.* New York: Harper and Row.

European Union Center of North Carolina. (2008). *The EU's Demographic Crisis.* Retrieved from www.unc.edu/depts/europe/business_media/mediabriefs/Brief9-0803-demographic-crisis.pdf.

Fenger, K., Braveman, B., & Kielhofner, G. (2008). Work-related assessments: Worker Role Interview and Work Environment Impact Scale. In B. J. Hemphill (ed.), *Assessments in Occupational Therapy Mental Health: An Integrative Approach,* 2nd ed (pp. 187–202). Thorofare, NJ: Slack.

Finlayson, M., & Braveman, B. (2005). Understanding and applying the principles of evidence-based practice to the management of occupational therapy services. In B. Braveman (ed.), *Leading and Managing Occupational*

Therapy Services: An Evidence-Based Approach (pp. 1–22). Philadelphia: F.A. Davis.

Ghose, A. K., Majid, N., & Ernst, C. (2008). *The Global Employment Challenge*. Geneva: International Labour Office.

Gordon, D. (2009). The history of occupational therapy. In E. B. Crepeau, E. S. Cohn, & B. A. Boyt Schell (eds.), *Willard and Spackman's Occupational Therapy*, 11th ed. (pp. 202–215). Baltimore: Lippincott, Williams & Wilkins.

Haworth, T. (2008). Events in the Development of Disability Policy. Careers education and workforce programs. State of Michigan website. Retrieved from www.michigan.gov.

Hill, R. B. (2005). History of work ethic. The Work Ethic Site. Retrieved from www.coe.uga.edu/workethic/.

Hotchkiss, J. L. (2004). Growing part-time employment among workers with disabilities: Marginalization or opportunity (Rep. No. Third Quarter 2004). Federal Reserve Bank of America.

Inikori, J. E. (2002). *Africans and the Industrial Revolution in England*. New York: Cambridge University Press.

International Labour Organization. (2008). Global employment trends for women 2008: More women enter the workforce, but more than half of all working women are in vulnerable jobs. Retrieved from www.ilo.org/global.

Jacobs, K., & Baker, N. A. (2000). Lesson 1: The history of work-related therapy in occupational therapy. In B. L. Kornblau & K. Jacobs (eds.), *Work: Principles and Practice—A Self-Paced Clinical Course from AOTA* (pp. 1–11). Bethesda, MD: American Occupational Therapy Association.

Johansson, C. (2006). The business of ergonomics. OT Practice Online.

Kaplan, D. (2008). The definition of disability—Perspective of the disability community. World Institute on Disability. Retrieved from www.peoplewho.org/debate/ kaplan.htm.

Kielhofner, G. (2008). *Model of Human Occupation: Theory and Application*. Baltimore: Lippincott, Williams & Wilkins.

Kielhofner, G. (2009). Emergence of the contemporary paradigm: A return to occupation. In *Conceptual Foundations of Occupational Therapy*, 4th ed. (pp. 41–56). Philadelphia: F.A. Davis.

King, P. M., & Olson, D. L. (2009). Work. In E.B. Crepeau, E. S. Cohn, & B. A. Boyt Schell (Eds.), *Willard & Spackman's Occupational Therapy*, 11th ed. (pp. 615–632). Baltimore: Lippincott, Williams, & Wilkins.

Kuhn, P., & Lozano, F. (2005). *The Expanding Work Week? Understanding Trends in Long Work Hours among U.S. Men, 1799–2004*. Cambridge, MA: National Bureau of Economic Research.

Mather, M., & Adams, D. (2007). The crossover in female–male college enrollment rates. Population Reference Bureau website. Retrieved from www.prb.org/Articles/2007/CrossoverinFemaleMaleCollegeEnrollmentRates.aspx.

Meager, N., Bates, P., Dench, S., Honey, S., & Williams, M. (1998). *Employment of Disabled People: Assessing the Extent of Participation*. London: Department for Education and Employment.

Mick, A., & Wolff, K. (2008). Our working history. Yale New Haven's Teacher's Institute. Retrieved from www.yale.edu/ynhti/.

Moore-Corner, R. A., Kielhofner, G., & Olson, L. (1998). *Work Environment Impact Scale Version 2.0*. Chicago: Model of Human Occupation Clearinghouse.

National Center for Health Statistics (2008). U.S. mortality drops sharply in 2006, latest data show. Centers for Disease Control: National Center for Health Statistics. Retrieved from www.cdc.gov/nchs/PRESSROOM/08newsreleases/mortality2006.htm.

National Organization on Disability. (2007). 2007 NOD Annual Report: National EmployAbility Partnership. National Organization on Disability. Retrieved from www.nod.org/index.cfm?fuseaction=Page.ViewPage&PageID=1572.

O'Brien, K. (2006). Dutch found to be most computer literate in the world. *International Herald Tribune*. Retrieved from www.nytimes.com/2006/02/21/technology/21iht-pew.html.

Rand Corporation. (2007). The future at work—Trends and implications. Retrieved from http://rand.org/pubs/research_briefs/RB5070/index1.html.

Reynolds, S., Ridley, N., & Van Horn, C. E. (2005a). *A Work-Filled Retirement: Workers' Changing Views on Employment and Leisure*. New Brunswick, NJ: Rutgers University, John J. Heldrich Center for Workforce Development.

Reynolds, S., Ridley, N., & Van Horn, C. E. (2005b). *Worktrends: Americans' Attitudes about Work, Employers, and Government*. New Brunswick, NJ: Rutgers University, John J. Heldrich Center for Workforce Development.

Ross, J. (2007). *Occupational Therapy and Vocational Rehabilitation*. Hoboken, NJ: Wiley.

Society for Human Resource Management. (2007). *The 2007–2008 Workplace Trends List: The Top Trends according to SHRM's Special Expertise Panels*. Alexandria, VA: Society for Human Resource Management.

Toossi, M. (2004). *Labor Force Projections to 2012: The Graying of the U.S. Workforce* Washington, DC: U.S. Bureau of Labor Statistics.

Tracy, B. (2007). Good question: Why do Americans work so much? Rand Corporation website. Retrieved from http:// wcco.com/topstories/good.question.work.2.367101.html.

Trupin, L., & Yelin, E. (2003). Impact of structural change in the distribution of occupations and industries on the employment of persons with disabilities in the U.S., 1970–2001. Disability Research Institute: University of Illinois at Urbana–Champaign. Retrieved from www.dri.uiuc.edu/research/p03-01c/p03_01c_w_figures_tables.pdf.

U.S. Bureau of Labor Statistics. (2008a). American time use survey summary. Retrieved from www.bls.gov/news.release/atus.nr0.htm.

U.S. Bureau of Labor Statistics (2008b). Number of jobs held, labor market activity, and earnings growth among the youngest baby boomers: Results from a longitudinal survey summary. Retrieved from www.bls.gov/news.release/nlsoy.nr0.htm.

U.S. Department of Justice Civil Rights Division. (2006). Americans with Disabilities Act: Questions and answers. Retrieved from www.ada.gov/q&aeng02.htm.

U.S. Department of Labor. (2000). Futurework: Trends and challenges for work in the 21st century. *Occupational Outlook Quarterly, 44*, 31–37.

U.S. Department of Labor (2007). *News: Bureau of Labor Statistics Employment Projections 2006–2016*. Retrieved from www.bls.gov/news.release/archives/ecopro_12042007.pdf.

U.S. Department of Labor: Office of Disability Employment Policy. (2008). Business ownership: Cornerstone of the American dream. Retrieved from www.dol.gov/odep.

U.S. Senate Special Committee on Aging. (2008). Senators react to SSA-OIG Report. Retrieved from http://aging.senate.gov/record.cfm?id=300183.

Vaknin, S. (2007). Workaholism, leisure and pleasure. The Work Ethic Site. Retrieved from http://samvak.tripod.com/leisure.html.

W.W. Norton & Company. (2008). The Renaissance in Europe. Norton Anthology of World Literature Websource. Retrieved from www.norton.com.

Waldrop, J., & Stern, S. S. (2003). Disability status: 2000-census 2000 brief. Washington, DC: U.S. Census Bureau.

Weber, M. (2002). *The Protestant Ethic and the Spirit of Capitalism.* New York: Routledge.

World Health Organization. (2004). *The World Health Report 2004—Changing History.* Geneva, Switzerland: World Health Organization.

Glossary

A **knowledge worker** is a modern-day worker who works with and produces *information* as a product.

The occupational therapy profession's **domain** comprises those areas of human experience in which occupational therapy practitioners offer assistance to others.

Occupations are activities of everyday life, named, organized, and given value and meaning by individuals and a culture. Occupation is everything people do to occupy themselves, including looking after themselves . . . enjoying life . . . and contributing to the social and economic fabric of their communities.

Onsite work programs seek to return injured workers to work as quickly as possible and to provide intervention at the worksite by involving the worker in real-life, real-job work occupations.

The **social model of disability** defines disability as a dominating attitude by professionals and others, inadequate support services when compared with society generally, as well as attitudinal, architectural, sensory, cognitive, and economic barriers, and the strong tendency for people to generalize about all persons with disabilities overlooking the large variations within the disability community.

Resources

Rand Corporation

www.rand.org

The Rand Corporation is a nonprofit institution that helps improve policy and decision making through research and analysis. Its website includes recent data on trends in the workplace and in the workforce.

United States Department of Labor

www.dol.gov

The Department of Labor fosters and promotes the welfare of job seekers, wage earners, and retirees in the United States by improving their working conditions; advancing their opportunities for profitable employment; protecting their retirement and health-care benefits; helping employers find workers; strengthening free collective bargaining; and tracking changes in employment, prices, and other national economic measurements. The DOL website also includes information on statistics and trends in the workforce.

Society for Human Resource Management

www.shrm.org

The Society for Human Resource Management (SHRM) is the world's largest association devoted to human resource management. Representing more than 250,000 members in over 140 countries, SHRM serves the needs of HR professionals and advances the interests of the HR profession. Its website includes resources on research related to the workforce as well as resources devoted to trends and forecasting.

2

Development of the Worker Role and Worker Identity

Brent Braveman

Key Concepts

The following are key concepts addressed in this chapter:
- Developmental theories of career development are consistent with a life-span approach to human development.
- Occupational identity, occupational competence, and occupational adaptation are important constructs related to work success.
- The *medical model* and *social model* are two models of disability that define disability differently and have implications for approaching occupational therapy intervention in work-related services.

Case Introduction

Craig is a 28-year-old black male referred to a work readiness program designed to help adults struggling with obtaining and maintaining employment. Craig spent some of his adolescence struggling with mental illness and was admitted to a psychiatric facility several times. He dropped out of high school at age 15 and spent the next few years using and selling drugs. At age 22, he entered a drug rehabilitation program, and after two failed attempts, he successfully entered recovery and has been "clean" since. He has become substantially adherent with the recommendations of his psychiatrist, including the use of psychotropic medications. He passed his General Education Development (GED) test at age 23 and spent the next few years moving from one part-time job to another. He reported that he was typically fired within the first 2 weeks of employment because he was chronically late to work.

In the initial interview with Craig, he explained that he previously participated in four different vocational preparation programs and had been "dismissed" from each because he was chronically late for programming. When asked why he was late to work or daily programming, he had difficulty articulating the reason. He stated, "Well, I always go to bed planning to be on time. Every night I say, 'Not again, tomorrow I am going to have it together,' but then I get up the next morning and everything falls apart, and somehow I just end up late. I don't mean to be late. I really want to be on time. I *really* want to work and do a good job. I am not a bad person, and once I get there, I work hard. Nobody has ever said that I am not a hard worker or that I don't do a good job; they just fire me because I get there late."

In reviewing records from previous vocational preparation service providers, Craig's therapists typically noted that at first they were optimistic about Craig's potential and his skills; however, the prior documentation also noted that he "lacked the motivation to participate as evidenced by his tardiness" and "Craig just does not seem to care enough about working to show up on time." The discharge report from the most recent program in which Craig was involved stated, "Craig states that he is highly motivated to obtain and maintain employment but is irresponsible and clearly *not* motivated. He has been 30 minutes or more late to programming 80 percent of the time. When Craig decides it is time to become serious about working, we would be happy to have him back to our program.

Introduction

Chapter 1 introduced the evolution of work from early Greek and Roman civilizations to modern times and reviewed occupational therapy's involvement as a profession in work-related practice. It highlighted the changes that have occurred over time in the nature of work itself as well as the resulting changes in the workplace and the influences on today's workers, who themselves are changing. The processes by which children and adolescents are introduced to work and the role of workers in our society have also changed over the last two centuries. This is especially true in industrialized nations. The assumption that young men would help their farmer fathers until they were 21 persisted in rural America up to the early 19th century (Kett, 1978). It was not until the early 20th century that children in upper-class families were excused from labor to devote time to education and leisure. While the involvement of children and adolescents in basic support of a family's day-to-day existence through farming or manual labor continues in many less developed nations, the expectation exists in industrialized nations that childhood and adolescence are a time to focus on education and exploration of the world. Thus it is through school and other childhood experiences that children learn about work and what it means to be a worker.

The focus of Chapter 2 is on vocational development across the life span and the development of an identity as a worker. While the focus of this text is primarily on paid and volunteer work in adults, it is helpful to understand the development of work-related capacities and skills in childhood and adolescence. Chapter 7 describes in depth the services provided to adolescents, including transition services offered under the Individuals with Disabilities Education Act (IDEA), in U.S. school systems. These services include a coordinated set of activities for a child with a disability that "is designed to be within a results-oriented process, that is focused on improving the academic and functional achievement of the child with a disability to facilitate the child's movement from school to post-school activities, including postsecondary education, vocational education, integrated employment (including supported employment), continuing and adult education, adult services, independent living, or community participation" (U.S. Department of Education, 2006). Chapter 8 focuses on work and older adults.

This chapter introduces concepts related to the development of a worker role and an identity as a worker. The major theories of vocational and career development are presented. You learn ways of thinking about how impairment and disability affect an individual's identity and sense of competence as a worker and of thinking about people who may not develop a strong worker identity in the first place.

Vocational Development Across the Life Span

Developmental perspectives on careers recognize that vocational development constitutes a lifelong process from infancy through childhood, adolescence, adulthood, and old age affected by both personal and contextual factors (Hartung, Porfeli, and Vondracek, 2005). This perspective is consistent with contemporary *life-span views* of development addressed in modern occupational therapy curricula. A life-span approach to development (1) views human development as never ending, (2) views development as a result of continuous interaction between an individual and his or her environment, (3) recognizes that development is not stable and that developmental events may arise and take center stage at various points throughout a person's life and then fade into the background, and (4) recognizes individuals as active in their own development. This perspective is also reflected throughout this text, recognizing that occupational therapy practitioners may provide work-related services or services to promote the development of occupational performance to support prevocational and vocational exploration to persons of almost every age.

As early as the second year of life, children begin to acquire the basic skills needed to function within their social and cultural environments. By age 5, children are able to move and explore their environments with considerable independence, should be open to learning and able to communicate with peers and adults, and are largely independent in activities of daily living (Cronin and Mandich, 2005). The critical cognitive, memory, and reasoning skills that allow children to enter and participate in classroom settings are also typically developed by this age.

Younger children base their perceptions about work on a mix of fantasy and actual observations of adults working, and these perceptions are processed and supported by their cognitive skills, which develop throughout childhood, adolescence, and into adulthood. It is widely recognized that no other theorist has impacted thought on cognitive development like Jean Piaget. Piaget (1977) described four major stages in cognitive development: (1) sensorimotor, (2) preoperational, (3) concrete operational, and (4) formal operational. These stages are described in Box 2.1. Contemporary theorists suggest that it is most appropriate to describe cognitive development in ways that recognize flexibility and variability and do not rely on rigid or fixed stages. Moreover, researchers point out that children are not always consistent in their performance of tasks within a particular stage of development. More recent educational research has found that up to 40 percent of college freshmen are either in transition between concrete and formal operations or lacking formal operational skills entirely (Anderson, 2003). Sutherland (1999) found that half of all U.S. adults function at a concrete operational level.

For young children, involvement in family activities such as helping with meal preparation and grocery shopping and in household chores such as cleaning their room or caring for pets not only prepares them to be responsible adults in general but also provides them an opportunity to develop basic work habits and skills (Fig. 2.1). Participation in such activities teaches children that other people have expectations of them and that performance

---

Box 2.1 Jean Piaget's Stages of Cognitive Development

1. Sensorimotor (birth to about age 2):
Children learn about themselves and their environments through motor and reflex actions. Thought derives from sensation and movement. Children learn they are separate from their environment and that people and things continue to exist even when they cannot be seen or heard.

2. Preoperational (begins about the time the child starts to talk to about age 7):
As language develops, children begin to use symbols to represent objects and can better process information about people and objects that are not immediately present. At this stage, children are temporally oriented to the present and have difficulty conceptualizing time. Thinking is influenced by fantasy, and children are not yet able to understand that others think differently about situations than they do. Play becomes increasingly imaginary and moves from simple make-believe to plots to more complex scenarios and games with sophisticated rules. At this stage, they can play teacher, firefighter, or nurse.

3. Concrete (about first grade to early adolescence):
During this stage, accommodation increases and children develop the ability to think abstractly and to make rational judgments about concrete or observable phenomena, which in the past they needed to manipulate physically to understand.

4. Formal operations (adolescence):
In the final stage of cognitive development, children no longer require concrete objects to make rational judgments and are capable of hypothetical and deductive reasoning. Thinking is no longer tied to events that can be observed, and adolescents at this stage can think hypothetically and use logic to solve problems.

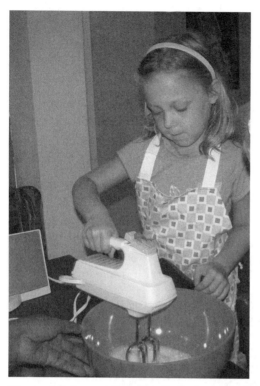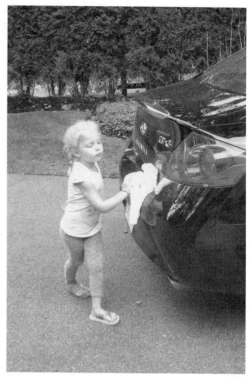

Figure 2.1 Ava and Alana develop basic work habits and skills by helping with chores around the house such as baking brownies or helping to wash the family car.

in daily activities is often evaluated and rewarded. Of course, much of the learning for young children occurs during play, which might be thought of as the primary "job" for a child. Early play is reality based and children imitate the actions of adults and objects are used for their intended purposes. For instance, a ruler is used to measure things rather than imagining it to be a sword or magic wand. Later, children begin to incorporate fantasy into play, which allows them to mentally experiment with new roles and situations in safe environments (Cronin and Mandich, 2005). These new roles often include imitating and mentally exploring work roles to which they are exposed. The creativity fostered during this play supports performance in both structured and nonstructured play in middle childhood, including playground free time, involvement in first hobbies, and formal and informal group games and sports.

Since the advent of a life-span approach to human development, life-span development theorists, including Erikson (1968); Ginsberg, Ginsburg, Axelrad, and Herma (1951); Havighurst (1964); Super, Savickas, and Super (1996); and Vondracek (2001), have acknowledged childhood as an important formative period in career development. However, Porfeli, Erik, Hartung, and Vondracek (2008) note that even today, some researchers and the general public tacitly accept the view that childhood is a period of fantasy and play and that consequently the importance of childhood as a period of vocational development has been downplayed. Instead of accepting this view, they propose a model of vocational development that casts middle childhood as the dawn of vocational development and includes those core constructs and mechanisms that presumably represent the essential antecedents of adolescent vocational development. They are in agreement with Savickas (2002), who stated, "Rather than conceiving of childhood as a passive, quiescent period disconnected from the whole of life-span vocational development, childhood should be viewed as a period of active precursory engagement in the world-of-work to develop initial concern about the future, control over one's life, conceptions about career decision making, and confidence to make and implement career choices."

> *Rather than conceiving of childhood as a passive, quiescent period disconnected from the whole of life-span vocational development, childhood should be viewed as a period of active precursory engagement in the world-of-work to develop initial concern about the future, control over one's life, conceptions about career decision making, and confidence to make and implement career choices." (Savickas, 2002)*

The model of vocational development proposed by Porfeli and colleagues spans middle childhood to late adolescence and is summarized in Table 2.1. The model highlights the impetus for vocational development in three stages of development: (1) middle childhood, (2) late childhood and early adolescence, and (3) middle adolescence to late adolescence.

In middle childhood (ages 6–10), children in industrialized nations are greatly influenced by participation in formal education in school systems, and children gain and

Table 2.1 Vocational Development From Childhood to Late Adolescence

Stage of Development	Causes	Mechanism	Outcomes
Middle childhood	• Curiosity • Industry • Aptitudes, abilities, and learning • Contextual affordances and constraints • Sex roles	• *Emerging* sense of personal aptitudes, abilities, and interests and awareness of work • *Emerging* sense of personal agency	• *Developing* awareness of work in relation to an *emerging* sense of self • *Emerging* sense of personal agency
Late childhood to early adolescence	• Exploration and learning with *little* reflection upon the self	• Exploration and learning with *limited* reflection upon *emerging* sense of self	• Exploration and learning with *extended* reflection upon *developing* sense of self in context
Middle to late adolescence	• *Emerging* awareness of work influenced by personal exposure and cultural stereotypes • *Emerging* sense of personal and vocational interests, aspirations, and expectations	• *Developing* awareness of work in relation to an *emerging* sense of self, which includes a sense of educational and vocational interests, aptitudes, values, emotions, and aspirations • *Emerging* sense of personal agency, which includes a sense of personal capabilities and contextual affordances and constraints	• *Developing* awareness of work in relation to a *developing* sense of self as an active agent defined by one's capabilities and affordances and barriers within the family, school, and peer contexts • *Developing* sense of personal agency • Postsecondary educational choices and tentative career plans

Porfeli, Erik, Hartung, and Vondracek, 2008. Reprinted with permission of the National Career Development Association.

experience considerably more independence as they spend longer periods of time away from home. During this time, the focus of energies is not only on formal academic preparation (reading, mathematics, and science) but also on expanding social networks and social interaction skills. Cronin and Mandich (2005) identified some of the typical educational goals for children in the age range of 6 to 10; see Box 2.2.

Middle childhood is also a time of increasing expectations for children, and while these expectations are focused on occupational performance in the home and school, many of the habits and skills that children develop support later work performance. Self-management skills develop such that children can manage both personal hygiene and toileting, follow schedules and routines in the home and classroom, and function more independently in a variety of community settings. Basic work habits such as initiating a project, staying focused and on task, and enduring in the face of minor frustration not only promote educational success but are also basic habits of industry needed for vocational success. In middle childhood, children begin to spend more time out of the home and develop broader social networks that are separate from the family and increasingly tied to their developing identity. The social and communication skills that develop during this time are also pivotal in preparation for later communication and negotiation in the workplace.

In middle childhood, children develop an emerging awareness of work influenced by personal exposure and by cultural stereotypes and an emerging sense of personal and vocational interests, aspirations, and expectations. These changes are primarily driven by external forces as natural curiosity drives children to interact with the world and develop an emerging awareness of work (Porfeli, et al., 2008). They are increasingly exposed to various forms of work in educational settings and in popular media including television and the Internet. They also begin to have the cognitive capacity to more fully process the work experiences of those with whom they interact, including family members and other role models. They understand more fully the conversations that they hear in which their parents, grandparents, and siblings talk about their work, including the frustrations, benefits, and rewards. For example, they may hear and begin to understand a parent who talks about the difficulties of managing both a busy work life and a busy home life and understand that working can have both upsides and downsides.

In late childhood to early adolescence, young persons develop an emerging sense of personal aptitudes, abilities, and interests; an awareness of work; and an emerging sense of personal agency and influence on their world. These changes are also driven by external forces as adolescents are increasingly exposed to the world and work including educational and vocational opportunities, but they process these experiences with limited self-reflection. At this age, they may begin to receive increased messages from others about the need to attend to their own futures. The encouragement and support, or lack thereof, to do well in school and other activities may have an impact on their perception of their identity and self-worth and on what role work may hold in their futures.

Box 2.2 Goals of Typical Schools for Children 6 to 10

- Master the basic skills of reading, writing, language development, and mathematics.
- Develop positive relationships with their peers and adults.
- Learn to deal in a mature way with their emotions.
- Explore and pursue interest in the arts and sciences.
- Develop into a physically fit and healthy individual.
- Promote the moral and civic values of their community.

(Cronin and Mandich, 2005)

Knowledge about occupations (used in this instance to mean a type of employment) and about self-in-occupations is found to be well developed by age 10 or 11 (McGee and Stockard, 1991). The earlier loosely integrated understanding of work roles based on fantasy and observation typically gives way by this age to a more realistic understanding of adult work, including gains in knowledge about job salaries and training requirements. By early adolescence, children begin to understand that work is interpreted differently by different adults and that there are varying levels of responsibility, effort required, and reward given for different forms of employment. As teenagers, adolescents become aware of potential negative aspects of work, such as dissatisfaction; schedule demands; and competing demands between work, family, and leisure interests. During this time, they begin to compare their own abilities to those required by different forms of work and grow increasingly aware that they must soon make decisions about education, training, and the type of work they hope to perform as adults.

As children become adolescents, they move from concrete operational thinking to formal operational thinking at around 10 to 12 years of age. During concrete operational thinking, children conceptualize the work they see but do not imagine the *behind the scenes* work that occurs. For example, they might admire the coach of a local sports team and be impressed by his or her actions on the field or court, but they are not aware of the hours of paperwork and preparation, meetings, or menial tasks that come with the job. However, as children become adolescents and formal operational thinking begins, they become more aware of the complexities involved in working and occupations, such as training, wages, and job satisfaction.

In middle to late adolescence, adolescents begin to develop an awareness of work that is much more connected to an emerging sense of self. These changes continue to be driven by external forces as adolescents explore the world and work but are now marked by increased self-reflection. They begin to see themselves as active individuals and agents of personal change defined by their capabilities and affordances and barriers within their family, school, and peer contexts (Porfeli, et al., 2008). The extent to which they perceive that they can impact their environments *and* their futures is further influenced by the experiences of family and peers. The primary developmental tasks related to work that are typically experienced in adolescence are summarized in Box 2.3.

An adolescent who is exposed to positive role models, who has experienced academic and vocational success, and who receives encouragement and support that they too can achieve success may begin to make concrete connections between the actions of today and a future role as a worker. However, those who do not have such role models or who receive negative messages about working or their likelihood of success may be less inclined to focus on achievement in the classroom or to explore vocational and career opportunities. Jordan and Pope (2001) examined which variables and aggregates of variables in the developmental histories of young persons studied from birth influenced their knowledge of

---

Box 2.3   Work and Development Tasks in Adolescence

- Explore their identity.
- Develop societal roles.
- Build relationships and social networks.
- Explore and deepen interests.
- Develop their social and problem-solving abilities.
- Obtain feedback about skills and capacities.

occupations in the adolescent years. They concluded that "adolescents' knowledge of occupational information is a determinate process; the developmental progression begins at birth with family socioeconomic level and proceeds in a manner in which perinatal social class, the cognitive maturity of the child and, to a lesser degree, that of the mother are major influences." Their findings highlight the influence that the environment has on what children and adolescents learn about working in today's society.

While many adolescents in the developing world struggle to attend school while actively participating in farming, selling "street goods," or other activities to support their families, in industrialized nations adolescents' entry to the formal workforce often means departure from school or at least decreased attention to academic success. Some parents living in poorer circumstances may perceive that they have little choice in deciding whether their children should work and may trade off immediate economic returns (their children's wages) with longer-term goals such as preparation for advanced education or for vocational training (Zimmer-Gembeck and Mortimer, 2006). In middle- and upper-class families, adolescents may choose to work for a variety of reasons, including increased independence; saving for a valued possession or goal, such as a car or computer or higher education, or participation in social activities.

Seventh grade appears to be a common and major transition point to paid work outside of the home and therefore could be considered a turning point in vocational exploratory behavior. By seventh grade, children often report some regular paid work experience outside of the home, including babysitting, yard work such as mowing lawns, or other manual labor (Hartung, et al., 2005), although the employment participation patterns of adolescents have varied in the United States over the last few decades as economic conditions have changed. In 1979, Goldstein and Oldham reported that 33 percent of teenagers reported working for an organization, 36 percent reported a work commitment of at least 7 hours per week, and 25 percent reported multiple types of work experiences. In 2000, the estimated labor force participation for 16- to 17-year-olds was 68.5 percent (75.3% for males, 62.1% for females), resulting in more than 6 million employed adolescents in the United States (Runyan, et al., 2007). However, in 2008, a report by the Center for Labor Market Studies at Northeastern University cited a 60-year historical low point for summer teen employment of 32.7 percent (Sum, Khatiwada, McLaughlin, and Palma, 2008). This downturn in adolescent employment was connected to rising unemployment in the United States and poorer economic conditions.

Zimmer-Gembeck and Mortimer (2006) point out that both the advantages and disadvantages to working as an adolescent should be weighed. The number of hours a teen works may be a key variable. As teenagers approach later adolescence, working has the potential to positively influence vocational identity, promote the process of learning to set and achieve personal goals, promote exploration of interests in work training and career paths, provide experiences that build confidence and competence in work skills, and provide exposure to diverse employment settings. Working also provides exposure to a range of adults and role models outside the family and school.

However, while the benefits of work for adolescents in terms of the development of lifelong skills to support self-determination and self-sufficiency are considerable, the potential negative outcomes must also be considered, and there is debate regarding the appropriate balance of work and school as the importance of formal education increases. Dangers other than distraction from school and academic success have also been noted. Runyan and colleagues (2003) conducted a cross-sectional survey of teens in the retail and service sectors and noted that "teens are exposed to multiple hazards, use dangerous equipment despite federal prohibitions, and work long hours during the school week. They also lack consistent training and adult supervision on the job." Higher rates of smoking and alcohol consumption have also been reported in teens who work a higher number of hours

(Paschall, Flewelling, and Russell, 2004; Ramchand, Ialongo, and Chilcoat, 2007). A 2003 report published by the Canadian Ministry of Industry summarized a number of research studies that correlated increased number of hours worked with an increased likelihood of dropping out of school (Bushnik, 2003).

While much of this text focuses on work-related services within the United States, the variability of experience for children and adolescents around the world is important to note as we become more globally connected and as the United States becomes more culturally diverse. This is true for both the value of education and the experience of adolescents with work. For example, in Germany, blue-collar work is viewed differently than in the United States, and more pride is taken in success in technical vocations. Adolescent apprentices in Germany learn a craft or trade and obtain certification to enter the same field upon completion of a coordinated school and work sequence. Zimmer-Gembeck and Mortimer (2006) cite a report by Fullarton that notes that in some parts of Australia, the existence of different tracks in secondary school necessitate that young people (and their families) consider their future fields of study as early as grades 8 and 9. In India, only 62 percent of children entering school at age 6 finish all 5 years of primary school. Among teenagers (10–19 years), one-third are illiterate. Verma and Sraswathi (2002) described the diversity of child employment in India: "Children work in agriculture, mines, in the match and fireworks industries, cigarette manufacturing, diamond polishing, handicrafts, carpet weaving, and glass factories. They are also employed as gas station attendants and in restaurants: Adolescents on the streets resort to rag-picking, begging, shoe-shining, selling balloons and fruits and vegetables."

It is also worth noting that considerable variability exists even in the United States. Heckman and LaFontaine (2008) noted that America is becoming a polarized society. While proportionately more American youth are going to college and graduating than ever before, at the same time, proportionately more are failing to complete high school. The levels and trends in the true high school graduation rate have been hotly debated in the popular press. Depending on the data sources, definitions, and methods used, the U.S. graduation rate has been estimated to be anywhere from 66 to 88 percent in recent years—an astonishingly wide range for such a basic statistic. The range of estimated minority rates is even greater—from 50 to 85 percent.

In the United States, late adolescence is focused on either transitioning directly to the workplace if a teenager fails to complete high school or does not pursue vocational training or college or to advanced education in a college, university, or technical school. Enrollment in degree-granting institutions has increased markedly in the United States and since the mid-1980s, more women than men have been graduating from these institutions. Between 1995 and 2005, overall enrollment increased by 23 percent. The number of young students has been growing more rapidly than the number of older students, but this pattern is expected to shift: by 2016, a 15 percent increase in enrollments of people under 25 and a 21 percent increase in enrollments of people 25 and over are projected (U.S. Department of Education National Center for Education Statistics, 2008). As with the U.S. population at large, the number of minority students (including Hispanics, Asian or Pacific Islanders, and black) enrolled in colleges has also increased. Multiple factors have driven higher college enrollments, including the changing status of the economy (higher rates of unemployment mean more high school graduates go on to more education or training), increasing requirements for obtaining some jobs or entering some professions (such as the move to postbaccalaureate education for occupational therapy), and the assumption that college graduates earn a higher income than those with only a high school education.

Defining the transition from adolescence to adulthood is difficult. While we can describe the physical and cognitive changes that occur during adolescence, such as the maturation of body systems and the move to formal operations and abstract thinking, defining clear-cut changes in roles and responsibilities is more difficult. Is the 20-year-old who lives in her own apartment, attends college part time, and works part time but receives financial assistance from her parents and eats dinner at their home several times a week while her mother does her laundry an adolescent or an adult? What about the 17-year-old single mother working full time and living with a multigenerational family that helps to care for her child? Or the 28-year-old son with a graduate degree who is employed full time but who still lives at home?

While shifts in the paths to adulthood have become more varied, making a decision about the work one will perform as an adult or the career one will pursue remains a major landmark in the transition from adolescence to adulthood. According to the U.S. Department of Labor, approximately 68 percent of U.S. adults participated in paid employment in 2009 (U.S. Bureau of Labor Statistics, 2009). This figure does not include persons performing nonpaid labor such as home or child care and those working for cash and not paying payroll taxes. Theories to explain the process of selecting a career or type of work continue to be researched and developed, and an awareness and understanding of these theories is most helpful especially for the occupational therapy practitioner working with adolescents or young adults. The most common of these theories are described in the next section.

Models of Career Exploration and Development

Career development theories have primarily been developed within the last century. *Vocational guidance*, which was the foundation for career development counseling, started in the early 1900s. Frank Parsons (1854–1908) is widely recognized as the "father of vocational guidance" and in 1909 published one of the first books on vocational guidance. Early theories of vocational development focused on the content of career choice, such as the characteristics of individuals, and became known as *trait* and *factor* theories (Patton and McMahon, 2006a). Later theories focused more on the process and stages of career development and became known as development theories. Most recently, theorists have focused on *constructivist perspectives* with an emphasis on context and cultural diversity and self-construction and development (Guichard and Lenz, 2005). A few models of career exploration, development, and vocational choice are presented next.

Ginzberg, Ginsburg, Axelrad, and Herma's Developmental Theory (1951)

Developmental theory proposes that vocational choice is influenced by four factors: (1) the reality factor, such as constraints in the world of work; (2) the influence of the educational process on the range of future opportunities available to an individual; (3) the emotional factor, which relates to the interaction between an individual and his or her work environment and the resulting work satisfaction or dissatisfaction; and (4) individual values as they relate to work (Patton and McMahon, 2006c). The theory further proposes individuals pass through three stages starting in preteen and ending in young adulthood: (1) fantasy, (2) tentative, and (3) realistic. In the fantasy stage, the child fantasizes about any possible occupational choice that may be influenced by family, popular media, and imagination. Through this process, children identify occupations and activities that match their interests, and these can be related to future career choices. Beginning in late childhood and continuing through mid-adolescence, young persons further explore and define their values, interests, and abilities in relation to occupational choice. The realistic stage, spanning from mid-adolescence through young adulthood, has three substages: exploration, crystallization, and specification. In the exploration stage, the adolescent begins to restrict choice on the basis of personal likes, skills, and abilities. In the crystallization stage, an occupational choice is made. In the specification stage, the individual pursues the education required to achieve his or her career goal.

The work of Ginzberg and colleagues continues to be highly influential in career development today. The primary criticisms are related to the linear nature of the theory, a common criticism with most *stage* theories; underconsideration of nonwork factors such as gender, personal and family relationships, and dynamics; the limited consideration of social class, economics, and the influence of culturally bound values on the workplace. The theory has also been criticized for its heavy focus on earlier developmental years. Others suggest that models such as Ginzberg's simply need to be updated as society evolves, and thus Ginzberg's model remains relevant if allowing for current cultural evolutions and the more constructivist view of career development assumed today.

Super's Theory of Vocational Development (1954)

The works of Super and Ginzberg and colleagues are closely related and are both described as *developmental* theories. Super's theory of vocational development identifies six life and career development stages. The six stages, approximate age ranges, and primary development tasks are presented in Table 2.2. As with most stage theories, considerable variability occurs among individuals in the age at which stages are experienced, the duration of a given stage, the significance of the stage, and the possibility that the stage will recur. Recurrence is common with adults who change careers, such as the many older or "nontraditional" students who enter occupational therapy educational programs.

Super's theory places an emphasis on the relationship between self-concept and choice of work and career. Vocational self-concept is specifically related to participation in work and vocational activity. Zunker (1994) stated that vocational self-concept "develops through physical and mental growth, observations of work, identification with working adults, general environment, and general experiences. As experiences become broader in relation to awareness of the world of work, the more sophisticated vocational self-concept is formed."

Super's work has been criticized for inadequate focus on women, persons of color, and the poor (Brown, 1990). Further, with changes in the demographics of the workforce, including an increasing number of older workers who may continue to work part time well

Table 2.2 | Super's Theory of Vocational Development

Stage of Vocational Development	Approximate Ages	Developmental Task
Crystallization	14–18	Developing and planning a tentative vocational goal based on general knowledge in adolescence
Specification	18–21	Developing a focused vocational goal as one prepares for adulthood and enters college, training, or work
Implementation	21–24	Training for and obtaining specific employment
Stabilization	24–35	Working and confirming one's career or vocational choice
Consolidation	36–54	Advancing in one's career
Readiness for retirement	55 and over	Preparing for separation from the workforce and for retirement

into late life or even start new careers in later life, this theory as originally proposed may have limited utility.

Holland's Career Typology (1959)

Holland's career typology theory is grounded in what he calls modal personal orientation, or a developmental process established through heredity and the individual's life history of reacting to environmental demands. More simply put, individuals are attracted to a particular occupation that meets their personal needs and provides them satisfaction, and the extent to which an individual is successful at his or her career depends on the goodness of this fit. The theory addresses personality *in* environments. The theory rests on four assumptions:

1. Persons can be categorized as one of the following personality types: realistic, investigative, artistic, social, enterprising, or conventional.
2. There are six modal environments: realistic, investigative, artistic, social, enterprising, and conventional.
3. People search for environments that let them exercise their skills and abilities, express their attitudes and values, and take on agreeable problems and roles.
4. Behavior is determined by an interaction between an individual's personality and the environments in which he or she operates.

Holland's theory has been particularly influential on the development and use of interest inventories in the field of vocational guidance and counseling, including the *Strong–Campbell Interest Inventory* (Campbell and Borgen, 1999). Holland's theory has influenced how vocational counseling and assistance have been delivered around the globe, and it continues to be a major influence today.

The strongest criticisms of this theory are based on gender bias because females tend to score in three personality types (artistic, social, and conventional). Holland attributes this to societal expectations that channel females into female-dominated occupations. If this is true, we may see a shift in how women score as the role of women in the workplace continues to change. The theory is also criticized for not adequately addressing the career needs of certain racial and ethnic groups, although Holland himself cautioned that "age, gender, social class, physical assets or liabilities, educational level attained, intelligence and influence" may affect successful application of his theory (Patton and McMahon, 2006a).

Lent, Brown, and Hackett's Social Cognitive Career Theory (1987)

Social cognitive career theory (SCCT) is an integrative theory of academic- and career-related interests, choice, performance, and satisfaction, and it extends Bandura's social cognitive theory to career choice and behavior (Bandura, 1989). It proposes that career choice is influenced by the beliefs that individuals develop and refine through four major sources: (1) personal performance accomplishments, (2) vicarious learning, (3) social persuasion, and (4) physiological states and reactions. These four sources affect the career development process as individuals develop skills and abilities for specific work and experience feedback based on their success or failure. Through these experiences, individuals' self-efficacy or belief in future continued work success is developed, and they are more likely to pursue activities and make career choices that relate to their expectation of success. As children and adolescents age and have increasing success and failure experiences, they can begin to narrow their focus toward successful ventures, and these attempts help them to create a specific career path. The extent to which persons anticipate that they will be rewarded for their successful vocational activities influences their perception of the importance of those activities and the continued likelihood of further participation.

The theory recognizes that environmental influences such as from peer, family, and other social groups affect our perception of the probability of success of the vocational choices we make. When perceived barriers to success are low, we may be more likely to anticipate success, which in turn reinforces a particular career path. However, if we perceive that the barriers are significant and may lessen our chance of success, we may be less likely to make continued career choices in that direction. By adolescence, most of us have a well-developed sense of our skills and abilities and what we perceive ourselves to be "good at." We can also connect our perceived capacities to various career choices. The SCCT differs from most career theories in its dynamic nature. Through its focus on the role of the self-system and the individual's beliefs, the inherent influence of social and economic contexts are addressed.

Systems Theory Framework (STF) of Career Development

The STF of career development views career development as a process affected by a variety of influences indentified over time by researchers and proponents of the theory (Patton and McMahon, 2006b). The term influence was deliberately chosen by the developers of the STF as a dynamic term that reflects both content and process components of earlier career theories. Content influences include (1) intrapersonal variables such as personality and age and (2) contextual variables that comprise both social influences, such as family, and environmental/societal influences, such as geographic location. The process influences include recurring interaction (both within the individual and between the individual and the context), change over time, and chance.

The individual system is at the core in the STF approach and includes a range of intrapersonal influences such as gender, interests, age, abilities, personality, and sexual orientation. In terms of systems theory, the individual is a system in its own right; however, an individual as a system does not live in isolation but as part of a much broader contextual system. Occupational therapy practitioners are likely to be familiar with systems theory because of its influence in the development of occupational therapy conceptual practice models, such as the model of human occupation (MOHO), that recognize that a person's volition, habituation, performance capacity, and environmental factors must be considered in assessment and intervention (Kielhofner, 2008).

The broader contextual system in which the individual operates includes the social system and the environmental/societal system. The social system refers to family members, teachers, peers, and other persons with whom the individual interacts. The individual and the social system both operate within the environmental/societal system. While the environmental/societal system clearly has a direct impact on career development, the influence of the individual and the social system should not be overlooked. Geographic location or socioeconomic circumstances may directly influence the career development opportunities available to the individual (McMahon, 2005).

Occupational Identity, Occupational Competence, and Occupational Adaptation

The career development theories just reviewed might provide explanation for the choices we make about the type of work we pursue and *what we do* as a worker. As occupational therapy practitioners, we recognize that our occupational choices (choices about which familiar and important everyday occupations we perform) are closely tied to our sense of *who we are*—or our identity (Christiansen and Townsend, 2010). Most people think about themselves in several ways, and these various perspectives often are tied to the roles they occupy and the life contexts in which they operate. In occupational therapy literature, the term *occupational identity* is defined as "a composite sense of who one is and wishes to become as an occupational being generated from one's history of occupational participation" (Kielhofner, 2008).

> *In occupational therapy literature, the term occupational identity is defined as "a composite sense of who one is and wishes to become as an occupational being generated from one's history of occupational participation." (Kielhofner, 2008)*

The various components of an individual's identity can be conceptualized as tied to the roles that he or she fulfills. Most of us perform multiple roles across our lives, and we may adopt new roles, abandon roles, or move in and out of a role across our lifetimes. For example, we adopt the role of parent upon having a child. We may leave the role of student or worker behind when we complete our education or retire. However, we may also return to school later in life or reenter the workforce and once again adopt the role of student or worker. And, although we may not perform the associated occupations of the role each and every day, those of us who are parents most likely see themselves within that role no matter how old or independent their children become.

To help understand this a bit more, think about how you answer the request, "Tell me about yourself." A common response might begin by listing the various roles that you occupy. For instance, you might say, "Well, I am a student, and a spouse, and a tennis player." When other persons recognize and respond to us as occupying a particular role with its associated status in society (Fig. 2.2), and we begin to see ourselves and our actions reflected in the attitudes and expectations of others in regard to this role, we

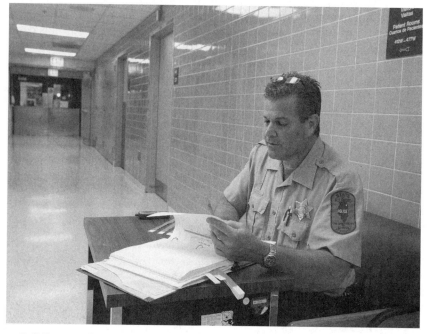

Figure 2.2 Some worker roles, such as a police officer, provide a strong and recognizable personal identity and an associated status in society.

might say that we have *internalized* that role. Kielhofner (2008) defines an internalized role as "the incorporation of a socially and/or personally defined status and a related cluster of attitudes and behaviors." Working typically carries with it a positive status in our society that reflects a level of responsibility, self-sufficiency, and maturity. Typically, adults are expected to adopt the worker role in some fashion and contribute in some manner to maintaining their own independence and to the functioning of society at large.

MOHO is cited liberally throughout this text because of its relevance for understanding work as an area of occupation within our lives. MOHO is an occupational therapy conceptual practice model that seeks to explain the factors that influence the adoption and performance of occupational behavior. Three related and important concepts to the current discussion of the worker role and identity are *occupational identity*, *occupational competence*, and *occupational adaptation*. Occupational identity has to do with the subjective meaning of one's occupational life. The major components of occupational identity are listed in Box 2.4.

Occupational competence is "the degree to which one sustains a pattern of occupational participation that reflects one's occupational identity" (Kielhofner, 2008). Occupational competence has to do with putting one's occupational identity into action. The major components of occupational competence are listed in Box 2.5.

Occupational adaptation is, according to Kielhofner, "a positive occupational identity and achieving occupational competence over time in the context of one's environment." MOHO views that all occupational behavior, including work performance, is influenced by the following:

- Volition: Patterns of thoughts and feelings about oneself as an actor in one's world that occur as one anticipates, chooses, experiences, and interprets what one does.
- Habituation: Internalized readiness to exhibit consistent patterns of behavior guided by habits and roles and fitted to the characteristics of routine temporal, physical, and social environments.
- Performance capacity: The ability to do things provided by the status of underlying objective physical and mental components and corresponding subjective experience.
- Environment: Particular physical and social features of the specific context in which one performs an activity that impacts what one does and how it is done.

Box 2.4 Major Components of Occupational Identity

- One's sense of capacity and effectiveness for doing.
- What things one finds interesting and satisfying to do.
- Who one is, as defined by one's roles and relationships.
- What one feels obligated to do and holds as important.
- A sense of the familiar and routines of life.
- Perceptions of one's environment and what it supports and expects.

(Kielhofner, 2008)

Box 2.5 Major Components of Occupational Competence

- Fulfilling the expectations of one's roles and one's own values and standards for performance.
- Maintaining a routine that allows one to discharge responsibilities.
- Participating in a range of occupations that provide a sense of ability, control, satisfaction, and fulfillment.
- Pursuing one's values and taking action to achieve desired life outcomes.

(Kielhofner, 2008)

To apply the concepts of occupational identity, occupational competence, and occupational adaptation, let's return briefly to the case illustration introduced at the start of this chapter. You met Craig, who failed at several attempts to complete vocational preparation programs due to an inability to arrive on time and who had been fired from multiple jobs for the same reason. Despite this, Craig claims to be highly motivated to attend and complete a vocational preparation program and to be successful at work. In fact, in further discussions, Craig talks about the success he has had as a worker, albeit limited, with pride. What might we say about Craig's occupational identity, occupational competence, and occupational adaptation based on what we know?

Because Craig continues to attempt to integrate work into his daily routine, recognizes society's messages and values as well as the positive status associated with being a worker, and continues to feel a sense of obligation to pursue working, we might say that Craig has internalized the role of "worker" to some extent. While his identity may be further crystallized with increased vocational success and may be at risk if he continues to fail, Craig sees working as part of who he is and the person he wishes to become, even if his experiences to date do not fully leave him with a positive self-image. However, because Craig has experienced great difficulty in putting his identity as a worker into sustained action, we might describe his level of occupational competence as low. He is not yet fulfilling typical expectations and standards for performance as an adult worker; is not maintaining a routine that allows him to meet all of his responsibilities; is not participating in a range of occupations that provide an adequate sense of ability, control, satisfaction, and fulfillment; and consequently is not achieving his desired life outcomes. We might also describe his level of occupational adaptation as low. Despite his struggle to create and solidify an identity as a worker, he has not yet achieved a sustained level of competence in that role.

Craig typifies one type of client sometimes seen by occupational therapy practitioners in work-related practice: a client who is working to establish an occupational identity as a worker and to develop a level of occupational competence that allows the client to meet internal and external expectations for occupational performance and to obtain a satisfactory level of occupational adaptation. However, occupational therapy practitioners often encounter clients who have a significant work history, who have established a solid occupational identity as a worker at some point in their lives, and who may have been highly successful as a worker but are now experiencing a challenge due to an impairment or disability. The next section of this chapter discusses the impact of impairment or disability on individuals' identity as a worker. Many of the other chapters focus on specific strategies for assessing areas of work performance and on intervention with clients in various work-related settings.

Conceptualizing Challenges to Occupational Identity, Competence, and Adaptation

Workers can face a myriad of challenges to occupational performance. Examples include an acute musculoskeletal injury such as a hand, shoulder, or back injury or more chronic or cumulative disorders such as carpal tunnel syndrome. Others may face longer-term challenges such as mental illness, multiple sclerosis, spinal cord injury, or head injury. A growing number of workers face challenges associated with more subtle changes that accompany age, such as decreased endurance or vision or hearing impairment.

You might be thinking there is a big difference between an acute injury that will likely be remediated (e.g., by surgery and a period of physical therapy) and a spinal cord injury or mental illness that will require longer-term attention and intervention and may never be "cured." And if so, you are correct. Before examining specific cases of the impact of challenges to occupational performance and an individual's worker role and identity, it is helpful to understand how these challenges are often conceptualized or categorized.

One way to conceptualize these challenges is to draw on concepts presented by the World Health Organization (WHO) in the *International Classification of Functioning, Disability and Health*, or ICF (2008). The ICF provides a standard language and framework for the description of health and health-related states, including both short- and long-term challenges to occupational performance. The WHO (2002) describes the ICF as "a classification of health and health-related domains—domains that help us to describe changes in body function and structure, what a person with a health condition can do in a standard environment (their level of capacity), as well as what they actually do in their usual environment (their level of performance). These concepts have been embraced by the occupational therapy profession and other health professions and are reflected widely in the revised *Occupational Therapy Practice Framework: Domain and Process*, 2nd edition (AOTA, 2008).

Figure 2.3 illustrates the model of disability that underlies the ICF, which views disability and functioning as outcomes of interactions between *health conditions* (diseases, disorders, and injuries) and *contextual factors*. The diagram identifies the three levels of human functioning classified by ICF: (1) functioning at the level of body or body part, (2) functioning at the level of the whole person, and (3) functioning of the whole person in a social context. Disability therefore involves dysfunction at one or more of these levels: impairments, activity limitations, and participation restrictions (WHO, 2002). Definitions of each of the components of the model presented in Figure 2.3 are included in Box 2.6.

Another important way to conceptualize major challenges to occupational performance is to consider *models of disability*. Two proposed models are the *medical model* and the *social model* of disability. The basic tenets of these models are incorporated into the ICF. The medical model views disability as a characteristic or feature of the person and

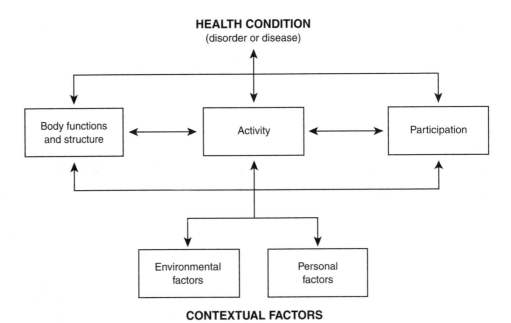

Figure 2.3 A model of disability as a basis for the ICF. (Adapted from World Health Organization, 2002.)

Box 2.6   Key Terms from the International Classification of Functioning, Disability, and Health

---

- Body functions are physiological functions of body systems (including psychological functions).
- Body structures are anatomical parts of the body such as organs, limbs, and their components.
- Impairments are problems in body function or structure, such as a significant deviation or loss.
- Activity is the execution of a task or action by an individual.
- Participation is involvement in a life situation.
- Activity limitations are difficulties an individual may have in executing activities. Participation restrictions are problems an individual may experience in involvement in life situations.
- Environmental factors make up the physical, social, and attitudinal environment in which people live and conduct their lives.

(World Health Organization, 2002)

holds that the underlying cause of decreased occupational performance or disability is the disease, trauma, or other health condition. In this model, disability is addressed via medical or other intervention focused on correcting the underlying problem. The model assumes that if the underlying problem is fixed or cured, the disability will automatically be alleviated.

The social model of disability views disability as a socially created construct or problem rather than as a characteristic or trait of the individual. From this perspective, alleviating disability requires environmental, systems, or political solutions or interventions. The underlying cause of disability is seen as a mismatch between the individual and the physical or social environment as a result of the attitudes or other characteristics of the social environment. According to this model, the negative effects of disability may be alleviated by interventions aimed at changing the environment and decreasing the gap in person–environment fit. For example, under the Americans with Disabilities Act (ADA), workers with disabilities may request *reasonable accommodations*, which are changes or adjustments in the work environment or sometimes in the work itself that make it possible for an otherwise qualified employee with a disability to perform the essential duties or tasks required of a job. Chapter 16 provides an in-depth discussion of the ADA. From a social model of disability perspective, we might ask, "If a person with a disability who has a fatiguing illness is provided the reasonable accommodation of taking more frequent breaks and being paid for fewer hours is able to fulfill all the essentials functions of the job, is that person disabled by his or her condition?" Strictly from the perspective of the social model of disability, the answer is no, at least in regard to the job and work environment, because there is no longer a mismatch between the person and his or her environmental demands.

While both the medical and social models of disability have aspects that can be useful in understanding challenges to occupational performance, they both also have limitations that prevent either from adequately addressing the full range of situations in which occupational therapy practitioners operate. As noted by the WHO (2008), "Disability is a complex phenomena that is both a problem at the level of a person's body and a complex and primarily social phenomena. Disability is always an interaction between features of the person and features of the overall context in which the person lives, but some aspects of disability are almost entirely internal to the person, while another aspect is almost entirely external. In other words, both medical and social responses are appropriate to the problems associated with disability; we cannot wholly reject either kind of intervention."

Now that you have been introduced to a few ways of conceptualizing challenges to occupational identity, competence, and adaptation, we return to the discussion of these constructs in regard to the worker role. The extent to which impairment or disability may interfere with occupational performance and challenge a worker's occupational identity, competence, and level of occupational adaptation depends on a number of factors, including the following:

- Has the individual previously developed a strong sense of occupational identity and competence as a worker upon which to draw?
- At what level can the challenge to occupational performance be characterized (e.g., impairment, activity, or participation)?
- Does the individual anticipate that the impairment or disability is temporary or permanent, and does he or she expect increased participation in the future?
- How severe an impact on occupational performance does the individual perceive the impairment or disability to be?
- Are there adequate social and environmental supports upon which the individual can draw to remediate or adapt to limitations to facilitate improved occupational performance?

These are just a few of the questions that must be answered in order to best assess and intervene in work-related practice. Later chapters in this text present strategies to assist you in answering these and other questions. However, it may be helpful to your understanding of the concepts in this chapter to see them applied to real-life cases. Let's return to our discussion of Craig and introduce another occupational therapy client, Halina, to illustrate how an individual with a disability can respond to challenges to occupational performance.

To begin with, we need to question what else we might learn about Craig and his situation to understand all of the factors affecting his success at obtaining and maintaining employment. We have information about his volition (i.e., motivation for work) and his competence, but what else do we need to know? For example, what are the societal and economic issues that he and other persons with disabilities face? Should we consider Craig a person with a disability? We might seek the answers to these questions, among others:

- What stigma is associated with being an adult with a limited work history and a history of substance abuse?
- What issues do employers face when considering hiring a person with a disability? What might be on an employer's mind when evaluating Craig?
- What is the current political economy? Is this a particularly good or bad time to consider special requests from employees or potential employees?
- What systems issues may make it difficult for Craig to stay in a job? Does he receive Social Security Income (SSI) and the associated health benefits that might be affected if he earns an income?
- What supports might Craig need to pursue his interests and succeed? Might the stress of working on a permanent basis influence his psychiatric condition?
- What are Craig's rights in the interview, training, and orientation and in employment processes?

Finding the answers to these questions is useful to the occupational therapy practitioner in guiding Craig and the employer in making decisions that are fair and legal to both parties.

Halina is a 50-year-old Polish immigrant who moved to the United States with her family when she was 11 years old. She had a mild stroke 2 years ago and has been unemployed since then. She recently enrolled in a work-readiness program. She had a strong work history prior to her cerebrovascular accident (CVA), having worked in customer service since graduating from high school. During the initial interview, Halina presents with a strong sense of volition and identity as a worker. However, she also states that "I really think I *could* be working, but there is so much to think about and so many things to figure out, I am considering just giving it all up and seeing if I can stay on disability." Before proceeding with Halina's case, stop reading for a moment and answer the following questions:

• Why do you think that Halina is not working? Can you identify several possible contributing factors?
• What more do you need to know? How might you start to assess Halina's strengths and limiting factors?
• What might you do to support both Halina *and* a potential employer?

As you work with Halina in the program, you administer and score the Worker Role Interview (WRI), which assesses Halina's psychosocial capacity for return to work (see Chapter 11 for an in-depth description of the WRI). You also complete assessments of Halina's cognitive and perceptual strengths, her motor capacities, and her functional abilities to complete some of the typical work tasks that she would perform, such as using a computer.

Through your evaluation, you have learned the following about Halina:

• Halina has normal cognitive and perceptual functioning and is able to independently complete routine work tasks despite minimally decreased coordination and some motor impairment in her right upper extremity.
• Halina has significant aphasia that causes her to slur her words, and she shares that others have interpreted this as her being cognitively impaired or even drunk. A customer had even called and "reported her" to her supervisor.
• Halina made a previous attempt to return to her old job but did so with no accommodations to work tasks and with no assistance or support. She states that it "fell apart" after just a few weeks, and she quit because she assumed she was about to be fired.
• Halina shares that she felt her previous employer was supportive overall but "just did not know what to do, and neither did I."

Following the assessment process, occupational therapy intervention focuses on exploring Halina's options for working and particularly the types of reasonable accommodations she might explore under the ADA. A volunteer experience confirms that Halina is highly motivated, as she arrived early each day for her shift and readily volunteered to stay late and come in extra days. Her volunteer supervisor confirms that Halina was able to complete basic computer functions with little difficulty and showed no signs of a cognitive or perceptual deficit that would interfere with working.

Despite becoming more confident in her potential and more comfortable around "coworkers," Halina remains very concerned about her aphasia and how customers and a boss in a "real job" would react to her speech. She remains hesitant to return to competitive employment even though she now has support and is aware of the options to request that her employer provide reasonable accommodations.

As you continue to work with Halina, you contact several companies that provide customer service to persons over the phone and the Internet and seek guidance and suggestions from their human resource offices. You learn that pursuing a job where Halina could work in customer service by "chatting online" with customers might be a good option both to accommodate for Halina's aphasia and because of the flexibility to work varied hours and from her home. After you discuss these options with Halina, she decides to contact her prior employer, who agrees to provide a positive reference after learning why Halina originally left the company. He also is able to give Halina some leads on companies that provide Internet customer service and often have open positions. By looking beyond challenges caused by the direct impact of Halina's stroke and examining the larger environment and factors influencing Halina's decision making, you successfully help Halina to explore options not previously considered.

By looking beyond challenges caused by the direct impact of Halina's stroke and examining the larger environment and factors influencing Halina's decision making, you successfully helped Halina to explore options not previously considered.

Chapter Summary

This chapter provided a description of vocational development across the life span but with an emphasis on earlier development during childhood and adolescence. Many of the other chapters focus on adults, and Chapter 8 focuses specifically on older adults. Factors that influence how children and adolescents come to learn about work and to develop and pursue vocational interests were explained. A number of the major models related to theories of career exploration and development were also introduced and discussed.

You were introduced to the important concepts of occupational identity, occupational competence, and occupational adaptation, as presented in the model of human occupation. Understanding the relationship between identity and competence will be of great importance as you begin to consider the factors that can influence whether or not a client obtains employment or returns to work following the onset of impairment or disability.

Finally, several methods of conceptualizing challenges to occupational performance were introduced and discussed. The ICF was introduced, and its influence on the occupational therapy profession was explained. Two models of disability (the medical model and the social model) were explained, and the advantages and disadvantages of each model were highlighted. Two case presentations illustrated many of these important concepts.

The next chapter explores some of the cultural influences on work and working as you read about work around the world and cultural perspectives on work and vocational rehabilitation.

Case Resolution

As part of the evaluation process with Craig, the occupational therapist administered a number of assessments, including an interview combining the Occupational Performance History Interview (OPHI-II) and the Worker Role Interview (WRI).[1] In addition to collecting a comprehensive work history, the therapist administered an Occupational Questionnaire. Through these assessments, the occupational therapist gained an in-depth understanding of Craig's view of his history, his true level of motivation to work, and what might be behind Craig's problems with getting to work or vocational preparation programming on time.

Craig validated much of what was documented in his records. He admitted that he was often late musing, "I'll be late for my own funeral, I guess." He told a similar story to that reflected in his history, as portrayed in program documentation, with one

---

[1]The assessments mentioned in the case resolution are all based on MOHO and are presented in later chapters. Additional information can be found in the list of resources at the end of the chapter.

exception. He consistently commented how much he wanted to work and to be independent and to care for himself. He noted the feelings of inadequacy and shame that he felt because he could not hold a job long enough to prove his abilities and to earn a living and become self-sufficient. He also worried about discrimination that might accompany the stigma often associated with a history of mental illness.

Upon reviewing the Occupational Questionnaire, an assessment designed to show the occupations that a client completes on a typical weekday and weekend day and their meaning and value to a client, the occupational therapist noted something interesting. Craig seemed to be spending an inordinate amount of time in the morning preparing for his day. In addition, there were times throughout the day that Craig simply could not account for. The therapist investigated further and found that Craig struggled with some basic daily routines and had never seemed to develop simple habits and organizational skills like focusing on one daily living task at a time. Because of the way Craig structured his day, it took him much longer than he planned to complete even the simplest tasks, which in turn caused him to be late. Rather than assuming that Craig was not motivated, the therapist assumed that Craig lacked habits and skills that he could learn to improve his occupational performance.

Over the following 2 months, Craig worked diligently with this therapist to implement a number of strategies to improve his organization and timeliness. In his eighth week, he successfully arrived to the work-readiness program on time 4 out of 5 days. Moreover, Craig and his occupational therapist met with the director of a vocational training program and reviewed his history and recent accomplishments. The director was impressed by what he called Craig's "obvious drive to be successful as a worker" and agreed to accept Craig in the program on a part-time basis while Craig and his occupational therapist continued to work to improve his competence in his basic organizational skills.

While earlier practitioners had given up on Craig because they assumed that he lacked the motivation to complete vocational training and obtain a job, the occupational therapist looked deeper. Because the therapist understood that a client's level of occupational adaptation comprises both occupational identity and competence, the therapist assessed these areas. The therapist discovered that Craig had a high level of volition to become a worker but lacked the basic habits and skills to allow for adequate occupational competence.

References

American Occupational Therapy Association. (2008). Occupational therapy practice framework: Domain and process, 2nd ed. *American Journal of Occupational Therapy, 62*, 625–683.

Anderson, D. E. (2003). *Longitudinal study of the development and consequences of formal operations and intellectual flexibility*. Meadville, PA: Allegheny College. (ERIC Document Reproduction Service No. ED481115).

Bandura, A. (1989). Social cognitive theory. In R.Vasta (ed.), *Annals of Child Development. Vol. 6. Six Theories of Child Development* (pp. 1–60). Greenwich, CT: JAI Press.

Brown, D. (1990). Summary, comparison, and critique of the major theories. In D. Brown & L. Brooks (eds.), *Career Choice and Development* (pp. 338–363). San Francisco: Jossey-Bass.

Bushnik, T. (2003). Learning, earning, and leaving: The relationship between working while in high school and dropping out (Rep. No. Catalogue no. 81-595-MIE—No. 004). Ottawa, Canada: Culture, Tourism and the Centre for Educational Statistics.

Campbell, D. P., & Borgen, F. H. (1999). Holland's theory and the development of interest inventories. *Journal of Vocational Behavior, 55*(1), 86–101.

Christiansen, C. H., & Townsend, E. A. (2010). *Introduction to Occupation: The Art and Science of Living,* 2nd ed. Upper Saddle River, NJ: Pearson Education.

Cronin, A., & Mandich, M. (2005). *Human Development and Performance throughout the Lifespan*. Clifton Park, NY: Thomson/Delmar Learning.

Erikson, E. E. (1968). *Youth and Crisis*. New York: Norton.

Ginsberg, E., Ginsburg, S. W., Axelrad, S., & Herma, J. L. (1951). *Occupational Choice: An Approach to a General Theory*. New York: Columbia University Press.

Goldstein, B., & Oldham, J. (1979). *Children and Work: A Study of Socialization*. New Brunswick, NJ: Transaction Books.

Guichard, J., & Lenz, J. (2005). Career theory from an international perspective. *Career Development Quarterly, 54*(1), 17–28.

Hartung, P. J., Porfeli, E. J., & Vondracek, F. W. (2005). Child vocational development: A review and reconsideration. *Journal of Vocational Behavior, 66*(3), 385–419.

Havighurst, R. J. (1964). Youth in exploration and man emergent. In H. Borow (ed.), *Man in a World at Work* (pp. 215–236). Boston: Houghton Mifflin.

Heckman, J. J., & LaFontaine, P. A. (2008). The declining American high school graduation rate: Evidence, sources, and consequences. National Bureau of Economic Research. Retrieved from www.nber.org/reporter/2008number1/heckman.html.

Jordan, T. E., & Pope, M. L. (2001). Developmental antecedents to adolescents' occupational knowledge: A 17-year prospective study. *Journal of Vocational Behavior, 58*(2), 279–292.

Kett, J. F. (1978). Curing the disease of precocity. *American Journal of Sociology, 84*(1), S183–S211.

Kielhofner, G. (2008). *Model of Human Occupation: Theory and Application.* Baltimore: Lippincott, Williams & Wilkins.

McGee, J., & Stockard, J. (1991). From a child's view: Children's occupational knowledge and perceptions of occupational characteristics. In S. Cahill (ed.), *Sociological Studies of Child Development: Perspectives on and of Children* (pp. 113–136). Greenwich, CT: JAI Press.

McMahon, M. (2005). Career counseling: Applying the systems theory framework of career development. *Journal of Employment Counseling, 42*(1), 29–38.

Parsons, F. (1909). *Choosing a Vocation.* Boston: Houghton Mifflin.

Paschall, M., Flewelling, R., & Russell, T. (2004). Why is work intensity associated with heavy alcohol use among adolescents? *Journal of Research on Adolescence, 34*(1), 79–87.

Patton, W., & McMahon, M. (2006a). *Career Development and Systems Theory: Connecting Theory and Practice,* 2nd ed. Rotterdam: Sense Publishers.

Patton, W., & McMahon, M. (2006b). Systems theory framework of career development. In *Career Development and Systems Theory: Connecting Theory and Practice,* 2nd ed. (pp. 195–223). Rotterdam: Sense Publishers.

Patton, W., & McMahon, M. (2006c). Theories focusing on process. In *Career Development and Systems Theory: Connecting Theory and Practice,* 2nd ed. (pp. 49–75). Rotterdam: Sense Publishers.

Piaget, J. (1977). *The Development of Thought: Equilbration of Cognitive Structure.* New York: Viking Press.

Porfeli, E. J., Erik, J., Hartung, P. J., & Vondracek, F. W. (2008). Children's vocational development: A research rationale. *Career Development Quarterly, 57*(1), 25–37.

Ramchand, R., Ialongo, N., & Chilcoat, H. D. (2007). The effect of working for pay on adolescent tobacco use. *American Journal of Public Health, 97*(11), 2056–2062.

Runyan, C. W., Schulman, M. J., Dal Santo, J., Bowling, J. M., Agans, R., & Ta, M. (2007). Work-related hazards and workplace safety of U.S. adolescents employed in the retail and service sectors. *Pediatrics, 119*(3), 526–534.

Savickas, M. L. (2002). Career construction: A developmental theory of vocational behavior. In D. Brown (ed.), *Career Choice and Development,* 4th ed. (pp. 149–205). New York: Wiley.

Sum, A., Khatiwada, I., McLaughlin, J., & Palma, S. (2008). *The Historically Low Summer and Year Round 2008 Teen Employment Rate: The Case for an Immediate National Public Policy Response to Create Jobs for the Nation's Youth.* Boston, MA: Center for Labor Market Statistics at NorthEastern University.

Super, D. E., Savickas, M. L., & Super, C. M. (1996). A life-span, life-space approach to career development. In D. Brown & L. Brooks (eds.), *Career Choice and Development: Applying Contemporary Theories to Practice,* 3rd ed. (pp. 197–261). San Francisco: Jossey-Bass.

Sutherland, P. (1999). The application of Piagetian and neo-Piagetian ideas to further and higher education. *International Journal of Lifelong Education, 18*(4), 286–294.

U.S. Bureau of Labor Statistics. (2009). Employment situation summary. Retrieved from www.bls.gov.

U.S. Department of Education. (2006). Building the legacy: IDEA 2004. Retrieved from http://idea.ed.gov/explore/view/p/,root,regs,300,A,300%252E43.

U.S. Department of Education National Center for Education Statistics (2008). Fast facts. National Center for Education Statistics. Retrieved from http://nces.ed.gov/fastFacts/display.asp?id=98.

Verma, S., & Saraswathi, T. S. (2002). Adolescence in India: Street urchins or Silicon Valley millionaires? In B. B. Brown, R. Larson, & T. S. Saraswathi (eds.), *The World's Youth: Adolescence in Eight Regions of the Globe* (pp. 104–140). New York: Cambridge University Press.

Vondracek, F. W. (2001). The developmental perspective in vocational psychology. *Journal of Vocational Behavior, 59*(2), 252–261.

World Health Organization (WHO). (2002). *Towards a Common Language for Functioning, Disability and Health: ICF the Classification of Functioning, Disabilty and Health.* Geneva, Switzerland: World Health Organization.

World Health Organization (WHO). (2008). International Classification of Functioning, Disability and Health home page. Retrieved from www.who.int/classifications/icf/site/icftemplate.cfm.

Zimmer-Gembeck, M. J., & Mortimer, J. T. (2006). Adolescent work, vocational development and education. *Review of Educational Research, 76*(4), 537–566.

Zunker, V. G. (1994). *Career Counseling: Applied Concepts of Life Planning.* Pacific Grove, CA: Brooks/Cole.

Glossary

Internalized roles are the incorporation of a socially and/or personally defined status and a related cluster of attitudes and behaviors.

International Classification of Functioning, Disability, and Health (ICF) is a classification of health and health-related domains that help us to describe changes in body function and structure, what individuals with a health condition can do in a standard environment (their level of capacity), as well as what they actually do in their usual environment.

Occupational adaptation is a positive occupational identity and achieving occupational competence over time in the context of one's environment.

Occupational competence is the degree to which one sustains a pattern of occupational participation that reflects one's occupational identity.

Occupational identity is a composite sense of who one is and wishes to become as an occupational being generated from one's history of occupational participation.

Resources

America's Career Resource Network

www.acrnetwork.org

A network of state and federal organizations that provide information, resources, and training on career and education exploration funded by a grant from the U.S. Department of Education.

Human Development and Performance throughout the Lifespan by Anne Cronin and Marybeth Mandich (Clifton Park, NY: Thomson/Delmar Learning, 2005). A resource on human development from an occupational therapy perspective.

Model of Human Occupation Clearinghouse

www.moho.uic.edu/assessments.html

Information on assessments.

World Health Organization

www.who.int/en/

Information on the *International Classification of Functioning, Disability, and Health.*

3

Work Around the World
Cultural Perspectives on Work and Vocational Rehabilitation

Supriya Sen and Brent Braveman

Key Concepts

The following are key concepts addressed in this chapter:
- An exponential rate of change in technologies and communications has contributed to workers becoming more globally connected and therefore more influenced by cultures around the world.
- The prevailing cultural values of the society in which a person or group lives often guides the types of work values pursued.
- A successful return-to-work outcome is dependent on work goals based on the individual's culture, values, and cultural *frame of reference*.
- Becoming a culturally competent occupational therapy practitioner requires application of a *process-oriented model* of cultural competence that includes knowing, doing, and becoming.
- Awareness of the employer's level of cultural sensitivity, practices, policies, and commitment to acceptance of diversity at a workplace, demonstrated by a client's supervisor and coworkers, has an impact on the return-to-work or vocational rehabilitation process.
- Culture and diversity affect both verbal and nonverbal communication, which can have a significant impact on the delivery of work-related services.
- Cultural factors must be considered in selecting an assessment, administering the assessment, and interpreting the information to assure a culturally accurate perspective.

Case Introduction

Maria, a 29-year-old Hispanic female, worked as a machine operator. A metal platform weighing approximately 100 pounds hit Maria in the head, neck, and shoulder while she was at work. She sustained bruising to the right cheek and began experiencing headaches with visual changes, including seeing black spots through the right eye.

At the time of the accident, she reported burning and stabbing pain radiating from the left side of her neck down her shoulder to the left fourth and fifth digits. She also reported pain in the left cheek, left ear, and behind the left eye. She complained of numbness and occasional tingling of the forearm. She was off work for 4 months, during which time she received physical therapy, and then returned to work without restrictions to activity.

Maria reaggravated the injury while at work and stopped working again. A magnetic resonance imaging (MRI) study revealed she had herniated disks at the cervical level. Subsequently, she was referred to physical therapy for her cervical spine and occupational therapy for the resulting upper extremity problems, including pain in her left arm, weak grip strength, and decreased functional mobility of her left upper extremity.

Introduction

In many ways, the world we live in is becoming an ever-smaller place, and we are more globally connected than ever before. One of the most significant influences on globalization has been the emergence of information technologies such as personal and laptop computers, e-mail, the Internet, cell phones and other wireless technologies, and voice-over-Internet protocol (VOIP). These technologies have opened up a new world which allows people who never before had access to each other to communicate rapidly, accurately, easily, and remotely, often using a wireless connection.

The Internet is one of the most powerful tools for communication and information sharing across the world. Channels of communication are evolving so quickly that it is sometimes difficult to keep up with the options available. In the 1980s, documents were mailed, faxed, or hand-delivered in hard copy; today, documents can be e-mailed to multiple recipients simultaneously with just a computer keystroke. Other technologies enable people in various locations to hold live meetings via videoconferencing, using the Internet with audio-video technologies, and even to share tasks such as creating and editing documents in real time from their homes or offices.

Today, occupational therapy practitioners throughout the world can easily communicate and collaborate with each other, with clients, and with other professionals. This advent in communication and information technologies also allows consumers of occupational therapy services to obtain information about a range of products and services so that they have more choices. Occupational therapy practitioners around the world are breaking new ground in work-related research and interventions and creating new initiatives to help occupational therapy consumers lead more productive and fulfilling lives. The availability and convenience of communication and information technologies supports improvement and innovation in research and intervention within the occupational therapy profession as well as the dissemination of information to consumers worldwide.

Because of the exponential rate of change occurring in today's world, the influence of our new global economy on migration patterns and trade between countries has increased substantially, resulting in dramatically increased diversity in the workplace and workforce. These changes have important implications for occupational therapy practitioners and the work-related services they deliver. For example, during the last half of the 20th century, the U.S. population grew dramatically more racially and ethnically diverse (U.S. Bureau of Labor Statistics, 2002). By 2050, about 53 percent of persons living in the United States will be non-Hispanic white; 16 percent will be black; 23 percent will be Hispanic; 10 percent will be Asian and Pacific Islander; and about 1 percent will be American Indian, Eskimo, and Aleut. The fastest-growing racial groups will continue to be the Asian and Pacific Islander population. The U.S. Bureau of Census projected that the Asian and Pacific Islander population will have expanded to over 12 million, or double its current size, by 2010, triple by 2020, and more than five times its current size, to 41 million, by 2050 (U.S. Census Bureau, 2008). Thus, it is imperative that occupational therapy practitioners understand, appreciate, and become familiar with concepts of (1) the different values and beliefs that persons from various cultures may hold and (2) the importance of developing cultural awareness, sensitivity, and competence in implementing the occupational therapy process with diverse populations. Understanding and integrating these concepts and skills into everyday practice can influence not just the quality of services provided by practitioners but also the client's perceptions of the services they receive. These perceptions in turn can influence the motivation for and level of participation in work-related services and other rehabilitation as well as the resulting vocational outcomes.

> *AOTA has identified work and industry as one of the six Centennial Vision focus areas where occupational therapy practitioners have great potential to provide expert services.*

The American Occupational Therapy Association's (AOTA) Centennial Vision incorporates the significance of a "globally connected and diverse workforce" in its vision for 2017 (AOTA, 2008). AOTA has identified work and industry as one of the six Centennial Vision focus areas where occupational therapy practitioners have great potential to provide expert services (Fig. 3.1). Specific opportunities identified as emerging areas of practice are ergonomics evaluations, injury prevention, and consultation regarding interpretation and application of legislation relating to disability management in the workplace (e.g., in the United States, this legislation is called the Americans with Disabilities Act).

The International Labor Organization (a tripartite United Nations agency that brings together governments, employers, and workers of its member states in common action to promote decent work throughout the world) has developed a *Code of Practice for Managing Disability in the Workplace* (Westmoreland & Buys, 2004). It is evident that disability management is viewed on a global basis as a primary solution to the economic and human costs of injury and disability in the workplace. Australia and Canada are examples of countries where occupational therapy practitioners are employed to ensure early intervention with workers for injury prevention and rehabilitation. The Canadian Association of Occupational Therapists (CAOT) reports an increase in the number of occupational therapy practitioners who work closely with employers, employees, and unions to prevent work-related injuries and reduce on-the-job stress (CAOT, n.d.). Deen, Gibson, and Strong (2002) reported that occupational therapy practitioners in Australia played an active role in prevention, assessment, and rehabilitation services in occupational rehabilitation. Note that work injury management is referred to by different terms in different countries; for example, in the United States, it is commonly called industrial rehabilitation, while in Australia and Canada, it is called occupational rehabilitation.

Given the new level of global connectedness and that occupational therapy practitioners are increasing their involvement in disability management in the workplace, occupational

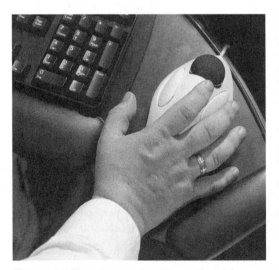 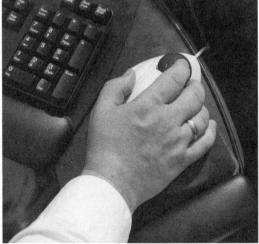

Figure 3.1 Emerging practice areas such as injury prevention and ergonomics will provide ongoing opportunities for occupational therapy practitioners around the globe in the coming decades.

therapy practitioners will benefit from gaining a greater understanding of differing cultural perspectives on *work* and *working*. While much of occupational therapy practice in the United States is embedded in Western values and influences, it is moving toward more culturally diverse and sensitive practice. Evidence suggests a shift in the occupational therapy paradigm over the last two decades as awareness of cultural concerns and the wider context in which occupational therapy operates has been raised (Awaad, 2003). More emphasis is being placed on needs-based program planning driven by culturally informed assessment. In addition, we recognize that by considering the wider social environment in which people exist, we can improve intervention, advocacy, and reevaluation of therapy goals. The *Occupational Therapy Practice Framework: Domain and Process,* or OTPF (AOTA, 2008), identifies culture as one of the six possible contextual and environmental features that influence occupational performance. The OTPF defines the cultural context as "customs, beliefs, activity patterns, behavior standards, and expectations accepted by the society of which the client is a member. It includes ethnicity and values as well as political aspects, such as laws that affect access to resources and affirm personal rights. It also includes opportunities for education, employment, and economic support."

It is important to recognize that increased global connectedness and growing diversity has implications for occupational therapy practice, including the use of culturally sensitive assessment tools, intervention strategies that recognize cultural and gender influences, and culturally sensitive communication skills that encourage full participation of clients, employers, and sometimes coworkers. To further understand how cultural awareness and sensitivity applies in the context of *work rehabilitation,* we discuss the concept of *work values* and how these values affect work goals and the resulting work outcomes within the context of cultural differences and expectations.

Work Values

Chapter 1 discussed the meanings and functions of work, and these concepts are keys to understanding work-related occupational therapy intervention. The varying interpretations of work held by different cultures and the wide range of work that humans perform in today's world also have important implications for occupational therapy practice. For the occupational therapy practitioner to collaborate effectively with clients, he or she must help the client to identify rehabilitation and vocational goals that meet the client's specific needs while appreciating the client's cultural perceptions of work. For example, if working gives a client a feeling of being connected with society as a whole and a sense of purpose in life, a different set of intervention strategies is required than for the client who perceives working solely as a means to earn an income and who does not attach any other meaning or expectations to working.

How is the meaning of work in the life of individuals influenced by prevailing cultural value priorities? To answer this question, researchers have attempted to define the construct of *work values*. The term *work values* typically refers to the goals or rewards people seek through their work, and these values can be grouped into four broad categories, presented in Table 3.1 (Schwartz, 1999).

The prevailing cultural values of the society in which the person or group lives often guides the types of work values pursued. For example, the pursuit of *power* values is likely to be more acceptable in the United States, where the cultural emphasis is on getting ahead through active self-assertion (Schwartz, 1999). However, the pursuit of power and its use as a motivator are likely to be less acceptable and perhaps arouse individual opposition in

Table 3.1 Four Categories of Work Values

Work Values	Meaning
Intrinsic values	Personal growth, autonomy, interest, and creativity
Extrinsic values	Pay and security
Social values	Contact with people and contribution to society
Power values	Prestige, authority, and influence

countries such as Sweden or Finland, where *egalitarian* values (the principle that all people are equal and deserve equal rights and opportunities) are more important. As a result, there is no single type of work goal that is likely to be most effective for a productive and satisfactory rehabilitation outcome across all cultures. Thus, for an occupational therapy practitioner, goals established to address a client's motivation during the rehabilitation process are more effective if they are compatible with the prevailing cultural emphasis of the workplace and the personal cultural context of the chosen value system. Elizur, Borg, Hunt, and Istvan (1991) proposed that values in a work context are any entity (i.e., object, behavior, and/or situation) on which a group places high worth or importance. When they compared work values among managers, employees, and students in eight countries—the United States, China, Korea, Taiwan, Israel, Germany, Holland, and Hungary—they found that work values are embedded into the broader sociocultural and technological conditions that influence performance. For example, Hungarian respondents rated supervisor recognition, meaningful work, and pay considerably higher than the Chinese, who considered contribution to society as very important but pay and other material outcomes as quite unimportant. Lack of appreciation of such differences in work values could confound the occupational therapy practitioner's ability to objectively approach the therapeutic milieu and interact with a client from a different culture.

Feldman, Ah Sam, McDonald, and Bechtel (1980) suggested another construct important to understanding differences in work values that they called *frames of reference.* It is important to note that frames of reference, as used here, does not hold the same meaning as commonly used in occupational therapy theory and practice. Feldman and colleagues describe frames of reference as standards against which the outcomes of work are judged and are thought to be partially a product of culture. Examples of outcomes of work include salary, benefits, recognition of good work, and rewards for meeting productivity guidelines. Several factors determine an individual's frame of reference, including culture, past experience, social class, and community characteristics; in turn, the frame of reference strongly influences satisfaction with work outcomes. For example, when New Zealanders (European ancestry) and Polynesians (Maori and Pacific Islanders) were asked what they considered important job outcomes, the Polynesians subscribed to the notion of *particularism,* which is the exchange of rewards on the basis of personal needs, such as love, service, or status. The New Zealanders, on the other hand, viewed the *universalistic* exchanges such as money, goods, or information as more significant and relevant to their needs.

Another dimension to the manner in which people perceive their world and behave is an adherence to a collective or individualistic value system. Table 3.2 includes examples of personal characteristics and behavioral indicators of these value systems.

Implicit in the U.S. rehabilitation system are *individualistic* values, which assume that individuals can express their emotions and can advocate for themselves or assert their rights. Rehabilitation policies and practices, including assessments, programs, supports, and success criteria, are based on these assumptions. For some individuals who

Table 3.2 Collectivist and Individualistic Value Systems

Cultural Concepts	Personal Characteristics	Behavioral Indicators
Individualism	• Self-expression • Assertiveness • Self-advocacy • Self-realization	• Communicating dissatisfaction with services • Holding a different view of services than views of family unit or community • Focus on the individual's unique set of talents and potential
Collectivism	• Individual's existence is inseparable from family and community • Self-interests are sacrificed for those of the family or larger group • Group activities are dominant	• Individual may not accept transportation and work outside his or her community • Supports to achieve self-sufficiency not welcomed

embrace strong family interdependence rather than individual independence, these assumptions will most likely pose conflicts in rehabilitation theory and practice. For example, many persons with disabilities desire assistive technology, vocational rehabilitation, and other services, but depending on their cultural values, they may want them for different reasons.

The United States, Australia, United Kingdom, and Canada are examples of countries that have culturally diverse populations. A culturally diverse population includes a wide range of aspects of life, such as values, dietary habits, beliefs about sexual orientation and gender roles, and religious beliefs, to name just a few. These aspects of diversity can interact to affect the outcomes of participation in work-related intervention and rehabilitation. The following is an example of the relation between religion and work affecting work values and the resulting work outcome expectation, in this case the outcome of "hard work." Niles (1999) compared work-related beliefs in a Westernized country (Australia) with the traditional Protestant work ethic with a non-Western, predominantly Buddhist country (Sri Lanka). In these two contrasting cultural and religious settings, they concluded that most religions and cultures have a common concept of a *work ethic* when it is defined as a commitment to hard work and to excellence. However, the outcomes of hard work, such as success, are not perceived similarly by both cultures. *Success* was presented to participants as the concept that "anyone able and willing to work hard had a good chance of succeeding and overcoming obstacles." Australians endorsed the sentiment that hard work led to success, but Sri Lankans did not perceive a direct relationship between hard work and success. They valued self-reliance and independence rather than the outcome of success. This example highlights the importance of an occupational therapy practitioner's ability to recognize the patient's work ethics during the rehabilitation process.

A successful return-to-work outcome is dependent on work goals based on the individual's work value frame of reference. This is true because the person's perception or experience of prior work outcomes as well as anticipated future work outcomes influences his or her motivation to engage in rehabilitation and to establish return-to-work goals. The client's abilities or deficits postinjury also influence perceptions of work outcomes. To encourage participation and to motivate the client, the occupational therapy practitioner must recognize and acknowledge the frame of reference that guides the return-to-work goals by engaging in culturally sensitive client-centered goal setting and intervention strategies.

To encourage participation and to motivate the client, the occupational therapy practitioner must recognize and acknowledge the frame of reference that guides the return-to-work goals by engaging in culturally sensitive client-centered goal setting and intervention strategies.

Work values and how these values affect return-to-work goals and the resulting vocational outcomes within the context of cultural differences and expectations are discussed throughout this chapter. It is apparent that a work culture is influenced by the work values that are held within that culture. These culture-specific work values are shaped and defined by such factors as personal experiences, religion, politics, and economic success and hardships, and have important implications for delivery of occupational therapy services. Successful application of this knowledge and awareness of differing work values cannot be realized in practice without thorough understanding of the concepts of *cultural awareness* and *cultural competency*.

Cultural Awareness and Cultural Competence

In the United States, multicultural and minority populations are growing quickly. Over the next 50 years, the population of the United States will grow by nearly 50 percent, from about 275 million in the year 2000 to an estimated 394 million people in 2050. Immigration will play the largest role in the growth of the U.S. population through midcentury. Growth rates of both the Hispanic and the Asian and Pacific Islander populations may exceed 2 percent per year until 2030. Concurrent with these shifts in population is a growing trend to shift the delivery of health care from hospitals to community settings. It is even more important in nonmedical settings for occupational therapy practitioners to be sensitive to their clients' values, attitudes, beliefs, and behaviors if they wish to provide effective interventions. Occupational therapy is concerned particularly with occupations and roles in daily living, and these tend to be highly culture specific.

Occupational therapy practitioners engage in work-related practice because work is part of daily living for most people and has intrinsic role value attached to it. Practitioners interact with clients and their family, coworkers, employers, physicians, payers, and other allied health-care providers. The occupational therapy practitioner must be culturally competent to ensure that evaluation of the client, intervention strategies, and communication ensure the best service most suited to the client.

Before discussing cultural competency, it is helpful to understand the terms *culture* and *cultural competence*. Suarez-Balcazar and Rodakowski (2007) define *culture* as an integrated pattern of behaviors, norms, and rules shared by a group and involving their beliefs, values, expectations, worldviews, communication, common history, and institutions; they define *competence* as having the capacity to function effectively. Betancourt, Green, Carrillo, and Ananeh-Firempong (2003) define a *culturally competent health-care system* as one that acknowledges and incorporates at all levels the importance of culture, assessment of cross-cultural relations, vigilance toward the dynamics that result from cultural differences, expansion of cultural knowledge, and adaptation of services to meet culturally unique needs. They also use *sociocultural barriers* to refer to social factors (e.g., socioeconomic status, environmental hazards, supports/stressors, and cultural factors such as health beliefs and values) that lead to differential treatment and varying quality of care.

Understanding people's diverse cultures, values, traditions, history, and institutions is not simply political correctness: it is integral to eliminating health disparities and providing high-quality care. Culture shapes the experiences, perceptions, and decisions of individuals as well as how they relate to others. Culture influences the way people respond to health-care services and preventive interventions and impacts the way clinicians deliver those services. For example, in a culturally diverse country such as the United States, occupational therapy practitioners should display awareness of and sensitivity to diverse client populations and their culturally influenced work values and beliefs to enable positive health behaviors, which includes vocational rehabilitation outcomes.

Culture permeates every clinical encounter in occupational therapy. The occupational therapy practitioner and the person seeking services each bring their own personal and familial cultural backgrounds to the encounter. The context in which services are provided adds yet another layer of culture (Munoz, 2007). Suarez-Balcazar and Rodakowski (2007) recognized the importance of understanding the external and internal factors, also called diversity factors, that play out in the cultural encounter. They suggest that if occupational therapy practitioners acknowledge their own diversity factors and recognize how they feel about or react to others who have different diversity factors, they will embrace the process of critical awareness. Many of these diversity factors are listed in Box 3.1.

Understanding cultural competence, which Campinha-Bacote (2002) describes as a process and not an event, requires that a practitioner understand five key concepts. The model called "the process of cultural competence in the delivery of health-care services" describes these concepts, and Table 3.3 lists them. All five concepts must be addressed and/or experienced in order to engage in the process of achieving cultural competence (Campinha-Bacote, 2002).

To be effective in work-related practice, occupational therapy practitioners have to establish a rapport with the worker and must identify sociocultural barriers that could mitigate the therapeutic process. Suarez-Balcazar and Rodakowski (2007) propose using a process-oriented model of culturally responsive caring (Fig. 3.2), originally described by Munoz in 2002. This model defines three distinct dimensions of cultural competence: (1) *knowing*—learning about one's own culture and that of others (e.g., your family's place of origin, traditions, history of immigration, values, and belief system; your client's ethnicity); (2) *doing*—engaging in multicultural experiences (e.g., attending a wedding, religious ceremony, or other event that is unique to a particular culture and different from the way you would celebrate that same event); and (3) *becoming*—developing an understanding of others who are different from you (e.g., seeking social and informal interactions with a variety of ethnic groups and engaging in a culture-specific community event).

Box 3.1 Diversity Factors

1. Ability/disability, which could be visible or hidden
2. Family and community support
3. Oppression experience, which could influence a person's knowledge of rights and services or sense of entitlement
4. Socioeconomic status
5. Religion, which can influence beliefs and values
6. Education
7. Acculturation
8. Immigration status
9. Urbanicity
10. Sexual orientation

Table 3.3 The Process of Cultural Competence in the Delivery of Health-Care Services

Concept	Explanation
Cultural awareness	Self-examination of cultural and professional background
Cultural knowledge	Process of seeking and obtaining a sound educational foundation about diverse cultural and ethnic groups
Cultural skill	Ability to collect relevant cultural data regarding the client's presenting problem as well as accurately performing a culturally based assessment
Cultural encounters	Process that encourages the health-care provider to directly engage in cross-cultural interactions with clients from culturally diverse backgrounds
Cultural desires	Motivation of the health-care provider to *want* rather than *have* to engage in the process of becoming culturally aware, culturally knowledgeable, culturally skillful, and familiar with cultural encounters

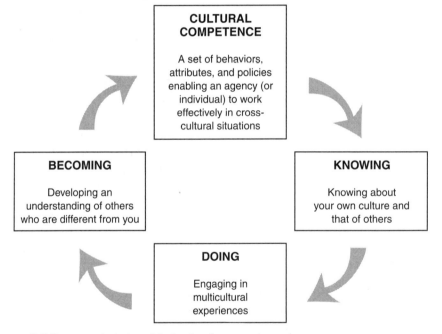

Figure 3.2 Process-oriented model of culturally responsive caring.

The process-oriented model is an ongoing process of evolving into a more competent practitioner by combining critical awareness, knowledge, and skills and putting them into practice. Suarez-Balcazar and Rodakowski acknowledge that culture does not stay the same and that it is not possible or necessary to know about all cultures to appreciate the concept of cultural competency. Becoming culturally competent is a reflective process: practitioners must be open to learning about other cultures and willing to engage in the process.

Occupational therapy theory traditionally embraces the Western society notion of productivity and mastery in which individuals are frequently defined by their work role and success is strongly emphasized (Krefting and Krefting, 1991). Occupational therapy practitioners regard occupational performance, functional ability, and meaningful and/or purposeful activity as having intrinsic therapeutic value and thus focus their assessment

Table 3.4 Culturally Competent Occupational Therapy Practice

Guidelines	Explanation
Qualities of the therapist	Openness to examination of assumptions and beliefs and the possibility of personal change
Awareness of the sociocultural environment	Intervention planning and implementation should consider cultural norms of clients and their social groups, such as socially acceptable and expected behavior, customs and traditions, and personal factors such as work ethic, gender, age, race, and religion
Individual focus in assessment	The individual's personal schema, societal roles, and expectations of therapy should guide the occupational therapy assessment, and the practitioner considers the client's attitudes toward work, leisure, and productive occupation
Analysis of activities	The value and importance of specific work and other occupations to clients and their social groups (as well as society at large) are considered along with cultural norms in choosing activities to include in intervention
Approaches to treatment	Focusing on the functional ability (rather than symptomatology) gives the therapist a cultural advantage in choosing appropriate theory and models to guide intervention. Goal setting should be culturally sensitive and reflect the priorities of the client

and treatment on these areas (Kinebanian and Stomph, 1992). All of these areas are sensitive to cultural interpretation; therefore, culturally aware occupational therapy practitioners are better equipped than others to provide culturally appropriate service.

To achieve cultural awareness in practice, Hopton and Stoneley (2006) suggest a three-part process that echoes the process-oriented model. First, the occupational therapy practitioner must reflect on personal values and assumptions before working with a client from a different culture, especially as occupational therapy has evolved from a Western middle-class perspective and the values and norms of culture underpin the profession (Awaad, 2003). Second, the practitioner needs to be aware of sociocultural factors that include beliefs, religion, diet, and dress so as not to cause offense or suggest inappropriate activities. Showing sincere interest by sharing with the client about his or her culture equalizes power and avoids reinforcing stereotypes; it also allows the client to make choices within a cultural framework. Finally, occupational therapy practitioners' awareness of culture can be enhanced by education and training during graduate school. Knowledge about culture could become more engrained throughout occupational therapy education and training by increasing an emphasis on social sciences such as sociology, anthropology, and geography. This leads to the question, What is a culturally competent occupational therapy practice? Awaad (2003) suggests five guidelines, highlighted in Table 3.4 along with examples of applying them in a work rehabilitation context.

Cultural Competency in the Workplace

As highlighted earlier in this chapter, cultural competency can be defined and explained using several models. Collectively, these definitions suggest that cultural competence is a complex, multidimensional construct that integrates cognitive, affective, and behavioral components (Munoz, 2007). One of the goals of this chapter is to discuss the relevance of cultural diversity in the workforce and the need for cultural competency in employers, managers, and vocational rehabilitation specialists. Diversity poses many challenges to employers because diverse populations bring different attitudes, perceptions, motivations, and needs to the workplace. It also encompasses ethnicity, gender, age, religion, and sexual preference considerations for individuals in the workplace and their employers. Riccucci (1997) reported that in the 1990s organizations developed "cultural awareness" training programs to embrace the anticipated demographic shift in ethnicity. However, most of the initiatives were driven by federal mandates (e.g., against sexual harassment and reasonable accommodation) and, while important, addressed only a fraction of diversity concerns and issues.

Rubaii-Barrett (1993) concluded that managers need to be better trained to understand and appreciate that levels of satisfaction among employees are not necessarily related only to the factors that the managers consider important. Ethnicity and cultural values play a role as well. Managers must move beyond recognizing and acknowledging issues of cultural diversity and develop skills and practices that increase satisfaction and performance in a workforce of mixed cultural and ethnic heritage.

During the rehabilitation process, the occupational therapy practitioner should also consider the level of cultural awareness and competency practiced by the client's current or potential employer. Occupational therapy practitioners are often involved in negotiating return-to-work options with employers on behalf of clients. They are also responsible for providing vocational counselors information about clients' physical functional status and work goals. Thus, a good match between a client's return-to-work goals and a company's cultural awareness and competency is often the key to a successful return to work. Awareness of the employer's level of cultural sensitivity, practices, policies, and commitment to acceptance of diversity at a workplace and demonstrated by a client's supervisor and coworkers will have an impact on the return-to-work or vocational rehabilitation process. Table 3.5 describes the continuum of cultural competency in the workplace.

Table 3.5 Continuum of Cultural Competency in the Workplace

Level of Competency	Explanation
Cultural destructiveness	Attitudes, policies, practices, and structures that are destructive to a cultural group: • Policy of gender-specific jobs • Inequality in salary based on gender or assumptions based on stereotypes
Cultural incapacity	Lack of capacity to respond effectively to culturally and linguistically diverse groups: • Practices that may result in discrimination in hiring and promotion • Disproportionate allocation of resources that may benefit one cultural group over another • Subtle messages that some cultural groups are neither valued nor welcomed • Lower expectations for some cultural, ethnic, or racial groups
Cultural blindness	• All people are viewed as the same • Little value placed on training • Little diversity among personnel • Policies and personnel that encourage assimilation • Institutional attitudes that blame consumers for their circumstances (families or individuals)
Cultural precompetence	• Commitment to human and civil rights • Hiring practices that support a diverse workforce • Tendency for token representation on governing boards • No clear plan for achieving organizational cultural competence • Expressly values the delivery of high-quality services and supports culturally and linguistically diverse populations

Table 3.5 Continuum of Cultural Competency in the Workplace—cont'd

Level of Competency	Explanation
Cultural competency	• Mission statement • Implement specific policies and procedures • Recruit, hire, and maintain a diverse and culturally and linguistically competent workforce • Dedicate resources for both individual and organizational self-assessment of cultural and linguistic competence • Practice principles of community engagement that result in the reciprocity
Cultural proficiency	• Employ staff and consultants to liaise with consumers with expertise in cultural competency standards • Actively pursue resource development • Advocate with and on behalf of populations who are traditionally underserved

Adapted from Duran et al., 2001.

Ideally, a culturally competent or proficient work environment responds to and fosters differences in values, beliefs, and behaviors. Return-to-work goals made by a culturally competent practitioner can be confounded if the workplace policies and practices pertaining to cultural diversity are not a good fit for the client.

Being culturally competent also includes proficiency in cultural communication techniques, which encompasses a wide range of skills that facilitate the therapeutic process between the services provider and those receiving the services. Language barriers can influence why people use or do not use health services, why they are limited to employment opportunities, or why they cannot advocate for themselves when faced with these challenges. The next section of this chapter elaborates on the differences in communication styles across cultures and the implications of linguistic barriers to providing culturally competent care.

Culture and Communication

As the demographics of the United States change, the ability to provide optimal occupational therapy intervention will increasingly rely on skills in communicating with clients from diverse backgrounds. Table 3.6 describes the population and race distribution with percentage of disability by race compiled from the 2000 census.

According to the 2000 census, 31.8 million U.S. residents, or 14 percent of the total population, spoke a language other than English at home. Spanish was the most frequently spoken language, followed by French or Creole, German, Chinese, and Italian. Approximately 4.5 million Americans spoke an Asian or Pacific Island language. In some states, the percentages of those speaking a language other than English at home were significantly higher than the national average (36% in New Mexico, 31% in California, and 20% each in Arizona, Hawaii, New Jersey, New York, and Texas). If trends shown in the 2010 census mirror the earlier census, the population of the United States will rise to 438 million in 2050, from 296 million in 2005, and 82 percent of the increase will be due to immigrants, some of whom speak a language other than English.

Communication is of primary importance in providing rehabilitation services. Communicating cross-culturally presents unique challenges to occupational therapy practitioners. These challenges must be understood, and strategies to overcome communication barriers

Table 3.6 Population and Race Distribution With Percentage of Disability by Race

Race	% Total Population	% With a Disability
European American	69.13	19.7
Hispanic/Latino American	12.55	15.3
African American	12.06	20.0
Asian American	3.73	9.9
American Indian	0.74	21.9
Two or more races	1.64	
Other	0.17	

Adapted from U.S. Census Bureau, 2000.

must be integrated into everyday practice. The primary challenges in effective cross-cultural communication are knowledge, awareness, and sensitivity to differences in both verbal and nonverbal communication.

Verbal Communication

According to the Center for International Rehabilitation Research: Information and Exchange (CIRRIE), Americans place heavy emphasis on the preciseness of words and expect them to be exact and technical (Jezewski and Sotnik, 2001). American conversation is dependent on what is said more than on what is not said. When description is lengthy, the American listener often becomes restless and impatient and generally does not value emotions in conversations. They tend to emphasize factual, logical communication; emotions assume a secondary role to logic and facts. This style of verbal communication is categorized as *low-context communication*. This characterization is more easily understood if we examine Hall's concepts of high- and low-context cultural factors in communication.

To distinguish communication styles among cultures, the anthropologist Edward T. Hall (1976) proposed a set of parameters to help situate cultures along a dimension spanning from the high-context/low-content category to the low-context/high-content category. Würtz (2005) used Hall's parameters to demonstrate that when customizing a website to appeal to a different culture, it is not enough merely to translate the text: the overall communication strategy should be appropriate to the audience as well. She demonstrated that communication patterns today still resonate with the cultural dimensions proposed by Hall decades ago.

Hall observed that meaning and context within communication are inextricably bound with each other and suggested that, to understand communication, we should look at meaning and context together with the code (i.e., the words themselves). By context, he referred to the situation, background, or environment connected to an event, a situation, or an individual. In a *high-context culture,* many contextual elements help people understand the rules for communicating. As a result, much is taken for granted. This can be very confusing for a person who does not understand the "unwritten rules" of the culture. In a *low-context culture,* very little is taken for granted. While this means that more explanation is needed to fully understand communication, it also means there is less chance of misunderstanding, particularly in the presence of a third party. High-context communication draws on physical aspects as well as the time and situation in which the communication takes place and the relationship between the people communicating. The closer the relationship, the more high-context the communication tends to be, drawing on the shared knowledge of the communicating parties. Face-to-face communication in high-context cultures is characterized by an extensive use of nonverbal strategies for conveying meanings. These strategies usually take the shape of behavioral language, such as gestures, body language, silence, proximity, and symbolic behavior, while conversation in low-context cultures tends to be less physically animated with the meaning depending on content and the spoken word. Table 3.7 describes some differences in communication between high- and low-context cultures, according to Hall.

To further elaborate Hall's parameter's, LeBaron (2003) suggested asking the following questions to understand the distinction between high-context and low-context communication: (1) Do I tend to "let my words speak for themselves," or do I prefer to be less direct, relying on what is implied by my communication (low-context communication)? (2) Do I prefer indirect messages from others, and am I attuned to a whole range of verbal and nonverbal cues to help me understand the meaning of what is said (high-context communication)? For example, an American occupational therapy practitioner may simply state to a Japanese client "No, you can't receive services tomorrow." To a recent Japanese immigrant, this logical, factual statement may be interpreted as rude and uncaring. There are as many as 16 ways to say "no" in Japanese, many of which are used to avoid embarrassing the person to whom the reply is directed. This example highlights the importance of occupational therapy practitioners understanding the context in which information is verbally communicated to culturally diverse consumers.

Nonverbal Communication

Another form of cross-cultural communication important for occupational therapy practitioners to be aware of is nonverbal communication, also commonly called *paralinguistics*. Nonverbal communication is an integral component of everyday communication and holds added importance in cultures where high-context communication patterns prevail. Some key factors to understanding nonverbal communication are *personal space, gestures, eye contact,* and *silence*.

Preferences for personal space vary across cultures. In communication, personal space is the distance individuals want between themselves and others at any given time, and this comfort zone is culturally determined. For instance, Americans feel most comfortable with approximately 3 to 4 feet of personal space (Jezewski and Sotnik, 2001). People from the Middle East stand closer for conversations with colleagues than Americans do. In a practitioner–client situation, a Middle Eastern client may interpret the distance placed by an American therapist as cold or uncaring. Such a client might not take the therapist seriously because of the nonverbal communication conveyed simply by the distance the therapist stands from the client.

Table 3.7 High- and Low-Context Cultures

Factor	High-Context Culture	Low-Context Culture
Overtness of messages	Many covert and implicit messages with use of metaphor and reading between the lines	Many overt and explicit messages that are simple and clear
Use of nonverbal communication	Much nonverbal communication	More focus on verbal communication than body language
Expression of reaction	Reserved, inward reactions	Visible, external, outward reaction

Gestures, including hand gestures, body movements, and facial expressions, are also culturally prescribed and affect communication cross-culturally (Jezewski and Sotnik, 2001). Hand gestures can easily be misinterpreted. In the United States, for example, using the index finger with the arm extended toward another person generally means "come here," but it is offensive in some Asian countries because the same gesture is used only to call an animal. Another easily misinterpreted hand gesture is the thumbs-up. In the United States, it means "that's great," but in Greece, it means "get stuffed," which has an altogether different connotation. Initial greetings between people also differ among ethnic groups: a firm handshake (United States), an embrace (South America), a kiss on each cheek (France), a bow (Japan). In some cultures, crossing one's legs while sitting facing another is impolite.

The amount of eye contact during conversation varies cross-culturally. Americans maintain eye contact while speaking or listening to another person because, in U.S. culture, it signals interest in the conversation, while lack of eye contact is perceived as disinterest or preoccupation. In other cultures, maintaining eye contact may be perceived as a sign of disrespect. Lowering the eyes during conversation or other interaction can be a sign of respect, especially when one party is perceived to have higher status or greater knowledge, as is sometimes the case in client–practitioner relationships.

The use of silence also varies across cultures. In the United States, very little silence is tolerated during conversation. Americans usually become uncomfortable during a lull in conversation (Jezewski and Sotnik, 2001). However, Asian cultures value silence: it is perceived as a sign of thoughtful respect, affirmation, or cooperation.

Understanding differences in verbal and nonverbal communication among cultures creates open lines of communication. People's different communication styles reflect deep philosophies and worldviews that are the foundation of their culture. Understanding these allows the practitioner to get one step close to being a culturally competent communicator. Table 3.8 describes nine strategies for effective cross-cultural communication.

Table 3.8 Strategies for Effective Cross-Cultural Communication

Strategy	Effective Cross-Cultural Communication
Ask questions	• Develop cultural knowledge • Stretch your understanding of a person's group or culture
Listen actively	• Learn to listen to what is being said and not what you want to hear • Test for understanding by asking questions and restating what was said
Think twice	• Avoid culturally insensitive language and behaviors
Respect differences	• Recognize cultural differences in verbal and nonverbal communication styles and other global concepts (time, silence, family, etc.)
Be honest	• Share your experiences honestly • Acknowledge any discomfort, hesitation, or concerns you may have
Avoid stereotyping	• Do not cast your assumptions in stone • Instead, use generalizations as a starting point to make good communication decisions
Recognize the complexity of communication	• Pay attention to multiple channels of communication; many barriers exist between the source and receiver • Practice two-way communication

Table 3.8 Strategies for Effective Cross-Cultural Communication—cont'd

Strategy	Effective Cross-Cultural Communication
Be flexible	• Alter your communication strategies as the situation necessitates • Choose appropriate channels
Distinguish perspectives	• Understand and carefully consider various points of views

Adapted from New York–New Jersey Public Health Training Center, 2008.

Gender, Culture, and Work

Popular stereotypes often conceptualize what men and women look for in their jobs and work life. Beliefs about differences can foster gender discrimination and segregation in the workplace. De Vaus and McAllister (1991) examined the extent to which men and women look for different things from their work, measured by *intrinsic* and *extrinsic* work values (see Table 3.1) and the degree to which they exhibit different levels of job satisfaction. Using closely comparable data collected in nine Western European countries, they found that overall, men place greater value than women on both intrinsic and extrinsic work values and are somewhat more satisfied than women with their jobs. However, they only considered Western countries. In contrast, Itzhaky and Ribner (1999) found that immigrant women who chose to work in their new country had significantly higher levels of job satisfaction and commitment to the workplace than did men. They attributed this to the possibility that these women, who had been acculturated to the role of homemaker, now found themselves in a new environment of paid employment that gave them a sense of responsibility not only to family but to the new context of the workplace.

Two broad approaches may explain gender differences in work values. First, the *gender socialization model* proposes that observed differences in work values (e.g., women have greater concern for social aspects of their work, whereas men are concerned with pay and career advancement) reflect how men and women are socialized differently. Second, the *social structural model* proposes that observed differences in work values reflect men's and women's differential access to the reward structures (e.g., women tend to work in lower status positions that typically offer relatively little opportunity for career advancement). However, the assertions of these models have been challenged as the female labor force in the United States and generally in the world has increased over the years. As of 2003, women accounted for 51 percent of the U.S. population and comprised 60 percent of the labor force. The bureau estimates that by 2050, non-Hispanic whites will constitute a little more than half the population (53%), with the number of Hispanics growing to approximately 23 percent and of blacks to approximately 16 percent. This data implies that women from ethnic backgrounds with different gender-role attitudes and behaviors will comprise a large sector of the U.S. female workforce (U.S. Census Bureau, 2008). Roehling, Jarvis, and Swoope (2005) suggest that ethnicity impacts gender-role and acculturation differences in work experiences. Traditional values often dictate whether a woman continues to be responsible for the home and family even while working for pay outside of the home. For example, Hispanic women who are relatively new to the United States have fewer and different cultural models than their American counterparts to inform their management of work life and home life when they enter the workforce. They must rely on more traditional gender-based arrangements of work and home tasks (child rearing is primarily the mother's responsibility) while living in the dominant American culture. The overload of responsibility often leads to very stressful situations that negatively influence social interactions and health. Even though the study looked at experiences of the Hispanic, black, and white women in the United States and did not include Asians or Middle Eastern women, we can assume that issues related to gender-role behavior and acculturation apply to women from any ethnic background. Factors such as job security, working hours, opportunity for advancement, and feeling of accomplishment can also influence work value preference.

The Meaning of Disability Across Cultures

Occupational therapy practitioners interact with people with varying degrees of impairment, challenges to occupational performance, and disability, and practitioners often face the challenge of accessing institutions and services that meet their clients' needs. Further confounding the challenge is that the clients' perception of their own disability is influenced by their cultural beliefs and values and by what they perceive are important activities for them to be able to execute, including community participation, return to work, and daily living activities. Disability is understood and defined in different ways by different cultures. In a Western culture like the United States, for instance, one way of defining disability is through the laws and regulations at national, state, and local levels. For example, the ADA, implemented in 1990, defines *disability* as the following:

> *With respect to an individual, the term "disability" means (A) a physical or mental impairment that substantially limits one or more of the major life activities of such individual; (B) a record of such impairment; or (C) being regarded as having an impairment. A person must meet . . . at least one of these three criteria to be an individual with disability under the Act. (Equal Employment Opportunity Commission and the U.S. Department of Justice, 1991)*

Scholars, researchers, and health-care providers have suggested that this definition is narrow and is based on Western faith in science. As mentioned earlier, the meaning of disability is influenced by cultural beliefs and values of consumers and service providers. Foreign-born populations or resident Americans from a non-Western culture may view disabling conditions, causal factors, and related services differently than do mainstream Americans. Americans with a European heritage may attribute the cause of disability to factors such as disease or genetic disorders; for them, acknowledging a disability is acceptable, and outside intervention is generally desirable. Individuals who are foreign born or who have a non-European heritage may not hold these opinions about disability. For example, in the Southeast Asian community, Buddhism and Hinduism are the predominant religions. Their principles stipulate that each person is responsible for his or her actions. Southeast Asians adhere to *karma,* a belief that an individual's present life is determined by what he or she has done, right or wrong, in a previous existence. Therefore, they accept a perceived misfortune, such as disability, as predestined. This comparison highlights that concepts such as a disability in occupational therapy are not generalizable across cultures. For example, the goal of independence might not be desirable to some clients from the Asian community. If interdependence is the norm within a family, then the occupational therapist may need to analyze how decisions are made in the family, focusing on the shift in roles and incorporating the family's views and expectations in the occupational therapy process.

Disability in the Mexican culture may be viewed either as an act of God or as a punishment for a wrongdoing (Santana and Santana, 2001). Physical disability is more accepted than mental disability. In Yucatan, Mexico, the native language of Zapotec does not even have a word for disability, and there are no retirement homes, nursing homes, or homes for people with disability. In India, persons with disabilities constitute a highly marginalized group. Many families are reluctant to report disability in view of the prevailing negative attitudes toward people with disability. Like Mexicans, Indians view the cause of disability as punishment for past deeds. Also, environmental barriers are so severe in India that most people with disabilities are unable to participate in public activities.

Understanding such differences in the meaning of disability across cultures has serious implications for occupational therapy practitioners. It allows the profession to implement standards in practice and academic learning and to reflect acceptance and understanding of cultural diversity within the context of differing notions of disability. Knowledge of, skills in, and sensitivity to cross-cultural variables are necessary for occupational therapy practitioners to be effective.

Culture and Assessments of Work Performance

Cultural competency and awareness among occupational therapy practitioners is critical to their growing recognition and involvement in the health-care industry. In addition to continuing their own progression of cultural competency, practitioners must make sure the tools they use adhere to cultural considerations:

• Are the evaluation tools used during the assessment process in work-related practice valid across various cultures and populations?
• Are the interpretations of these tools culturally sensitive?
• Are the interventions specific to the person and his or her cultural context?

The OTPF (AOTA, 2008) identifies six aspects of occupational therapy's domain, listed in Box 3.2. These six aspects interact to influence the client's engagement in occupations, participation, and health. Occupational therapy practitioners and the person seeking occupational therapy bring their own personal and familial cultural interpretations and expectations to all six aspects of the occupational therapy domain. In work rehabilitation, a culturally competent practitioner recognizes that the process of occupational therapy service delivery involves facilitating interactions between the client and the domain aspects relevant to the client's cultural context in order to help the client reach the desired health outcomes, return-to-work goals, or alternative vocational goals.

In work rehabilitation, a culturally competent practitioner recognizes that the process of occupational therapy service delivery involves facilitating interactions between the client and the domain aspects relevant to the client's cultural context in order to help the client reach the desired health outcomes, return-to-work goals, or alternative vocational goals.

Box 3.2 Six Aspects of Occupational Therapy's Domain	
1. Areas of occupation	**4.** Performance patterns
2. Client factors	**5.** Context and environment
3. Performance skills	**6.** Activity demands

(AOTA, 2008)

The OTPF describes the occupational therapy process as a dynamic occupation and client-centered process that involves ongoing interaction among evaluation, intervention, and outcomes. The evaluation process consists of the *occupational profile* (information about the client's needs, problems, and concerns about work performance) and *analysis of occupational performance* (collecting and interpreting information using assessment tools designed to observe, measure, and inquire about factors that support or hinder work performance). The intervention process consists of an *intervention plan* (selected occupational therapy approaches and types of intervention), *intervention implementation* (putting the plan into action), and *intervention review* (reevaluating and reviewing the intervention plan, the effectiveness of its delivery, and outcomes). Occupational therapy practitioners working in industrial rehabilitation use a variety of assessments during each of the three processes, some of which are based on occupational therapy practice models and some on other health-related fields.

The various work assessments used to determine the psychosocial, physical, environmental, cognitive, and perceptual factors that impact a person's ability to work are described in later chapters. The next section of this chapter discusses the influence of culture on assessment and the implications for selecting and administering an assessment and interpreting the results in a culturally competent manner. Many assessments and evaluation tools used in the health-care setting are based largely on the sociocultural norms of white, middle-class populations (Fig. 3.3). These tools have overwhelmingly incorporated Western values, ethics, theories, and standards. They are not always appropriate for ethnic and culturally diverse populations, and the interpretation of their results may lead to nonoptimal treatment approaches.

The variety of assessments and related evaluation tools used in the practice of industrial rehabilitation range from review of medical and vocational records to informal interviews of the client, family, and employer, as well as observations of work practices of the client at the worksite and standardized and nonstandardized evaluation tools. Examples of some of these tools are listed in Table 3.9. Choosing the right assessment or evaluation tool must be guided by the outcome and relevance of that tool to the ultimate goal of the client. For example, if the goal is to assess the physical demands of a job the client intends to apply for, a job analysis is the most appropriate assessment. A job analysis identifies the physical demands of the job, the skill level required, the physical environment of the job, communication requirements, safety requirements, and tools that must be operated. A culturally competent practitioner then determines whether the client can communicate in English if that is the primary language spoken, and if not, whether an interpreter is available. Language barriers can be a serious concern because safety instructions are often in English in American workplaces. If the client cannot read the safety instructions over machinery, then his or her personal safety can be compromised. Common language is also necessary for social cohesiveness in the workplace.

Language and cultural issues are of great concern in the cross-cultural adaptation process of an assessment. For example, consider the *disability of arm, shoulder, and hand*

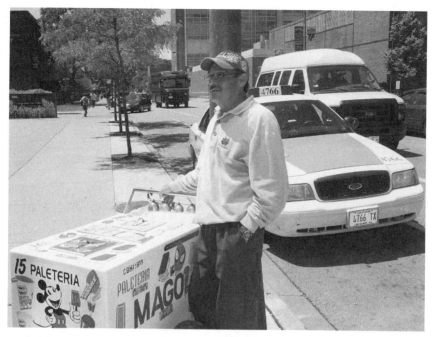

Figure 3.3 Immigration between countries is a global phenomenon, and language and other cultural barriers can present challenges to the occupational therapy practitioner in assuring culturally competent intervention.

Table 3.9 Examples of Assessment and Evaluation tools

Factors to Assess	Examples of Assessment and Evaluation Tools	Impact of Culture
Physical • Strength • Endurance • Range of motion • Flexibility/agility • Posture	Numerous tools are available to measure an individual's physical behavior: • Manual muscle testing • Dynamometry (e.g., Jamar hand grip dynamometer) • Fine and gross hand manipulation evaluations (e.g., Perdue Pegboard) • Goniometers to measure range of motion of joints • Rapid Upper Limb Assessment (RULA) measures hand and arm movements and related postures during a certain activity to predict risk of work-related upper limb disorders (e.g., repetitive upper limb involvement in an assembly task) • DASH (disabilities of the arm, shoulder, and hand) outcome questionnaire is available in several languages	These assessments and evaluations are generally pure measurements of the human body and are not influenced by a person's culture. However, participation by a client during some of these assessments could be influenced by culture (e.g., a female might not want to be touched by a male therapist). Culturally competent practitioners will modify their behavior to respect the client's needs
Environment • Noise • Light • Temperature • Work surface heights • Equipment/tools • Social	Various measurement tools and observation techniques help assess environment: • Measure light intensity with lux meter • Measure temperature with thermometer • Measures work surface heights with tape measure • Photograph or document tools being used • Observe work practice and document physical count of employees	A client's culture will not influence assessment/evaluation of the environment. These are pure measurements and can be performed in any cultural context

(table continues on page 72)

Table 3.9 Examples of Assessment and Evaluation tools—cont'd

Factors to Assess	Examples of Assessment and Evaluation Tools	Impact of Culture
Psychosocial • Values • Interests • Work role • Work habits • Perception of work environment • Motivation for work	There is a dearth of assessments and evaluation tools specific to industrial rehabilitation that address these factors in the absence of cultural biases of the client and the evaluator. • Work Environment Impact Scale (WEIS): a semistructured interview designed to gather information on how individuals experience and perceive their work environment. This instrument has good psychometric properties. It measures a single construct of work environment impact, can be culture free, and is readily learned • Worker Role Interview (WRI): a semistructured interview that obtains valuable information about the psychosocial capacity of workers with a range of physical and psychosocial diagnoses to return to work. It is a psychometrically sound instrument across cultures and diagnoses	A person's culture can influence all of these factors, as discussed in the chapter

(DASH), which is an upper extremity outcome measure commonly used by occupational therapy practitioners that has been translated into several languages. It assesses the symptoms and functional status of clients with upper limb conditions. A systematic review of cross-cultural adaptation of the DASH by Alotaibi (2008) highlighted the relevance of cultural norms and activities that can be culture specific. For example, when adapting the DASH to German, "playing Frisbee" was removed from the list of recreation activities because it is uncommon in Germany. Cultural norms can be a key factor in determining attitudes toward answering certain items. For example, in the Chinese culture, DASH questionnaire item 21, "sexual activities," was believed to be invasive of their cultural norms. Gender roles are viewed differently in different cultures and may affect how items are interpreted. For example, in the Armenian culture, cooking is believed to be a woman's task. Therefore, the majority of men did not answer item 4, "preparing a meal," on the Armenian DASH because cooking was less relevant as an activity of daily living (Alotaibi, 2008).

The Work Environment Impact Scale (WEIS) and the Worker Role Interview (WRI), based on the model of human occupation, are two more examples of assessment tools commonly used by occupational therapy practitioners. The WEIS is a semistructured interview designed to gather information on how individuals experience and perceive their work environment. This instrument has good psychometric properties and measures a single construct of work environment impact, is valid across cultures, and is readily learned. The WRI is also a semistructured interview and obtains valuable information about the psychosocial capacity of workers with a range of physical and psychosocial diagnoses to return to work. It is a psychometrically sound instrument across cultures and diagnoses. The interview questions are designed to generate data relevant to the individual and should be administered in a culturally sensitive manner. Ultimately, it is the responsibility of the practitioner to make the client feel comfortable by respecting the client's cultural norms related to personal space, gender requirements, verbal and nonverbal language, work values, and work roles.

Vocational Rehabilitation and Culture

Occupational therapy practitioners play an important role in the vocational rehabilitation process. Return to work is a recognized goal of work rehabilitation, and in the absence of a vocational rehabilitation specialist, the task of addressing vocational issues often falls upon the occupational therapy practitioner. This is appropriate, because occupational therapy practitioners understand the relationship of the individual's medical condition, functional abilities, and psychosocial status with work demands (Stuckey, 1997). An increasing number of people are requesting occupational therapy intervention aimed specifically at return to work, especially in countries where occupational therapy practitioners have a high profile in work rehabilitation and vocational rehabilitation (e.g., the United Kingdom, Canada, Hong Kong, and Australia). Return-to-work interventions usually include analysis of work skills, the practice of work-related tasks, advice on graded return, adaptations to the workplace or job, and communication with the employer (Main and Haig, 2006). In the United Kingdom, the College of Occupational Therapists, a wholly owned subsidiary of the British Association of Occupational Therapists (BAOT), launched its rehabilitation strategic goals in November 2008. The aim is to steer the College and its members to ensure service users, employees, and employers have access to occupational therapy within all vocational rehabilitation services.

Over the past two decades, occupational therapy literature has confirmed the profession's contribution to the management of occupational injuries. Jundt and King (1999) identified that occupational therapists in the United States were prolific in providing prevention, assessment, and rehabilitation services for managing occupational injuries. A study by Lo (2000) on work rehabilitation programs in Hong Kong also revealed substantial growth in occupational therapy's role in the area over the past decade. However, evidence suggests that individuals from minority cultures may underutilize vocational rehabilitation services in the United States.

The Vocational Rehabilitation Act of 1973 (Title V) was put in place to correct the problem of discrimination against people with disabilities in the United States. The U.S. Vocational Rehabilitation (VR) system, although slightly different in each state, shares similar dominant cultural aspects. A review of contemporary VR legislative content, funding processes, policies, and practices confirm the cultural values of individualism and independence discussed earlier. Table 3.10 includes some examples of the effect that the values of individualism have on vocational rehabilitation principles.

The VR system is regulated by legislation, so services are regulated by the associated rules and statutes of each legal jurisdiction. The system is outcome and placement driven (Jezewski and Sotnik, 2001). Success is defined as the quickest route to being placed in paid employment. Successful cases typically consist of individuals who believe in the

Table 3.10 Effects of Individualism on Vocational Rehabilitation Principles

Individualism	Principles of Vocational Rehabilitation
Self-determination: individuals control personal situation	Consumers set their own rehabilitation goals and are self-advocates
Success is defined in terms of professional achievement of the individual	Employment is successful rehabilitation
Person is unique and independent	Self-sufficiency is an ideal outcome

Adapted from Jezewski & Sotnik, 2001.

same values, can be readily employed, and are English speaking. This is contradictory to the provision of culturally responsive services to people from diverse backgrounds.

In late 1999, the Congress ratified the Ticket to Work and Work Incentive Improvement Act (TWWIIA). This legislation represents a significant opportunity for increasing the employment of people with disabilities. The TWWIIA provides for two landmark measures that have the potential to enable millions of Americans with disabilities to join the workforce. The first is the creation of the Ticket to Work Program, administered by the Social Security Administration (SSA). This program modernizes employment-related services offered to Americans with disabilities. Through the Ticket to Work Program, individuals with disabilities can receive job-related training and placement assistance from an approved provider of their choice. This provision enables individuals to go to providers whose resources best meet their needs, including going directly to employers. The second measure expands health-care coverage so that individuals with disabilities may become employed without fear of losing their health insurance. The objective of the Ticket to Work Program is to work with businesses, state vocational rehabilitation agencies, and other traditional and nontraditional service providers to prepare individuals with disabilities for work and link them with employers who want to hire qualified employees.

The legislation has meant new opportunities for occupational therapy practitioners who are qualified to assist with return-to-work transitions. They have expertise in assessing clients, work environments, and modifications, and they can work with individuals and/or employers to facilitate employment. Occupational therapy practitioners can teach work-related personal skills, coaching people in the work habits and attitudes needed to get and keep employment. They can also refer clients to other service providers through the Ticket to Work Program. The legislation allows clients with disabilities to go beyond traditional state vocational rehabilitation programs and obtain employment support services through networks of private providers. Occupational therapy practitioners can assist clients in selecting the most appropriate provider and ensure that the provider understands the client's work goals.

Culturally competent occupational therapy practitioners can be a valuable resource as a liaison between clients and vocational rehabilitation providers. They can ameliorate culturally appropriate communication between clients and vocational counselors. For example, they can inform vocational counselors or service providers about clients' views of disability, ensuring that client expectations are understood by providers and that clients are referred to providers who have the resources to deal with culture-specific needs.

Chapter Summary

Occupational therapy practice in work-related services and industrial rehabilitation is a growing field worldwide. The last two decades have seen a significant increase in occupational therapy literature that addresses issues relating to culture and cultural differences and the importance of understanding ourselves as therapists in an attempt to avoid ethnocentric practice. This chapter described the importance of considering culture in the provision of occupational therapy services in work-related services and industrial rehabilitation. It discussed how the meaning of work in the life of individuals is influenced by prevailing cultural norms and the challenges that immigrant and ethnic workers have to deal with when faced with health problems or work-related injuries and the subsequent rehabilitation process. The concept of work values was explained in the context of an individual's cultural background.

Definitions and models of cultural competency were discussed in depth with the aim of providing occupational therapy practitioners techniques on developing new cultural competency skills or improving on existing skills. Practical strategies for effective cross-cultural communication were presented (Table 3.8) because communication is of primary importance in providing occupational therapy services.

The significance of a culturally competent occupational therapy practitioner was further highlighted by examples of clinical and workplace utilization of appropriate culturally sensitive work assessments and evaluation tools, followed by a discussion of the valuable contribution of occupational therapy practitioners in vocational rehabilitation.

Culture presents itself in every clinical encounter in occupational therapy. People practice healthy habits, define illness, and seek assistance to deal with their health problems universally, but they are guided by their cultural norms. This chapter provided an insight to the importance of practicing culturally sensitive and culturally competent occupational therapy, as culture is profoundly and inextricably tied to matters of health and health care.

Case Resolution

Although Maria's occupational therapist was only mildly fluent in Spanish, she utilized family members and interpreters to supplement her skills, which allowed for efficient verbal communication and prevented misunderstandings. During the assessment and evaluation processes, the therapist utilized relevant and culturally sensitive tools. The initial client interview was completed in Spanish. A job analysis of Maria's work space and tasks was completed, and a functional capacity evaluation was performed to determine her physical functional abilities. The occupational therapist chose to administer the Worker Role Interview to determine psychosocial variables influencing work success and the Work Environment Impact Scale to assess how the characteristics of the work environment affected Maria's work performance.

The occupational therapist identified the following issues during the evaluation:

- Maria's English proficiency was limited because Spanish was her native language.
- She was a single mother with two children, ages 9 and 5.
- She was a recent immigrant with no college education and had taken the first job she was able to attain and perform.
- Maria's employer accepted her work-related injury under the company's workers' compensation insurance and was paying for her medical expenses.
- Maria had limited social support. Her primary source was the local church that she attended.
- She was unfamiliar with the workers' compensation process and depended on her employer and friends to guide her through the process.
- Her family physician was a doctor recommended to her by her social network. He was of Hispanic origin and spoke Spanish. Maria was satisfied with the care he had given her and her two children. However, he was not involved with her medical care for her work-related injury, and an orthopedic clinic recommended by her employer was treating her.
- Maria was very concerned about her ability to return to her current job, and she feared job loss if she was unable to meet her job demands. She was unsure about alternative vocational prospects because of her limited education, language barriers, and lack of job experience.

As part of the occupational therapy intervention, the occupational therapist also interviewed Maria's employer about her return-to-work options and the company's expectations of Maria when she returned to work. She referred Maria to a vocational counselor, as Maria was not able to return to her normal job, and her current employer did not have alternative job options. The employer's insurance paid for ongoing medical care and vocational counseling services.

The occupational therapist in this case engaged in work-related practice that was culturally sensitive. Her compensation for her full ability to communicate in the client's native language ameliorated possible misunderstanding by the client about her rehabilitation process. She sought to understand Maria's fears and concerns about

(case study continues on page 76)

the rehabilitation process and fully explored Maria's return-to-work options. The therapist acted as a liaison between the employer and the client to clarify any miscommunication between them and to educate the employer about the importance of supporting a culturally sensitive work environment (e.g., the use of an interpreter and displaying safety signs in languages relevant to the workers). The therapist used assessment and evaluation tools aimed at capturing the client's unique cultural perspective about work roles, habits, work environment, and expectations. The therapist was able to advocate for the client, which resulted in Maria's receiving appropriate vocational rehabilitation.

References

Alotaibi, N. M. (2008). The cross-cultural adaptation of the disability of arm, shoulder and hand (DASH): A systematic review. *Occupational Therapy International, 15*(3), 178–190.

American Occupational Therapy Association (AOTA). (2008). AOTA's Centennial Vision. American Occupational Therapy Association website. Retrieved from www.aota.org.

Awaad, T. (2003). Culture, cultural competency and occupational therapy: A review of literature. *British Journal of Occupational Therapy, 66*(8), 356–362.

Betancourt, J. R., Green, A. R., Carrillo, J. E., & Ananeh-Firempong, O. (2003). Defining cultural competence: A practical framework for addressing racial/ethnic disparities in health and health care. *Public Health Reports (Washington, D.C.: 1974), 118*(4), 293–302.

Campinha-Bacote, J. (2002). The process of cultural competence in the delivery of healthcare services: A model of care. *Journal of Transcultural Nursing, 13*(3), 181–184.

Canadian Association of Occupational Therapists (CAOT). (n.d.). Current trends affecting occupational therapy. Retrieved from www.caot.ca/default.asp?pageid=291.

Deen, M., Gibson, L., & Strong, J. (2002). A survey of occupational therapy in Australian work practice. *Work, 19,* 219–230.

De Vaus, D., & McAllister, I. (1991). Gender and work orientation: Values and satisfaction in Western Europe. *Work and Occupations, 18*(1), 72–93.

Duran, D. G., Pacheco, G., Epstein L. G.; U.S. Health Resources and Services Administration, Bureau of Primary Health Care; U.S. Office of Minority Health; Substance Abuse and Mental Health Services Administration; National Alliance for Hispanic Health. (2001). *Quality health services for Hispanics: The cultural competency component.* Washington, DC: Department of Health and Human Services, 2001.

Elizur, D., Borg, I., Hunt, R., & Beck, I. M. (1991). The structure of work values: A cross-cultural comparison. *Journal of Organizational Behavior, 12*(1), 21–38.

Feldman, J. M., Ah Sam, I., McDonald, W. F., & Bechtel, G. G. (1980). Work outcome preference and evaluation: A study of three ethnic groups. *Journal of Cross-Cultural Psychology, 11*(4), 444–468.

Freedman, R. I., & Fesko, S. (1996). The meaning of work in the lives of people with significant disabilities: Consumer and family perspectives. *Journal of Rehabilitation, 62*(3), 49.

Hall, E. T. (1976). *Beyond Culture.* New York: Doubleday.

Hopton, K., & Stoneley, H. (2006). Cultural awareness in occupational therapy: The Chinese example. *British Journal of Occupational Therapy, 69*(8), 386–389.

Jezewski, M. A., & Sotnik, P. (2001). *The rehabilitation service provider as culture broker: Providing culturally*

competent services to foreign-born persons (CIRRIE Monograph Series). Buffalo, NY: Center for International Rehabilitation Research, Information and Exchange.

Jundt, J., & King, P. M. (1999). Work rehabilitation programs: A 1997 survey. *Work, 12,* 139–144.

Itzhaky, H., & Ribner, D. S. (1999). Gender, values and the work place: Considerations for immigrant acculturation. *International Social Work, 42*(2), 127–138.

Kinebanian, A., & Stomph, M. (1992). Cross-cultural occupational therapy: A critical reflection. *American Journal of Occupational Therapy, 46*(8), 751–757.

Krefting, L., & Krefting, D. (1991). Leisure activities after a stroke: An ethnographic approach. *American Journal of Occupational Therapy, 45*(5), 429–436.

LeBaron, M. (2003). *Bridging Cultural Conflicts: A New Approach for a Changing World.* San Francisco: Jossey-Bass.

Lo, E. K. S. (2000). Demographic study on occupational therapy work rehabilitation programs in Hong Kong hospital authority. *Work, 14,* 185–189.

Main, L., & Haig, J. (2006). Occupational therapy and vocational rehabilitation: An audit of an outpatient occupational therapy service. *British Journal of Occupational Therapy, 69*(6), 288–292.

Munoz, J. P. (2007). Culturally responsive caring in occupational therapy. *Occupational Therapy International, 14*(4), 256–280.

Niles, F. S. (1999). Toward a cross-cultural understanding of work-related beliefs. *Human Relations, 52*(7), 855–867.

Riccucci, N. M. (1997). Cultural diversity programs to prepare for work force 2000: What's gone wrong? *Public Personnel Management, 26*(1), 35–41.

Roehling, P. V., Jarvis, L. H., & Swoope, H. E. (2005). Variations in negative work family spillover among white, black and Hispanic American men and women: Does ethnicity matter? *Journal of Family Issues, 26*(6), 840–865.

Rubaii-Barrett, N. (1993). Minorities in the majority: Implications for managing cultural diversity. *Public Personnel Management, 22*(4), 503–519.

Santana, S., & Santana, F. O. (2001). *An introduction to Mexican culture for rehabilitation service providers* (CIRRIE Monograph Series). Buffalo, NY: Center for International Rehabilitation Research Information and Exchange.

Schwartz, H. S. (1999). A theory of cultural values and some implications for work. *Applied Psychology, 48*(1), 23–47.

Stuckey, R. (1997). Enhancing work performance in industrial settings: A role of occupational therapy. *British Journal of Occupational Therapy, 60*(6), 277–278.

Suarez-Balcazar, Y., & Rodakowski, J. (2007). Becoming a culturally competent occupational therapy practitioner. *OT Practice, 12*(17), 14–17.

U.S. Bureau of Labor Statistics. (2002). *Monthly Labor Review.* Vol. 125, No. 5.

U.S. Census Bureau. (2008). Population profile of the United States: National population projections. Retrieved from www.census.gov/population/www/pop-profile/natproj.html.

Westmoreland, M. G., & Buys, N. (2004). A comparison of disability management practices in Australian and Canadian workplaces. *Work, 23,* 31–41.

Würtz, E. (2005). A cross-cultural analysis of websites from high-context cultures and low-context cultures. *Journal of Computer-Mediated Communication, 11*(1), article 13. Retrieved from http://jcmc.indiana.edu/vol11/issue1/wuertz.html.

Glossary

Culture is an integrated pattern of behaviors, norms, and rules that are shared by a group and involve their beliefs, values, expectations, worldviews, communication, common history, and institutions.

Cultural context is the customs, beliefs, activity patterns, behavior standards, and expectations accepted by the society of which the client is a member. It includes ethnicity and values as well as political aspects, such as laws that affect access to resources and affirm personal rights.

Paralinguistics are nonverbal elements of communication, such as personal space, gestures, eye contact, and silence.

Work values are the goals or rewards people seek through their work and are grouped into four broad categories: intrinsic, extrinsic, social, and power.

Work value frames of reference are standards against which the outcomes of work are judged and are thought to be partially a product of culture.

Resources

Model of Human Occupation Clearinghouse (Assessments)

www.moho.uic.edu/assessments.html

Social Security Administration Ticket to Work

www.yourtickettowork.com

U.S. Department of Health and Human Services: Health Resources and Services Administration. Cultural Competence Resources for Health Care Providers

www.hrsa.gov/culturalcompetence

"Becoming a Culturally Competent Occupational Therapy Practitioner" by Y. Suarez-Balcazar and J. Rodakowski. *OT Practice, 12*(17), 14–17, 2000.

Cultural Competence in Health Education and Health Promotion by M. A. Perez and R. R. Luquis (San Francisco: Jossey-Bass, 2008).

4 Occupational Therapy Conceptual Practice Models and Related Knowledge to Support Work Practice

Jenica Lee

Key Concepts

The following are key concepts addressed in this chapter:

- The use of conceptual practice models is important in providing a framework for decision-making and supporting an evidence-based approach to practice.
- The theoretical frameworks discussed in this chapter are classified into two types of knowledge: occupational therapy knowledge and related knowledge.
- By combining the use of conceptual practice models, therapists can achieve a more holistic and effective approach to understanding and treating the worker.

Case Introduction

Mr. Wallace is a 50-year-old man who suffered a stroke 5 weeks ago that left him with upper extremity weakness, slight memory deficits, and bowel incontinence. He lives with his wife and two daughters who are both attending college. Before the stroke, he worked as a foreman for a commercial construction company for 15 years. He made significant progress during his stay in in-patient rehabilitation, and he looks forward to returning home. Unknown to anybody, Mr. Wallace is getting depressed and feels trapped in a disabled body. Although he expresses interest in returning to his former employer, he does not think he can return to work. He is worried his coworkers might react awkwardly to his physical impairment, and since he has difficulty with incontinence, he fears that he might have accidents at work. Because of his cognitive and physical deficits, Mr. Wallace is doubtful that he can still perform his job requirements effectively. Outpatient therapy now is focused on ensuring his successful transition from hospital to home and investigating the possibilities of returning to work.

Introduction

This chapter discusses the theories most often used in occupational therapy work-related practice. The primary tenets of each theory or model is identified, and their relevance to work-related intervention is explained. Examples of the application of each theory or model to a specific work problem or setting highlight the importance of evidence-based practice. Examples of how to translate research and evidence to practice further support the need for familiarity with a range of theories and the importance of the development of competencies to support an evidence-based approach to practice. The concepts of a "scholarship of practice" and striving to become "practice scholars" set the stage for the remainder of the chapter.

Types of Knowledge Defined

As you learned in Chapter 1, occupational therapy practitioners have played an active role in the delivery of prevention, assessment, and management of occupational injuries since the profession's inception (Deen, Gibson, and Strong, 2002; Gainer 2008). Like all professional groups, occupational therapy practitioners draw on their conceptual, theoretical, and professional paradigms to guide their clinical reasoning process and actions (Kielhofner, 2004; Mattingly and Fleming, 1994; Tornebohm, 1985). Each individual's professional paradigm is shaped by the integration of theoretical knowledge, skills, and experiences (Kielhofner 2009; Schell, 2009). In work-related practice, practitioners encounter a wide range of occupational problems, so it is common to use multiple practice models to guide their clinical decision-making. The theoretical frameworks discussed in this chapter are classified into two main types of knowledge, following Kielhofner's (2009) taxonomy:

1. *Occupational therapy knowledge,* which includes conceptual practice models developed in the domain of the field and reflects the nature, purpose, and value of occupational therapy practice.
2. *Related knowledge,* which includes theories, concepts, and techniques developed from other fields but also incorporated in occupational therapy practice.

Theoretical knowledge, which is formally organized into "conceptual practice models" (Kielhofner, 2009) provides a systemic way to understand the nature of the occupational challenges faced by clients as well as justify the types of services to provide them. Each practice model is developed from a specific perspective and contains information to address a specific phenomena or problem. In work-related practice, practitioners encounter a wide range of occupational problems, so it is common to use multiple practice models to guide their clinical decision-making.

Related knowledge is not developed within occupational therapy but is selected for its relevance to occupational therapy practice. Related knowledge is developed in other fields, such as public health and psychology, and is used to complement conceptual practice models.

Theoretical knowledge, which is formally organized into "conceptual practice models" (Kielhofner, 2009) provides a systemic way to understand the nature of the occupational challenges faced by clients as well as justify the types of services to provide them.

Evidence-Based Knowledge

It is the occupational therapy practitioner's ethical responsibility to base his or her clinical decision-making on evidence-based knowledge. It is important for practitioners to choose the practice model most fitting for context and situation of the client and equally important to critically evaluate the existing research base of these theoretical frameworks, as they inform the value and effectiveness of these models. Doing so ensures that the interventions and clinical approaches based on these theories are most effective for the clients. Numerous formal theoretical models have been published in the area of work-related practice, but only the models that are most widely used and validated by scientific study are addressed in this chapter.

This chapter serves as a beginning to increase the reader's understanding of the state of theory and provides an overview of relevant theoretical frameworks developed within and outside of occupational therapy in the area of work-related practice.

Occupational Therapy Conceptual Practice Models in Work-Related Practice

Of the contemporary occupation-based models, evidence shows that two have most successfully been applied in work-related practice: the Canadian model of occupational performance and engagement and the model of human occupation. These models are broad in scope, and each offers a unique perspective to explain the relationship between the human, occupation, and the environment. The key concepts of each model, technologies for application, and the research base of each model will now be further discussed.

Canadian Model of Occupational Performance and Engagement (CMOP-E)

Formerly called the Canadian model of occupational performance (CMOP), this model began as a process designed to identify guidelines for occupational therapy practice in Canada (Kielhofner, 2004). Through continued refinement of the model, the most recent version has expanded to include the concept of engagement. These developments are reflected in name change to CMOP-E (Townsend and Polatajko, 2007).

Key CMOP-E Concepts

This model seeks to explain influences among the dimensions of occupational performance and engagement through three main concepts:

• Person
• Environment
• Occupation

The dynamic interaction of these three components results in occupational performance and engagement (see Fig. 4.1). As depicted in the model, the person is at the center to highlight the client-centered perspective and is composed of three performance components: cognitive, affective, and physical. Spirituality is at the core of the person to reflect the human essence that shapes the values and beliefs of the individual. A person's spirituality is influenced by the environment and ultimately influences his or her choice to engage in specific occupations (CAOT, 1997; 2002). The *person* is connected to the *environment* and occupation occurs as interactions between persons and their environments. The environmental context is unique to each individual and has four dimensions: cultural, institutional, physical, and social. The concept of *occupation* connects the person and environment and is further classified into three occupational purposes: self-care, productivity, and leisure.

Applying CMOP-E in Practice

According to the CMOP-E, occupational challenges arise when any change or imbalance occurs in any part of the person–environment occupation interaction. Occupational therapy intervention based on this model uses the process of "enablement" to restore balance or improve the transactions among the person, occupation, and environment. Although specific details of the therapeutic process are not explicitly stated in the model, a general guideline of enabling approaches are mentioned and involve collaboration with clients to facilitate autonomy and opportunity for positive change (Townsend and Polatajko, 2007).

The Canadian Occupational Performance Measure (COPM) is a semistructured interview developed to apply the model (Law, et al., 1994). It is designed to help client and therapist identify problems in areas of self-care, productivity, and leisure. The COPM is also used to facilitate identification of priorities for therapy and can be used as an outcome measure. Box 4.1 illustrates how the CMOP-E can be used in an industrial rehabilitation setting.

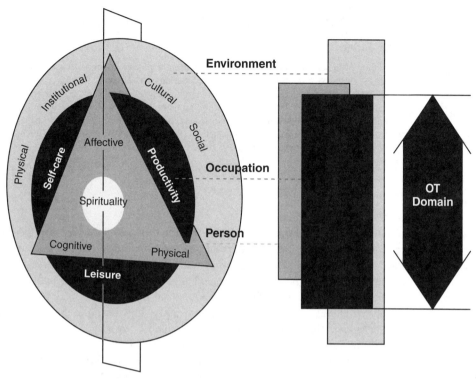

Figure 4.1 Canadian model of occupational performance and engagement. Reprinted from Polatajko, Townsend, and Craik (2007).

Box 4.1 CMOP Case Example: Client-Centered Approach

A clothing manufacturing company recently implemented a new line of equipment to increase quality and production and to ultimately expand the business. Operation of these new machines requires the worker to stand for prolonged periods, and as a result, many employees began complaining about back, shoulder, and neck problems (physical component) and had to leave work because of their injuries. An occupational therapist was hired to help employees adjust to the new work processes and to assist those who were unable to work to return to work.

Using the CMOP-E, the occupational therapist identified the person-related issues, workplace environment, and work processes (occupation) environment that contributed to the occupational performance problems.

Person-Related Issues

Employees expressed dissatisfaction in the lack of transition time and support to change from sitting to standing positions. All injured employees wanted to return to work but felt anxious and questioned their ability to stand without reaggravating their problems (affective component). Some injured workers have been with the company for 20 years and have developed a strong identity and bond with the company: they cannot imagine working elsewhere (spirituality component).

Occupation-Related Issues

Current workstations require employees to work in standing rather than sitting positions.

Environment-Related Issues

Employees are now required to operate new equipment in standing rather than sitting positions (institutional component). A cultural shift is also required: before the changes, employees manufactured the clothes more manually and now must accept the change and adapt to the new working position and machine operation (cultural component).

(box continues on page 82)

Box 4.1   CMOP Case Example: Client-Centered Approach—cont'd

Intervention

Resolution of the performance issues in this situation required a collaborative approach among the managers, employees, and therapists. Recommendations for achieving the organization's goals of enabling the occupational performance included employee involvement in the decision-making process and development and delivery of education programs to prevent and reduce work injuries. Involving the employees in the decision-making process helped facilitate their transition to the new culture and work environment. Employees were educated on the use of healthy workplace practices for occupations requiring standing, which ultimately helped them return to work and helped reduce workplace injuries for the company.

CMOP-E Research Base

Over 100 studies have been published related to this model, but most of the published research has focused on the development and examination of the assessment tool, COPM, rather than the model. The COPM has undergone extensive research in many different occupational therapy practice situations, but about one-tenth of the published studies are specific to work (Bedell, 2008; Clarke, 2003; Corr and Wilmer, 2003; Harper, Stalker, and Templeton, 2006; Herzberg and Finlayson, 2001; Ingvarsson and Theodorsdottir, 2004; Sloan, Winkler, and Callaway, 2004). Psychometric properties including clinical utility, validity, and responsiveness were studied in many of the papers. The results were very positive, demonstrating support for the reliability and validity of the COPM (Chan and Lee, 1997; Cup, Scholte op Reimer, Thijssen, and van Kuyk-Minis, 2003; McColl, Paterson, Davies, Doubt, and Law, 2000).

The CMOP-E practice model can be used to facilitate a client-centered approach to understanding how person and environmental factors affect the occupational performance and full engagement of the worker. We now discuss another established occupational therapy conceptual practice model used widely in work-related practice, the model of human occupation.

Model of Human Occupation

The model of human occupation (MOHO), first published in 1980, is an occupationally oriented theory to guide practice (Kielhofner, 2008). It seeks to explain work behavior and challenges as a function of four components:

- Volition
- Habituation
- Performance capacity
- Environment

The MOHO is frequently used to guide work-related interventions and programs (Ingvarsson and Theodorsdottir, 2004; Jackson, Harkess, and Ellis, 2004; Kielhofner, Braveman, Fogg, and Levin, 2008; Mentrup, Niehaus, and Kielhofner, 1999). Evidence shows that it is the most widely used occupation-based model in the United States and internationally (Brown, Rodger, Brown, and Roever, 2005; Lee, Taylor, Kielhofner, and Fisher, 2008; NBCOT, 2004; Wikeby, Pierre, and Archenholt, 2006).

Key MOHO Concepts

Volition is the process by which persons are motivated toward and choose what they want to do. Volition includes the worker's values, interests, and personal causation (e.g., beliefs about personal capacity and efficacy). Value is what the worker holds as important or the meaningfulness of the person's job. Personal causation is the worker's sense of competence and effectiveness in the work environment. Interests are what the worker finds enjoyable and satisfying as a result of participation in work. Together, these characteristics of volition are critical to clients' decision-making about returning to work and to their ability to succeed at work (Ásmundsdóttir, 2004; Ekbladh, Haglund, and Thorell, 2004; Scheelar, 2002).

Habituation structures behavior into the recurrent patterns that make up the routines and rhythms of everyday life. Two components of habituation, internalized roles and habits, provide regularity and order to what people do and how they do it. Internalized roles refer to a person's sense of identity both as a worker and in roles outside of work (e.g., husband, parent, coach), and they shape the individual's attitudes and behaviors. Habits, then, influence how people perform routine activities, use time, and behave. In a work setting, because of habits, people intuitively know when the work shift is over or what step follows when performing a familiar work task. Together, a person's ability to recognize work role expectations and his or her habits are supports to work success (Corr and Wilmer, 2003; Kielhofner, et al., 2004).

Performance capacity, or an individual's underlying ability to do things, is determined by the status of both physical (e.g., musculoskeletal and cardiopulmonary) and mental or cognitive components that are involved in work. Although performance capacity is an important element in the MOHO framework, the theory does not directly address it because a number of other established practice models (e.g., tests of strength, range of motion [ROM], endurance from the biomechanical model) objectively measure these performance components. These other models are discussed later in the chapter.

Nevertheless, according to the MOHO framework, performance capacity provides the basis for skilled performance. When capacity is used in actual performance, it is manifest as skills. Skills are defined as goal-directed actions that make up the actual performance and have been shown in literature to correlate with return to work after injury (Braveman, Helfrich, Kielhofner, and Albrecht, 2004; Kielhofner, et al., 2004). The MOHO identifies three types of skills: motor, process, and communication/interaction skills.

The final MOHO concept, the *environment,* is conceptualized as including both physical (e.g., arrangement, accessibility, sensory qualities of workspace) and social (e.g., coworker interactions, work schedules, supervisor communication, and family support) characteristics that relates to both inside and outside the work situation. These environmental characteristics are interdependent with the person factors and can create either opportunities or constraints for the individual. The degree of fit between the worker characteristics (e.g., values, roles, performance capacity) and the work environment characteristics determines whether the impact is positive or negative.

The successful interplay of these four components or the match between the worker's values, interests, personal causation, abilities, and environmental context over time brings about positive occupational identity and occupational competence (Fig. 4.2). Together these make up occupational adaptation.

Applying MOHO in Practice

According to the MOHO, problems in occupational adaptation arise when there is maladaptive change in the worker's motivation, lifestyle, performance, and/or environment. For a worker with an injury or longstanding disability to return to work, changes and adaptation in any of these factors are required. The MOHO conceptual practice model can be used by occupational therapy practitioners to understand how these factors may impact the person's ability to work or return to work.

Many resources, including assessments, manuals of MOHO-based work programs, and case examples have been developed to apply the model to work settings and work-related practice. To date, 21 assessments are available for use with this model, but four of them are specifically developed for use in work rehabilitation contexts; they include the Worker Role Interview (WRI), Work Environment Impact Scale (WEIS), the Dialogue

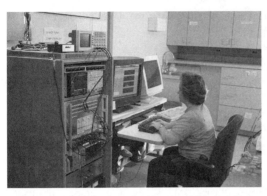 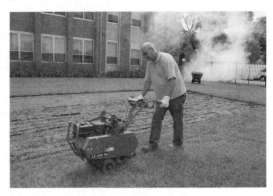

Figure 4.2 Two workers perform very different types of work but are both influenced by values, interests, and personal causation (volition); internalized roles and habits (habituation); their abilities (performance capacity); and their environments.

about Ability Related to Work (DOA), and Assessment of Work Performance (AWP). The latter two assessments are fairly new MOHO-based instruments being developed in Sweden (Linddahl, Norrby, and Bellner, 2003; Sandqvist, Gullberg, Henriksson, and Gerdle, 2006; Sandqvist, Tornquist, and Henricksson, 2006). Table 4.1 summarizes some characteristics of these assessments. Additionally, several other MOHO assessments (the Occupational Performance History Interview [OPHI], the Occupational Self-Assessment [OSA], and the MOHO Screening Tool [MOHOST]) have been used in work programs (Forsyth and Kielhofner, 2008; Kielhofner, et al., 2008; Levin, Kielhofner, Braveman, and Fogg, 2007).

In addition, four comprehensive work-related programs have been developed on the basis of the MOHO. These include programs designed for inpatient and outpatient

Table 4.1 Characteristics of MOHO-Based Work Assessments

Assessment	Administration	Purpose	Population
Worker Role Interview (WRI)	• Semistructured interview and rating scale • Has three interview formats for workers with recent injuries/disabilities, for clients with chronic disabilities, and for combining the WRI with the Occupational Circumstances Assessment Interview and Rating scale	• Assesses impact of personal causation, values, interests, roles, habits, and perception of the environmental on potential for obtaining or returning to work • Provides clients an opportunity to express attitudes and opinions toward work, gives new direction to goal setting in a work program, provides a clear structure for formatting reports, and can assess a person's abilities • The WRI helps therapists to better understand workers' concerns, develop positive rapport, identify inconsistencies between the worker's perceptions and objective evidence, and precisely identify barriers to return to work that need to be addressed	• Clients with physical or mental disabilities, including those with longstanding illness or disability who have limited work histories

Table 4.1 Characteristics of MOHO-Based Work Assessments—cont'd

Assessment	Administration	Purpose	Population
Work Environment Impact Scale (WEIS)	• Semistructured interview and rating scale	• Assesses features in the work environment that support or impede performance, satisfaction, and well-being. • Used to identify needed workplace accommodations	• Clients experiencing difficulty on the job whose work is interrupted by an injury or illness
DOA: The Dialogue about Ability Related to Work	• Client self-assessment and professional observation in Swedish and English	• Assesses influence of volition, roles, physical ability, and communication and interaction skills on work ability	• Clients with psychiatric and psychosocial problems
Assessment of Work Performance (AWP)	• Observation-based performance rating scale	• Assesses motor, process, communication, and interaction skills within a work activity	• Any client experiencing a work-related problem

Visit the MOHO website for additional information: www.uic.edu/depts/moho/.

psychiatric service, a community-based daily program, and two community-based programs. These vocational programs are applied across diverse populations from all over the world, including persons with physical, cognitive, and psychiatric disabilities and persons with a variety of social challenges such as substance abuse, felony convictions, homelessness, and domestic violence. Table 4.2 provides more detailed information about these programs. Box 4.2 illustrates how the MOHO practice model is used in a work rehabilitation setting.

Table 4.2 MOHO-Based Work Programs

Program	Purpose and Resources
Employment Options Program (EO)	• A four-phase vocational rehabilitation program developed to support persons living with HIV/AIDS to develop skills related to volition, habituation, and performance capacity to increase work potential • The EO manual (www.moho.uic.edu/images/EO%20Manual.pdf) outlines program content, which includes strategies and methods for assessment, intervention protocols, and program evaluation
Enabling Self-Determination (ESD)	• A four-phase intervention, developed through collaboration with clients and caretakers, to support individuals with HIV/AIDS to return to work and/or other productive roles • The ESD manual (www.uic.edu/depts/moho/images/ESD Manual Final.pdf) outlines program content, which includes strategies and approaches to assessment, goal setting and managing routines, developing competence, and achieving community and work participation
Work Readiness Program	• A community-based vocational treatment program for people with chronic disabilities; it meets 5 days a week, giving individuals an opportunity to explore and develop work skills and habits over a period of time • Protocols of the different skills groups (e.g., daily living skills, communication and interactions skills, and work skills) are described in a detailed manual (www.uic.edu/depts/moho/programs and interventions/workreadiness.html)

(table continues on page 86)

Table 4.2 MOHO-Based Work Programs—cont'd

Program	Purpose and Resources
Work Rehabilitation in Mental Health Program	• The program manual outlines the development and implementation of work programs in inpatient and outpatient psychiatric settings; protocols of vocational groups and job clubs and their related activities are also included in the manual (www.uic.edu/depts/moho/programs%20and%20interventions/workrehabilitation.html)

Visit the MOHO website for additional information: www.uic.edu/depts/moho/.

Box 4.2 MOHO Case Example: Looking Beyond Functional Capacity

Jordan is a 50-year-old laborer who sustained a back injury from a motorcycle accident 5 months ago. He works for a wholesale seafood company, and his line of work requires repetitive manual lifting (20–70 lb) and operation of a forklift. When he returned to work, he found his job increasingly difficult. The increased sales of the company required Jordan to stock and move heavier loads of product, and he subsequently reinjured his back. Jordan has been absent from work for 6 months, and the Worker Role Interview was used to assess his potential for return to work.

Volition

Jordan exhibited a decreased sense of efficacy but still expressed a strong commitment to return to work. He expressed fear and questioned his ability to work at the seafood company again. At this point, he was not sure how much he could lift and carry. Having been doing this job for 20 years, Jordan is not sure what other line of work he can do. He mentioned that he has worked at similar places but that "this was the best job I've ever had." He mentioned that the job pays well, and he enjoys working with all his coworkers. He also enjoys fishing with his coworkers once a month, but he has not done that since his injury. He feels pretty "useless" at the moment because he is not doing anything or providing for his family.

Habituation

Consistent with his values, Jordan expressed strong identification with being a worker. He also mentioned how the injury has impacted his role as the family provider and husband. He said he can no longer help his wife with certain household and garden chores, like mowing the lawn and shoveling the snow. He said that he would like to be able to return to those roles at some capacity.

Prior to his injury, Jordan had well-organized habits. He always showed up to work on time and rarely missed work. He completed all his work tasks in a timely manner and had enough energy to participate in his leisure and home activities outside of work. However, since his injury, his routine has deteriorated dramatically. Watching TV is now his main daily activity. The current lack of routine and habits contributes to his feelings of ineffectiveness and deconditioned health status.

Performance Capacity

This factor was assessed using a musculoskeletal evaluation and a work capacity evaluation that included performance of functional tasks. These assessments revealed significant performance limitations (e.g., lifting, squatting, carrying, reaching, pushing), and Jordan's current level of performance do not meet the job demands. Other limitations, including pain, limited ROM in the spine, and reduced physical endurance also negatively impact Jordan's ability to perform at his current job.

Environment

Jordan perceived the physical work environment as inflexible and nonaccommodating to his needs. For example, since the injury, he needed to vary his body positioning more than is possible at work. Jordan also mentioned that his supervisor is supportive and tried to reassign tasks among his coworkers so that Jordan can perform fewer heavy lifting tasks. However, Jordan senses some disapproval from his coworkers, who seem to not fully understand the impact of the injury on Jordan's ability to perform.

Box 4.2   MOHO Case Example: Looking Beyond Functional Capacity—cont'd

Intervention

The WRI provided the therapist an understanding of how Jordan's current volition, habituation, and work environment would impact his ability to return to work. Identifying issues in these areas enabled the therapist to provide a comprehensive rehabilitation program that went beyond the physical reconditioning goals to facilitate progress and positive outcome. The therapist shared with Jordan his situation and her proposed treatment plan. She recommended that Jordan test his work capability in a realistic environment that would also match his interests. With support, Jordan agreed to begin work practice at a local motorcycle repair shop, where the span of work included a wide variety of motorcycle repairs and grounds maintenance. They chose this workplace because the work matched Jordan's interests.

This work practice period facilitated Jordan to redevelop his habits and structure his daily routines. He also developed a better awareness of his work abilities and limitations. In addition, he was taught proper body mechanics and pain management strategies that helped him to feel more confident about his work abilities. Within 2 months of completing his work hardening program, he returned to his previous job on a part-time basis.

Further information about these work-related programs and assessments can be obtained through the MOHO Clearinghouse website: www.uic.edu/depts/moho/. The MOHO Clearinghouse is a not-for-profit organization directed by Dr. Gary Kielhofner and serves as a center of international communication for clinicians, students, and scholars to share information and experiences about MOHO. The MOHO Clearinghouse website provides up-to-date information, resources, and evidence reference lists of the work programs and assessments just discussed.

MOHO Research Base

The MOHO has an extensive research base. Since its conception 30 years ago, MOHO is the topic of close to 400 publications, 45 of which are specific to work-related practice (Fig. 4.3). The existing empirical base includes evidence related to the dependability and utility of work-based assessments as well as evidence supporting the development, implementation, and outcomes of MOHO-based work programs (Braveman, 2001; Corner, Kielhofner, and Lin, 1997; Kielhofner, et al., 2008; Norbby and Linddahl, 2006; Paul-Ward, Braveman, Kielhofner, and Levin, 2005; Sandqvist, et al., 2008).

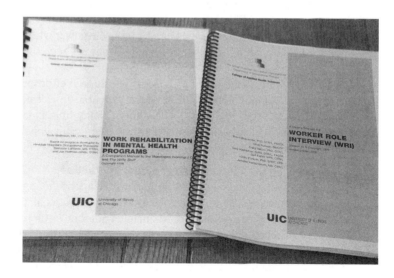

Figure 4.3 Numerous published descriptions of MOHO-based programs, such as the *Work Rehabilitation in Mental Health Programs,* and over 20 MOHO-based assessments, such as the Worker Role Interview, are available.

The MOHO practice model is a useful framework to understand how both psychosocial and environmental factors impact a worker with a work-related disability. Although the two most widely used occupation-based models with the largest empirical base are introduced in this chapter, other occupation-based conceptual models have been developed and can be used to guide assessment and intervention in the area of work practice (Baum and Christiansen, 2005; Schkade and McClung, 2001). The few models discussed in this chapter serve as initial steps to orient the reader to both evidence-based and occupation-based theories in work rehabilitation. The practitioner is encouraged to use clinical judgment when selecting the most appropriate practice model. The following sections introduce other theories developed outside the field of occupational therapy but used to guide work-related practice.

Biomechanical Model

In work rehabilitation and work-related practice, occupational therapy practitioners often use adjunct knowledge from the biomechanical model to address occupational issues due to impairments in body structure and functions, including decreased strength, limited ROM, and poor endurance. For example, this model underlies much of the approach to physical assessment of the worker discussed in Chapter 12. The theoretical foundations of the biomechanical model are based on reductionistic principles of kinetics and kinematics, which involve the study of forces and their effect on how the body accomplishes body movement (James, 2003; Kielhofner, 2004). Such knowledge provides an understanding of the pathology resulting from disease or trauma (e.g., work injury) in the musculoskeletal system, peripheral nervous system, integumentary system, or cardiopulmonary system.

Key Biomechanical Concepts

According to the biomechanical model, the capacity for functional motion includes three domains:

• Joint ROM
• Muscle strength
• Physical endurance

Joint ROM is the amount of movement that is possible at a joint. The range of possible movement at a particular joint is dependent on both the anatomy and the elasticity of the soft tissues (e.g., connective tissue, muscle, skin) surrounding that joint. Trauma or disease to the joint structures or surrounding tissues can decrease the amount of motion at that joint and limit occupational functioning (Trombly and Radomski, 2002).

Muscle strength is the degree of muscle power when movement is resisted from either weight or gravity. Tension produced by muscles serves to stabilize and produce movement at the joint.

Physical endurance is the ability to sustain effort or intensive activity. It is related to both cardiopulmonary and muscular function. Impairment in any of these three areas—ROM, strength, endurance—may significantly limit the movement(s) required to perform work activities, which results in decreased occupational performance. Using this model allows the practitioner to identify and directly address biomechanical deficits.

Applying the Biomechanical Model in Practice

Extensive technology exists to support the application of this model. Typical assessments of biomechanical impairments used by occupational therapy practitioners include the goniometer to measure ROM, manual muscle testing to measure strength, and timed test of repetitions or how long the person can perform an activity before fatigue to measure endurance.

In addition to these basic assessments of strength and endurance, several kinds of more complex evaluation systems are often used in work-related practice, including the VALPAR

Component Work Samples (VCWS) system and Functional Capacity Evaluation (FCE) (Gibson and Strong, 2002; Jundt and King, 1999; Radomski and Latham, 2007). The VALPAR system consists of a wide range of work samples simulating different job tasks to measure specific performance skills (e.g., ROM, problem-solving, stamina, and mobility). The FCE is another comprehensive assessment that objectively measures physical capacities such as strength, posture, gait, sensation, and reflexes. These physical properties are measured during work-related tasks, such as lifting, sitting, and standing. The literature base concerning both of these assessment tools continues to grow, but existing research suggests good validity and reliability of these instruments (Innes, 2006; Jackson, et al., 2004). See Chapter 12 for more information on the physical assessment of the worker.

Interventions based on the biomechanical approach are also clearly outlined in existing literature. Treatment within this model focuses on preventing impairments or restoring physical capacity by decreasing impairments through structured programs of graded physical conditioning/strengthening exercises, functional tasks, and simulated work activities. Remediation of physical deficits is also known as work conditioning (Radomski and Latham, 2007). If a client's physical capacity cannot be fully restored, compensatory strategies to treatment may be used. Consider a typist diagnosed with de Quervain's disease caused by overuse of the thumb and wrist. This condition causes tendon pain in the thumb and wrist, swelling, and possible decreased strength and endurance. During the acute phase of the disease, preventative strategies may be employed; for example, an orthotic splint may be prescribed to immobilize the joint to prevent further damage to the tendons. Immobilization may also help reduce swelling and promote tendon healing. Compensatory strategies, including teaching the client modified ways of typing and how to use a dictation device, may allow the client to continue working. When the swelling decreases, the occupational therapist can employ restorative strategies, including exercises to bring back the normal ROM and strength of the hand and thumb.

Work hardening is a multidisciplinary treatment program designed to maximize an individual's capacity to return to work. This program usually follows work conditioning, and not only does it aim to improve physical capacity, it also addresses other aspects that may determine a person's ability to return to work, such as psychosocial, communication, safety, and productivity components. Because work hardening is aimed at a specific job, intervention usually involves work simulation and specific work tasks (Kielhofner, 2004; Radomski and Latham, 2007).

Research related to the biomechanical model is substantial. Existing empirical knowledge generally supports the validity and positive outcomes of biomechanical-based assessments and interventions used in work rehabilitation (Lieber, Rudy, and Boston, 2000). For example, several studies lend support to work hardening as effective programs to facilitate return to work for disabled workers (Baker, et al., 2005; Krause, Dasiner, and Neuhausel, 1998). Since biomechanical-based treatment often incorporates rote exercise, many studies have looked at the efficacy of exercise-based interventions related to return-to-work outcomes. Results from these studies support that rote exercise was effective in restoring physical capacity, reducing pain, and increasing endurance, thereby facilitating clients' return to work (Karjalainen, et al., 2004; Michener, et al., 2001).

Related Knowledge

While occupation-based models provide the basis for knowledge used in practice, there are always situations in which occupational therapy practitioners must draw on knowledge outside of the field to further guide the main holistic elements of occupational therapy practice. For example, in providing services to a client who lost a limb because of a work injury, the occupational therapy practitioner may draw on the medical model to address or monitor the healing process (e.g., infections, pain management). Because the client is likely to have difficulty coping emotionally with an amputation, the therapist also may draw on psychodynamic principles. As this example illustrates, understanding occupational and human behavior requires us to combine different types of knowledge.

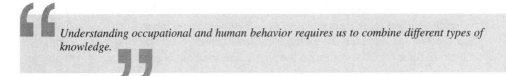

Understanding occupational and human behavior requires us to combine different types of knowledge.

Readiness for Change Model

While the MOHO model may be an appropriate choice to address potential psychosocial issues a worker may face, the occupational therapy practitioner may also consult knowledge related to the readiness for change model to further assess how psychological and/or social factors motivate learning or impact the worker's behavior. The readiness for change model, also known as the transtheoretical model (TTM) or the "stage model," conceptualizes behavior change as a five-stage process or continuum related to a person's readiness to change: precontemplation, contemplation, preparation, action, and maintenance (Franche, Corbiáere, Lee, Breslin, and Hepburn, 2007; Prochaska, Redding, and Evers, 1997). People are thought to progress through these stages at varying rates, often moving back and forth along the continuum a number of times before attaining the goal of maintenance. The five stages as they relate to return to work are described in more detail in the next section.

Key TTM Concepts

In the first stage of change, the *precontemplation* phase, the injured worker does not make any initiating behaviors to support return to work. For a person with a serious injury, work goals are put aside, and the physical process is the main priority at this stage. The *contemplation* phase begins when the worker starts to recognize the benefits of change or starts to consider return to work as a possible goal. The worker considers the pros and cons of returning to work but does not take any concrete steps to do so. The worker is ready and makes a commitment for change in the third stage, *preparation* for action. In this phase, the worker begins to take small actions and is receptive to action-oriented help from external sources (e.g., workplaces, health-care providers) to reach the return-to-work goal. The fourth stage of change is *action*. The worker is fully engaged in return-to-work goals and usually has gone back to work in some capacity. Although the worker is more responsive and displays increased self-efficacy and motivation to tackle work issues, he or she is also at high risk for relapse or unemployment due to potential barriers. In the *maintenance* stage, the worker employs specific skills to face high-risk situations that can trigger a relapse to behaviors that interfere with successful return to work. For example, he or she is consistent with exercise regimens, maintains a positive mood, and engages in behaviors that help ensure continued employment.

Applying the TTM in Practice

According to the TTM, tailoring interventions to match a person's readiness for change or stage of change is essential. For example, for people who are in the first or second stage and are not yet contemplating or committing to return to work, the occupational therapy practitioner may use strategies such as consciousness raising to increase the person's awareness about work and help the individual to articulate what specific barriers and benefits he or she may encounter regarding work (Prochaska, 1994). Once the worker advances to later stages and expresses commitment to return to work, then the occupational therapy practitioner can use strategies such as establishing a support system or rewards system to facilitate continued positive behavior.

The Readiness for Return-to-Work (RRTW) scale is a newly developed instrument to assess stage of readiness to return to work. Initial research supports its relevance as a return-to-work evaluation and points to continued research on the instrument to further establish its validity in a work context (Franche, et al., 2007).

The TTM model has strong empirical support and has been used to guide a variety of health issues, including smoking cessation (Prochaska, Velicer, DiClemente, and Fava, 1988), drug addiction (Prochaska, et al., 1994), and pain management (Keefe, et al., 2000). The model's application to work rehabilitation is relatively recent, so its evidence base is still being established.

Psychiatric Rehabilitation Model

Work plays a central role in the rehabilitation of individuals, including those with mental illness, and the psychiatric rehabilitation (PsyR) model is one theoretical framework that can be used to increase employment potential and address work issues faced by persons with mental illness. The foundation of the PsyR model reflects a biopsychosocial approach, integrating principles of physical rehabilitation and techniques commonly used in psychotherapy (Farkas and Anthony, 1989).

Key PsyR Concepts

The rehabilitation of persons with physical and psychiatric disorders follows a four-stage framework to understand the nature and course of disease: (1) pathology, (2) impairment, (3) disability, and (4) handicap. Table 4.3 defines the four elements and provides examples of rehabilitation strategies associated with each stage as it relates to work. Like physical rehabilitation, psychiatric rehabilitation usually begins when the pathology and impairments of the acute stage stabilize. When functional limitations imposed by psychiatric impairments result in decreased social role performance and/or work incapacity, the individual is said to have a disability. A disability occurs when a person's limitations place him or her at a disadvantage relative to others in society (Farkas and Anthony, 1989; Liberman, 1988). Disadvantage may occur through stigma and discrimination, as when employers are reluctant to hire persons with mental illness and when society does not provide appropriate accommodations and compensation for their impairments or disabilities.

Applying the PsyR Model in Practice

The clinical practice of psychiatric rehabilitation consists of two intervention strategies: skill development (e.g., teaching specific work behaviors) and environmental resource development. These strategies are guided by the basic principle of rehabilitation: providing the disabled person the needed skills and environmental supports increases the person's ability to participate and perform in his or her desired roles, thereby reducing his or her impairment, disability, or handicap (Farkas and Anthony, 1989; Liberman, 1988).

Specific modules and formal vocational rehabilitation programs have been developed for skills training, and many of these approaches involve simple advice, coaching, and modeling (Liberman, 1988; Pratt, Gill, Barrett, and Roberts, 2007). Many of these skills training approaches are well documented; current evidence in general supports their efficacy to increase coping and competence of chronic mentally ill patients in the areas of living and employment (Anthony and Liberman, 1986).

When restoring vocational functioning through skills training is limited, rehabilitative efforts focus on environmental and supportive interventions. For example, clients with severe, chronically disabling disorders, such as schizophrenia, may be unable to reestablish specific impaired or lost skills required for a job. Environmental approaches such as supported

Table 4.3 Stages in the Rehabilitation Model of Chronic Mental Disorders

Stage	Pathology	Impairment	Disability	Handicap
Definition	Lesions or abnormalities in the central nervous system caused by agents or processes responsible for the etiology and maintenance of the biobehavioral disorder	Any loss or abnormality of psychological, physiological, or anatomical function (resulting from underlying pathology)	Any restriction or lack (resulting from an impairment) of the ability to perform an activity in the manner or within the range considered normal	A disadvantage for a given individual that limits or prevents the fulfillment of a role that is normal (depending on age, sex, social, cultural factors) for that individual
Example(s)	Brain tumors or infections etiologically linked to psychotic symptoms	Positive or negative symptoms of schizophrenia (delusions, anhedonia)	Deficient social skills	Homelessness; unemployment
Interventions	Laboratory and radiographic tests	Syndromal diagnosis; pharmacotherapy; hospitalization	Functional assessment; skills training, social support	National and state vocational rehabilitation policies; community support programs

Reprinted from Liberman (1986). In the public domain.

employment (SE) in such cases is a viable strategy to support persons with severe disabilities to participate in work roles. SE is an individualized approach to help persons achieve integrated employment. SE services provide training, support, and supervision (e.g., job coaching) to the worker in selecting, obtaining, and maintaining employment (Pratt, et al., 2007). Research related to SE continues to grow, and existing research provides substantial evidence that SE services have achieved significantly better employment-related outcomes than other vocational rehabilitation services (e.g., day treatment programs) (Bond, 2004; Lehman, et al., 2002; Mueser, et al., 2004).

In addition to skills and support strategies, interventions at a societal/systems level are established to remove handicaps faced by persons with chronic mental illness. Examples include key legislations such as the Vocational Rehabilitation Act of 1973, Targeted Job Tax Credit, and the Americans with Disabilities Act, all of which have been instrumental in developing vocational accessibility and opportunities for people with mental illness (Liberman, 1988).

Integration of these approaches to intervention is most often required to bring about an optimal outcome. The emphasis on the types of intervention varies with the nature of the disorder and should be decided on a per client basis. Nevertheless, concepts and strategies from the PsyR model may be an effective complement for rehabilitation professionals to use when treating clients with mental illness.

Social Model of Disability

The social model of disability is a progressive political concept that takes on a unique perspective in defining disability. In contrast to the medical model in which problems related to disability are located within the individual, this model conceptualizes disability as a by-product of societal, social, and environmental barriers. To illustrate this concept, consider the following examples:

- Aisha was discharged from the company because of a rumor that she is HIV-positive. She did not have a functional impairment but was treated as if she did.
- Hector is an experienced assistant manager of a convenience store who has a prominent facial scar. He was passed over for promotion to store manager because the owner believed that customers and vendors would not want to look at this person.
- Paula, who has mild mental retardation, is qualified and hired to work as a bagger at a local grocery store. She is the breadwinner of her family. Although she would like to work full time, she cannot do so because she will lose her supplemental disability benefits.
- Ming, who has a spinal cord injury and uses a wheelchair, cannot return to his former work because the building where he used to work is not wheelchair accessible.

These examples illustrate how disability is not rooted in the disabled person's physical, emotional, sensory, or cognitive impairment but rather in discrimination and social processes created in society. Consideration of these aspects of this model allows the occupational therapy practitioner to further understand the experiences of work disability and look beyond physical factors related to the disability. Application strategies of the social model of disability include barrier removal, education to remove prejudice, and advocacy (Kielhofner, 2004).

Policy directives such as the Americans with Disabilities Act (1990), now in existence for almost two decades, have greatly influenced occupational therapy work-related practice as agents for social change to better protect the worker with disabilities and provide resources in better managing employment (Batavia and Schriner, 2005). Because this model is a relatively new discipline, the theoretical base is still undergoing development. Regardless, the social model of disability offers another important perspective on disability and thus an appropriate model to consider when exercising best-practice occupational therapy in the area of work-related practice.

Scholarship of Practice

Each model discussed previously integrates theory, research, and practice. Although each model differs in level of development in these areas, they all reflect the scholarship of practice. That is, the knowledge base that is generated through research for each of these models directly informs practice, and subsequent questions derived in practice are addressed through scholarship. Thus, development of knowledge under a scholarship of practice tradition should grow out of partnerships among the researchers, practitioners, and clients (Kielhofner, 2005).

Despite the importance of theory and research in occupational therapy practice, current practice is still not strongly grounded in theory, occupation, and evidence. Findings suggest that occupational therapy practitioners are often unable to identify or articulate the occupational therapy theories behind their practice (Elliot, Velde, and Wittman, 2000; Javetz and Katz, 1989). Some studies have identified literature that focuses more on issues of scholarship than on implications for practice as a major barrier to using theory in practice (Kielhofner, 2005). Therefore, the scholarship of practice approach to the development and dissemination of knowledge is one solution to narrowing the gap between research and practice.

> *No single model can be used alone but must be used together to provide a holistic picture of the biological, psychosocial, and environmental circumstances that influence a worker's capacity for employment.*

Chapter Summary

This chapter examined a subset of evidence-based occupational therapy conceptual practice models and related knowledge useful to guide work-related practice. Theoretical knowledge in this practice area is drawn from both in and outside the field of occupational therapy. No single model can be used alone but must be used together to provide a holistic picture of the biological, psychosocial, and environmental circumstances that influence a worker's capacity for employment. Furthermore, these approaches are most effective when combined and most consistent with best-practice occupational therapy.

Case Resolution

Several conceptual practice models were used to guide the assessment and intervention process with Mr. Wallace. Using the MOHO framework, the occupational therapy practitioner evaluated the motivational and emotional state of the client. Mr. Wallace expressed interest in going back to work, but his residual impairments from the stroke negatively affected his sense of competence. The MOHO also helped orient the therapist to his feelings of control loss and fear of failure when returning to work. Related knowledge from the stage theory helped the therapist determine Mr. Wallace's readiness to return to work. His current attitude and motivation level reflected the stage of contemplation, which was characterized by his ambivalence about the matter. Active listening strategies, creating opportunities to further discuss this possibility of return to work, helped Mr. Wallace gain insights about the specific barriers he might encounter when returning to work. Meanwhile, physical capacity issues (e.g., upper extremity weakness, bowel incontinence) were addressed through biomechanical intervention principles. Compensatory strategies such as the use of diapers eliminated his fear of coping with incontinence at work. Continued improvement in the areas of his physical capacity and function in the home helped improve his psychological state. He felt more confident in his abilities and more hopeful about returning to his former worker role.

At this point, aware of Mr. Wallace's improvement in personal causation and commitment to return to work, the occupational therapist performed a job evaluation using the WRI and FCE to better understand his job demands as a foreman. Results indicated that his job is not physically taxing but intellectually demanding. As foreman, he must handle all aspects of onsite personnel management, which requires organizational skills, memory, and problem-solving. At times, but seldom, he is required to assist the laborers in manual activity, which may involve heavy lifting and using tools and require strong grasp and fine dexterity to manipulate objects. Because of his residual upper extremity weakness and slight memory issues, he will not be able to return to his former job at full capacity. Employing an advocacy approach, the occupational therapist negotiated with the employer for several reasonable work environment modifications and adjustments to Mr. Wallace's job requirement so that he could safely resume work. Mr. Wallace is now back at work part time, where his performance is closely monitored by his supervisor and occupational therapist.

References

Anthony, W. A., & Liberman, R. P. (1986). The practice of psychiatric rehabilitation: Historical, conceptual, and research base. *Schizophrenia Bulletin, 12*(4), 542–559.

Ásmundsdóttir, E. E. (2004). The worker role interview: A powerful tool in Icelandic work rehabilitation. *Work, 22*(1), 21–26.

Baker, P., Goodman, G., Ekelman, B., & Bonder, B. (2005). The effectiveness of a comprehensive work hardening program as measured by lifting capacity, pain scales, and depression scores. *Work, 24*(1), 21–31.

Batavia, A. I., & Schriner, K. (2005). The Americans with Disabilities Act as engine of social change: Models of disability and the potential of a civil rights approach. *Policy Studies Journal, 29*(4), 690–702.

Baum, C. M., & Christiansen, C. H. (2005). Person-environment occupational performance: A conceptual model for practice. In C. Christiansen, C. M. Baum, & J. Bass-Haugen (eds.), *Occupational Therapy:*

Enabling Function and Well-Being, 3rd ed. (pp. 243–266). Thorofare, NJ: Slack.

Bedell, G. (2008). Balancing health, work, and daily life: Design and evaluation of a pilot intervention for persons with HIV/AIDS. *Work, 31*(2), 131–144.

Bond, G. R. (2004). Supported employment: Evidence for an evidence-based practice. *Psychiatric Rehabilitation Journal, 27*(4), 345–359.

Braveman, B. (2001). Development of a community-based return to work program for people with AIDS. *Occupational Therapy in Health Care, 12*(3), 113–121.

Braveman, B., Helfrich, C., Kielhofner, G., & Albrecht, G. (2004). The experiences of 12 men with AIDS who attempted to return to work. *Israel Journal of Occupational Therapy, 13,* E69–E83.

Brown, G., Rodger, S., Brown, A., & Roever, C. A. (2005). Comparison of Canadian and Australian paediatric occupational therapy practice: Theory, assessments, and interventions. *Occupational Therapy International, 12*(3), 137–161.

Canadian Association of Occupational Therapists (CAOT). (1997). *Enabling Occupation: An Occupational Therapy Perspective.* Ottawa: CAOT Publications ACE.

CAOT. (2002). *Enabling Occupation: An Occupational Therapy Perspective* (rev. ed.). Ottawa: CAOT Publications ACE.

Chan, C. C. H., & Lee, T. M. C. (1997). Validity of the Canadian Occupational Performance Measure. *Occupational Therapy International, 4*(3), 229–247.

Clarke, C. (2003). Clinical application of the Canadian model of occupational performance in a forensic rehabilitation hostel. *British Journal of Occupational Therapy, 66*(4), 171–174.

Corner, R., Kielhofner, G., & Lin, F. L. (1997). Construct validity of a work environment impact scale. *Work, 9*(1), 21–34.

Corr, S., & Wilmer, S. (2003). Returning to work after a stroke: An important but neglected area. *British Journal of Occupational Therapy, 66*(3), 186–192.

Cup, E. H., Scholte op Reimer, W. J., Thijssen, M. C., & van Kuyk-Minis, M. A. (2003). Reliability and validity of the Canadian Occupational Performance Measure in stroke patients. *Clinical Rehabilitation, 17*(4), 402–409.

Deen, M., Gibson, L., & Strong, J. (2002). A survey of occupational therapy in Australian work practice. *Work, 19*(3), 219–230.

Ekbladh, E., Haglund, L., & Thorell, L. (2004). The Worker Role Interview: Preliminary data on the predictive validity of return to work clients after an insurance medicine investigation. *Journal of Occupational Rehabilitation, 14*(2), 131–141.

Elliott, S. J., Velde, B. P., & Wittman, P. P. (2002). The use of theory in everyday practice: An exploratory study. *Occupational Therapy in Health Care, 16*(1), 45–62.

Farkas, M. D., & Anthony, W. A. (1989). *Psychiatric Rehabilitation Programs: Putting Theory into Practice.* Baltimore: Johns Hopkins University Press.

Forsyth, K., & Kielhofner, G. (2008). Communication and documentation. In G. Kielhofner (ed.), *A Model of Human Occupation: Theory and Application,* 4th ed. (pp. 407–441). Baltimore: Lippincott Williams & Wilkins.

Franche, R., Corbiáere, M., Lee, H., Breslin, F. C., & Hepburn, C. G. (2007). The readiness for return-to-work (RRTW) scale: Development and validation of a self-report staging scale in lose-time claimants with musculoskeletal disorders. *Journal of Occupational Rehabilitation, 17*(3), 450–472.

Gainer, R. D. (2008). History of ergonomics and occupational therapy. *Work, 31*(1), 5–9.

Gibson, L., & Strong, J. (2003). A conceptual framework of functional capacity evaluation for occupational therapy in work rehabilitation. *Australian Journal of Occupational Therapy, 50*(2), 64–71.

Harper, K., Stalker, C. A., & Templeton, G. (2006). The use and validity of the Canadian Occupational Performance Measure in a posttraumatic stress program. *OTJR: Occupation, Participation and Health, 26*(2), 45–55.

Herzberg, G., & Finlayson, M. (2001). Development of occupational therapy in a homeless shelter. *Occupational Therapy in Health Care, 13*(3), 133–147.

Ingvarsson, L., & Theodorsdottir, M. (2004). Vocational rehabilitation at Reykjalundur Rehabilitation Center in Iceland. *Work, 22*(1), 17–19.

Innes, E. (2006). Reliability and validity of functional capacity evaluations: An update. *International Journal of Disability Management Research, 1*(1), 135–148.

Jackson, M., Harkess, J., & Ellis, J. (2004). Reporting patients' work abilities: How the use of standardised work assessments improved clinical practice in Fife. *British Journal of Occupational Therapy, 67*(3), 129–132.

James, A. B. (2003). Biomechanical frame of reference. In E. B. Crepeau, E. S. Cohn, & B. A. Boyt Schell (eds.), *Willard & Spackman's Occupational Therapy,* 10th ed. (pp. 240–242). Philadelphia: Lippincott Williams & Wilkins.

Javetz, R., & Katz, N. (1989). Knowledgeability of theories of occupational therapy practitioners in Israel. *American Journal of Occupational Therapy, 43*(10), 664–675.

Jundt, J., & King, P. M. (1999). Work rehabilitation programs: A 1997 survey. *Work, 12*(2), 139–144.

Karjalainen, K., Malmivaara, A., Mutanen, P., Roine, R., Hurri, H., & Pohjolainen, T. (2004). Mini-intervention for sub-acute low back pain: Two-year follow-up and modifiers of effectiveness. *Spine, 29*(10), 1069–1076.

Keefe, F. J., Lefebvre, J. C., Kerns, R. D., Rosenberg, R., Beaupre, P., Prochaska, J., et al. (2000). Understanding the adoption of arthritis self-management: Stages of changes profiles among arthritis patients. *Pain, 87*(3), 303–313.

Kielhofner, G. (2004). *Conceptual Foundations of Occupational Therapy,* 3rd ed. Philadelphia: F.A. Davis.

Kielhofner, G. (2005). Scholarship and practice: Bridging the divide. *American Journal of Occupational Therapy, 59*(2), 231–239.

Kielhofner, G. (2008). *A Model of Human Occupation: Theory and Application,* 4th ed. Baltimore: Lippincott Williams & Wilkins.

Kielhofner, G. (2009). *Conceptual Foundations of Occupational Therapy,* 4th ed. Philadelphia: F.A. Davis.

Kielhofner, G., Braveman, B., Finlayson, M., Paul-Ward, A., Goldbaum, L., & Goldstein, K. (2004). Outcomes of a vocational program for persons with AIDS. *American Journal of Occupational Therapy, 58*(1), 64–72.

Kielhofner, G., Braveman, B., Fogg, L., & Levin, M. (2008). A controlled study of services to enhance productive participation among persons with AIDS. *American Journal of Occupational Therapy, 62*(1), 36–45.

Krause, N., Dasiner, L., & Neuhauser, F. (1998). Modified work and return to work: A review of the literature. *Journal of Occupational Rehabilitation, 8*(2), 113–139.

Law, M., Baptiste, S., Carswell, A., McColl, M. A., Polatajko, H., & Pollock, N. (1994). *Canadian Occupational Performance Measure,* 2nd ed. Toronto: CAOT Publications ACE.

Lee, S. W., Taylor, R. R., Kielhofner, G., & Fisher, G. (2008). Theory use in practice: A national survey of therapists who use the model of human occupation. *American Journal of Occupational Therapy, 62*(1), 106–117.

Lehman, A. F., Goldberg, R., Dixon, L. B., McNary, S., Postrado, L., Hackman, A., et al. (2002). Improving employment outcomes for persons with several mental illnesses. *Archives of General Psychiatry, 59*(2), 165–172.

Levin, M., Kielhofner, G., Braveman, B., & Fogg, L. (2007). Narrative slope as a predictor of work and other occupational participation. *Scandinavian Journal of Occupational Therapy, 14*(4), 258–264.

Liberman, R. P. (ed.). (1986). Psychiatric rehabilitation. *Schizophrenia Bulletin (Special Edition), 12*(4).

Liberman, R. P. (1988). *Psychiatric Rehabilitation of Chronic Mental Patients.* Washington, DC: American Psychiatric Press.

Lieber, S., Rudy, T., & Boston, J. R. (2000). Effects of body mechanics training on performance of repetitive lifting. *American Journal of Occupational Therapy, 54*(2), 166–175.

Linddahl, I., Norrby, E., & Bellner, A. (2003). Construct validity of the instrument DOA: A dialogue about ability related to work. *Work, 20*(3), 215–224.

Mattingly, C., & Fleming, M. H. (1994). *Clinical Reasoning: Forms of Inquiry in a Therapeutic Practice.* Philadelphia: F.A. Davis.

McColl, M. A., Paterson, M., Davies, D., Doubt, L., & Law, M. (2000). Validity and community utility of the Canadian Occupational Performance Measure. *Canadian Journal of Occupational Therapy, 67*(1), 22–30.

Mentrup, C., Niehaus, A., & Kielhofner G. (1999). Applying the model of human occupation in work-focused rehabilitation: A case illustration. *Work, 12*(1), 79–92.

Michener, S. K. W., Olson, A. L., Humphrey, B. A., Reed, J. E., Stepp, D. R., Sutton, A. M., et al. (2001). Relationship among grip strength, functional outcomes, and work performance following hand trauma. *Work, 16*(3), 209–217.

Mueser, K. T., Clark, R. E., Haines, M., Drake, R. E., McHugo, G. J., Bond, G. R., et al. (2004). The Hartford study of supported employment for persons with severe mental illness. *Journal of Consulting and Clinical Psychology, 72*(3), 479–490.

National Board for Certification in Occupational Therapy (NBCOT). (2004). A practice analysis study of entry-level occupational therapist registered and certified occupational therapy assistant practice. *OTJR, Occupation, Participation and Health, 24*(2), S1-S3.

Norrby, E., & Linddahl, I. (2006). Reliability of the instrument DOA: Dialogue about ability related to work. *Work, 26*(2), 131–140.

Paul-Ward, A., Braveman, B., Kielhofner, G., & Levin, M. (2005). Developing employment services for individuals with HIV/AIDS: Participatory action strategies at work. *Journal of Vocational Rehabilitation, 22*(2), 85–93.

Polatajko, H. J., Townsend, E. A., & Craik, J. (2007). Canadian model of occupational performance and engagement (CMOP-E). In E. A. Townsend and H. J. Polatajko (eds.), *Enabling Occupation II: Advancing an Occupational Therapy Vision of Health, Well-Being, and Justice through Occupation* (p. 23). Ottawa: CAOT Publications ACE.

Pratt, C. W., Gill, K. J., Barrett, N. M., & Roberts, M. M. (2007). *Psychiatric Rehabilitation,* 2nd ed. Burlington, MA: Elsevier Academic Press.

Prochaska, J. O. (1994). Strong and weak principles for progressing from precontemplation to action on the basis of twelve problem behaviors. *Health Psychology, 13*(1), 47–51.

Prochaska, J. O., Redding, C. A., & Evers, K. E. (1997). The transtheoretical model and stages of change. In K. Glanz, F. M. Lewis, & B. K. Timmers (eds.), *Health Behavior and Health Education, Theory Research and Practice,* 2nd ed. (pp. 63–91). San Francisco: Jossey-Bass.

Prochaska, J. O., Velicer, W. F., DiClemente, C. C., & Fava, J. (1988). Measuring process of change: Application to the cessation of smoking. *Journal of Consulting and Clinical Psychology, 56*(4), 520–528.

Radomski, M. V. & Latham C. A. (2007). *Occupational Therapy for Physical Dysfunction,* 6th ed. Baltimore: Lippincott Williams & Wilkins.

Sandqvist, J. L., Gullberg, M. T., Henriksson, C., & Gerdle, B. (2008). Content validity and utility of the Assessment of Work Performance (AWP). *Work, 30*(4), 441–450.

Sandqvist, J. L., Tornquist, K. B., & Henricksson, C. M. (2006). Assessment of work performance (AWP): Development of an instrument. *Work, 26*(4), 379–387.

Scheelar, J. F. (2002). A return to the worker role after injury: Firefighters seriously injured on the job and the decision to return to high-risk work. *Work, 19*(2), 181–184.

Schell, B. A. (2009). Professional reasoning in practice. In E. B. Crepeau, E. S. Cohn, & B. A. Schell (eds.), *Willard & Spackman's Occupational Therapy,* 11th ed. (pp. 314–327). Baltimore: Lippincott Williams & Wilkins.

Schkade, J. K., & McClung, M. (2001). *Occupational Adaptation in Practice: Concepts and Cases.* Thorofare, NJ: Slack.

Sloan, S., Winkler, D., & Callaway, L. (2004). Community integration following severe traumatic brain injury: Outcomes and best practice. *Brain Impairment, 5*(1), 12–29.

Tornebohm, H. (1985). *Reflections on Practice-Oriented Research.* Goteborg, Sweden: University of Goteborg.

Townsend, E. A., & Polatajko, H. J. (2007). *Enabling Occupation II: Advancing an Occupational Therapy Vision for Health, Well-being & Justice through Occupation.* Ottawa: CAOT Publications ACE.

Trombly, C. A., & Radomski, M. V. (2002). *Occupational Therapy for Physical Dysfunction.* Baltimore: Lippincott Williams & Wilkins.

Wikeby, M., Pierre, B. L., & Archenholtz, B. (2006). Occupational therapists' reflection on practice within psychiatry care: A Delphi study. *Scandinavian Journal of Occupational Therapy, 13*(3), 151–159.

Resources

OTworks.Ca

www.caot.ca/default_home.asp?pageid=2398

To obtain more information about the CMOP-E and other work-related resources, visit Canada's resource site for occupational therapists.

Model of Human Occupation Clearinghouse

www.uic.edu/depts/moho/

To obtain more information about the model of human occupation and its related work programs and assessments, visit the Model of Human Occupation Clearinghouse website or consult the most recent edition of the MOHO text: Kielhofner, G (2008). *A Model of Human Occupation: Theory and Application,* 4th ed. Baltimore: Lippincott Williams & Wilkin.

Resources to Learn More About Social Model of Disability

The Social Model of Disability: Europe and the Majority World, C. Barnes and G. Mercer, eds. (Leeds: Disability Press, 2005).

Understanding Disability: From Theory to Practice by M. Oliver (Basingstoke: Macmillan, 1996).

The Social Model of Disability, Wikipedia: The Free Encyclopedia (2001). http://en.wikipedia.org/wiki/Social_model_of_disability.

5 Professional Roles
Occupational Therapist and Occupational Therapy Assistant Collaboration in Work-Related Practice

Arlene Kinney and Debora Oliveira

Key Concepts

The following are key concepts addressed in this chapter:
- The number of occupational therapy assistants has increased greatly over the last century along with the increasing demand for occupational therapy services.
- Effective interaction between the occupational therapist and occupational therapy assistant can lead to collaboration and a professional partnership that results in higher quality occupational therapy intervention.
- Trust and respect, communication, and responsibility and accountability are keystones of effective therapist–assistant partnerships.

Case Introduction

 Ruth is a woman in her late 70s who has battled chronic rheumatoid arthritis for most of her life. The disease disabled and deformed her small frame to the extent that she has to live in a long-term rehabilitation hospital. Surprisingly, Ruth was assigned to a work hardening program following her initial occupational therapy interview. John is a father of five who suffered a low back injury working as a baggage handler for an airline, and Kevin injured his low back lifting a 50-pound box while at work in a manufacturing company. Like many people across America, both John and Kevin have families that depend on them. Ruth, John, and Kevin share the common goal of returning to work. While their conditions and treatment settings differ, the focus of rehabilitation for each of them is on work hardening. While all three clients are similar in terms of diagnostic categories, the roles and relationships of the occupational therapists and the occupational therapy assistants vary in each case. This chapter explores these roles and relationships and how they may vary according to client needs. Both occupational therapists and occupational therapy assistants must be open to variations of duties and scope of patient treatment.

These three cases were selected to highlight the effectiveness and variability of the professional collaboration between occupational therapists and occupational therapy assistants. The cases are used throughout the chapter to highlight the occupational therapy partnership during each stage of intervention and provide the reader with ideas and suggestions for developing a productive occupational therapy practitioner partnership.

In addition, information related to the history of the occupational therapy assistant in the profession, the dynamics of supervision and the supervisory challenges facing this partnership, and the need for the assistant level of practice to continue to secure opportunities in the area of work hardening are presented throughout the chapter.

Introduction

Occupational therapists, at some point in their practice, are likely to have to supervise and collaborate with an occupational therapy assistant. This relationship can be complex and influenced by the expectations of each practitioner, his or her level of prior experience, and how roles are delineated, among other factors. For example, consider the experience of this chapter's author. When she began working as an occupational therapist, she had little knowledge of what an occupational therapy assistant's duties entailed. She had not had any exposure to occupational therapy assistants during her fieldwork experience. In one of her first jobs, she had an eye-opening experience. The director of rehabilitation took her and another occupational therapy practitioner to complete an initial visit with a female patient who had a 20-year history of multiple sclerosis (MS). After introductions were made, the director asked both practitioners about the wheelchair modifications needed for this patient. As a new graduate unfamiliar with MS, she clumsily stumbled through the brainstorming effort, mentioning all the pads and cushions she could think of for each part of the patient's body that came in contact with the wheelchair. She assumed that, at minimum, safety and prevention of ulceration were necessary. The other practitioner's turn proved to be both humbling and enlightening. The practitioner easily mentioned specific adaptations, including brand names and costs, that the author had not considered. The more items she mentioned, the more the author's admiration and embarrassment grew. This second practitioner was an occupational therapy assistant with 10 years of clinical practice under her belt and the department's "expert in wheelchair modification." The author was in awe of her knowledge and learned to never underestimate the value of an assistant.

The director of rehabilitation used a unique strategy to convey the lesson, and it was delivered with the precision of a surgeon's scalpel. Since that time, the experience has served as a reminder of the valuable daily contributions occupational therapy assistants make to patient treatment. The circumstances under which therapist–assistant relationships begin vary greatly, yet the expectation is that it matures into a "partnership" (AOTA, 2006). *Partnership, collaboration,* and *alliance* are terms used throughout the literature to define the relationship between the occupational therapist and the occupational therapy assistant.

The Historical Ascent of the Occupational Therapy Assistant Role

The need for expansion of occupational therapy services has been consistent since the era of the reconstruction aids, which demanded rapid training of personnel (Sladyk and Ryan, 2005). Occupational therapists needed to increase service delivery, which required entrusting the care of patients to personnel who could be trained in providing treatment (Hirama, 1994; Holland-Carr, 2005). Treatment methods in the early years of the profession largely meant crafts and activities that enabled patients to learn a productive skill they could use as a means of employment or to earn a living. During that period, work hardening appeared as a core construct of occupational therapy practice. The possibility of the patient's return to gainful employment appeared as a clear and essential goal for patient treatment in occupational therapy despite the setting of practice.

Occupational therapists were able to entrust patient treatment to personnel with lower levels of education largely because, at the core, they trusted the "occupation" in occupational therapy. The supervising therapist was always in the clinic planning, regulating, and supervising patient engagement, and occupational therapy assistants served an efficient role in providing the activities and occupation-centered treatment that the occupational therapist designed. The trust in delegating treatment was also possible because the therapist could see the occupational outcome—the skill acquisition the patient had experienced and developed (Quiroga, 1995)—as tangible evidence of patient success.

During the latter half of the century, the professional contributions made by occupational therapy assistants was well documented in professional literature (Hirama, 1986; Punwar and Peloquin, 2000; Sladyk and Ryan, 2001). The technical level of practice was mastered, and new educational initiatives emerged, enabling the assistant level of practice to flourish. The timeline that reflects the professional progression of the assistant level can be found in the fourth edition of Ryan's text, *Occupational Therapy Assistant: Principles, Practice Issues and Techniques,* and in the American Occupational Therapy Association (AOTA) archives in Bethesda, Maryland. Some major events in this timeline include:

- 1949—The approval of the first one-year training programs for assistants.
- 1958—The establishment of a grandfather clause.
- 1960—The certification of over 300 assistants with the grandfather clause.
- 1968—Several assistants served in AOTA committees.
- 1973—The career mobility plan enacted by AOTA whereby assistants could become therapists by passage of the certification exam.
- 1975—An award of excellence created for the assistant level.
- 1977—First national certification administered to assistant level.

Since 1977, the assistant level has grown as part of AOTA, and occupational therapy assistants have contributed to the growth of the association and the profession by serving on committees, on the AOTA Board of Directors, in state association leadership, on state regulatory and licensing boards, and by receiving recognition for publications, service provision, and meritorious effort. AOTA recognizes the contributions assistants have made to the profession by enabling advocacy and representative positions in the association. Some of these positions are highlighted in Table 5.1.

> *Since 1977, the assistant level has grown as part of AOTA, and occupational therapy assistants have contributed to the growth of the association and the profession by serving on committees, on the AOTA Board of Directors, in state association leadership, on state regulatory and licensing boards, and by receiving recognition for publications, service provision, and meritorious effort.*

As medical stays diminished and intervention became more acute, the relationship between the supervising therapist and the assistant evolved in response to these contextual demands. Therapists have needed to respond to a multitude of forces demanding attention in the medically acute work environment. The therapist's responsibilities now often encompass administrative, management, and research duties. "Limited time and scheduling conflicts" are just a few of the forces that challenge the supervisory process (Toto and Hill, 2001, pp. 209–212). In response to these pressures, the relationship between therapists and assistants has not gone unscathed; it has been riddled with conflicts in terms of scope of practice.

Historically, the relationship between both professionals was labeled initially as needed and cooperative and later as abrasive and problematic (Hirama, 1994). Challenges to role delineation and the need to develop and document clinical competencies exist at every level of practice. The need for supervision both at the clinical and administrative

Table 5.1 Timeline of the Occupational Therapy Assistant (OTA) in the Occupational Therapy Profession

Year	Event
1949	Approved first-year training program for assistants
1958	First essentials and guidelines established for approved educational program for OTAs
1959	First OTA education program established in Massachusetts
1960	Grandfathered in for certification of over 300 assistants
1967	First OTA meeting held at AOTA conference
1968	OTAs served on several AOTA committees
1973	Career mobility for OTAs enabling them to become occupation therapists by passing certification examination
1977	First national certification examination administered to assistants
1982	Career mobility plan terminated
Ongoing	OTAs recognized for service, publications, serving on boards, and meritorious service

levels does not disappear when the demands of the work environment increase; on the contrary, this is when the supervisory effort is needed most. State professional licensure boards are actively committed to clarify language that can help regulate the supervisory process. Hirama discussed the increased need for supervision in several functions of the assistant level of practice. These issues continue to hold attention and seem to remain unresolved in the national discourse. The value and contributions the assistant level offers the occupational therapy profession has prepared us to face the challenges we are currently experiencing, with the clear understanding that the assistant role not only is needed but also is advantageous for our profession.

The growth of the occupational therapy profession continues to create a demand for assistant-level practitioners. Statistical reports maintained by AOTA indicate that both professional roles have continued to grow during the century. In 1962, there were approximately 5,923 occupational therapists and 761 occupational therapy assistants, a ratio of 7.7:1 (Ryan, 2005). According to Shaun Conway, director of credentialing services for the National Board for Certification of Occupational Therapists, of the more than 180,000 certified occupational therapy practitioners in the United States in 2010, 130,655 were occupational therapists and 54,578 were occupational therapy assistants, a ratio of 2.4:1 (Conway, e-mail message to author, January 6, 2010). This data demonstrates a dramatic increase in the number of professionals at the assistant level. Today, assistants work in a variety of settings, historically with almost 50 percent of them working in skilled nursing facilities. In nursing homes, many assistants find opportunities to become directors of rehabilitation, which is an additional avenue for professional growth. They have also successfully moved into administrative positions as activity directors, business owners, and entrepreneurs. These instances highlight the skills of these practitioners and their leadership in providing services to patients, organizations, and communities. It also begs the profession to question, Who would be responsible for providing these leadership roles and duties if occupational therapy assistants were not available? These roles would definitely be awarded to other professionals. The supervisory process related to the relationship between the therapist and the assistant levels must be clarified and honored for both to succeed and for the profession to continue its advancement.

The Nature of the Occupational Therapist–Occupational Therapy Assistant Supervisory Relationship

The terms *partnership* and *collaboration* (employed by AOTA to describe the relationship between an occupational therapist and an occupational therapy assistant) imply a degree of equality in a relationship that the term *supervision* negates. Supervision acknowledges a chain of command, one in which the supervisee requires the approval of the supervisor. According to the AOTA Standards of Practice (2006), it is incumbent upon the occupational therapist to supervise and approve every aspect of service delivery in occupational therapy. State licensure laws often require that supervision be documented and tend to define minimal specifications of what the supervisory process entails. State statutes vary widely regarding supervisory guidelines for the occupational therapist–occupational therapist assistant relationship (see Table 5.2). For example, Florida state law defines supervision as the "control . . . providing both initial direction . . . and periodic inspection of . . ." (Florida Legislature, 2010). Supervision implies that the occupational therapist must ensure the occupational therapy assistant is competent in each technique, intervention strategy, and service delivery issue and has ultimately approved these interventions.

The method in which competency is established may vary by setting. *Competency* means the ability to effectively perform a specific skill set and implement it in practice. Competency and supervision imply oversight and training. Supervision in occupational therapy practice entails establishing competency measures for the assistant, yet it also entails responsibility and accountability by both the supervisor and the supervisee. In accordance with professional ethics, once competency is established, an honor code is assumed in which the supervisee will continue to perform as deemed competent. This is a paramount assumption in which the occupational therapy assistant transitions from a purely supervisory relationship to a partnership and collaborative relationship with the supervising therapist. Once initial competence is established, the assistant has demonstrated the ability and skills to be entrusted and responsible with their duties. Assistants often have exceeded the initial competency requirements and developed mastery and excellence in practice. A skilled, competent assistant is an excellent asset yet can also become a professional liability if not supervised properly. This is where oversight becomes an important element in the professional relationship. A competent assistant seeks oversight of his or her practice to ensure reliability and validity of service. Oversight goes beyond the initial training and mastery of skills and beyond basic supervision of productivity. Oversight ensures professional development, including clinical reasoning, ethical, and professional development.

Ultimately, the responsibility for service delivery and supervision remains with the occupational therapist (in accordance with AOTA and state practice laws) whose chief responsibility is to oversee service. The amount and type of supervision can vary with the years of experience and the skills and competencies of the occupational therapy assistant. As suggested earlier, *partnership* and *collaboration* may imply that there is equality in the relationship, yet this can only be acquired through respect and knowledge (Schoen, 2006). The supervising therapist must have a keen understanding of the assistant's competencies, must respect the assistant as a person of integrity, and must know the assistant can be relied on to follow through with directions. Respect and knowledge are earned through the process of supervision. As both partners come to understand their knowledge base, the therapist–assistant relationship evolves from a purely supervisory one into a partnership and a true collaboration. Both partners have a clear understanding of their duties and responsibilities. Both partners trust each other in advancing the profession through service provision and professional credibility and integrity.

Table 5.2 Comparison of Three States and Practice Acts Guiding Supervision

State	Practice Acts
Florida	Supervision means responsible oversight and control, with the licensed occupational therapist providing both initial direction in developing a plan of treatment and periodic inspection of the plan implementation.
	Such plan of treatment shall not be altered by the supervised individual without prior consultation with, and the approval of, the supervising occupational therapist. The supervising occupational therapist need not always be physically present or on the premises when the assistant is performing services; however, except in cases of emergency, supervision shall require the availability of the supervising occupational therapist for consultation with and direction of the supervised individual.
Illinois	A certified occupational therapy assistant shall practice only under the supervision of a registered occupational therapist. Supervision is a process in which two or more persons participate in a joint effort to establish, maintain, and elevate a level of performance and shall include the following criteria:
	(1) To maintain high standards of practice based on professional principles, supervision shall connote the physical presence of the supervisors and the assistant at regularly scheduled supervision sessions.
	(2) Supervision shall be provided in varying patterns as determined by the demands of the areas of patient/client service and the competency of the individual assistant. Such supervision shall be structured according to the assistant's qualifications, position, level of preparation, depth of experience, and the environment within which he/she functions.
	(3) The supervisors shall be responsible for the standard of work performed by the assistant and shall have knowledge of the patients/clients and the problems being discussed.
	(4) A minimum guideline of formal supervision is as follows:
	(A) The occupational therapy assistant who has less than one year of work experience or who is entering new practice environments or developing new skills shall receive a minimum of 5% on-site face-to-face supervision from a registered occupational therapist per month. On-site supervision consists of direct, face-to-face collaboration in which the supervisor must be on the premises. The remaining work hours must be supervised.
	(B) The occupational therapy assistant with more than one year of experience in his/her current practice shall have a minimum of 5% direct supervision from a registered occupational therapist per month. The 5% direct supervision shall consist of 2% direct, face-to-face collaboration. The remaining supervision shall be a combination of telephone or electronic communication or face-to-face consultation.
	(C) Record Keeping. It is the responsibility of the occupational therapy assistant to maintain on file at the job site signed documentation reflecting supervision activities. This supervision documentation shall contain the following: date of supervision, means of communication, information discussed, and the outcomes of the interaction. Both the supervising occupational therapist and the occupational therapy assistant must sign each entry.
Michigan	No relevant regulations.

Florida Legislature, 2010; Illinois Occupational Therapy Practice Act, 2005; State of Michigan, 2010.

> *As both partners come to understand their knowledge base, the therapist–assistant relationship evolves from a purely supervisory one into a partnership and a true collaboration.*

Dynamics of the Supervisory Relationship

All partnerships and collaborative efforts are bound by intrapersonal and interpersonal dynamics. Intrapersonal issues of self-esteem, self-confidence, temperament, values, beliefs, and attitudes can influence the nature of the supervisory relationship. Interpersonal issues related to communication styles, ability to relate to authority figures and subordinates, work ethics, and expectations all affect the relationship. AOTA defines the parameters of the occupational therapist–occupational therapy assistant relationships with three key points: "trust and respect, communication, and responsibility and accountability" (Campbell, 1998, pp. 135–136). Partnerships defined by dyadic interactions pose additional threats and complexities, so both parties must be aware of their interpersonal styles and needs and how these impact the partnership. Dyadic relationships are at most risk for generating complex emotions because of their potential for intimacy or lack thereof.

Partners need to explore how trust and respect, communication, and responsibility and accountability are evidenced in their supervisory relationship. Even more important, they must explore how their interpersonal styles and dynamics are expressed in the work relationship in order to build an effective partnership. Preestablished expectations held by the supervising therapist and the assistant regarding role delineation and responsibilities may affect the partnership. Take, for example, a situation in which an entry-level therapist with a master's degree is partnered to work with and supervise an expert-level assistant. In this situation, the assistant may perceive the newly graduated therapist as a threat to his or her achieved level of seniority and expertise; the newly graduated therapist may perceive the experienced assistant as intimidating because of his or her clinical experience or, conversely, as a subordinate at his or her beck and call. Specific role delineation responsibilities and duties are necessary to ensure proper guidelines of supervision are followed in clinical practice. Any interpersonal dynamic that emerges, other than the full collaborative clinical partnership, hinders the advancement of the profession altogether.

At any level, the therapist–assistant relationship is likely to be productive when the patient is at the center of the work agenda. When both practitioners can place the interpersonal and intrapersonal issues aside and focus on the patient, the relationship may evolve into a productive one. The work agenda should always remain occupation based and focused on client-centered practice and research. To the degree that both professionals are focused on this outcome, occupational therapy as a profession advances. It is ultimately the therapist's responsibility, as the supervising partner, to manage the nature and focus of the relationship. An assistant who is focused on developing occupational-based treatment interventions and seeking supervision proactively provides a positive sign that the partnership is a professional and productive one (Fig. 5.1).

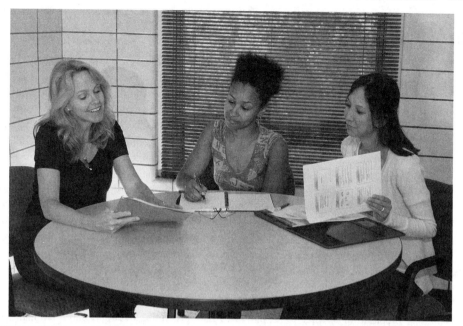

Figure 5.1 Occupational therapists and occupational therapy assistants develop partnerships through demonstration of trust and respect, communication, and responsibility and accountability.

Occupational Therapist–Occupational Therapy Assistant Relationship in Work Hardening

In 1985, AOTA published the "Guidelines for Work Hardening," which defined the domain and the process for this area of practice (Fenton and Gagnon, 2003). The occupational therapist–occupational therapy assistant role delineation outlined in the work hardening guidelines echoes the wording found in the current occupational therapy official documents (Schoen, 2006). The following section of this chapter describes occupational therapist–occupational therapy assistant role delineation in work hardening in an attempt to shed light on this professional relationship. While work hardening is utilized as a specific example, parallel delineations exist in other areas of work-related services. Case examples are employed to analyze the fundamental elements that can foster the collaborative work between these two professionals at each stage of intervention. It is important to note that while the three case studies discussed occur in different treatment settings, all address the same therapeutic goal of return to work. As we have seen in other chapters, work hardening is defined through the therapeutic goal of return to work and can be offered in many settings. In a demographic study conducted by Wyrick, Niemeyer, Ellexson, Jacobs, and Taylor (1991), work hardening programs were found as a service affiliated with practice settings across the health-care continuum, from acute-care hospitals to private practice. Work hardening seems to transcend specific clinical settings to be defined by clients' needs and treatment goals. Occupational therapists easily recognize the importance of work hardening as a key occupational area of function for independence.

Role Delineation

Both occupational therapists and occupational therapy assistants are responsible for upholding occupational therapy values and principles, legal and ethical standards, and philosophical foundations of the profession. The standard makes a clear distinction about supervision: the occupational therapist supervises and is responsible for the implementation and monitoring of all aspects of occupational therapy practice. The occupational therapy assistant requires a supervisor at all levels of clinical practice and in all settings where they practice clinically. The assistant is responsible for implementation of treatment as agreed to by the supervising therapist. An occupational therapy assistant must show distinct professional skills in order to move through discrete levels of supervision. Yet many facilities do not have policies to define how assistants progress through these levels of supervision. The vague language defining levels of supervision may cause confusion about role boundaries and overall misinterpretations of occupational therapist–occupational therapy assistant roles across facilities and areas of practice.

At present, no specialty certification exists for work hardening. Evidence demonstrates that while work hardening has become highly specialized, "the majority of practicing work hardening therapists did not obtain their knowledge through academic preparation" (King, 1992, p. 849). Many practicing occupational therapists are attracted to work hardening in part because it represents the basic values of the profession: work- and occupation-centered practice. There is a realistic link between the injured worker's functional capacity and the realistic simulation of tasks, which mandates the required use and implementation of activity analysis (King, 1992). Yet occupational therapy practitioners may acquire specialty certifications for methodologies and treatments used in work hardening. For example, physical agent modalities and ergonomics certifications are just two of a wide variety of skill sets required of an occupational therapy practitioner in a work hardening setting. The occupational therapy assistant is qualified to gain these certifications in accordance with and following state regulations. Most of the skills needed to perform competently in work hardening, however, can be acquired through experience and on-the-job training. Many of the skills are integrated into fundamental learning in the occupational therapy academic curriculum, including activity analysis, kinesiology, muscle testing, energy conservation techniques, and work simplification. Despite the academic preparation and qualifications of the assistant for work hardening, King's 1991 study profiled 251 therapists in work hardening of which only one was an assistant and 99 percent were therapists. Little has changed since King conducted this work.

Screening, Evaluation, and Reevaluation

The assessment and evaluation process involves multiple issues that the occupational therapist is best qualified to address. The work hardening evaluation represents a person-environment-occupation model and requires the therapist to establish measures for all three domains. These domains applied to the current *Occupational Therapy Practice Framework: Domain and Process* reflect the client's occupational skills, context, patterns, and activity analysis (AOTA, 2008a). The therapist must complete a thorough evaluation of all client factors; measures of all occupational skill levels including cognitive, neuromuscular-skeletal, emotional, perceptual, and sensory; and an evaluation of the client's values, beliefs, and attitudes related to work (AOTA, 2008b). The therapist must also evaluate and assess the work environment, including an "on-site evaluation when necessary to develop a breakdown of job tasks and critical job demands" (AOTA, 1986, p. 842). Finally, the therapist must complete an activity analysis of the specific job and modifications that would enable the client to perform the task with greater proficiency. This three-part assessment and evaluation of the client's person-environment-activity requires critical thinking and clinical reasoning. An occupational therapist is best suited to complete such an inclusive and thorough evaluation. According to the AOTA Standards of Practice, an occupational therapy assistant can prove competency in administering standardized assessment instruments and would greatly benefit the work agenda by assuming some evaluation duties.

We return now to discussion of Ruth, John, and Kevin, who were introduced at the beginning of the chapter.

Ruth: Long-Term Rehabilitation Focused on Work Hardening

Ruth, a retired 78-year-old Jewish mother and grandmother, was stricken with rheumatoid arthritis in her 20s. Now in her senescence, she was barely able to straighten two fingers because the systemic disease had deformed her small, frail body. The only physical description for this lively woman, full of hutzpah, was that of a human knot. She sat in her wheelchair unable to accommodate any part of her body into postural alignment due to the contractures in all her joints.

After the initial introductions and determining that "nothing really worked," she was asked to voice her occupational goal: "What would you like to do that you can't?" Without hesitation, Ruth answered, "I want a job!"

"Let's try that again. You're retired, you've worked your entire life, now let's do something for fun: a craft? a hobby?" the occupational therapist asked, hoping that Ruth would respond to the reality orientation offered. "Lady, you asked, and that's my answer. I want a job; if it's the last thing I do in the world, I want to be working!" Those words resonated in the therapist's head because they were the least expected reply. There was a moment of silent contemplation as the therapist considered dozens of ethical questions, and finally she considered the look in Ruth's eyes. Was her goal realistic? Was it possible? Ruth's spunk, her attitude, her heart, and her spirit of human dignity that refused to be broken settled on the therapist. She thought, *Who am I to question that spirit and that willpower?* "Okay, you've got it. That will be your goal; we will see how far we can get to find you a job." The deal was sealed with a handshake even as the therapist questioned her ability to help Ruth accomplish this goal. The occupational therapy assistant looked at the therapist with eyes that questioned her response.

As the formal evaluation proceeded, the range of motion assessment proved taxing for Ruth because each joint could barely be moved and could not reach a functional range. The occupational therapy assistant helped document the ranges as they moved cautiously through the upper extremities. She was assigned to complete a standardized pegboard and manual dexterity test. The findings were reported, and an analysis of the results was developed. Both practitioners worked as a team, critically inspecting the data in terms of functional potential. For example, Ruth would need an electric wheelchair for mobility, but what modifications would be required for her to manage it independently? These and other questions were anticipated with the evaluation results.

John: Outpatient Workers' Compensation

John, a 34-year-old Alaskan Native, was working as a baggage handler when he injured his back lifting a deceptively heavy package from a small plane. John was the sole provider for his family and living in the small community of Nome, Alaska, a town on the edge of the Bering Sea where life is harsh and expensive. John's paycheck provided for basic living expenses, and he performed subsistence activities such as hunting caribou, gathering berries, and fishing to make ends meet.

His employer assisted him in submitting a workers' compensation claim, and John immediately went to the community's only hospital. The physician who evaluated John concluded that he had sprained muscles in his lower back, and no additional tests were ordered. He was instructed to stop work and rest until he felt able to return to work. John followed the doctor's instructions, using only over-the-counter medication for pain relief. After 2 weeks, he was still in severe pain. When John returned to the hospital, an MRI was ordered, which identified a herniation in his lower back between the fourth and fifth lumbar disks. John continued to be seen regularly by his physician, who prescribed pain medication, and he received periodic treatment by a physical therapist.

Three months later, John was sent to Anchorage for additional medical treatment because he was still experiencing back pain and unable to work. He was seen at a clinic that specialized in spinal injuries. Extensive testing was performed, and it was determined that he would benefit from the clinic's work hardening program. John agreed to complete a 6-week program because he was eager to return to work and a normal family life.

John was flown 539 miles from Nome to Anchorage and put up in a hotel where he was to reside for the 6 weeks of his program. On the first day of the program, the occupational therapist performed an initial evaluation and targeted areas that needed improvement. John, the occupational therapist, and the occupational therapy assistant discussed his evaluation together so that the team was in agreement on the assessment and goals. The assistant explained the details of the program to John, stressing the importance of his attendance and how communication among everyone was vital to achieve the best outcome. John needed to know that he could approach her or the occupational therapist about anything so that modifications could be made for optimal participation.

Kevin: Outpatient Workers' Compensation

Kevin was a 38-year-old employee at a large manufacturing company in the Northeast. He injured himself at work lifting a 50-pound box. He complained of low back pain and was diagnosed with lower lumbar pain. He had been out of work for 3 months and was referred to occupational therapy for a work capacity evaluation and work hardening.

The occupational therapist and occupational therapy assistant both greeted Kevin when he arrived at the outpatient clinic. He first had a musculoskeletal examination by the physical therapist and then began his work capacity evaluation. The occupational therapist went over the critical demands of his job as listed in his job description. A physical capacity evaluation was initiated.

The occupational therapy assistant was responsible for explaining how to rate his pain and had him assess his status after each activity. The occupational therapist continued the assessment until Kevin's capabilities and limitations were established. The physical therapist, occupational therapist, and occupational therapy assistant all met to discuss Kevin's plan of care, and the assistant was assigned to monitor his work hardening program. She briefed Kevin on the expectations for a work hardening program and worked with him on a schedule. She also informed him that the occupational therapist would be sending a weekly report to his workers' compensation provider regarding his progress in the program. She stressed the importance of compliance with the program.

It is evident in all three cases that the assistant was delegated duties by the therapist that facilitated the team effort and continuity of patient care. During the evaluation and assessment phase, the occupational therapy assistant may complete standardized assessments as proven competent and can educate the patient and family about the treatment process. The assistant can also document findings and initiate the therapeutic alliance so that patient care is viewed as a team effort. All three cases demonstrate how the assistant can assume different roles and duties as assigned by the supervisor.

Intervention and Intervention Planning

The key function in the occupational therapy assistant's job description is to implement treatment as directed by the occupational therapist. It is incumbent upon the occupational therapist to establish an outline of the treatment plan according to occupational therapy principles and professional clinical judgment and expertise. It is fundamental to the function of the team that each member maintain open communication to understand the degree of expertise each professional offers. Each practitioner has levels of expertise founded in education and accrued over years of clinical practice. The recognition that each partner has varying degrees of competency and expertise in in his or her area establishes the foundation of respect, a key element in a productive relationship.

It is during intervention planning that the occupational therapist–occupational therapy assistant alliance ideally cements to form a truly collaborative partnership. Each professional offers his or her repertoire of skills, knowledge, and experience with the singular purpose of planning an intervention that best serves the patient. Over time, this planning session lays the groundwork for professional development, mutual respect, and creative collaboration.

> *It is during intervention planning that the occupational therapist–occupational therapy assistant alliance ideally cements to form a truly collaborative partnership. Each professional offers his or her repertoire of skills, knowledge, and experience with the singular purpose of planning an intervention that best serves the patient.*

When the occupational therapist shares the evaluation results and identifies the patient's goals and how each goal should be addressed, both members of the partnership can begin to formulate an array of possible treatment activities. Some specific treatment issues are easily identified, especially those within the preparatory level of the treatment continuum. Identifying purposeful and occupation-based activities requires more critical analysis and brainstorming reflecting the uniqueness in each patient's case. Yet what a delight to brainstorm within the occupational therapist–occupational therapy assistant relationship, as two professionals share their perspectives and ideas to develop customized activities.

The occupational therapist has to manage the treatment plan, the timing of activities, the degree of complexity of these activities, the introduction of adaptive equipment, the management of resources, and the discharge. Ultimately, the guardianship of the profession has the supervising therapist's signature. The occupational therapy assistant becomes the right hand in the therapy process, allowing the occupational therapist to move safely into other responsibilities as the implementation is carried through. The therapist entrusts the assistant with his or her patient for safekeeping and care. The ability to perform these duties is foundational to the development of trust, respect, and accountability in the professional relationship. Both the occupational therapist and the occupational therapy assistant must communicate what they are critically thinking and clinically reasoning in regard to patient care. When this communication is open, honest, and nonjudgmental, effective planning and use of resources can be promoted, problems anticipated and prevented, duplication of service avoided, and affiliations cemented.

Types of interventions used for the development of a work hardening treatment plan (AOTA, 2008a) include preparatory methods such as physical agent modalities, splints, pain management, and physical body conditioning through exercise, to name a few. Purposeful activities may include circuit training and work simulation, energy conservation, ergonomics, job analysis for restoration of specific performance skills, and work simulations. Occupation-centered activities may include work hardening, education for stress management, determining reasonable accommodations to work site, job coaching, and transitional work development. An occupational therapy assistant can complete many of these treatment interventions after demonstrating competency and when supervised by an occupational therapist.

Intervention Planning With Ruth: Long-Term Rehabilitation

During the occupational therapist–occupational therapy assistant treatment planning meeting, which included Ruth, reality would set in. The assistant listened patiently as the therapist presented Ruth's case, summarized her evaluation results, and discussed her goals. Ruth's return-to-work goal seemed lofty, but the occupational therapist advocated for the patient. She suggested referral to a sheltered workshop, training in the use of an electric wheelchair, and mastery of a graded one-step task, all with environmental accommodations within Ruth's reach. The therapist's arguments were just enough to convince the occupational therapy assistant to join the effort in Ruth's journey. As they sat down to discuss the details and explore possible problems, solutions, and activities, the partnership began to reveal itself. Their mutual focus, motivation, and effort formed a synergy that fueled the creative process of intervention planning. This positive energy was felt by all, including Ruth.

Ruth started arriving for therapy punctually every afternoon. She completed all simple, one-step, repetitive tasks with the diligence and pride anticipated of a person with such high work ethics. The occupational therapy assistant developed a multitude of tasks for Ruth to complete. Whether it was drying cups and spoons or separating sheets of papers into three different colored stacks or adding numbers on a calculator, no task was small for Ruth's pincer grasp (her most functional skill). The occupational therapy assistant developed a sign-in page so that Ruth could be held accountable for punctuality and attendance, just as in a real work environment.

Learning how to drive the electric wheelchair posed a problem because Ruth had never before driven. Ruth was extremely resistant, and the occupational therapy assistant asked the occupational therapist for help with this important goal. The first day that Ruth finally sat in the wheelchair, she required little instruction to master the task, and then she took off like the roadrunner. With time, other patients began calling her the unit "mayor" because she was the unofficial ruler of her kingdom. She knew everyone, she ran daily errands to the gift shop, she policed the halls and alerted patients of incoming visitors— she grew wings.

Ruth's treatment continued with increases in her endurance for task completion, fatigue management, adaptive strategies lessons, and joint protection. Slowly she felt she was returning to work, reconnecting to her valuable role and occupations.

The occupational therapy assistant developed many of these work tasks, but when questions about the patient's functional ability to complete the task arose, she consulted the occupational therapist. Developing work samples for such a disabled patient proved challenging, yet working together, it felt more like a tag team, brainstorming ideas and arriving at solutions in order to enable patient function. Often, the therapist or assistant would arrive in the morning with a good idea for Ruth, yet what seemed like a good idea needed to be refined and adapted to match her skill level. The patient usually arrived at the clinic asking, "What do you have for me to do today?" and would leave saying, "I did it!"

Intervention Planning With John: Outpatient Workers' Compensation

John began the 6-week program with 4 hours in the clinic. The occupational therapist had given the occupational therapy assistant detailed instructions, and they collaborated on a daily program for John. The activities were initially light cardiovascular exercise, stretching, core stabilization exercises, body mechanic drills, aquatic therapy, and relaxation techniques. The assistant instructed John on all of the activities and monitored him at all times. When John began his 6 weeks, there were six other participants who were at various stages of the program. It was important that the occupational therapy assistant maintain good group dynamics and keep each patient in his or her own individual exercise regime.

The occupational therapist, occupational therapy assistant, and John met weekly to discuss his progression and any concerns. On numerous occasions, John said that he was slightly depressed because he did not have his family close to him for support. The therapist and assistant worked together with the airline John had worked for to obtain free tickets for his wife to come visit him for a few days during the program. This greatly improved John's general mood and attitude. (Today, computer technology enables families to communicate through webcamming and online virtual social networks, so family separation may be less of an issue.)

Throughout the remaining program, John's hours of participation increased to 6 hours a day and then finally to 8 hours for the final 2 weeks of treatment. The occupational therapy assistant worked closely with John to help re-create different tasks of his job, and the job description obtained by the occupational therapist provided additional information. Lifting drills were progressed as tolerated with emphasis on good body mechanics. The LIDO WorkSET was used to increase John's grip strength.

John maintained good attendance throughout the program. He was a little shy and did not always initiate conversations even when he was experiencing problems. The occupational therapy assistant and the occupational therapist realized that part of this hesitancy was not uncommon among Alaskan Natives and often initiated dialogue. This cultural issue was respected and understood by both practitioners. John had some exacerbations of his back pain occasionally, and a TENS unit was used with good results. The occupational therapist agreed that this would be a good modality for pain relief and, after the approval of John's attending physician, had the assistant order one for John to have permanently. The occupational therapy assistant's concern for the patient's mood during task completion alerted them to the need to address family involvement, which eventually moved the patient's treatment in a positive direction. This keen observation, developed through the therapeutic alliance, served the patient's care and also enhanced the professional respect within the therapist–assistant relationship.

Intervention Planning With Kevin: Outpatient Workers' Compensation

Kevin began his work hardening program as scheduled. He was seen four times a week for 4 hours each visit. The occupational therapy assistant initiated a walking, standing, and mild lifting program outlined by the occupational therapist. She provided modeling for proper body mechanics and simple pain-relief methods, such as stretching and heat.

At first, Kevin rated his pain as a 10 on a scale of 1 to 10 every time he began a new activity. The occupational therapy assistant told him he needed to go to the emergency room when he was a 10, and he quickly reduced the pain number to an 8. She also noted any inconsistencies in Kevin's performance. She reported to the occupational therapist on a daily basis, and they noted that the inconsistencies were adding up.

The occupational therapist and the occupational therapy assistant were concerned that Kevin was magnifying his symptoms. The assistant determined that his exaggerated response to any activity was not due to any secondary gain but to fear of increasing his pain. He had a bad experience during the acute phase of his injury and was very concerned about reinjuring himself. It became critical that the assistant develop a trusting relationship with Kevin so that he could progress through the program without fear. The initial plan was altered so that the assistant could incorporate activities into the program that Kevin enjoyed, such as woodworking, which she adapted to increase his standing tolerance. In a short time, Kevin no longer exaggerated his pain and began to coach the other clients in work hardening on how to fill out the pain form.

In summary, the occupational therapy assistant's forte is in treatment implementation. A well-developed and discussed treatment plan enables any competent assistant to follow the plan, develop and create treatment options when needed, and identify the need for changes. In the case studies presented, the assistant's observations and clinical reasoning helped develop treatment activities and work samples and alerted the team to the need for changes of pace in the treatment focus. The therapist's oversight of the treatment process supports or clarifies the assistant's clinical impressions. As these instances prove effective for patient outcome, the professional relationship between both practitioners is secured. As both practitioners plan the treatment and support each other during the implementation phase, the relationship grows stronger. When treatment planning becomes a collaborative effort, the assistant's understanding of clinical issues increases, which enables focused observations and stronger reasoning for treatment implementation (Fig. 5.2). As the assistant demonstrates the ability to clinically reason treatment and its impact on overall patient care and outcomes, the therapist is free to assume more administrative and managerial duties.

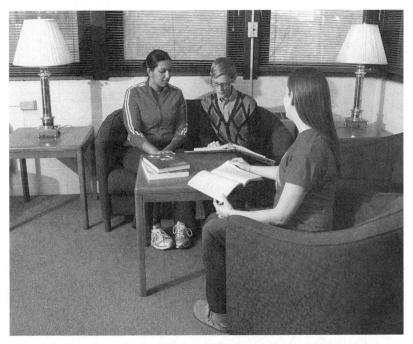

Figure 5.2 Occupational therapy assistants play an integral role in identifying options for planning and implementing occupational therapy intervention.

Intervention Outcomes

Determining when to stop treatment is closely scrutinized by payers such as insurance companies and by providers, especially in medical model settings. Some patients may be seen by occupational therapy for extended periods of time, and others may be followed by occupational therapy intermittently for several years because of their degree of lifestyle maladjustment and high-risk behaviors. An occupational therapist has to weigh both ethical and legal issues and operate within the realistic parameters of patient benefits. Return-to-work treatment may entail advocacy issues because the patient may require additional time for adjustment to the worksite or additional accommodations that the employer may refuse to grant. The therapist may need to advocate for continued rehabilitation supports or network with state and local agencies in order to successfully reintegrate the patient into the work environment.

Outcomes With Ruth: Long-Term Rehabilitation

Ruth's first visit to the sheltered workshop proved to be productive; several tasks had potential for her workstation. After a lengthy discussion, the team settled on packaging poker chips into boxes. A small setup enabled the chips to fall into Ruth's desktop, where she could easily position them into the colored sequence inside the box for closing. The occupational therapy assistant quickly understood what was required and stepped in to demonstrate to the vocational team how to adapt the environment so that the patient could easily master the task. As Ruth assembled her first box of poker chips, a great smile overtook her face; she was hired. It was agreed that after the last visit to the workshop, discharge was in order.

Approximately 2 years later, Ruth's daughter informed the team of Ruth's death. She noted how often Ruth mentioned the therapists who gave her the ability to work and remain productive until her dying days. She wanted the team to know that Ruth always said that, even in a hospital and ridden with her disabling illness, she still had found a life worth living.

Outcomes With John: Outpatient Workers' Compensation

Upon completion of his work hardening program, John underwent standardized testing performed by the occupational therapist. After evaluating all of the information using the Blankenship system, the occupational therapist recommended that John could return to work at a job requiring medium to heavy strength. This recommendation, along with a comparison to the job analysis, supported the conclusion that continued employment at the airline would be possible. John's attending physician received these results and agreed that John could return to his job.

Outcomes With Kevin: Outpatient Workers' Compensation

After an 8-week work hardening program, Kevin returned to work part time. The occupational therapy assistant went to his workplace to ensure he was using the lifting techniques outlined in his program. He stated his back still flared up to a 4 on the pain scale, but he was able to do his work and looked forward to returning to full time. The therapeutic relationship that the assistant had developed with the client was evident in his willingness to work toward his goals. The teamwork demonstrated by the physical therapist, occupational therapist, and the occupational therapy assistant allowed Kevin to progress to return to work and take control of his pain.

In each case, the occupational therapy assistant proved a valuable asset for termination of treatment and transition into the workplace. Assistants can recommend and develop task-environment modifications, they can complete worksite inspections, and they can support the achievement of patient goals. In addition, the depth of the relationship with the patient requires therapeutic use of self to enable a positive transition as the patient completes treatment. The assistant is trained to use self therapeutically to enable a positive termination process.

Chapter Summary

The number of occupational therapy assistants has grown dramatically over the last century, as has the demand for occupational therapy intervention. Occupational therapy assistants have become an integral part of the occupational therapy profession and have adopted roles as leaders, administrators, managers, and business owners. In addition to these key roles, occupational therapy assistants continue to play a critical role in the provision of occupational therapy services.

While the occupational therapist has clear responsibility for oversight of intervention and supervision of the occupational therapy assistant, an effective partnership and true collaboration can be developed through trust and respect, communication, and responsibility and accountability. Occupational therapy assistants contribute to the occupational therapy process, including intervention planning, intervention, and occupational therapy outcomes.

Case Resolution

 Patients like Ruth, John, and Kevin demonstrate a team effort to return a person to meaningful employment. The occupational therapist and the occupational therapy assistant in these instances were an integral part of the treatment plan and its implementation. Ruth was not ignored in the client-centered approach and was happy at the end of her life because she was engaged in productive work. John, motivated to return to gainful employment for his family's sake, was understood and respected by his therapists. Kevin, fearful of pain and therapists in general, developed a trusting relationship with the occupational therapy assistant, which allowed him to take advantage of a program that enabled him to return to work.

Both the occupational therapist and the occupational therapy assistant worked together to continually assess the status of the client and to develop strategies to achieve the clients' goals. The therapist valued the observations and recommendations of the assistant, and the assistant reported concerns to the therapist to further the therapeutic process.

Ruth, John, and Kevin all benefited from the collaborative effort of the occupational therapist–occupational therapy assistant team. The skills and knowledge of both professionals were an important component of the delivery of services, client intervention and progress, and overall treatment outcome.

References

American Occupational Therapy Association (AOTA). (1986). Work hardening guidelines. *American Journal of Occupational Therapy, 40*(12), 841–843.

American Occupational Therapy Association (AOTA). (2006). Guidelines for supervision, roles and responsibilities during the delivery of occupational therapy services. In W. Schoen (ed.), *Reference Manual of the Official Documents of the American Occupational Therapy Association, Inc.*, 11th ed. (pp. 173–179). Rockville, MD: AOTA Press.

American Occupational Therapy Association (AOTA). (2008a). Occupational therapy practice framework: Domain and process, 2nd ed. *American Journal of Occupational Therapy, 62*, 625–683.

American Occupational Therapy Association (AOTA). (2008b). OT services in work rehabilitation. Retrieved from www.aota.org/Practitioners/PracticeAreas/Work/Fact-Sheets/35205.aspx.

Campbell, K. (1998). Forging OTA-OT partnerships that work. In T. Black & K. Eberhardt (eds.), *The Occupational Therapy Assistant Resources for Practice and Education* (pp. 135–136). Bethesda, MD: AOTA Press.

Fenton, S., & Gagnon, P. (2003). Work activities. In E. Blesedell-Crepeau, E. Cohn, & B. Schell (eds.), *Willard and Spackman's Occupational Therapy,* 10th ed. (pp. 342–346). Philadelphia: Lippincott Williams & Wilkins.

Florida Legislature. (2010). Regulation of Professions and Occupations. Title XXXII, Chapter 468.201–225. Retrieved from http://leg.state.fl.us/statutes.

Hirama, H. (1986). *Occupational Therapy Assistant: A Primer,* rev. ed. Baltimore: Chess Publications.

Hirama, H. (1994). Should certified occupational therapy assistant provide occupational therapy services independently? *American Journal of Occupational Therapy, 48*(9), 840–843.

Holland-Carr, S. (2005). The occupational therapy assistant heritage: Proud and dynamic. In K. Sladyk & S. Ryan (eds.), *Ryan's Occupational Therapy Assistant: Principles, Practice Issues, and Techniques,* 4th ed. (pp. 14–23). Thorofare, NJ: Slack.

Illinois Occupational Therapy Practice Act. (2005). 2005 Illinois Code, Chapter 225 Professions and Occupations 225 ILCS 75. Retrieved from http://law.justia.com/codes/illinois/2005/chapter24/1314.html.

King, P. (1992). Profiling the work hardening therapist: Education and experience. *American Journal of Occupational Therapy, 46*(9), 487–489.

Punwar, A., & Peloquin, S. (2000). *Occupational Therapy Principles and Practice,* 3rd ed. Philadelphia: Lippincott Williams & Wilkins.

Schoen, W. (2006), *Reference Manual of the Official Documents of the American Occupational Therapy Association, Inc,* 11th ed. Bethesda, MD: AOTA Press.

Sladyk, K., & Ryan, S. (eds.). (2005). *Ryan's Occupational Therapy Assistant: Principles, Practice Issues and Techniques,* 4th ed. Thorofare, NJ: Slack.

State of Michigan. (2010). Occupational therapist and occupational therapy assistant required state licenses. Retrieved from www.michigan.gov/statelicensesearch/0,1607,7-180-24786_24826-81550—,00.html.

Toto, P., & Hill, D. (2001) Successful OT-OTA partnerships: Staying afloat in an ea of ethical challenges. In T. Black & K. Eberhardt (eds.), *The Occupational Therapy Assistant Resources for Practice and Education* (pp. 209–212). Bethesda, MD: AOTA Press.

Wyrick, J., Niemeyer, L. O., Ellexson, M., Jacobs, K., & Taylor, S. (1991). Occupational therapy work-hardening programs: A demographic study. *American Journal of Occupational Therapy, 45*(2), 109–112.

Quiroga, V. (1995). *Occupational Therapy: The First 30 Years 1900–1930.* Bethesda, MD: AOTA Press.

Resources

Guidelines for Supervision, Roles, and Responsibilities During the Delivery of Occupational Therapy Services

http://www.aota.org/Practitioners/Official/Guidelines/36202.aspx

This document is available for AOTA members on the AOTA website and contains four sections that direct the delivery of occupational therapy services: General Supervision, Supervision of Occupational Therapists and Occupational Therapy Assistants, Roles and Responsibilities of Occupational Therapists and Occupational Therapy Assistants During the Delivery of Occupational Therapy Services, and Supervision of Occupational Therapy Aides.

OTA Leadership Development Toolkit

http://www.aota.org/Practitioners/Resources/OTAs/OTA-Leadership.aspx

Resources for professional development for the occupational therapy assistant developed by the American Occupational Therapy Association.

An Overview of Occupational Therapy Work-Related Service Settings and Populations

Chapters 6 through 10 provide an introduction and overview of some of the most common populations and settings in which occupational therapy work-related services occur. Chapter 6 focuses on work-related services for persons with developmental delay and provides an introduction to *supported employment,* which is also discussed in other chapters of the text in relationship to other consumer populations. Chapter 7 continues some themes presented in Chapter 6 but specifically addresses occupational therapy work-related services provided under the Individuals with Disabilities Education Act (IDEA) in school systems and transition services provided to persons 18 to 21 years of age. Chapters 8 and 9 review relevant issues and approaches to working with older adults and with people with mental health concerns. Some persons who desire to enter or return to work may not achieve that aim, and others may need safe and secure opportunities to develop work skills or explore their capacity to work; Chapter 10 discusses how occupational therapy practitioners may use volunteer and leisure activities in therapeutic intervention.

6

Supported and Alternative Employment
Developmental Disabilities and Work

Ricardo C. Carrasco, Susan Skees Hermes, and Betsy B. Burgos

Key Concepts

The following are key concepts addressed in this chapter:

- History and evolution of work intervention with individuals with developmental disabilities leading to state-of-the-art intervention practices.
- Theoretical frameworks that facilitate practice for work programs in developmental disabilities.
- Resources for developing and evaluating best practices with children, adolescents, and adults with developmental disabilities.
- Key issues faced by occupational therapy managers and practitioners.
- Impact of technology in work development and participation.
- Current, best, and evolving practices in the area of work for persons with developmental disabilities.

Case Introduction

Joey and Benjie have been friends for a while, attending a special education school in an urban area in the Philippines. Fortunately, their families can afford the tuition required for them to attend a private school for people with developmental disabilities. Unfortunately, others like them in the community, but without the same resources, stay home each day, and family members take turns supervising them in their daily routines.

Today, just as on other days, the two young men sat awkwardly at their school desks, obviously too small for their 18-year-old frames, and joined others from ages 3 to 21 for the morning circle song. Needless to say, Joey and Benjie looked out of place in the classroom and did not feel very motivated. After the song, they ate their morning snack at the desks, which seemed to get smaller each time they moved. Snack time was followed by the day's lessons, a dip in the pool during physical education class, and lunch served by the school cafeteria. Occasionally, if severe behavior problems arose in the classroom, the school psychologist supported the special education teachers with behavior-management techniques. At the end of the day, their chauffeurs picked them up, and the two rejoined their respective families.

Day after day, they went through the same routine of "academic programs" but without preparation for the world of work. Joey, Benjie, and their classmates followed the same routine they had been performing for most of their lives until the school hired an occupational therapist as a program director. The occupational therapist collaborated with the staff in expanding the existing shop program into a sheltered workshop. The goal was to provide training and supported employment for students who were old enough and who possessed sufficient physical, cognitive, and psychosocial abilities to participate. The school consulted with the Cultural Center of the Philippines' paper-making expert, who taught the shop, and an art teacher to learn how to make paper from natural fibers, such as pampas grass, which was abundant around the school property (Fig. 6.1). Equipped with inexpensive mold and deckles; safe, natural chemicals; a steam press; and their new-learned skills, the teachers converted a section of

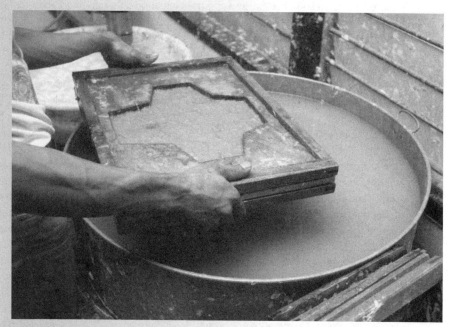

Figure 6.1 Papermaking at a Filipino sheltered workshop. An individual lifts a mold and deckle to trap the processed natural fibers from the slurry that will dry to become a handmade paper envelope.

the woodworking and art shop for the project. The teachers then selected appropriate "workers" and oriented them to how they would spend most of their school day at "work." The workers learned about how they would be required to go shopping as a group for materials, work together to make papers and other products, and then sell the goods they produced. This was in 1979.

Today, the sheltered workshop continues to make handmade organic stationery, note cards, and envelopes, accepting orders from local area businesses. The students receive pay equivalent to their hard but fun and productive work. On-the-job training through the independent living skills program now also includes training for office, restaurant, commercial kitchen, janitorial, laundry, car wash, supermarket, and post office work. Educational services at the center continue for children 4 to 14 years of age, with the option to continue the independent living skills program and learning to earn money on their own.

Evolution of Work Intervention for Individuals With Developmental Disabilities: From Need and Legislation to State-of-the-Art Intervention Practices

Sheltered Workshop vs. Supported Employment and Related Nomenclature, Legislation Brief, and History

Controversy over the care of people with developmental disabilities and intellectual challenges has existed for over a century (Wysocki and Neulicht, 2004), and early founders of the occupational therapy profession, such as George Barton, William Rush Dunton, and Eleanor Clarke Slagle, addressed this issue by promoting appreciation for the therapeutic value of work intervention (described in Chapter 1). Key legislative acts in the

United States and other countries support occupational therapy work interventions (described in Chapters 1, 16, and 17). Today's occupational therapy practitioners identify work as an area of specialized practice, and an appreciable body of work, defensible conceptual frameworks, and consistent terminology are developing in the area of developmental disabilities work intervention in particular.

Work interventions in occupational therapy date back to curative and leisure groups among the mentally ill and the return-to-work programs for wounded World War I soldiers through some form of "occupational therapy" pioneered by Eleanor Clarke Slagle, then a social worker. Through their personal and professional experiences, George Barton and William Rush Dunton laid the foundation for using occupation in retraining and adjustment toward re-employment (Quiroga, 1995). After contracting tuberculosis and experiencing a cerebrovascular accident, Barton established Consolation House in New York as a vocational entity and community-based workshop for the ill and disabled. Dunton spearheaded occupational therapy interventions for psychiatric patients, insisting on workday planning that promoted the development and maintenance of work habits. Around the same time, the Civilian Vocational Rehabilitation Act (Smith-Fess Act of 1920, Pub.L. 66-236) defined rehabilitation to mean returning to gainful employment after disability. The series of enactments before and after this act paved the way for vocational rehabilitation services in schools, industry, and commercial establishments and, as necessary, in private homes on an individual basis. The contributions of people like Barton, Dunton, and Sagle together with legislative support offered occupational therapists opportunities to engage in what was then called prevocational programming in sheltered and curative workshops (Jacobs, 1992).

Current Approaches to Supported Employment

From work skills training to supported employment, transitional jobs, and supported jobs, occupational therapy practitioners can apply their expertise in different types of work interventions for individuals with developmental disabilities. Current approaches to supported employment include the following:

- Supported employment at sheltered workshops (commonly called community rehabilitation facilities) involves skills training and work adjustment with the goal of paid work in the community. The training is usually for routine and low-paying work. Supported employment in sheltered workshops has been severely criticized because of its limited carryover. For example, rates of transition to sustained independent employment were found to be very low after 2 years (Bellamy, Rhodes, Bourbeau, and Mank, 1986).
- Individual placement of a worker by a training or rehabilitation agency refers to competitive employment accompanied by one-on-one support from a job coach for the duration of the employment at the facility. Training and negotiation for employment usually precede the placement.
- Enclaves are groups of no more than eight persons with severe disabilities under the supervision of a full-time supervisor. Work in enclaves is usually integrated in an industrial or corporate setting.
- Mobile work crews involve contracted work by groups of as many as eight workers who travel to worksites in the community under the supervision of a full-time supervisor.
- Entrepreneurial business employment is work in private enterprises that serve as subcontractors or prime manufacturers. These businesses employ groups of no more than eight supported workers for the additional purpose of integrating supported workers with persons without disabilities.
- Transitional employment is paid work for integrated businesses or industries on a part-time and temporary basis while the worker continues to receive other support or training services.

- Supported jobs integrate supported employees into a job site, although wages are below minimum; the pay scale is usually based on productivity, and workers receive continuous training and advocacy from a support coach.

Work Skills: Development Across the Life Span

Infants become adults, and infant play evolves into adult work and leisure skills. Early in life, infants learn about their bodies as they relate to both human and nonhuman environments, and the brain creates neuronal models of how that body becomes the tool for navigating space, managing materials, interacting with other humans, and participating in purposeful activities in different contexts and cultures (Fig. 6.2). Developmental play and relationships create work-related themes through repetition, leading to positive work concepts and attitudes. Through their active imagination and natural curiosity, preschoolers role-play novel, pretend, and routine home chores. Children of school age learn through intensified academic expectations to attend to and persist at tasks to satisfactory completion. Their participation in group activities such as team sports promotes the ability to be a good sport and to be a contributing member with other peers (Fig. 6.3).

> *Developmental play and relationships create work-related themes through repetition, leading to positive work concepts and attitudes.*

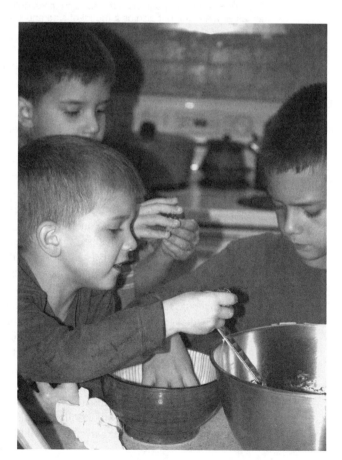

Figure 6.2 Children learn work skills through engagement in daily living activities.

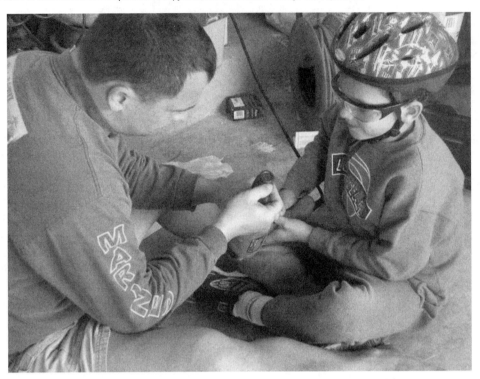

Figure 6.3 A school-age child learns about assembly work and safety from his father who serves as a mentor, but also as a model of safe and skilled work behavior.

Adolescents tackle their first jobs and model work behaviors from the adults in their life, both at home and in the community, but also start exploring possibilities for future careers. If the young adult leaves home to go to college, serious consideration and action for work preparation occurs, sometimes coupled with the opportunity to develop a lifetime partnership. In other cases, the young adult dives directly into the world of work because of family business ties, natural gifts or talents, employment opportunities, or financial necessity.

Adulthood comes with increased emphasis on productivity and opportunities for career advancement but can also give rise to serious work transitions such as unemployment, illness, and other challenges. As individuals reach retirement age, they decide how to continue productivity and pursue leisure activities through continued employment or volunteer opportunities in the community.

This typical development happens naturally, almost like a choreographed dance between nature and nurture. However, this is not the case for persons with developmental disabilities. Persons with developmental disabilities face physical, cognitive, emotional, and social challenges that present obstacles to smoothly developing work skills for independence. Because of these challenges, individuals with developmental disabilities follow a different trajectory that is mostly dictated by the context of home, school, and related services they receive. Their development is commonly tracked in the following stages: (1) early intervention and school from birth to 21 years, (2) work and family period from 22 to 64 years, and (3) retirement at 65 years and older (Florida Developmental Disabilities Planning Council, 2005). Occupational therapy practitioners play an important role in providing opportunities during these life stages and in developing the necessary skills for play and work opportunities as well as educating families about the possibilities, albeit realistically limited in comparison to typical, for the evolving worker with developmental disabilities.

Prevocational and Work Opportunities in and After School in Developmental Disabilities

The evolution of legislation for the education of individuals with disabilities goes beyond academic outcomes and inclusion in school settings: in particular, the 2004 revision of the Individuals with Disabilities Education Act (IDEA) provides for transition planning. However, the role of occupational therapy in life skills training has been viewed as limited by special education and behavioral specialists at middle and high school levels, in part because the role of occupational therapy in schools has historically been an accountability model for educationally relevant but not vocationally relevant services. This is an area where occupational therapy practitioners can reclaim a vital role in work development in the schools.

But what happens after age 21? In the United States, over 40 percent of individuals with disabilities, ages 18 to 64, who are capable of working if provided some type of accommodations, are unemployed (Dick and Golshani, 2008). This represents more than 9 million people. The most common cause for this situation is lack of adequate academic preparation and training to pursue possible positions. In the past, a contributing factor was the lack of accessible educational programs for competitive professions. However, advancements in technology and an increase in the number of specialized organizations have improved services to many people.

Since the 1973 Section 504 of the Vocational Education Act and the 1990 Americans with Disabilities Act (ADA) were approved, they have supported vocational education and training for adults with developmental disabilities (Luftig and Muthert, 2005). The Office of Special Education and Rehabilitative Services (OSERS) awarded grants to 47 states to develop employment programs that facilitate the transition from the educational setting to the working environment (transition services are described in depth in Chapter 7). In addition, OSERS created informational tools for consumers and businesses that can help them select the best working choices and prepare companies to employ people with disabilities. These efforts have resulted in increased employment of persons with disabilities over the past 20 years (Migliore, Mank, Grossi, and Rogan, 2007).

Among the many programs available today, great importance is given to vocational rehabilitation programs funded by the federal government with matching funding from the states. Created in 1920 with the approval of the Smith-Fess Act, these programs were the first federally authorized programs to facilitate the employment needs of persons with disabilities (Cassell, Mulkey, and Grubbs, 2005). According to public records, in 2008, close to 1 million individuals with disabilities sought assistance from vocational rehabilitation programs (American RehabACTion, 2010). Due to increased demand in recent years, many vocational programs have even been forced to develop waiting lists for people who apply for these services.

Other programs and organizations that educate and advocate for the workforce development of individuals with disabilities include the National Council on Independent Living (NCIL), the Institute for a Competitive Workforce (ICW), and the American Association of People with Disabilities (AAPD). These programs and organizations also support sheltered workshops and supported employment settings and facilitate the transition of individuals into community-based employment by considering their work skills, interests, and attitudes (Schmidt and Smith, 2007).

Unfortunately, as previously noted, the nationwide unemployment rate for individuals with disabilities is noticeably higher than that of the typical population despite the increased development of supported and vocational employment programs. There is also a considerable discrepancy between the earnings of persons with disabilities and of the general and other minority populations (Schmidt and Smith, 2007). Some federal agencies that might assist individuals with these situations are listed in Table 6.1.

Table 6.1 Federal Resources on Employment of Individuals With Developmental Disabilities

Resource	Website	Description
Access Board	www.access-board.gov	The Access Board is an independent federal agency devoted to accessibility for people with disabilities. It operates with approximately 30 staff members and a governing board of representatives from federal departments and public members appointed by the president. Key responsibilities of the board include developing and maintaining accessibility requirements for the physical environment, transit vehicles, telecommunications equipment, electronic and information technology; technical assistance and training on these guidelines and standards; and enforcing accessibility standards for federally funded facilities.
DisabilityInfo.gov	www.disabilityinfo.gov	DisabilityInfo.gov is the result of a collaborative effort across multiple federal agencies in conjunction with the president's New Freedom Initiative. It contains information on civil rights, education, employment, housing, health care, technology, and transportation, among other subjects. The website is a one-stop source of government information relevant to people with disabilities, their families, employers, and service providers. Employers can specifically learn about sources for job candidates with disabilities at www.earnworks.com and about tax credits to offset the cost of accommodations, assistive technologies, and more at www.irs.gov/formspubs/article/0,,id=96151,00.html.
EmployABILITY	www.employ-ability.org	EmployABILITY is a California government program to create career empowerment for persons with disabilities.
Social Security Administration, Ticket-to-Work Program	www.yourtickettowork.com	Ticket-to-Work is a nationwide initiative administered by the Social Security Administration designed to increase job training and employment choices for individuals with disabilities. Employers that offer (or arrange for) job training, vocational rehabilitation (VR), support, retention or other types of job-related services, and assistance for individuals with disabilities can become Employment Networks and are eligible for compensation for services. Employers can directly provide or arrange for appropriate employment services, including job readiness, placement, VR, training and support, or retention services for individuals with disabilities.
Office of Special Education and Rehabilitative Services (OSERS)	www.ed.gov/about/offices/list/osers	OSERS is committed to improving results and outcomes for people with disabilities of all ages. OSERS provides a wide array of supports to parents and individuals, school districts, and states in three main areas: special education, vocational rehabilitation, and research
U.S. Department of Homeland Security (DHS)	www.ready.gov	The Department of Homeland Security hosts the Ready Business website, which features the Plan to Stay in Business, a series of emergency planning guidelines for employees. The site, accessible at www.ready.gov/business/plan, offers guidance for addressing the needs of people with disabilities in emergency planning, evacuation, and recovery.

Table 6.1 Federal Resources on Employment of Individuals With Developmental Disabilities—cont'd

Resource	Website	Description
U.S. Department of Justice, Americans with Disabilities Act (ADA) home page	www.usdoj.gov/crt/ ada/adahom1.htm	This Department of Justice website provides information and technical assistance on the ADA, which prohibits discrimination and ensures equal opportunity for persons with disabilities in employment, state and local government services, public accommodations, commercial facilities, and transportation.
U.S. Department of Labor, Office of Disability Employment Policy (ODEP)	www.dol.gov/odep	ODEP provides national leadership to increase employment opportunities for adults and youths with disabilities while striving to eliminate barriers to employment. Employers can find examples of best practices and guidance on how to account for the needs of people with disabilities in the workplace, including their safe evacuation from the workplace during emergencies.
U.S. Equal Employment Opportunity Commission (EEOC)	www.eeoc.gov	EEOC enforces Title I and Title V of the ADA, prohibiting employment discrimination on the basis of disability in the private sector and state and local governments. In 2002 and 2003, the EEOC conducted a series of ADA workshops for small businesses. These workshops included information on tax incentives and community resources.
U.S. Small Business Administration (SBA)	www.sba.gov	The SBA's ADA page (www.sba.gov/ada) supports the ADA, which guarantees equal opportunity for individuals with disabilities in public accommodations, employment, transportation, state and local government services, and telecommunications. SBA also has published a 15-page illustrated guide, *ADA Guide for Small Businesses*, available at www.sba.gov/ada/smbusgd.html (HTML) or www.sba.gov/ada/smbusgd.pdf (PDF), that presents an overview of some basic ADA requirements for small businesses that provide goods and services to the public. It offers guidance on how to make services accessible and how tax credits and deductions may be used to offset costs incurred in accommodations. In addition, the SBA has launched Business.gov at www.business.gov, a resource to help businesses navigate government rules and regulations and get access to information on the employment of people with disabilities.
Workforce Recruitment Program	www.dol.gov/odep/ programs/workforc.htm	Coordinated by the U.S. Department of Labor and the U.S. Department of Defense, the Workforce Recruitment Program provides summer work experience, and in some cases full-time employment, for students with disabilities. The program develops partnerships with other federal agencies and businesses. Each year, recruiters develop a database of approximately 1,500 qualified students that employers can use to recruit interns.

Adapted from U.S. Department of Education, 2007.

Work Opportunities for Aging Individuals With Developmental Disabilities

As with the general population, the life span and productive performance of people with developmental disabilities has increased significantly over the past decades (Boyd, 1997; Jacobsen and Wilhite, 1999). The National Center for Birth Defects and

Developmental Disabilities (NCBDDD; www.cdc.gov/ncbddd/index.html) reports that all 50 U.S. states as well as the District of Columbia, Guam, Puerto Rico, and the Virgin Islands, have been developing health surveillance initiatives for people with disabilities since 2003. These efforts allow individuals with disabilities to remain healthy and to live in private residences within their community. It also shows positive trends toward health initiatives empowering independent living opportunities and more probable connections with familial employment and community resources as clients get older. Individuals with developmental disabilities who continue to reside with their parents may face relocating to a retirement community with their aging parents. Resources for supported employment may be limited in senior living communities, but opportunities for informal supervision and encouragement in limited-demand employment settings (e.g., retail or discount store as greeter or stock staff) close to their parents and their retired friends may exist.

Advances in health care have contributed to improved physical health for individuals with developmental disabilities, yet factors such as lack of health insurance, limited use of the health-care system, and higher rates of chronic conditions (e.g., diabetes, depression, elevated blood pressure and cholesterol, obesity, tooth loss, vision and hearing impairments) are noted in adults with disabilities. These factors combined with diminished opportunities for social participation (e.g., regular education classrooms, high school completion, employment, community-organized or employee-sponsored health and social events) and decreased adherence to recommended health behaviors (e.g., cardiovascular, strengthening, and flexibility activities; smoking cessation) impact quality of life as adults with developmental disabilities get older.

Despite supportive national and state policies, a nonrandomized study indicated that integrated employment continues to be out of reach for at least 24 percent of adults with intellectual or developmental disabilities, and this population continues to be served in facility-based programs (Migliore, et al., 2007). As funding sources shift and paid employment options shrink, the role of occupational therapy in assisting aging clients to participate in meaningful work roles requires broad application of occupational performance across the life span. However, even when adults with developmental disabilities are willing to seek employment, they are less likely than the general population to be employed. As a result, they tend to utilize income support programs or depend on family support more than other groups because, employed or not, their incomes are generally the poverty level (Schmidt and Smith, 2007; Yamiki and Fujiura, 2002).

Older individuals who are employed or involved in volunteer activities may experience cognitive and physical declines that can negatively affect their activities. Occupational therapy practitioners and other team members are challenged to collaborate on the design of intervention strategies to improve their occupation performance (Larson and Ellexson, 2005). Possible areas of intervention include environmental adaptation, identification of job coach, adaptation of work-related tasks, establishment of a social connection or support group, and ergonomic changes.

Carving a Niche for Work Participation by Individuals With Developmental Disabilities: Management and Practice Issues

Academically driven projects have for many years provided grant-funded or pro bono occupational therapy consulting services and intervention in sheltered workshops and various employment settings for individuals of all ages with developmental disabilities. The paradigm shift away from more traditional psychosocial services created new opportunities for occupational therapy practitioners to serve adults with developmental disabilities in employment venues. With the move in 2007 to graduate-level entry to the occupational therapy profession, these opportunities may continue to increase. As rising numbers of practitioners with master's degrees and doctorates enter practice, administrative positions, community-based programs, research programs, and grant-funded initiatives may flourish. Positions not necessarily identified with occupational therapy but that require academic or clinical experience in the work world may also offer avenues of employment for occupational therapy professionals. For example, consider the following case of an adult day training program in Central Florida, where the potential is high for an occupational therapy practitioner to work in program design, ergonomics, wellness, behavior regulation, and sensory processing.

A Day in the Life of an Individual Participating in an Adult Day Training Program

Felipe wakes up to the sound of his alarm clock in a group residential facility in downtown Orlando, Florida. He is surprisingly cheerful today. His work supervisor at the nonprofit agency told him they have a new contract to assemble goody bags for a local theme park. Happily and mindfully, albeit slowly, Felipe showers, shaves, and dresses for work with minimal supervision from the residential manager and aide. He eats breakfast with his seven roommates. A few of his roommates will attend a therapeutic arts program at the agency today. The rest will join Felipe and about 100 other individuals with various developmental disabilities, all between ages 21 and 65, at workstations, where they will stuff cloth bags with items to be given away at the theme park. The seven roommates pile into the van and head off to the "factory," as they affectionately call their workplace. When they arrive, they greet coworkers, friends, and staff. After a few instructions, they head to their assigned places at tables and, under the supervision of several staff, proceed with their work.

The setting looks like a mini-factory: each table is lined with chairs with adequate distance between workers for them to complete their tasks but close enough that they can pass finished bags to the next person in the assembly line. The workstation configuration also allows maximum visual supervision by the staff to assure quality of work.

Before long, it is lunchtime, and shortly afterwards, it is time to go home. This is a typical day for Felipe and the other individuals with developmental disabilities at this Central Florida adult day training center. Their contractual work varies. They sometimes assemble screws and other hardware into distribution packets, for example, or prepare promotional giveaways for a local drug store. In some cases, workers are divided into groups of three: one stuffs a bag with product, another weighs it for accuracy, and the third staples and places the bag into distribution boxes.

At the end of the pay period, each individual receives his or her pay according to work performed or hours worked based on Department of Labor guidelines. Other training and supported activities in the agency include enclaves, each with eight workers and a supervisor; at a local mall, the enclaves provide janitorial services or sell popcorn or collect tickets at the movie theater.

Not everybody has the opportunities that Felipe and his peers have at the adult day training center. As previously mentioned, this population faces high unemployment rates and sustained employment challenges. Many individuals with disabilities are willing to work but have limited social and work skills. And even though many employers may indicate the willingness to hire individuals with disabilities, communication issues often arise because the multiple public and private agencies providing resources can be overwhelming for the employer. In response to this issue, the Consortium for Employment Success (CES) model has been proposed to provide a single point of contact and coordinate services and communication for and from client and employer.

CES is a venue through which occupational therapy practitioners can utilize evidence-based best practice to support individuals with developmental disabilities in acquiring prevocational skills, engaging actively in acquiring work skills, and succeeding with transitional and supported employment to reach the goal of performing their work role with ultimate satisfaction. Occupational therapy practitioners are guided by the Occupational Therapy Practice Framework (OTPF) and AOTA's Centennial Vision. While it is not the taxonomy, theory, or model of occupational therapy, the OTPF guides occupational therapy practitioners in combining knowledge with evidence related to current and emerging occupations and occupational therapy practice (AOTA, 2008). Combined with the direction provided by AOTA's Centennial Vision for a practice that is diverse, global, evidence based, and powerful, the OTPF can empower occupational therapy practitioners to be on the forefront as change agents in creating opportunities for sustained employment for individuals with developmental disabilities.

Preprofessional and continuing education in work intervention for developmental disabilities is essential for best practice, but current offerings leave a lot to be desired. Likewise, job openings for occupational therapy positions in work intervention in developmental disabilities are very few. Within the occupational therapy literature and resources, however, many opportunities currently exist to participate in electronic updates through public and private agencies, such as the Virginia Commonwealth University Research and Training Center on Workplace Support and Job Retention, the Premier Source for Developmental Disabilities News, and the U.S. Department of Health and Human Services Administration on Developmental Disabilities (www.acf.hhs.gov/programs/add) as well as state-level councils on developmental disabilities (www.worksupport.com/training) and Disability Scoop (www.disabilityscoop.com).

Need for Literature and Research on Occupational Therapy Evidence-Based Interventions Across the Life Span

The expectation that interventions be evidence based has changed the health-care environment in the past decades, resulting in more effective clinical decision-making. Becoming informed about the best available evidence is crucial in selecting assessments and developing interventions for consumers in all health-care areas. This same expectation applies to occupational therapy practitioners who serve individuals with developmental disabilities. Such practitioners must be able explain why they recommend services and substantiate their clinical decisions. Evidence-based information is expected on both ends of the intervention spectrum, from referral to discharge and all the steps in between—all decisions must be informed and justifiable. Evidence must be relevant to the individual's chronological and/or developmental age, condition, family situation, and environment. Detailed information might include successful interventions, research outcomes, and effective technologies or services. Based on client information, the level of evidence (see Table 6.2) is determined and categorized according to its reliability (Cutting, 2008).

A wide array of literature is available from professional databases (e.g., MEDLINE [Medical Literature Analysis and Retrieval System Online], CINAHL [Cumulative Index to Nursing and Allied Health Literature], PubMed, OTDBase, OTSeeker), journals, and other publications. Clinicians also can obtain information about evidence-based practice from their professional association resource websites. Despite the increasing use of evidence-based practice in the area of rehabilitation, there is still a lack of research in work intervention with individuals with developmental disabilities, especially at levels 1 and 2 (Chronister, Torkelson, Chan, Rosenthal, and da Silva, 2008).

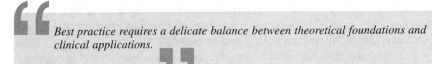

Best practice requires a delicate balance between theoretical foundations and clinical applications.

Table 6.2 Hierarchy of Evidence

Level 1	Strong evidence from at least one systematic review of multiple, well-designed randomized controlled trials
Level 2	Strong evidence from at least one properly designed, randomized, controlled trial of appropriate size
Level 3	Evidence from well-designed trials without randomization, single group pre-post, cohort, time series, or matched-case-controlled studies
Level 4	Evidence from well-designed nonexperimental studies from more than one center or research group
Level 5	Evidence from opinions of respected authorities, based on clinical evidence, descriptive studies, or reports of expert committees

Impact of Technology in Work Development and Participation

Jacob is a 27-year-old with congenital nystagmus and optical atrophy. He has limited central vision with peripheral blindness. Jacob works at a local manufacturing company as a computer applications specialist. He lives by himself in a downtown apartment and enjoys his job and social life with friends and family. Jacob's success is well earned. With the help of occupational therapy and other professionals, he learned daily living skills, job preparedness, how to use assistive technology, and how to advocate for himself.

While in middle school, Jacob was evaluated by an occupational therapist who recommended the use of assistive technology equipment (e.g., screen readers) to help Jacob use computers. He was introduced to the Internet with the help of JAWS for Windows (a screen-reading program that uses synthesized speech and can also output information in Braille) and enlarged key labels on the keyboard. During his last year of high school and first year of college, an adaptive technology specialist, who was an occupational therapist, helped Jacob learn how to use learning management systems (platforms for online classes), library databases, and electronic books. He was also trained in daily living skills and adaptive equipment for his home to promote independent living.

In some of the jobs Jacob had after graduating from college, his employers did not provide him with the equipment required to complete his job responsibilities, or they assigned him clerical duties that were unrelated to his academic preparation. Most of these situations occurred because the employers lacked knowledge about hiring people with disabilities. With the help of a job coach and his previous occupational therapist, Jacob learned to advocate for the minimal equipment necessary to complete his work. He also affiliated with governmental organizations that provided information about policies and rights of people with disabilities in the workforce.

Today Jacob volunteers at sheltered workshops, vocational schools, and training centers to help other people with disabilities accomplish what he did. He also participates at local assistive technology expositions, demonstrating the use of accessibility equipment for homes and computer access, trying to make an impact on other people's lives.

Before the 1990s, the services that enabled Jacob's progression through high school and college to gainful employment and independent living were unavailable to people with disabilities because there were no government support systems to address their specific needs. The passage of the ADA in 1990 raised a formal consciousness among Americans about the rights of the individuals with disabilities. The ADA was the first legal document that mandated equal opportunity in public places, employment, transportation, state and local government locations, and telecommunications (Hotchkiss,

2003). With the September 2008 amendments, the ADA now creates more demands on the public and especially on employers to meet the needs of people with disabilities.

In 1998, President Clinton signed the Workforce Investment Act, which includes Section 508 of the Rehabilitation Act Amendments mandating that when federal agencies create or use any type of electronic and information technology, they should guarantee access of the information to individuals with disabilities (Seale, 2006; U.S. Department of Labor, 1998). This section also includes access to public information from federal agencies, and failure to meet the standards can have legal consequences. In other parts of the world, similar laws are being passed.

New technologies impact the lives of many people with disabilities. Examples of new interfaces that increase access to information and services and enhance communication and interaction include eye gaze devices, switches, remote controls, integrated keyboards, adaptive software (word prediction, video conferencing with text captioning, enhanced optical character recognition, and speech-synthesis tools that read computer displays aloud or convert speech to text). In addition, government and educational organizations are working on a variety of new technologies to enhance the abilities of many individuals. For example, several universities teamed in 2008 to develop the DHH Cyber-Community in STEM project to advance students who are deaf or hard of hearing (DHH) in science, technology, engineering, and math (STEM) using technologies such as remote interpreters and captioners and multimedia classroom platforms (Aycinena, 2008). New technologies continue to improve the education, play, leisure, work, and activities of daily living experiences of persons with disabilities, helping them to be more productive participants in the community.

Technologies can change across the life span of individuals with developmental disabilities, but some of the tools selected in their childhood or adolescent years will continue to be useful in their adult life (Post, Hartmann, Gitlow, and Rakoski, 2008). For example, communications tools (e.g., computer keyboards and interface devices, augmentative communication devices) and EADLs (electronic aids to daily living to operate automatic door openers, TV, radios, etc.) might vary in design and sophistication as technology advances, but their functions remain the same (Fig. 6.4). Other tools, such as for activities of daily living (e.g., universal cuff, adaptive utensils and cups) and writing (e.g., pencil grips, mouth sticks) will likely not change.

The acquisition of technological devices will depend on the physical and cognitive needs of the individual. It will also depend on the individual's community and work involvement, which may dictate the types of accommodations needed. Computers, cell phones, and associated software are some of the technologies that may be adapted to meet a variety of visual, audio, and organizational needs. Computer software is available to assist individuals with planning (checklists, shopping lists, contacts lists), identifying coins and paper currencies, and word processing (e.g., Write Out Loud, IntelliTalk combined with word prediction software, e.g., WorkQ, EZ Keys for Windows). Portable assistant devices (e.g., Alpha Smart, PDAs, Blackberries) also facilitate communication and planning.

Virtual reality environments are also part of the new technology used with people with disabilities to improve life and work skills (Fig. 6.5). Simulated environments can assist to improve cognitive and social skills that can later be transferred to the real world. For example, studies conducted in the United Kingdom and Canada reveal that virtual environments can help children with developmental disabilities learn skills such as mailing letters at a post office, shopping in a supermarket, and following traffic signs in a virtual city (McComas, Pivik, and LaFlamme, 1998). Virtual reality is proving beneficial to persons with autism, especially using Second Life, a three-dimensional virtual world accessible on the Internet (Biever, 2007; Schmidt and Smith, 2008). As the younger population

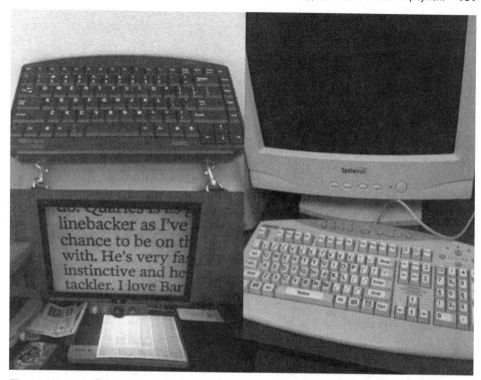

Figure 6.4 The PAC Mate Pocket PC with built-in JAWS (Job Access With Speech) screen-reading software (top left), the TOPAZ desktop video magnifier (bottom left), and a keyboard with enlarged key labels (right) are accessibility technologies that enable persons with disabilities to use computers and other electronic devices.

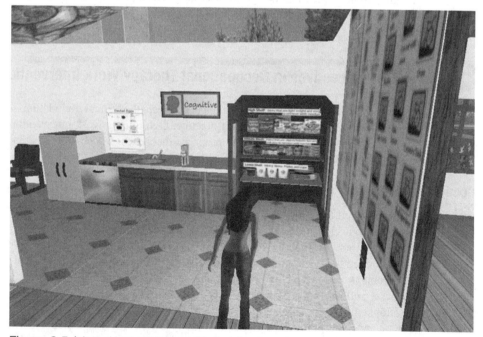

Figure 6.5 Adapted home in Second Life that demonstrates how to adjust a home for low vision and cognitive and mobility problems. This virtual home was created by Jefferson School of Health Professions–Occupational Therapy Department.

Table 6.3   Resources on Assistive Technologies

Resource	Website	Description
AbleData	www.abledata.com	This site provides information about assistive technology products.
Closing the Gap	www.closingthegap.com	Closing the Gap focuses on assistive technology for people with special needs.
Disability Online	www.disabilityonline.com	This website offers a Web link directory with sites that provide services and assistance for people with disabilities. It also has a social networking community with blogs, chat, polls, quizzes, and videos. Assistive technology equipment can be purchased at this site.
DO-IT	www.washington.edu/doit	Do-It is a program created by the University of Washington to facilitate the use of computers and networking technologies to increase independence, productivity, and participation of people with disabilities.

with developmental disabilities becomes familiar with these technologies, more of them may seek higher education and pursue paid employment and careers.

In the past decade, online learning enrollment in college has hit projected records. In the United States alone, over 3.5 million students were enrolled in some type of online course by 2006 (Allen and Seaman, 2007). Of this population, approximately 8 to 12 percent of students enrolled in U.S. universities had some type of disability (Sun and Wen, 2008). Many educational institutions are now dedicating effort to become part of a barrier-free information infrastructure. There is still a long way to go for the academic environments to provide a universal and accessible design to meet the needs of every individual, but technological advances are helping to achieve this goal (Table 6.3).

Theoretical Perspectives in Occupational Therapy Work Intervention

Best practice requires a delicate balance between theoretical foundations and clinical applications. Just as in other areas of practice, high-quality work interventions for developmental disabilities are based on appropriate theoretical frameworks to assure quality in assessment and interventions.

Occupational Behavior and Model of Human Occupation

To write about the continuum of play to work without referencing Mary Reilly is tantamount to ignoring the founder of the occupational behavior model that paved the way from the model of human occupation to the discipline now called occupational science. To introduce the occupational behavior model, Reilly defined occupational behavior as engagement in purposeful activities that occupy a person's time, reach satisfactory success, and are consistent with economic realities. Reilly saw the value of normal development along a continuum of childhood play for exploration to adult work for competence and productivity. Health is the result of a healthy balance between activity and rest supported by a healthy structure and predictable order through habits on a daily basis (Cole and Tufano, 2008).

Habit is a term used in many disciplines because it has numerous definitions. In occupational therapy, the concept of habits has experienced an evolution since the early 1900s, making it more specific to support the occupational performance of individuals (Christiansen, Baum, and Bass-Haugen, 2005). Habits are now defined as "specific, automatic behaviors" integrated into more involved patterns that allow individuals to perform in their daily activities (AOTA, 2008, p. 641; Kielhofner, Forsyth, Kramer, Melton, and Dobson, 2009).

Routines are a group of habits that guide individuals to develop activities in sequences or rituals. Routines provide stability and order during daily activities (Christiansen, Baum, and Bass-Haugen, 2005). For many individuals with developmental disabilities, habits and routines help them to develop the strategies and occupational adaptations necessary for work behaviors. Occupational therapy can help clients establish or maintain a routine during activities of daily living such as getting dressed, preparing meals, and using transportation. Life coaching is also provided by occupational therapy practitioners to empower individuals with the skills and self-confidence necessary to perform independently or with modified assistance in work environments.

Occupational Behavior and Model of Human Occupation (MOHO)

The MOHO (presented in detail in Chapter 4) is a practice model and frame of reference that attempts to explain how human occupation is motivated, patterned, and performed on the basis of three interrelated components: volition, habituation, and performance capacity within the environment. Core assumptions of MOHO expand on these concepts. Volition includes personal causation, values, and interests and refers to the motivation for occupation. Individuals' volition develops and changes as they interact with their physical and social environment; and they bring their volition and capacity to each new performance situation (Kielhofner, 2008; Kielhofner, et al., 2009).

Habits and routines assist individuals with developmental disabilities to form strategies and adaptations necessary for work. Occupational therapy practitioners can assist in establishing or maintaining routine daily living tasks such as getting dressed, preparing meals, and using transportation and can also help clients establish good work habits and routines. As clients with developmental disabilities age and transition between service providers and settings, many of the habits and routines supporting successful occupational performance are interrupted and may not generalize from one setting to another, such as from home to school or from school to work venues. Such changes may negatively affect the individual's motivation, performance patterns, and competency in self-care and work tasks.

Resources (i.e., Internet resources, intervention protocols, case examples) are available to guide the application of MOHO assessments and interventions that are applicable across practice areas, settings, and populations. Two interview assessment tools are the Worker Role Interview (WRI), which is routinely combined with the Occupational Circumstances Assessment Interview and Rating Scale (OCAIRS), and the Work Environment Impact Scale (WEIS). These can be combined with observational assessments such as the Assessment of Motor and Process Skills (AMPS), the Assessment of Communication and Interaction Skills (ACIS), and the Volitional Questionnaire (VQ) to get a clearer picture of clients' performance skills and patterns. Depending on the client's cognitive capacity, some pediatric assessments such as the Pediatric Volitional Questionnaire (PVQ), the Short Child Occupational Profile (SCOPE), and the Child Occupational Self-Assessment (COSA) may provide information to promote developmentally appropriate work adaptation and performance capacity for sheltered workshop participation (Kielhofner, 2008). More information on all of these assessments may be found at the Model of Human Occupation Clearinghouse website at www.moho.uic.edu.

MOHO helps in assessing, treating, and reevaluating by prioritizing client feedback and needs, uses a client-centered holistic approach, offers a strong base to rationalize interventions, and generalizes treatment goals across disciplines (Kielhofner, 2008). MOHO supports occupation-focused practice and many of the common issues individuals and groups dealing with developmental disabilities encounter (see Box 6.1). Examples of the difficulties that persons with developmental disabilities might experience in the work environments are unrealistic sense of abilities and/or lack of confidence for work, difficulty structuring time for work tasks, lack of work-role experience, and problems with processing and/or communication skills for work. The model can also be used as a framework for individual and program development in which four basic steps are undertaken: (1) needs assessment, (2) program planning, (3) program implementation, and (4) program evaluation (Kielhofner, 2008; Todorova, 2008). More information on developing programs is provided in Chapter 18.

Allen's Cognitive Model

The cognitive disability model predicts what an individual will realistically be able to do as well as the level of severity of functional limitation. It has been significantly influenced by Piaget's developmental cognitive theory, Anderson's information-processing theory, and the clinical work of Claudia Allen and colleagues assessing inferred mental processes based on the person's attention to environmental cues and observed verbal and motor behavior resulting in the person's ability to translate the cue into activity performance (Allen, Blue, and Earhart, 1995; Bruce and Borg, 2001). The Allen Cognitive Scales are hierarchical ordinal levels from a global or multicomponent perspective focusing on the sensory motor function associated with the stage identified necessary to guide voluntary motor action and behavior (Allen, 1985; Allen, Blue, and Earhart, 1995; Bruce and Borg, 2001; Levy, 1996).

Historically, the cognitive disablement model identified cognitive disability as "a restriction in voluntary motor action originating in the physical or chemical structures of the brain and producing observable limitations in routine task behavior" (Allen, 1985, p. 31; Bruce and Borg, 2001; Katz, 2006). Basic assumptions within the model begin with recognizing that

---

Box 6.1 Case Brief Using MOHO

Roy is a 33-year-old man with Down syndrome who worked at a fast-food restaurant in his suburban community. After a change in management at the restaurant and a move from his family home to a group home to be closer to his work, Roy began to refuse to perform routine tasks, showed a decline in ADL independence, and became emotional at work. The WRI and the WEIS were used to gather more information from Roy on his perception of work and on the factors that were influencing his work performance. The administration of these assessments also helped establish a therapeutic relationship to guide communication across settings to help identify Roy's work strengths and needs in resuming productive work performance. Use of the ACIS informed the occupational therapist about Roy's ability to communicate and interact at work and in his group home.

Although Roy's interests, values, and roles had stayed the same, the move to the group home setting and the new boss had impacted Roy's work habits and his perception of his work. Roy's limited ability to adapt to transitions and new circumstance combined with a breakdown in communication between the group home and the new manager were identified as factors contributing to his change in performance. New efforts were made to establish routines and support Roy's good work habits. Staff at the group home refocused on familiar supportive strategies to help Roy with routine ADLs. The worksite provided more opportunities for the manager to interact with Roy and for another coworker to model positive interactions with the new manager. Efforts were also focused on carrying over some of the structured strategies put in place from the group home for Roy to return to increased independence and performance at work.

cognition underlies nearly all aspects of individual performance and is a basic component and universal human trait. Our ability to interact, communicate with others, maintain autonomy and independence, and preserve our quality of life all depend on higher-order cognitive functions. By modifying activities appropriately, occupational therapy practitioners can optimize cognitively disabled individuals' capacities and compensate for their limitations to retain a sense of competence, comprehension, and control throughout the life span (Levy, 1996).

The continuum of function/dysfunction for an individual can be affected by shifts in internal stressors or external supports impacting observable work performance behaviors. Clients with developmental disabilities may have maximized cognitive capacity but can optimize function with more environmental adaptations to support their safety and process skills in a specific work setting. Conversely, they may exhibit temporary reduction in functional capacity if external supports that previously optimized their work performance are changed or strained.

The Allen Cognitive Battery consists of tools for evaluating attention, problem-solving, and learning in persons with cognitive restrictions. The Routine Task Inventory-Extended (RTI-E) addresses occupational performance in the areas of self-care, instrumental activities at home and in the community, social communication through verbal and written comprehension and expression, and readiness for work relations and performance. Assessment tools that might be used to support and gather more information on cognition include the Allen Cognitive Level Screen (ACLS), the Large Allen Cognitive Level Screen (LACLS), the Cognitive Performance Test (CPT), and the Allen Diagnostic Module (ADM).

Clients with developmental disabilities may have difficulty identifying safety hazards or social cues in the work environment; following verbal or written directions; communicating information about self, the environment, or others; and maintaining activities of daily living skills necessary for supported employment. They may need support through a hierarchy of sensory cues to attend while performing a task at any given cognitive level and will benefit from having an optimal fit between their cognitive capacity and the work task.

Although it has been associated with studies involving dementia in the geriatric client or cognitive changes in the mental health populations, the cognitive disabilities model is appropriate for use in sheltered workshop settings. Intellectual impairments of clients with development delays may be moderate to profound, and the Allen cognitive disability model may provide strategies to promote and support social, basic self-care, prevocational, and task skills. The occupational therapy practitioner identifies the activity demands and potential environmental modifications and supports indicated to maintain optimal safe functional level for successful participation in the identified activities of daily living and work context (Katz, 2006).

The Allen cognitive disability model has some limitations in occupational therapy practice: (1) variability in the theory constructs over time, (2) self-directed data collection with limited external research studies, (3) a small base of existing research, (4) lack of technology-driven neurobiological study correlations, and (5) lack of current primary research university or institute affiliation (Bruce and Borg, 2001). Although as life expectancy of individuals with developmental disabilities are extended, the Allen cognitive disability model may provide common cognitive language and environmental modifications from early prevocational and school assessments and transition information when clients reach an age or stage requiring more structured or extensive medical care in a facility familiar with the Allen model. Such consistency in care throughout a client's life may promote successful participation in nonpaid work tasks and reinforce optimal environmental cues for independence in self-care skills and volunteer and leisure activities in the extended care setting (see Box 6.2).

Box 6.2 Case Brief Using Allen's Cognitive Model

Eloise is a 28-year-old Hispanic female who attends a community sheltered workshop program and lives at home. Recently, a student occupational therapy club volunteered at the workshop with their fieldwork supervisor and realized Eloise was one of many who could benefit from an Allen cognitive assessment battery to help promote work skills.

Upon completion of the RTI II and an ACLS, Eloise was identified as functioning at 4.4, indicating that she could complete a goal and function in a familiar place with assistance to remove any safety hazards and solve any new problems in the environment. It was also determined in the hierarchy of information-processing supports that she performed best with visual cues, needed extra time to complete a work assignment, and would likely tolerate continuance work for only 2 to 4 hours. With this in mind, the staff at the sheltered workshop used a visual schedule and work assignment board; assisted Eloise with new tasks she wanted to try, providing support the first two or three times; and allowed her to perform familiar routine tasks such as loading or unloading light boxes of supplies or mail, as long as safety hazards were removed.

Biomechanical Frame of Reference

This frame of reference focuses on the development of physical skills that are incorporated from the increase of range of motion (ROM), strength, and endurance (James, 2003). The major focus of biomechanics applied to occupational therapy is to gain or regain occupational performance. To achieve this goal, individuals must learn to use affected body structures to enhance movement and stability.

Latella and Meriano (2003) proposed that the biomechanical approach assumes ROM improves through purposeful activities; that improved ROM, strength, and endurance enhance functional activities; that the body needs rest to heal; and that individuals must have an intact central nervous system to accurately measure ROM, strength, and endurance.

A continuum of function/dysfunction guides the evaluation process and identifies the abilities and deficits of individuals. The continuum encompasses the evaluation of ROM, head and trunk control, and functional skills during head and upper-extremity movements, mobility, feeding, and toileting (Colangelo, 1999).

Some examples of difficulties that persons with decreased ROM, endurance, and/or strength might experience in work environments include limited use of computers (keyboard, mouse) or other work-related equipment, inability to use wall-mounted time clocks, difficulty standing or sitting for prolonged periods, difficulty bending to pick up objects or lifting objects from different surfaces, or difficulty reaching objects in workstation.

Biomechanics-based intervention relates to the use of activities and exercises to prevent or decrease deficits (James, 2003). The use of the environment is also considered in the treatment. Some of the interventions in occupational therapy might include modifying tasks to increase or decrease complexity, splinting hands or wrists to reduce deformity or increase functional ROM, enhancing posture and function with ergonomic equipment, and adapting equipment and environment to promote performance (see Box 6.3).

Occupational therapy practitioners can find guidance for work-related intervention for people with developmental disabilities in existing conceptual practice models and frames of reference as well as through legislative and organizational supports.

> ### Box 6.3   Case Brief Using the Biomechanical Model
>
> Carlisle is a 25-year-old man with cerebral palsy who uses a manual wheelchair for mobility. He works at the admissions office of the local community college. Some of his job responsibilities include data entry, answering phones, and filing. Because of his decreased bilateral elbow and shoulder extension and decreased endurance, Carlisle initially had difficulties reaching objects in his workstation, filing documents in higher cabinets, and picking up the phone and maintaining it on his ear for conversations longer than 3 minutes. After an assessment of needs for work performance, his employer and consultant team made some adaptations to his work area. They rearranged all objects on his desk according to his reaching ratio and range of motion limitation and installed a height-adjustable desk with additional lower shelves on the wall. They provided him with a voice-activated speaker phone with an automatic dialing system that he could also access from his computer. His computer was adapted with a speech-recognition system with options for alternative keyboards and a trackball mouse to decrease hand movements. An accessible filing system was also installed with lower file drawers in vertical cabinets. After these modifications, Carlisle's job performance increased by 50 percent.

While the biomechanical approach continues to be used in occupational therapy, it is limited in that it does not incorporate motivation, psychosocial, emotional, or social aspects or rehabilitation (Foster, 2002). It is therefore used mostly in combination with other frames of references to provide a more holistic approach (James, 2003).

Chapter Summary

This chapter discussed supported and alternative employment opportunities for individuals with developmental disabilities. Case studies illustrated ways that occupational therapy practitioners can help this distinct population in their development through the life span, preparing them for productive, independent living.

Occupational therapy practitioners can find guidance for work-related intervention for people with developmental disabilities in existing conceptual practice models and frames of reference as well as through legislative and organizational supports. However, the profession continues to be challenged by the paucity of training opportunities and employment openings, limited occupational therapy literature and evidence, low employment rates among individuals with developmental disabilities, lack of knowledge among employers regarding occupational therapy services in prevocational training and work-related interventions in schools, and a shortage of supported and alternative employment settings.

All of these challenges point to the need for advocacy, interdisciplinary communication, education, and more research. The cases included in this chapter illustrated the first three challenges. In both settings, the occupational therapy practitioner had to take action in informing the settings about what occupational therapy can offer. In the case of the Filipino papermaking sheltered workshop, the occupational therapist seized the opportunity to turn existing shop and art programs into a training and supported employment project for the qualifying individuals. Using administrative and managerial insight, coupled with the skill to assess individuals and systems, the occupational therapist made a proposal for a sustainable program that would offer work opportunities for its existing and graduating clientele. The occupational therapist at the nonprofit adult day training center served as a consultant instead of a hired employee and made ergonomic and self-regulatory recommendations to the support staff for better lighting, group management, seating, sensory preparation, and behavior regulation techniques. Recommendations also included identifying funding to employ an occupational therapist to work with staff on developmentally appropriate activities for work training and other needed services at the agency, such as self-sustaining arts and crafts perhaps including papermaking, and a sheltered workshop with a gift shop where finished art work could be displayed and sold. Research and documentation are integral in furthering occupational therapy goals and can serve as a catalyst for other programs in other settings that serve individuals with developmental disabilities.

Case Resolution

 Today, Joey and Benjie continue to be friends. They live with their families; Joey with his aging parents, and Benjie with his oldest brother's family. Living with families is not unusual for people with developmental disabilities in the Philippines where most families prefer to take care of family members at home rather than send them to institutions. Joey and Benjie both lead happy and productive lives. Joey works for a company that provides the printing services for the sheltered workshop; he is part of an enclave from a rehabilitation center, and he assembles envelopes, cards, and other printed items before delivery. Benjie, on the other hand, did not stray too far from the sheltered workshop. He works as the shop assistant for the new teacher-manager, and loves teaching younger sheltered workshop clients "to do well like me," he says.

Once in a while, Joey comes to visit, and together they serve as good role models for their younger counterparts. They joke about "retiring" because they have seen their older siblings do that, but they both agree that they love what they do, and want to continue doing what they do for work. Besides, they say, "the money is good." The truth is, they are both approaching 50 years, and while they continue to be very healthy, they will have to face the realities of growing older with a developmental disability.

References

Allen, C. K. (1985). *Occupational Therapy for Psychiatric Diseases: Measurement and Management of Cognitive Disabilities.* Boston: Little, Brown.

Allen, C., Blue, T., & Earhart, C. (1995). *Understanding Cognitive Performance Modes.* Ormond Beach, FL: Allen Conferences.

Allen, I. E., & Seaman, J. (2007). Online Nation: Five Years of Growth in Online Learning. Retrieved from www.aln .org/publications/survey/pdf/online_nation.pdf.

American Occupational Therapy Association. (2008). Occupational therapy practice framework: Domain and process, 2nd ed. *American Journal of Occupational Therapy, 62,* 625–683.

American RehabACTion. Vocational Rehabilitation in the FY 2009 Budget. Retrieved from www.americ anrehabaction.org/conference/fy09budget.html.

Aycinena, P. (2008). Access for all. *Communications of the ACM, 51*(8), 12–13.

Bellamy, G. T., Rhodes, L. E., Bourbeau, P. E., & Mank, D. M. (1986). Mental retardation services in sheltered workshops and day activity programs: Consumer benefits and policy alternatives. In F. R. Rush (ed.), *Competitive Employment Issues and Strategies* (pp. 168–203). Baltimore: Brookes.

Biever, C. (2007). Let's meet tomorrow in Second Life. *New Scientist, 194*(2610), 26–27.

Boyd, R. (1997). Older adults with developmental disabilities: A brief examination of current knowledge. *Activities, Adaptation, and Aging, 2*(3), 7–28.

Bruce, M. A. G., & Borg, B. (2001). Cognitive disability frame of reference: Acknowledgement and limitations. In *Psychosocial Frames of Reference: Core for*

Occupation-based Practice, 3rd ed. (pp. 232–243). Thorofare, NJ: Slack.

Cassell, J. L., Mulkey, S. W., & Grubbs, L. R. (2005). *Rehabilitation Caseload Management: Concepts and Practice* (2nd ed.). New York: Springer.

Christiansen, C. H., Baum, C. M., & Bass-Haugen, J. (2005). *Occupational Therapy: Performance, Participation, and Well-Being,* 3rd ed. Thorofare, NJ: Slack.

Chronister, J. A., Torkelson, R., Chan, F., Rosenthal, D. A., & da Silva, E. (2008). The evidence-based practice movement in healthcare: Implications for rehabilitation, *Journal of Rehabilitation, 74*(2), 6–15.

Colangelo, C. A. (1999). Biomechanical frame of reference. In P. Kramer & J. Hinojosa (eds.), *Frames of Reference in Pediatric Occupational Therapy,* 2nd ed. (pp. 257–322). Baltimore: Lippincott Williams & Wilkins.

Cole, M. B., & Tufano, R. (2008). *Applied Theories in Occupational Therapy: A Practical Approach.* Thorofare, NJ: Slack.

Cutting, K. F. (2008). Should evidence dictate clinical practice or support it? *Journal of Wound Care, 17*(5), 216.

Dick, W., & Golshani, K. (2008). An accessibility lane on the information superhighway. *IEEE Multimedia, 15*(4), 22–26.

Florida Developmental Disabilities Planning Council. (2005). *Planning Ahead: A Handbook for Parents, Family Members, and Guardians of Individuals with Developmental Disabilities* (rev. ed.). Tallahassee: Florida Developmental Disabilities Council.

Foster, M. (2002). Theoretical frameworks. In A. Turner, M. Foster, & S. Johnson (eds.), *Occupational Therapy and Physical Dysfunction: Principles, Skills and*

Practice, 5th ed. (pp. 73–74). London: Churchill Livingstone.

Hotchkiss, J. L. (2003). *The Labor Market Experience of Workers with Disabilities: The ADA and Beyond.* Kalamazoo, MI: W. E. Upjohn Institute for Employment Research.

Jacobs, K. (1992). *Occupational Therapy: Work Programs and Assessment.* Boston: Little, Brown.

Jacobson, S. A., & Wilhite, B. C. (1999). Residential transitions in the lives of older adults with developmental disabilities: An ecological perspective. *Therapeutic Recreation Journal, 33*(3),195–208.

James, A. B. (2003). Theories derived from rehabilitation perspectives. In E. B. Crepeau, E. S. Cohn, & B. A. B. Schell (eds.), *Willard and Spackman's Occupational Therapy,* 10th ed. (pp. 240–242). Philadelphia: Lippincott Williams & Wilkins.

Katz, N. (2006). Routine Task Inventory–Expanded (RTI-E). Retrieved from www.allen-cognitive-network.org/index .php/allen-model/routine-task-inventory-expanded-rti-e.

Kielhofner, G. (2008). *Model of Human Occupation: Theory and Application,* 4th ed. Baltimore: Lippincott Williams & Wilkins.

Kielhofner, G., Forsyth, K., Kramer, J. M., Melton, J., & Dobson, E. (2009). The model of human occupation. In E. B. Crepeau, E. S. Cohn, & B. A. B. Schell (eds.), *Willard and Spackman's Occupational Therapy,* 11th ed. (pp. 446–461). Philadelphia: Lippincott Williams & Wilkins.

Larson, B., & Ellexson, M. (2005). Occupational therapy services in facilitating work performance. *American Journal of Occupational Therapy, 59*(6), 676–679.

Latella, D., & Meriano, C. (2003) *Occupational Therapy Manual for Evaluation of Range of Motion and Muscle Strength.* Clifton Park, NY: Thomson/Delmar Learning.

Levy, L. L. (1996). Cognitive integration and cognitive components. In K. O. Larson, R. G. Stevens-Ratchford, L. Pedretti, & J. L. Crabtree (eds.), *ROTE: The Role of Occupational Therapy with the Elderly,* 2nd ed. (pp. 573–596). Bethesda, MD: AOTA Press.

Luftig, R. L., & Muthert, D. (2005). Patterns of employment and independent living of adult graduates with learning disabilities and mental retardation of an inclusionary high school vocational program. *Research in Developmental Disabilities, 26*(4), 317–325.

McComas, J., Pivik, J., & LaFlamme, M. (1998). Current uses of virtual reality for children with disabilities. In Riva, G., Wiederhold, B., & Molinari (eds.), *Virtual Environments in Clinical Psychology and Neuroscience.* Amsterdam: IOS Press.

Migliore, A., Mank, D., Grossi, T., & Rogan, P. (2007). Integrated employment or sheltered workshops: Preferences of adults with intellectual disabilities, their families, and staff. *Journal of Vocational Rehabilitation, 26*(1), 5–19.

Post, K. M., Hartmann, K., Gitlow, L., & Rakoski, D. (2008). AOTA's Centennial Vision for the future: How can technology help? *Technology Special Interest Section Quarterly, 18*(1), 1–4.

Quiroga, V. A. M. (1995). *Occupational Therapy: The First 30 Years, 1900 to 1930.* Bethesda, MD: AOTA Press.

Schmidt, M. A., & Smith, D. L. (2007). Individuals with disabilities perceptions on preparedness for the workforce and factors that limit employment, *Work, 28*(1), 13–21.

Seale, J. K. (2006). *E-learning and Disability in Higher Education: Accessibility Research and Practices.* New York: Routledge.

Sun, Z., & Wen, J. (2008). Exploration of Chinese website accessibility evaluation model. *Proceedings of the IEEE International Conference on Computer Science and Software Engineering.* Jinhua, China, 1357–1360.

Todorova, L. (2008). Assessing employment needs of Bulgarian youths with intellectual impairments. *Occupational Therapy in Health Care, 22*(2–3), 77–84.

U.S. Department of Education. 2007. Disability Employment 101. Retrieved from www.ed.gov/about/offices/list/ osers/products/employmentguide/index.html.

U.S. Department of Labor (1998). Section 508, Rehabilitation Act. Retrieved from www.section508.gov/index .cfm?FuseAction=Content&ID=14.

Wysocki, D., & Neulicht, A. T. (2004). Work is occupation: What can I do as an occupational therapy practitioner? In Ross, M., & Bachner, S. (eds.), *Adults with Developmental Disabilities: Current Approaches in Occupational Therapy.* Bethesda, MD: AOTA Press.

Yamiki, K., & Fujiura, G. (2002). Employment and income status of adults with developmental disabilities living in the community. *Mental Retardation, 40*(2), 132–141.

Glossary

Cognitive employment is individual placement of a worker by a training or rehabilitation agency.

Community rehabilitation facilities (also known as sheltered workshops) are vocational programs supported by the government that provide training and work for people with developmental disabilities and mental retardation.

A **job coach** is a person trained to teach individuals with disabilities basic responsibilities required to perform a job.

Sheltered workshops (see community rehabilitation facilities).

Supported employment is a paid job at which the employee receives continuous training and advocacy from a support coach.

Resources

Rehabilitation Services Administration

Switzer Building
330 C Street, S.W.
Washington, D.C. 20202
(202) 205-9297

Administration on Developmental Disabilities

Department of Health and Human Services
200 Independence Avenue, S.W.
Washington, D.C. 20201
(202) 690-5504

Office of Disability Employment Policy

1331 F Street, N.W.
Washington, D.C. 20002
(202) 376-6200; (202) 376-6205 TTY/TTY

U.S. Department of Labor, Office of Disability Employment Policy

www.dol.gov/odep/archives/fact/supportd.htm

U.S. Department of Education Disability Employment 101

www.ed.gov/about/offices/list/osers/products/ employmentguide/index.html

7

The Younger Worker
Transition Services for the Adolescent and Young Adult With Special Needs

Navah Z. Ratzon, Edna Alon, Tamara Schejter-Margalit,
and Susan M. Cahill

Key Concepts

The following are key concepts addressed in this chapter:

- Adolescents and young adults with special needs are described as a population.
- Theoretical models commonly used with adolescents and youth to provide social, environmental, and cognitive support are presented and explained.
- Training processes that are successful with the adolescent and young adult population are presented and examples are provided.
- Legislation and policies that affect treatment of adolescents and young adults are discussed.
- Transition services and strategies to help the young adult with special needs to transition to work are presented.

Case Introduction

Gail is an 18½-year-old young adult with special needs who was born prematurely and diagnosed with left hemiplegia due to cerebral palsy. She has mild spasticity and is able to ambulate independently with slightly decreased stability. Increased tonus is observed in her left arm and leg during effort. Occupational therapy evaluation included the administration of assessments, observations in multiple settings, and frequent interviews with Gail, her family, and other team members. The following information was obtained about Gail through the evaluation process:

- *Psychological evaluation* revealed below average intellectual function (IQ = 71) with many gaps between potential and actual function.
- Her *occupational history* shows that Gail has the ability to attend to tasks and to persevere in the performance of occupations, but her level of function is inconsistent and is affected by frequently changing moods. In an interview, Gail states that she wants to work in competitive employment, but she cannot identify an interest in a specific type of work.
- An *occupational profile* was developed for Gail, and it revealed that she is independent in activities of daily living (ADL) and partially independent in instrumental activities of daily living (IADL). She does not participate in leisure activities beyond watching TV and playing computer games. At school, Gail reads and writes at a third-grade level, performs basic addition and subtraction, but has great difficulty with multiplication and division. She is verbally capable, but her speech is marked by stuttering. Her sensory functioning (vision, hearing, taste, and smell) is normal.
- Gail's *performance patterns* show that she often seeks support and assistance from others and develops an obsessive attachment to authoritative figures. She acts impulsively and has great difficulty adapting to new situations and to transitions from setting to setting. Gail has difficulty maintaining focus and is currently attending only approximately 50 percent of the center's activities.

During the evaluation process and the first months of intervention, the family was skeptical regarding the impact occupational therapy would have on Gail's outcomes, and therefore there was little cooperation.

Introduction

The focus of this book is primarily on work-related practice and services with adults. However, in Chapter 2 you learned about the process of vocational development across the life span. Occupational therapy practitioners often address work-related issues with adolescents and young adults, particularly as they relate to the transition from school life to the working world of adulthood. In the United States, the services provided by occupational therapy practitioners are guided by federal legislation and state and local policies. In other countries, such as Israel, laws against discrimination address, among other rights, equal employment opportunities for people with disabilities. Additionally, the new World Health Organization (WHO, 2008) framework for measuring health and disability has encouraged better work opportunities for adolescents and young adults with special needs throughout the world.

Adolescents and young adults with special needs face unique challenges as they transition to adulthood. The effectiveness of transition plans depends on the level at which an adolescent or young adult with special needs participates in the decision-making process and the transition process itself. The level of family involvement and the collaboration between the adolescent or young adult with the family and professional team are also important factors that impact the effectiveness of transition plans.

Children who require supportive services to make the transition into the typical roles and occupations of adolescence and young adulthood are commonly described as having *special needs.* These children require additional resources because of physical, sensory, cognitive, and learning challenges; mental health issues; and problems due to social, cultural, linguistic, or family factors (Varga-Toth, 2006). Special needs can be defined as either special health-care needs (e.g., therapy, medication, equipment, and physician care) or social services needs (e.g., case management and social security benefits) (Blomquist, 2006). This innovative resource-based definition of special needs has considerable support internationally because it stresses the adaptations that must be made to improve outcomes for children and adolescents with special needs rather than deficits "within" the individual (Varga-Toth, 2006). Throughout this chapter, when we speak of adolescents and young adults, it should be assumed that we are referring to that group of adolescents and young adults who have special needs.

The occupational therapy practitioner's role with the adolescent and the young adult has undergone extensive change in the past few decades. Modern society's legal and social processes are responsible for many of these changes. In the last 30 years, western countries have recognized the rights of people with disabilities and anchor these rights in actions, legislation, and regulations that promote equality. As a result, the emphasis in occupational therapy with this population has moved from providing remedial services to providing supportive services designed to help adolescents and young adults transition to adulthood.

> *In the last 30 years, western countries have recognized the rights of people with disabilities and anchor these rights in actions, legislation, and regulations that promote equality.*

With the growing implementation of legislation and policies against discrimination in western countries, a new horizon has opened for people with disabilities (Council of the European Union, 2000). Laws against discrimination imply, among other things, equal opportunities for employment for people with disabilities and foster new opportunities for those with special needs. Other chapters such as Chapter 16 (on the Americans with Disabilities Act) and Chapter 17 (on work incentives and health policy) describe these efforts in depth. Despite some variation in remedies in different countries, it is hoped that the process of integrating more people with disabilities into the workforce will accelerate and result in an increased need for occupational therapy services.

Legislative and Professional Courses of Action

In the United States, key civil rights legislation and court decisions related to employment practices include Title VII of the Civil Rights Act of 1964, Title I of the Americans with Disabilities Act of 1991 (ADA), and guidelines from the Equal Opportunity Commission (EEOC). Title I of the ADA prohibits employers from discriminating against a qualified individual with a disability if the individual with a disability can perform the essential functions of the job with or without reasonable accommodation. The ADA is discussed at length in Chapter 16. The EEOC provides enforcement guidelines on disability-related inquiries that prohibit any discrimination. In addition, the 2004 (Pub.L. 108-446) Individuals with Disabilities Education Improvement Act (IDEIA) supports helping adolescents transition to adult life. School districts in the United States are required to provide transition services to adolescents and young adults who are eligible for special education and related services such as occupational therapy. The purpose of transition services is to facilitate each student's transition from school to adult life through an individualized plan (IDEIA, Section 1401 [34]). The IDEIA requires that school teams have transition plans in place by the time students reach age 16.

Adolescents and young adults who are eligible for training services under Workforce Investment Act of 1998 (WIA) are guaranteed access to the full range of services provided by vocational rehabilitation without having to establish relationships with multiple agencies or case managers. According to the U.S. Office of Disability and Employment Policy (2000), the WIA:

- Improves transition programming by allowing vocational programs and employers to coordinate information and services to ensure accessibility at one-stop career centers.
- Provides options and resources for evaluations, career planning, job training, and job placement.
- Promotes access to information about career opportunities, financial assistance, and work-related trends.
- Offers skills training in several areas, including how to write a résumé and answer interview questions.

As you will learn in Chapter 16, the ADA ensures that individuals with disabilities are guaranteed civil rights and protections (EEOC, 2008). Under the ADA, employers cannot discriminate against qualified individuals on the basis of disability. According to the EEOC, qualified individuals are defined as those people who possess relevant skills, experience, and education to meet the essential job functions with or without reasonable accommodations. In addition, employers must demonstrate fairness and equity in all employment practices, including job application procedures, career advancement, and compensation.

An additional influence that has contributed to improvement in services for adolescents and young adults is the development of WHO's *International Classification of Function, Disability, and Health (ICF)* (2008). This framework for measuring health and disability was introduced in Chapter 2. The definitions included in this framework encourage a better understanding of the nonlinear correlations between impairment, disability, and handicap and recognition of the impact of nonmedical variables such as the environment and sociodemographic variables on the function of people with disabilities. According to the ICF, adolescents and young adults with special needs can have meaningful and independent lives by participating in normative everyday life activities, obtaining education, working, and being active members of their communities (Van Naarden Braun, Yeargin-Allsopp, and Lollar, 2006).

Professional teams have begun to integrate the ICF into their practice and to shift their attitudes regarding support of the full participation of adolescents and young adults with special needs in society in general and in work in particular. Occupational therapy practitioners are integral members of these professional teams because they can critically examine the relationship between the worker, the work itself, and the environment in which the work takes place. The enactment of new legislation combined with the understanding that children with special needs grow up to be adolescents who need vocational rehabilitation has led to a process focused on creating opportunities for young adults to achieve maximal participation.

Who Are Adolescents and Young Adults With Special Needs?

Limitations in participation and activity manifested during the developmental period (birth to 22 years) may have implications for success in the normative adult social roles of employment and education as well as the attainment of independent living and achievement of economic self-sufficiency (Van Naaden Braun, Yeargin-Allsopp, and Lollar, 2009; see Fig. 7.1). These limitations can be characterized as health factors, medically determinable physical factors (e.g., motor, sensory), or mental or behavioral impairment and can result in chronic conditions that might include functional limitations (Piek and Dyck, 2004).

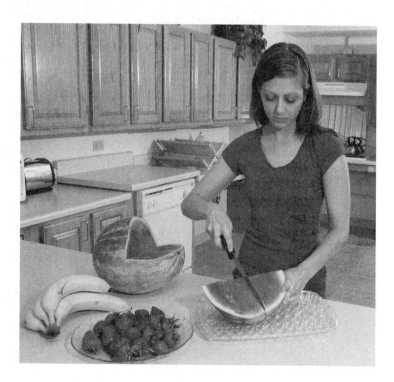

Figure 7.1 Many factors can contribute to the development of an adolescent or young adult with special needs.

Although health factors are hypothesized to influence limitations in activity and participation, limitations may not arise from health-related factors alone. Factors such as economic and social constraints (i.e., environmental factors in the ICF framework) may impose limitations beyond those attributable to specific physical, sensory, psychological, or intellectual impairments (Groce, 1999). Disabling factors like low socioeconomic status are of particular concern because adolescents and young adults with impairments are likely to experience less support in carrying out daily activities as a result of societal prejudice and discrimination (Kaye, 1997). Yet, non-health factors can act as enabling factors for those who have the adequate socioeconomic support (Ratzon, Ornoy, Greenbaum, Peritz, and Dulitzky, 1996).

The prevalence of children with special needs is difficult to determine because the etiology can be attributed to a variety of diagnoses and conditions, which include, but are not limited to, attention deficit-hyperactivity disorder (ADHD), motor skills disorders, intellectual disabilities, learning disorders, communication disorders, pervasive developmental disorder, and mental health disorders. The National Health Interview Survey in the United States (McManus, Newacheck, and Greaney, 1990), which included a nationally representative sample of 10,394 randomly selected noninstitutionalized young adults ages 19 to 24, reported that almost 6 percent of young adults have disabilities. Examining the prevalence of the different possible etiologies of conditions experienced by adolescents and young adults reveals a similar picture. The possible etiologies of adolescents and young adults with special needs are further highlighted in Box 7.1.

Box 7.1 Possible Etiologies of Adolescents and Young Adults With Special Needs

- *Attention deficit-hyperactivity disorder (ADHD)* is characterized by "prominent symptoms of inattention and/or hyperactivity-impulsivity that is more frequently displayed and more severe than is typically observed in individuals at a comparable level of development." ADHD has several subtypes, such as predominantly inattentive, predominantly hyperactive-impulsive, and combined. While reported prevalence of ADHD among school-aged children is estimated at 3 to 7 percent, data on the prevalence of ADHD in adolescence and adulthood are limited.
- *Motor skills disorder* includes developmental coordination disorder (DCD), which is characterized by "motor coordination that is substantially below that expected given the person's chronological age." While prevalence of DCD is estimated to be as high as 6 percent, data on prevalence of DCD in adolescence and adulthood are limited.
- *Mental retardation* is characterized by "significantly subaverage intellectual functioning (an IQ of approximately 70 or below) with onset before age 18 years and concurrent deficits or impairments in adaptive functioning." Different studies report different rates depending on definitions used, methods of ascertainment, and population studies.
- *Learning disorders* are characterized by "academic functioning that is substantially below that expected given the person's chronological age, measured intelligence, and age-appropriate education." Approximately 5 percent of students in public schools in the United States are identified as having a learning disorder.
- *Communication disorders* are characterized by "difficulties in speech or language and include expressive language disorder, mixed receptive-expressive language disorder, phonological disorder, stuttering, and communication disorder not otherwise specified." Prevalence estimates vary according to the diagnosis.
- *Pervasive developmental disorders* are characterized by "severe difficulties and pervasive impairment in multiple areas of development. These include impairment in reciprocal social interaction, impairment in communication, and the presence of stereotyped behavior, interests, and activities."
- *Borderline personality disorder's* essential feature is "a pervasive pattern of instability of interpersonal relationships, self-image, and affects and marked impulsivity that begins by early adulthood and is present in a variety of contexts." The prevalence of borderline personality disorder is estimated to be about 2 percent of the general population.

(American Psychiatric Association, 2000)

The rate of employment for young adults with special needs is lower than for young adults without special needs. The 2000 NOD/Harris Survey found that 32 percent of people with disabilities versus 81 percent of people without disabilities were working part time or full time; the 2004 NOD/Harris Survey found that only 35 percent of people with disabilities were working. This is approximately the same percentage as in 1986 before the ADA was enacted (Stapleton and Burkhauser, 2003). The same trend is seen among adolescents and young adults with special needs (Brown, Moore, and Bzostek, 2004). In studies of typical young adults, their working rate is only 44 percent (in year-round or summer employment) compared to 56 percent of all 19 year olds and 72 percent of 18 to 29 year olds. Of those who did not work, the majority (67%) wanted to work. Vocational rehabilitation services were used by 33 percent of the respondents, and among those who went through vocational rehabilitation, only 40 percent were working. The major concern of that study was that 26 percent of these young adults were not participating in any activity—not working, not in school, and not staying at home with children (Blomquist, 2006).

More optimistic data was presented by the U.S. Department of Education's Institute of Education Sciences and the National Center for Special Education Research in the 2005 National Longitudinal Transition Study-2, which reported that 75 percent of adolescents and young adults with special needs were employed at some point since they graduated high school and 56 percent were employed at the time of the interview (in comparison to 66% employment among a control group). In-depth analysis reveals that of the adolescents and young adults with special needs who were employed during a period of 1 to 4 years after leaving high school, 25 percent were employed 2 months or less, 31 percent were employed 2.1 to 6 months, 24 percent were employed 6.1 to 12 months. Only 21 percent were employed more than 12 months.

The Importance of Physical, Social, and Institutional Environments

During the 1990s, awareness of the importance of the environment progressed, and environmental aspects were increasingly integrated into the theory and practice of occupational therapy (Kielhofner, 2008). *Environment* refers to the external physical and social surroundings in which the client's daily life occupations occur (AOTA, 2008b). A person can only be understood across the life cycle in the context of his or her environment. For people with disabilities, the environment has special importance because it can enable performance or limit it. Enabling environments encourage participation and growth with normative function; limiting environments may increase dysfunction.

The American Occupational Therapy Association (AOTA) defines several types of environment in the Occupational Therapy Practice Framework: Domain and Process. The *physical environment* is the natural (geographic terrain, sensory qualities of environment, plants and animals) and built, nonhuman environment (buildings) and the objects in them (furniture, tools, devices) (AOTA, 2008a). As children encounter developmental milestones, the physical environment can influence their development and the actions of their adult caregivers (Evans, 2006).

Children with disabilities encounter environmental constraints that limit their active participation in daily life (Law and Dunn, 1993). Parents and other caregivers constantly adapt physical environments to accommodate their children with disabilities. Teachers, therapists, and other educators do the same in other environments. Service providers in schools have an ethical obligation, and in the United States are mandated, to adapt the environment so that children with special needs can take part in school activities on equal terms with other children. This means, among other things, that the premises must be physically accessible to children with restricted mobility, the outer environment must be adapted for restricted mobility, there must be individually tested technical aids, and the children's technical aids must function well in these environments (Prellwitz and Tamm, 2000).

The physical work environment is as influential to the success of the worker as the physical school environment is to the success of the student. Therefore, the same attitudes and approaches used to evaluate the fit between student and physical school environment should be applied to his or her new work environment. Guiding principles from ergonomics and universal design are helpful, but some work environments need special, individualized adaptations. Throughout the transition process, occupational therapy practitioners examine the influence on occupational performance of the physical environments in which the adolescent or young adult will function and recommend adaptations and enhancements to facilitate performance. They also examine how the social environment facilitates or restricts the adolescent's participation at work.

The *social environment* is constructed by the presence, relationships, and expectations of the persons, groups, and organizations with which the person has contact. The social environment includes the availability and expectations of significant individuals such as spouse, friends, and caregivers; relationships with individuals, groups, or organizations; and relationships with systems that are influential in establishing norms, role expectations, and social routines (AOTA, 2008b).

The social environment is a crucial influence on the occupational performance of adolescents and young adults. As children develop, families and caregivers who provide enabling environments promote the confidence, motivation, and strength to succeed. Special education settings can also be constructed so that their social environments are supportive. In addition to the academic knowledge, students learn what society expects from them (regular participation, timeliness, appropriate dress and behavior, following routines, etc.). Adolescents and young adults also learn how to interact effectively with people outside their family and home, such as teachers, classmates, friends, and others. A job coach and peers in the workplace are also components of the social environment. The occupational therapy practitioner can recommend changes in the social environment that help the adolescent or young adult meet demands for performance during a transition from school to work.

Continuity is needed throughout the process of transition (Bellini and Royce-Davis, 1999). To maintain continuity, professionals in special education and vocational rehabilitation settings should develop expertise in strategies specifically for adolescents and young adults, such as the use of transition-focused, person-centered planning tools (e.g., the McGill Action Planning System [MAPS] and Planning Alternate Tomorrows with Hope [PATH]; for more information, see Falvey, Forest, Pearpoint, and Rosenberg, 2003). It is important that professionals in these settings fully cooperate to maintain a synergistic effect in supports and processes developed to enable the occupational performance of the adolescent or young adult. Occupational therapy practitioners can be instrumental in assuring this continuity and in making necessary changes to environmental supports as the adolescent or young adult moves from one setting to another.

Context refers to a variety of interrelated conditions within and surrounding the client. They are often less tangible than the physical and social environments but nonetheless exert a strong influence on performance (AOTA, 2008b). The *cultural context* of most modern societies includes values supported by laws that affirm the personal rights of adolescents and young adults and afford increased access to resources and opportunities for education, employment, and economic support.

Occupational Characteristics and Needs of Adolescents and Young Adults

According to AOTA (2008a), occupational therapy practitioners collaborate with school-based transition teams to support young adults as they move from high school to adult life by completing the following tasks:

- Preparing young adults for new roles and routines.
- Providing education to parents and community stakeholders about young adults' needs.
- Facilitating vocational and independent-living skills development.
- Promoting self-determination.
- Facilitating social and community integration.
- Recommending assistive technology for work and living situations.

Occupational therapy practitioners are well prepared to assess how an individual's participation in daily occupations is influenced by performance skills and patterns and how these factors match with an activity's demands and with the context in which it takes place (AOTA, 2008a). The unique skills of occupational therapy practitioners make them valuable collaborators on transition teams and facilitate their ability to provide services in the areas of postsecondary education, employment, and community participation (Kardos and White, 2005; Orentlicher, 2007; Spencer and O'Daniel, 2005).

The unique skills of occupational therapy practitioners make them valuable collaborators on transition teams and facilitate their ability to provide services in the areas of postsecondary education, employment, and community participation.

Following a vocational assessment, occupational therapy practitioners deliver services in three ways: (1) direct service, (2) consultation to the transition team as challenges arise, and (3) education to employers and other key individuals about the nature of the client's needs and disability (Spencer and O'Daniel, 2005). Direct services are based on individualized transition goals, are occupation-based, and, whenever possible, should occur within the environment and context where the student will be employed. The team should consider the student's personal vocational goals, strengths, and needs when making decisions about potential employment opportunities and vocational skills instruction (Kohler and Field, 2003; McGlashing-Johnson, Agran, Sitlington, Cavin, and Wehmeyer, 2003; Michaels and Orentlicher, 2004; Orentlicher, 2007). Vocational instruction should take place in a context that is highly relevant to the skills being taught (Kohler and Field, 2003; Spencer and O'Daniel, 2005). Consultation services are also based on individualized transition goals and generally take place within context of transition teams. The purpose of consultative services is to help team members develop individualized accommodations or modifications and/or to design environments that are more supportive of the student with special needs. Education about an individual's specific needs and disability may also be provided to employers by occupational therapy practitioners.

Theoretical Models of Intervention With Adolescents and Young Adults With Special Needs

Occupational therapy practice with adolescents and young adults with special needs is based on a variety of conceptual practice models and related knowledge, as described in

Chapter 4. This chapter presents several models that are often used with adolescents and young adults to support transition from school to employment (Box 7.2). The first model is the transition support model, which is the one of the most commonly used models. Two other models presented in this chapter are the Canadian model of occupational performance and engagement (CMOP-E) and the dynamic interactional model of cognition. These two models are not unique in their application to adolescents and young adults.

Transition Support Model

For any young person, the transition from high school to adult life is a challenge. This challenge can be especially difficult for students with developmental or intellectual disabilities (Hughes, 2001). International research shows that high school is not necessarily a positive experience leading to a successful transition to adult life, especially in terms of unemployment, financial dependence, and the absence of meaningful social relationships (Bollingmo, 1997; Wagner, 1995). Hughes (2001) states that these findings were corroborated by international studies on students with disabilities. For example, research in Ireland, the Netherlands, Norway, the United Kingdom, and the United States reveals similar data with rates of 90 percent and above for unemployment and social uninvolvement among students with disabilities (Bollingmo, 1997; Felce and Perry, 1997; Korpel, 1996; Wagner, 1995; Walsh and Linehan, 1997).

To improve outcomes in the transition from high school to adult life, numerous models have been proposed and implemented, such as the work-study model, career education model, special needs model, bridges model, and community adjustment model (Whetstone and Browning, 2002). Of the models proposed, the most commonly used is the transition support model. The transition support model (Hughes, et al., 1997a; Hughes, Hwang, Kim, Killian, and Harmer, 1997b; Hughes, et al., 1997c; Hughes, et al., 2000) is empirically based on 113 studies that addressed transitional support, including a survey of researchers and field testing of the model, and has been supported by the identification of nearly 600 strategies by secondary school transition teachers.

Support in the transition support model is designed to meet the individual needs of students rather than to "fix" or "cure" them (Wehman, 2000). This approach is based on the belief that all people need support, but to different degrees and in different areas of life (Hughes, 2001).

One goal of the transition support model is to develop supports in the environment and includes the following components: (1) promoting social acceptance, (2) increasing environmental support, and (3) increasing social support. A second goal is to increase students' competence and includes (1) identifying and promoting student strengths, (2) increasing students' self-determination, (3) increasing students' choice and promoting decision making, and (4) promoting social interaction among students (Hughes, 2001).

Strategies for Promoting Social Acceptance

Employment opportunities for adolescents and young adults with special needs can be viewed on a continuum from opportunities with the least amount of social integration to opportunities with the most amount of social integration. Later in this chapter, we explain

---

Box 7.2 Theoretical Models Applicable for Adolescents and Young Adults With Special Needs

- Transition model support
- Canadian model of occupational performance and engagement (CMOP-E)
- Dynamic interactional model of cognition

the differences between traditional sheltered workshops and more contemporary vocational training models that emphasize social integration. Chapters 6 and 9 also include in-depth discussions of these models.

Strategies for promoting social acceptance are based on the principle that inclusion in the mainstream of life is a primary goal of transition services (Agran, Snow, and Swaner, 1999). *Social inclusion* may be defined as "fully participating in the interactions that occur within an environment to the same extent as other people do who are a part of that setting" and a situation in which "individual differences are accepted and individual competencies are maximized and supported" (Hughes and Carter, 2000; Hughes, et al., 1997a). Strategies for promoting social acceptance include involving teachers, employment specialists, and therapists to increase community awareness of people with special needs and improve access to information, services, and facilities.

Following are examples of strategies for promoting social acceptance:

- Introduce students with disabilities to music and fashion that is popular in their peer culture.
- Teach social skills (e.g., introducing one's self and terminating a conversation).

Strategies for Increasing Environmental Support

Strategies for increasing environmental support also include involving teachers, employment specialists, and therapists to increase community awareness of people with special needs and improve access to information, services, and facilities (Hughes, 2001).

An example from Gail's case illustrates this strategy. During therapeutic sessions in the occupational therapy department, a cognitive intervention was performed to improve Gail's functioning and to raise her awareness of her strengths, abilities, successes, and difficulties. The occupational therapist and Gail sought to identify strategies to help Gail circumvent her difficulties and to limit the negative impact of her emotional state on her occupational performance.

Strategies for Increasing Social Support

The amount of social support that students receive can influence the degree of success and satisfaction they experience as they transition from high school to adult life (Staub, Spaulding, Peck, Gallucci, and Schwartz, 1996). The principle goal of strategies for increasing social support is to create opportunities for social interaction and identify the degree of social support the student needs. The amount of social support differs among students, ranging from an occasional reminder to ongoing assistance or encouragement (Chadsey-Rusch and Heal, 1995; Schalock, et al., 1994). Support needs may change in different environments and over time. The role of occupational therapy practitioners is to assist students in acquiring social skills that enable them to access various environments and to educate family members, coworkers, and managers to offer assistance and social support to students.

Following are examples of strategies for promoting social support:

- Encourage the employer to schedule the student's breaks to coincide with a friendly and supportive coworker's breaks.
- Encourage the employer to schedule the student and his or her preferred coworkers on the same shifts.

Strategies for Identifying and Promoting Students' Strengths

The principal goal of these strategies is to emphasize students' strengths rather than weaknesses and move from a "deficit-based" education to a program that reflects the belief that all students can be maximally included in everyday school, work, and community environments (Walker, 1999). Occupational therapy practitioners can identify students' strengths by observing them in different environments (school, work, social activities) and by recording circumstances that promote the use of students' strengths. Information can be obtained from family members, peers, and others who see and meet the student on different occasions as well as from students themselves (Hagner and Sande, 1998). The practitioner can apply all of the information gathered to develop interventions that support full participation.

Following are examples of strategies for promoting students' strengths:

- Design environments that capitalize on strengths (e.g., post visual schedules and other visual reminders).
- Assign job tasks that match strengths (e.g., a student who is good at math can balance cash drawers).

Strategies for Increasing Students' Self-Determination

Self-determination is promoted to enable students to express their interests and preferences and to support students in carrying out their lifestyle choices, managing their daily lives, advocating for themselves, making decisions, and acting on their decisions (Wehmeyer and Bolding, 1999). The role of the occupational therapy practitioner is to help students improve their skills in occupations that demand decision-making and to teach them how to expand the spectrum of decisions.

Following are examples of strategies for increasing students' self-determination:

- Conduct preference assessments.
- Provide opportunities for students to make choices about the work tasks they will complete or the order in which they will complete them.
- Teach self-advocacy skills, such as asking for help when it is needed and declining to do another worker's job.

Strategies for Increasing Students' Choices and Decision-Making

The main objective of these strategies is to provide students the opportunity to make their own choices and decisions, such as what to wear, what to study, or where to live. Occupational therapy practitioners must be familiar enough with the student's interests and needs that they can present an array of opportunities for the student to choose from and can support the student in making decisions by himself or herself (Hughes, 2001).

Following are two examples that illustrate how the occupational therapy practitioner used strategies for promoting social support with Gail:

- During the nearly year-long intervention, Gail decided she wanted to work in the open market. She was encouraged to apply to a cooking course conducted in cooperation with a participating hotel.
- Throughout the intervention, Gail required enabling reinforcement and treatment of disabling factors that affected independence and everyday functioning. At the end of the process, Gail was able to travel independently using public transportation over long distances to get to the cooking course.

Strategies for Promoting Students' Social interaction

The goal of these strategies is to promote social skills that enable students to fit better into the social community, which includes peers, neighbors, and work colleagues. Occupational therapy practitioners can collaborate with students' worksite supervisors, teachers, and others by initiating social interactions that create opportunities to teach students social skills (Hughes, 2001). In Gail's case, she learned to accept the authority of her supervisors and the rules of the workplace. Gail also learned that when she received instructions from people who were not defined as her supervisors, she did not necessarily need to carry them out.

Canadian Model of Occupational Performance and Engagement (CMOP-E)

The CMOP-E and its application to work-related services were introduced in Chapter 4. A basic tenet of this model is that the values and beliefs of occupational therapy support the concepts of occupational performance and a client-centered approach. Consistent with this point of view, the main task of the occupational therapy practitioner is enabling occupational performance while involving the client in the choice, planning, and performance of tasks that the client defines as being meaningful in a specific environment. Occupational performance is recognized as a dynamic relationship among the person, environment, and occupation, with the person at the center (CAOT, 1997). Occupational performance refers to the client's ability to choose, organize, and satisfactorily perform personally meaningful occupations in the three areas of self-care, productivity, and leisure, according to the age and culture of the client (CAOT, 1997; Cresswell and Rugg, 2003). For example, Gail was fully involved in choosing the type of work she wanted to pursue. In the process of making the choice, Gail and the occupational therapist addressed the significance of the choice and discussed the pros and cons of the selection.

The three-dimensional structure of the CMOP-E shows the interdependence among the person, the environment, and the occupation. Change in any of these areas affects occupational performance and satisfaction achieved from performance of the occupation. Spirituality is at the core of the model and "resides in persons, is shaped by the environment and gives meaning to occupations" (CAOT, 1997). For example, when Gail's parents took the responsibility of helping her get to school, Gail's attendance improved, which in turn improved her task performance.

Dynamic Interactional Model of Cognition

Toglia's (2005) dynamic interaction model of cognition is based on neuropsychology, cognitive psychology, and social psychology. This model recognizes the interaction among the individual, task, and environment in determining cognitive function. Evaluation in the dynamic interaction model includes performance prediction, task performance, and performance evaluation. In the process of assessment, the occupational therapy practitioner uses cues and task alterations to identify the person's potential for change.

According to the model, intervention can focus on "changing the person's strategies and self-awareness; modifying external factors such as the activity demands and environment; or simultaneously addressing the person, activity, and environment to facilitate performance" (Toglia, 2005).

Toglia (1991, 2003) also described the multicontext treatment approach in which activities and situations are gradually changed but strategies and techniques remain constant. Training strategies suggested by Toglia (2005) include *anticipation* of obstacles and outcomes and the need for strategies and *self-prediction* of the level of difficulty and speed and accuracy of performance, which can be compared with self-evaluation after performance. At intervals during task performance, strategies such as *time monitoring, self-checking,* and *self-evaluation* can be used. *Self-questioning* can be facilitated by questions on a cue card. *Role reversal* is another recommended technique: the therapist performs the task with errors, and the client is asked to provide feedback.

Toglia (2005) suggested that transfer of learning can occur in different degrees on a horizontal continuum. Near transfers occur when an individual can perform activities that are similar. Intermediate transfers are activities that share some features with the original task. In far transfers, the activities are physically different from the original activity. Very far transfers are activities in which individuals can apply what they have learned in intervention to everyday occupations, such as work.

First-time exposure of an adolescent or young adult to work activities and occupations during the transition to a working life requires acquaintance with the tasks and the ability to predict the person's ability, performance, and learning experience. Transfer of learning can occur when the student can apply skills learned in school to everyday occupations, such as work.

Transition From the Educational to the Vocational System

As children with special needs make the transition into adolescence and young adulthood, they can require special resources because of physical, sensory, cognitive, and learning challenges; mental health issues; and problems related to social, cultural, linguistic, or family factors (Varga-Toth, 2006). Adolescence is fraught with issues related to identity and competence, particularly so for adolescents with special needs, because maturing physically according to chronological age does not necessarily assure personal maturation. Moving into adulthood requires independence in ADL and IADL skills, leaving the protected school environment for the work environment, and gradual experience in new social roles as an adult. Adolescents are expected to transition to act as "normative adults," which means becoming educated, productive, and independent (Van Naarden Braun, et al., 2006). Adolescents and young adults with special needs benefit from specialists who guide them through this period and provide intervention based on comprehensive and accurate evaluations. Occupational therapy practitioners have unique knowledge and skills to assist adolescents and young adults with the transition from school to adult life (Kemmis and Dunn, 1996; AOTA, 1998, 2008b).

This book emphasizes that the capacity to work is influenced by a wide range of factors—physical, cognitive, emotional, social, and others. In this regard, evaluating the adolescent or young adult with special needs is similar to evaluating clients in other areas of work-related services. However, there are also aspects of evaluation specific to adolescents and young adults, and care should be taken when using tools that are not specifically normed on this population. For example, many of the tests used with adolescents were developed for adults and include norms exclusively for adults (Betz and Nehring, 2007). This section reviews a number of evaluations that may be used as part of transition services, and Table 7.1 summarizes the evaluations.

Evaluations Commonly Used in Planning Transition Services

A well-planned transition from adolescence to young adulthood requires continuity between school life and work life. It requires educational planning focused on achieving the necessary knowledge, competencies, and training for success in a particular type of work that is appropriate to the needs of the adolescent or young adult. It is a spiral pathway involving ongoing evaluation of the student's qualifications and interests to find the proper occupational match for the specific stage the client has reached. This is followed by reevaluation to find an occupation that matches the next stage and prepares the adolescent or young adult for gaining the necessary competencies for that stage. A comprehensive evaluation process is ongoing and takes four forms: (1) evaluation of vocational interests and tendencies, (2) evaluation of performance skills, (3) evaluation of activity and participation (ADL/work), and (4) a work-based evaluation (on the job site).

Evaluation of Vocational Interests and Tendencies
One focus of evaluation where the occupational therapy practitioner may make a particular contribution is identification of the adolescent's or young adult's vocational interests

Table 7.1 Sample Assessments Used During Transition Services With Adolescents and Young Adults With Special Needs

Name of Assessment	Focus	Assessment Outcomes
Self-Directed Search Inventory (Holland, Fritzsche, and Powell, 1994; Holland, Powell, and Fritzsche, 1994)	Vocational interests	Provides a three-letter "Holland Code" based on six worker types: realistic, investigative, artistic, social, enterprising, and conventional. Each worker type corresponds to a set of worker characteristics and can be matched with specific types of occupations.
Canadian Occupational Performance Measurement (COPM) (Law, et al., 1998; McColl and Pollock, 2001)	Self-care, productivity, and leisure	Provides a measure of a client's self-perception of occupational performance in the areas of self-care, productivity, and leisure. Outcome measures of the COPM are the client's most important problems in occupational performance, a total score for performance, and a total score for the client's satisfaction of his or her ability to perform specified activities.
Occupational Performance History Interview II (OPHI II) (Kielhofner, et al., 2004)	Occupational adaption via three scales (occupational identity, occupational competence, and occupational behavior settings)	Provides an appreciation of a person's life history, the impact of disability, and the direction in which the person would like to take his or her life. Occupational identity, occupational competence, and occupational settings (environment) are explored and rated on separate scales. A life history narrative and a graphical narrative slope are created, giving clients the opportunity to reflect upon, continue, or remake life stories.
Worker Role Interview (WRI) (Braveman, et al., 2005)	Psychosocial capacity for work	Provides information on psychosocial and environmental factors affecting the likelihood that an injured worker or person with longstanding disability will return to work. Ratings are completed on16 items.
Feasibility Evaluation Checklist (FEC) (Matheson, Ogden, Violette, and Schultz, 1985)	Capacity to perform job functions	Scores are completed on 21 items in three areas: productivity, safety, and interpersonal behavior. Each item is scored in regard to the present feasibility for competitive employment and the potential for improvement.
Toglia Category Assessment (TCA) (Toglia, 1994)	Mental ability to establish and switch concepts	The TCA uses plastic utensils that can be sorted according to size, color, and type. It emphasizes qualitative aspects of performance and is based on dynamic interactional principles of testing. Detailed and systematic guidelines for facilitating performance through the use of cues are provided. The extent to which performance can be modified with cues provides information that can be directly used to choose and design an intervention program.
Behavioral Assessment of Dysexecutive Syndrome (BADS) (Wilson, Alderman, Burgess, Emslie, and Evans, 1996)	Executive functions	BADS is constructed to sample the range of problems commonly associated with dysexecutive syndrome in four broad areas: emotional or personality changes, motivational changes, behavioral changes, and cognitive changes. Each item is rated on a 5-point scale representing problem severity.

(table continues on page 154)

Table 7.1 Sample Assessments Used During Transition Services With Adolescents and Young Adults With Special Needs—cont'd

Name of Assessment	Focus	Assessment Outcomes
The Neurobehavioral Cognitive Status Examination (Cognistat) (Kiernan, Mueller, Langston, and Van Dyke, 1995)	Neurological health in relation to behavior	Describes performance in central areas of brain-behavior relations: level of consciousness, orientation, attention, language, constructional ability, memory, calculations, and reasoning. The subareas of language are spontaneous speech, comprehension, repetition, and naming. The subareas of reasoning are similarities and judgment. Exploration occurs through interactive behavioral tasks that rely on perception, cognitive processing, and motor skills.
Purdue Pegboard Test (PPT)	Fine and gross motor dexterity and coordination	The PPT measures dexterity for two types of activity: one involving gross movements of hands, fingers, and arms and the other involving "fingertip" dexterity. Five separate scores can be obtained with the PPT: right hand, left hand, both hands, right plus left plus both hands (R+L+B), and assembly.

and tendencies. This knowledge is crucial to creating an effective match between the client and the demands of an appropriate job.

One of the most widely used tools internationally is the *Self-Directed Search (SDS)* interest inventory developed by John Holland and designed to aid in the career decision-making process (Holland, Fritzsche, and Powell, 1994; Holland, Powell, and Fritzsche, 1994). The SDS has six scales based on Holland's career typology theory of career (discussed in Chapter 2). Holland described the six scales using a hexagonal model that categorizes people into six types: (1) realistic, (2) investigative, (3) artistic, (4) social, (5) enterprising, and (6) conventional. According to Holland, both people and careers can be classified into those six different types. People who choose careers that match their own type are most likely to be both satisfied and successful.

Occupational therapy practitioners often use the *Canadian Occupational Performance Measurement (COPM)* to help clarify students' volition and interests and self-perception of performance (Law, et al., 1998; McColl and Pollock, 2001). This assessment measures occupational performance on the basis of a client-centered approach to practice. It is a cross-cultural tool used for a variety of activities and participation in different populations (Carpenter, Baker, and Tyldesley, 2001; Egan, Dubouloz, Vallerand, and Robichaud, 2008; Kjeken, Slatkowsky-Christensen, Kvien, and Uhlig, 2004; Sewell, Singh, Williams, Collier, and Morgan, 2005; Verkerk, Wolf, Louwers, Meester-Delver, and Nollet, 2006). The COPM is administered in three sections corresponding to self-care, productivity, and leisure. It is scored for occupational performance and satisfaction with occupational performance.

The *Occupational Performance History Interview II (OPHI II)* is another assessment that provides insights into the vocational interests and tendencies of an adolescent or young adult (Kielhofner and Henry, 1988; Kielhofner, et al., 2004; Kielhofner, Mallinson, Forsyth, and Lai, 2001). The OPHI II is based on the model of human occupation (see Chapter 4) and is designed to assess the three underlying constructs of occupational adaptation: (1) occupational identity, (2) occupational competence, and (3) the impact of occupation behavior settings. The OPHI II uses a semistructured interview and has been shown to predict the likelihood of being employed or engaged in other productive activity (Levin, Kielhofner, Braveman, and Fogg, 2007).

The *Worker Role Interview (WRI)* is used during the initial assessment process as an adjunct to the typical physical and/or work capacity assessment and provides a measure of psychosocial capacity for working (Biernacki, 1993; Braveman, et al., 2005; Ekbladh, Haglund, and Thorell, 2004; Velozo, et al., 1999). When administering this assessment, the occupational therapist rates factors that support and affect successful return to work. Recommended questions to guide the interview are provided, and observations made during task performance and other aspects of the work capacity assessment are also used to guide scoring of 16 items. Research has demonstrated through Rasch analysis that these items assess the single construct of psychosocial capacity for return to work (Forsyth, et al., 2006).

Evaluation of Performance Skills: Motor, Cognitive, and Emotional Capabilities

The occupational therapy practitioner must thoroughly understand the specific task demands of the occupations performed in a given work setting. Identifying the physical, perceptual, and cognitive demands of a work setting requires specific evaluations of strength, motor coordination, finger dexterity, field of vision, concentration, memory, orientation, social interaction, and appropriate work behavior (see Fig. 7.2). This comprehensive evaluation is essential to identifying behavior that may require special attention during intervention (Reimer, D'Ambrosio, Coughlin, Fried, and Biederman, 2007; Johnson and Rosen, 2000; Stewart, Law, Rosenbaum, and Willms, 2001). Physical assessment of the worker is described in depth in Chapter 12, and cognitive and perceptual assessment is described in depth in Chapter 13. A few assessments commonly used in transition services are described briefly in the next few paragraphs.

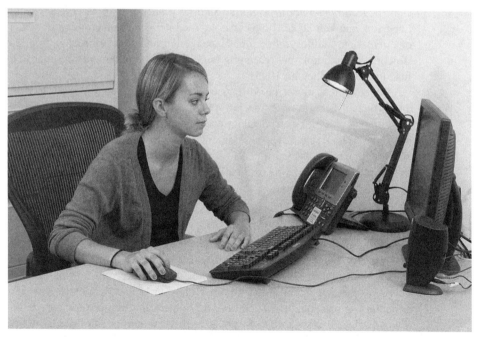

Figure 7.2 Transitional services help to provide the optimal experience for the adolescent and young adult with special needs.

The *Feasibility Evaluation Checklist (FEC)* evaluates behaviors pertaining to acceptability as an employee (Matheson, Ogden, Violette, and Schultz, 1985). It provides information about the ability to cope with basic requirements of work such as attendance, timekeeping, workplace tolerance, and accepting supervision. The FEC is measured by observation in an actual or simulated work environment, a supported work setting, or at a therapeutic workstation. The work environment must be structured to approximate the temporal demands of work, requiring regular daily attendance and adherence to a set schedule. Nonstandardized observations are also common in order to gain an impression about performance patterns such as time management, punctuality, proportion of time spent on work tasks and breaks, and sequence of work.

Standardized assessments are sometimes used for motor and cognitive performance skills, although few assessments are standardized specifically on the population of adolescents and young adults with special needs. When introducing the adolescent or young adult to work, occupational therapy practitioners typically already have access to some data, such as IQ test results and other evaluations administered in the educational setting. When there are specific job demands and specific information is needed, occupational therapists use evaluations such as the *Toglia Category Assessment (TCA)* (Toglia, 1994), a mental ability test that examines the ability of adults with brain injury or psychiatric illness to establish categories and switch conceptual sets. The test emphasizes qualitative aspects of performance and is based on dynamic interactional principles.

An executive function battery often used for such purposes is the *Behavioral Assessment of Dysexecutive Syndrome (BADS;* Wilson, Alderman, Burgess, Emslie, and Evans, 1996). This battery includes six subtests: (1) Temporal Judgment, (2) Rule Shift Cards, (3) Action Program, (4) Key Search, (5) Zoo Map, and (6) Modified Six Elements. The battery aims to predict problem-solving, planning, and organizational skills in everyday tasks and is used with a variety of diagnostic groups (Evans, Chua, McKenna, and Wilson, 1997; Norris and Tate, 2000; Wilson, et al., 1996).

The *Neurobehavioral Cognitive Status Examination,* or *Cognistat* (Kiernan, Mueller, Langston, and Van Dyke, 1995) assesses the intellectual functioning of adults in the areas of orientation, auditory attention, language (comprehension, recognition, naming), construction, calculation, and reasoning (similarities and judgment) in order to test cognitive function (Kiernan, et al., 1995).

Other typical motor performance skills such as strength, endurance, and dexterity are evaluated according to the job demands and the potential skills of the adolescent or young adult (Tuckwell, Straker, and Barrett, 2002). Many jobs require good manual dexterity. When functional assessment of the hand is needed, the *Purdue Pegboard Test (PPT)* can be used. It measures gross movements of hands, fingers and arms, and fingertip dexterity and was originally used to screen the dexterity of industrial workers. The PPT has been standardized for men and women of different ages and for different occupations (Tiffin, 1987).

Evaluation of Activity and Participation

The ICF (introduced in Chapter 2) was adopted by the WHO in 2008. It provides a conceptual framework and specific terminology that facilitates investigation of the consequences of developmental disabilities in young adulthood. According to this framework, activity limitations are an inability to carry out daily tasks independently and can range from difficulties in personal care, such as ADL, to difficulty in more complex activities, such as fixing meals and paying bills. By applying the ICF and measuring activity limitations as a dimension separate from that of impairment, we can test the general assumption that activity limitations in young adulthood do not inevitably arise from childhood impairment.

If applying the ICF framework, ADL and IADL are part of the performance domains evaluated when considering occupational characteristics and needs. For example, adolescents and young adults with special needs, like other workers, need to have proper dress and appearance, use transportation to get to and from work, and be able to do basic calculations in order to pay and get change. As far as daily activities, adolescents and young adults are typically considered along with adults, and usually there are no specific tools for adolescents. The *Functional Status Questionnaire (FSQ)*, a self-administered instrument that measures daily function (ADL, IADL, work, social interaction), is often used (Jett and Cleary, 1987). The *Daily Activities Checklist (DAC)* is a self-administered questionnaire as well. It is aimed more at populations with mental health problems who live in the community. It covers home activities, community-living skills, socialization, and quality of performance (Brown, et al., 1996).

Information from family members can help occupational therapists gain a comprehensive view of the client. The *Instrumental Activities of Daily Living Scale* is a questionnaire administered to a family member and gives information about independence in IADL, such as shopping, home duties, and public transportation (Lawton and Brody, 1969). Focused tests for ADL and IADL are used to evaluate specific problems. For example, the *Executive Functions Performance Test (EFPT)* assesses the level of assistance required when occupations involve executive functions (Baum, Morrison, Hahn, and Edwards, 2007). The *Modified Kitchen Task Assessment (M-KTA)* evaluates executive functions during the performance of kitchen tasks (Baum and Edwards, 1993).

Evaluations of functional capacity are sometimes needed during the transitional process in order to gain specific information about physically demanding jobs. A variety of functional capacity evaluations (FCEs) refer to work, and these evaluations are discussed in depth in Chapter 12. In the case of an adolescent or young adult, FCEs should be used with caution because many of these tests have norms exclusively for adults (Betz and Nehring, 2007). Some FCEs are tailored specifically to a population or to a specific diagnosis such as low back pain, and few adolescents and young adults within the special education system face these problems.

Onsite or At-the-Job Evaluation

We must be aware of limitations associated with standardized assessments; many may emphasize disability and identification of deficit rather than ability and identification of strengths. For some people with disabilities, it is preferable to carry out customized evaluations at the job site. Sometimes situational assessments in work settings, or *onsite evaluations,* allow the occupational therapy practitioner to obtain a more accurate picture of the client's capabilities. Such assessments enable more effective transition services and support (Kardos and White, 2005). In general, onsite evaluations are recommended as part of the evaluation process, and such evaluations are well established in a wide variety of therapeutic environments (Kardos and White, 2005; Spencer and O'Daniel, 2005). These evaluations can start while the adolescent or young adult is still at school, and they offer a way to bridge the gap between the therapeutic environment and a work setting. A particular strength of onsite evaluations is that they enable appropriate task analysis for the occupations involved in the specific type of work. A detailed task analysis of the specific job serves as the basis for creating the best match between a job and the person.

According to Koller (1994), this process involves several stages. The first stage is a task analysis of the job. The practitioner then provides "job teaching" in which a job coach teaches the job tasks as a process of evaluation. During this process, if the disability requires job modification or accommodations, whether physical or cognitive, they are offered to enable the new worker to better use his or her skills to meet the job demands.

The strategies are taught, and the new worker is trained to implement new approaches in the workplace as part of the evaluation. The last stage is empowerment, which is achieved by repeated training and positive reinforcement.

The large range of variability in physical, cognitive, emotional, and psychosocial conditions of the adolescent or young adult with special needs demands individualized evaluation and highly individualized methods of support. When standardized assessments are used, special biomechanical, physiological, and function norms must be applied (Phelps and Hanley-Maxwell, 1997). Nevertheless, standardized evaluations are often inappropriate for use with adolescents or young adults, and therefore nonstandardized and onsite evaluations are often used.

Intervention

An Overview

Historically, individuals with developmental disabilities lacked adequate vocational opportunities that included social integration. As late as the 1970s, a common view held that individuals with developmental disabilities needed to be protected and could only engage in work that involved routine and repetitive tasks (Kiernan, 2000). This view led to the cultivation of sheltered workshops. Sheltered workshops were and are segregated places where individuals with disabilities go to develop basic vocational skills (e.g., assembly and collating) and participate in daily work activities with other individuals with similar disabilities. Sheltered workshops are viewed as training centers for some adolescents and young adults with special needs who will then move on to more integrated and competitive vocational experiences. For others, a sheltered workshop may be considered an end goal (Kiernan, 2000). Current evidence suggests that adolescents and young adults with special needs, even those with significant cognitive impairments, who learn vocational skills in an integrated context have better outcomes than those with similar disabilities who do not (Jahoda, Kemp, Riddell, and Banks, 2008; White and Weiner, 2004).

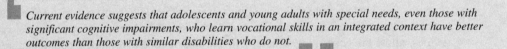

Current evidence suggests that adolescents and young adults with special needs, even those with significant cognitive impairments, who learn vocational skills in an integrated context have better outcomes than those with similar disabilities who do not.

Many adolescents and young adults with special needs, especially those with significant motor, cognitive, and communication needs, first receive vocational skills training in traditional classroom or school-based environments (White and Weiner, 2004). The purpose of providing services in this context is to ensure that necessary readiness skills are developed before the student enters the community setting (Rutkowski, Daston, Van Kuiken, and Riehle, 2006; White and Weiner, 2004). For example, a young adult with a significant intellectual disability and autism who has vocational goals related to obtaining a janitorial job in the community may first work on cleaning skills in his or her own classroom. The teacher and the occupational therapy practitioner may design opportunities and training experiences for the young adult to sweep and mop the floor, empty trash cans, or wash tables or desks. Another young adult with significant motor impairments might wish to work at a movie theater. This young adult might first learn to handle money and operate a cash register through simulated experiences in the classroom (see Fig. 7.3). While this

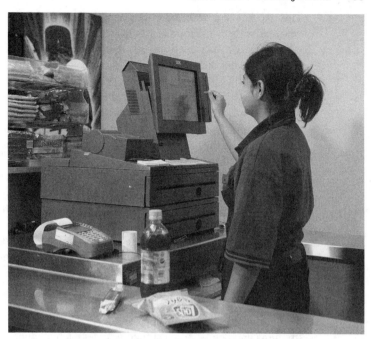

Figure 7.3 Simulated experience in the classroom can prepare the individual for independent work.

model emphasizes readiness, instruction is not provided in the natural working environment, and some of the skills may be lost by young adults who have difficulty generalizing their learning from one context to another (White and Weiner, 2004).

Another model of providing vocational training is the work-study model (Rutkowski, et al., 2006). This model combines traditional classroom instruction and work simulation strategies with opportunities to practice skills at a job site a few hours a week. Such an approach provides the young adult with an opportunity to experience work in a real-life setting to ensure that skills are generalized (King, Baldwin, Currie, and Evans, 2005). The adolescent or young adult is often accompanied by a job coach, and the onsite training occurs during off-peak hours. A job coach is a person hired by a community or educational agency to provide training and assistance in the work environment (ODEP, 1993). A job coach can use different strategies to foster success in the worker role. According to Ohtake and Chadsey (2001), these strategies include:

- Providing opportunities for the coworkers to autonomously provide support.
- Suggesting to coworkers that they support the adolescent or young adult with special needs in specific work occupations.
- Overseeing the support provided by coworkers.
- Providing opportunities for coworkers to provide instruction.
- Providing direct training with input from coworkers.
- Providing direct training without input from coworkers.

Job coaches have to balance the amount of support they provide with the adolescent's or young adult's needs and the coworkers' desire for involvement. The support provided by the job coach is dynamic and can be viewed on a continuum with the job coach providing more or less support as needed (Ohtake and Chadsey, 2001).

Job coaches also play a large role in supported employment settings. The purpose of supported employment is to facilitate the development of work skills for individuals with disabilities who, due to the nature of their impairments, are expected to require continuous or temporary support in order to perform the essential duties of their job (ODEP, 1993).

This type of setting is described in detail in Chapter 6. Adolescents and young adults who participate in supported employment opportunities report receiving higher wages, better benefits, increased job satisfaction, and more satisfying social outcomes than do individuals with disabilities who do not participate in supported employment opportunities (Jahoda, et al., 2008; White and Weiner, 2004).

Supported employment, also called integrated employment, is a form of competitive or paid employment, and such opportunities take place in the community (White and Weiner, 2004). Adolescents with disabilities can be matched to a community-based worksite where they work individually with their job coach or as part of a small team of individuals with disabilities. For example, several adolescents or young adults from the same vocational or educational agency might be employed by a hotel. Each of the individuals would have their own job, but they may possibly work in different departments (e.g., housekeeping and kitchen). A key feature of supported employment is the emphasis on natural supports. Natural supports include mentoring, training with coworkers without disabilities, opportunities to receive feedback from coworkers and site supervisors regarding job performance, and opportunities for socializing and developing relationships with coworkers (ODEP, 1993). Such natural supports are thought to assist the adolescent or youth with special needs with learning the culture of the workplace and increase the likelihood of job retention (Jahoda, et al., 2008).

Individualized transition plans take into account each student's unique profile of strengths and needs, are designed to meet each student's plans for the future, and generally include goals related to further education, community participation, and vocational development (Kohler and Field, 2003; Orentlicher, 2007). Family members, school personnel, and outside agency staff may support the student in working toward his or her transition goals. These individuals are also responsible for developing a summary of performance (SOP), which outlines the student's progress and current functioning in the areas of academics, functional skills, and vocational skills (Individuals with Disabilities Education Improvement Act of 2004, § 614 [c] [5] [B] [ii]).

Effective transition plans are student-centered, focused on student development, collaborative, and dependent on a high level of family involvement (Kohler and Field, 2003). Student-centered plans take into account the student's interests, personal goals, and dreams (Michaels and Orentlicher, 2004). School teams can use a variety of planning tools to collect information from students and their families, such as the MAPS (Vandercook, York, and Forest, 1989) and the PATH system (Falvey, et al., 2003). These systems help professionals to structure discussions with students and families to explore postschool outcomes and design individualized plans to meet these outcomes (Michaels and Orentlicher, 2004). In addition to student-centered planning, school teams are required to complete age-appropriate evaluations focused on education, training, independent living skills, and employment-related skills (Kardos and White, 2006).

The Training Process

Training clients for the transition from the educational setting to a work setting is a three-stage process (see Box 7.3) involving (1) knowledge acquisition; (2) group experiencing of work skills and cognitive, emotional, and behavioral processing; and (3) personal experience in a work environment and development of an occupational personality.

Stage 1: Knowledge Acquisition

In school, students receive individualized educational services in the least restrictive environment and are supported by professionals who have expertise in the area of special education. The opportunity to individualize educational services means that students can learn in an environment that suits their abilities while presenting a level of challenge or difficulty that is "just right."

Box 7.3   The Training Process

- *Knowledge acquisition:* The client learns about different work and work characteristics, policies related to the workplace, and behavioral norms at the workplace.
- *Group experience:* The client gains work skills and learns cognitive, emotional, and behavioral processing through work workshops and transitional workshop.
- *Personal experience:* The client experiences a work environment and develops an occupational personality by defining individual areas of occupation, finding the appropriate occupation and environment, and receiving guidance during the occupational experience.

The first stage in the transition to the work environment is introducing the adolescent or young adult to the various work-related programs. These programs are typically introduced by the teachers, occupational therapy practitioners, and other team members. Lessons about the work-related programs take place in the classroom and are complemented by videos, stories, and pictures. Additionally, when addressing behavior-related knowledge, the lessons are complemented with workshops and role-playing. In the course of the lessons, the educational staff connects the conceptual framework to the individual world of each student using examples from the student's private life.

The areas of knowledge that are part of these lessons can be divided into three components: (1) knowledge about different work and work characteristics, (2) knowledge about policies related to the workplace, and (3) knowledge about behavioral norms in the workplace. These components are described in Table 7.2.

Table 7.2   Knowledge Components of the Skills Acquisition Stage

Knowledge About Different Work and Various Work Characteristics

Characteristics of the physical environment	Logistics related to work, including the location of employment, distance from home, distance from other known places, etc.
	Size of the building where the work will take place
	Stimuli at worksite, such as temperature, noise, intensity of the light
	Other factors such as how the environment is organized and standards related to cleanliness
Characteristics of the human environment	Number of people at work and number of people involved in a work task
	Relationships among workers, including managers and coworkers
	Characteristics of coworkers, such as gender, age, interests
	Encounters with familiar and unknown people at work and encounters with peers and persons with authority
	Nature of the work as it relates to others, such as providing and receiving services
Content characteristics	Exposure to various work tasks (e.g., copying, packaging, answering phones, providing service, cooking, gardening, maintenance, data entry)
Characteristics of work requirements	Specific roles and responsibilities related to work (e.g., animal handling involves cleaning cages, not just interacting with animals)
	Expectations connected to specific work (e.g., maintaining confidentiality in hospital settings)

Knowledge About Policies Related to the Workplace

Work is different from school in that individuals do not necessarily stay with the same cohort or peer group as time goes on. Individuals are responsible for finding their own job and getting to and from their own workplace (with the assistance of the team as needed).

(table continues on page 162)

Table 7.2 Knowledge Components of the Skills Acquisition Stage—cont'd

The workplace is not a permanent place for life. People can choose to leave their workplace, and the workplace can choose to dismiss employees who do not meet expectations or for economic reasons.

People receive payment according to the amount of time they work and the function they fulfill. Full-time employment is generally based on an 8-hour workday. Some employees work only part time and therefore receive less pay.

The number of vacation days from work is usually fewer than the days off that are given in school. At most workplaces, employees need approval for taking vacation days and must notify the employer in advance of taking them.

Employees who receive a salary are often entitled to sick days. Workers who are employed on an hourly basis may not be eligible for sick days. Different places of employment have different procedures for excused absences from work. For example, some places of employment may require employees to call their supervisors to announce an absence, and others may require documentation from a physician related to the absence. Not following the workplace's procedures may result in docked pay or even termination.

Employees must meet the required schedules. This includes punching in and out on time and returning on time from breaks.

Information about methods related to job searching and networking.

Information and experience related to interviewing, writing résumés, and writing letters of resignation.

Knowledge About Behavioral Norms in the Workplace

The difference between the supports available at school and at the workplace and the need to manage certain responsibilities independently or with little assistance (e.g., managing transportation to and from work, arriving to work on time).

Expectations related to work schedules.

Expectations related to physical appearance. Dynamic activities can be used to teach adolescents and young adults that their physical appearance is their "business card." At this stage it is necessary to raise their awareness that their acceptance at work depends also on their physical appearance, which includes proper clothing, personal cleanliness, esthetics, and more.

Expectations related to interpersonal relationships (e.g., policies related to dating coworkers).

As part of the first stage, the team works with the students to define the concept of work and explore the various characteristics of work. The differences between various occupations are emphasized in the physical, cognitive, social, and emotional realms.

Adolescents and young adults may have little or no knowledge about the norms related to appropriate behavior in the workplace or various policies related to specific places of employment. Examples of the type of knowledge students need regarding workplace policies are included in Table 7.2.

In preparation to join the labor force, students must develop responsibility, initiative, independence, and greater self-discipline than is necessary in school. Moreover, they are exposed to a new type of interpersonal confrontations, including meeting people of different ages but the same status as theirs at work. Workers are responsible for their normative behavior. They must meet schedules and maintain a physical appearance that is appropriate for the work environment. Table 7.2 presents four types of examples of this knowledge.

Knowledge in these areas is generally acquired in dynamic workshops or lessons. The lessons are usually conducted by a teacher and a rehabilitation professional. Lessons are accompanied by exposure to various situations by means of stories, descriptions of various events, case studies, and dramatizations, which should be analyzed within the framework of the classroom. Cognitive and behavioral processing of the events makes it possible to define acceptable behavioral standards that can be used for better integration in the workplace.

Stage 2: Group Experiencing of Work Skills and Cognitive, Emotional, and Behavioral Processing

In parallel with knowledge and exposure, the adolescent or young adult must also experience the work environment as a means for personal and occupational study and growth. The school framework is different in many respects from the work environment. For example, coping at the workplace requires various skills that are fundamentally different from those used in the school environment, and therefore exposure to work experiences must be gradual. Different types of work spaces enable studying the necessary skills and how to function within these spaces. These include *work workshops* and *transitional workshops* (Devine and Koch, 2003).

Work workshops are provided within the school or rehabilitation framework. The workshop is usually conducted by a teacher or instructor who instructs and guides the adolescents and young adults in various work areas. Usually, each workshop deals with one or two specific occupations, and it is conducted in a room other than the classroom. With the help of assignments, participants learn independence on the job; responsibility; and development of self-regulation abilities, initiative, problem-solving, and more. The objective of the workshop is primarily the development of basic work habits that differ from study habits. Additionally, participants are exposed to a range of assignments and to various types of occupations. In schools in which there is only one workshop room, several occupations are usually handled in the same room. Adolescents and young adults also benefit from informal assessments conducted by an occupational therapy practitioner and the workshop instructor during various lessons. The objective of the assessment is to determine the differences between the existing requirements of a particular work task and the current functioning of the student as it relates to the skills necessary to complete the work task.

Transitional workshops are experiences provided outside the school or rehabilitation framework. These workshops usually involve a group of students who go together with a staff member (e.g., teacher, occupational therapy practitioner) from the school to a workplace. At the workplace, the students receive work-related instructions and must confront the new environment. If they experience difficulties, have questions, or cannot cope, they can receive support from the staff member with whom they are familiar. In a gradual and guided manner, the staff member coaches the student on how to independently and appropriately address other workers in the environment. In parallel with the experience, cognitive, behavioral, and emotional processing of the experience is conducted. The processing includes analysis of both the positive and problematic events that occur during the experience, with an attempt to teach the principles involved and to help students apply them for use in the future.

Transitional workshops can have diverse characteristics:

- *Projects that offer a limited time in which a group of students performs a certain task.* When the task is completed, the project ends. Examples are a packing project in preparation for an unusual event or the planting of a garden.
- *Permanent work that continues over time.* Examples are packaging projects that are ongoing or the maintenance of a garden.

- *Completing several different functions at a workplace.* Students arrive at the place as a group, accompanied by a teacher, an occupational therapy practitioner, a coach, or another team member. Each student has his or her own workstation. At the end of the day, students assemble as a group and return to school or go home.
- *Occupational training that integrates occupational experience in the studied area.* For example, the cooking course taken by Gail in the case introduction included a day of theoretical studies at the hotel. The teachers were professionals from the hotel and were joined by a special education teacher. In addition, the course required 3 days of work in the hotel's kitchens with an occupational therapy practitioner accompanying the practical study of the profession.

It is recommended to allow each student to have three experiences in various work environments, with assignments in different types of work settings to maximize the student's breadth of work skills. Each experience can last from 3 to 4 months to a full academic year.

Stage 3: Personal Experience in a Work Environment and Development of an Occupational Worker Role

In stages 1 and 2, adolescents and young adults with special needs typically are exposed to a variety of experiences and occupational fields within a class or group framework. They encounter a range of occupations in school and in transitional workshops. From this limited selection, they can choose the fields that were most closely aligned with their interests and strengths. The next step is the individual stage.

One of the main differences between the school and work environments pertains to leaving the supportive and protective framework of the classroom, with its peer group of corresponding age, and starting life individually and separately. At this stage, the intervention of the professional workers, especially of the occupational therapy practitioner, becomes more individualized and personal.

The beginning of this stage includes exposure to preferred areas of work. With this in mind, the adolescent or young adult and the occupational therapy practitioner collect all the personal information that has accumulated in the course of the vocational development process. In the process of this data collection, the adolescent or young adult is made aware of personal factors that are relevant to finding the best occupational match, which include the following:

- Areas of interest specific to working.
- Work environments that appear most appropriate and supportive of occupational performance, including both the physical and the social environment.
- The scope of employment or the number of days and hours most appropriate for the adolescent or young adult to work.

The next stage involves the adolescent or young adult and the occupational therapy practitioner presenting their findings to everyone involved in the transition plan, including family members (generally the parents), the program coordinator (teacher/social worker), and all the people who provided significant intervention services throughout the process.

Differences of opinion may occur among participants in the process. Resolving the oppositions and debating the various components of the program enables raising the awareness of the adolescent or young adult and serves as a good preparation for what is to follow.

At the end of this stage, the complete team (the adolescent or young adult, the family, and the rehabilitation/educational staff) devise a plan for finding a workplace where the student can attempt independent work. The choice involves the occupational area, the workplace, the scope of the employment, and the degree to which the environment is supported.

Finding the Appropriate Type of Work and Environment

The job search process is complex. It depends to a great extent on the job market, where the adolescent or young adult resides, and, naturally, on the specific field being sought. Different members of the team may be responsible for directing the job search, but however the responsibilities are dispersed, it is critical that the adolescent or young adult be involved with the process and understand the difficulty of finding work.

The occupational therapy practitioner and the adolescent or young adult together search for job opportunities using such sources as the newspaper, the Internet, and personal acquaintances. The prospective workplace is usually approached by one of the professionals.

The occupational therapy practitioner introduces the adolescent or young adult as a person with special needs and describes his or her abilities and skills without disclosing personal details and diagnoses. In general, at this stage, interested employers may need to explore legal aspects of hiring a young person with a disability, and the client is not involved in this step of the process. Initially, prospective employers should consider providing the adolescent or young adult with an experience in the open labor market for the sake of the experience, with limited working hours and days, limited variety and complexity of the tasks, and generally no pay. Gradually, the employer will be expected to assign more responsibilities, schedule increased working hours, and begin treating the adolescent or young adult like a regular employee.

Once the employer has agreed to the various terms, the occupational therapy practitioner and the adolescent or young adult set up a job interview. This interview also can serve as an opportunity for the client to tour the workplace. Prior to meeting with prospective employers, a résumé should be prepared and reviewed, and the adolescent or young adult should be prepared for the initial introduction and job interview. This can be accomplished in a group or individually with the occupational therapy practitioner and the teacher.

The occupational therapy practitioner should work with the adolescent or young adult on proper physical appearance for the interview, acceptable behavior, the limits of what is being disclosed in a job interview, and so on. Often the occupational therapy practitioner accompanies the client to the job interview and provides support as needed, such as negotiating a start date if a job offer is made. Each work opportunity and workplace must be treated differently, and all individuals involved must prepared for the unexpected and for events that may not go according to plans.

Guidance During the Work Experience

After an opportunity has been secured in an appropriate workplace, the adolescent or young adult, and often the employer, must be guided through the process of integrating the client into the workplace. Each party involved needs guidance to a different extent, and the professional providing the guidance (sometimes a job coach, other times the occupational therapist) must constantly adapt to the situation. It may be necessary for the guide to remain at the workplace to help mediate situations with other workers related to learning the job, becoming familiar with the site, coping with new people and a new place, and so on. The guide also provides support for the other workers and models how to interact with and provide feedback to the adolescent or young adult. Team members must be alert and sensitive regarding their presence at each workplace. At some worksites, it is appropriate to have close and personal contact with the adolescent or young adult on the first day; at other work sites, it is more appropriate to wait to follow up with the student after his or her initial orientation.

The adolescent or young adult and the occupational therapy practitioner meet regularly, and the frequency of these meetings is based on the individual's needs. The objectives of the meetings are to review the various events taking place at the workplace and in personal lives, to celebrate accomplishments, and to identify areas for support. The employer and the new worker may identify many difficulties arising during the initial orientation and training process. One of the main functions of the occupational therapy practitioner during this stage is to highlight successes and abilities and problem-solve strategies to reduce difficulties. If, for example, the young adult is doing an accurate job but not in a timely manner, the occupational therapist will highlight the accurate job and provide strategies for improving work pace. The therapist will then provide graded support and reinforcement until the expected pace is achieved.

The occupational therapy practitioner's function in addressing the difficulties faced by the adolescent or young adult at the workplace include analyzing the situation, identifying the source of the difficulty, and finding ways to match skills and abilities to work functions. The occupational therapy practitioner may then make recommendations related to the use of adaptive devices or equipment, the use of a compensation strategy to circumvent the difficulties, and alternative functions or technologies that better match the skills and abilities of the individual.

Over time and with success, the scope of employment is increased, and the degree of direct involvement by the occupational therapy practitioner is reduced. Visits to the workplace can then become less frequent, and the client is encouraged to seek support from the occupational therapy practitioner when new issues arise.

In the final stage, if the adolescent or young adult has been acclimated and accepted at the workplace, by agreement between the staff and the employer, he or she is hired as a regular employee. From this point on, the occupational therapy practitioner's follow-up is further reduced. Problem-solving at this stage can be handled in a group meeting with other adolescents and young adults in similar situations. However, some issues may arise that are of such significance that they require the team to go back and restart the process at the appropriate point. In the case of a mismatch, the team's primary function is to assist the adolescent or young adult in coping emotionally with this setback and cultivating a sense of hope and belief in future success.

It is important to note that even if there is a mismatch at the workplace or in a given job, and a change in workplace must be made, the repeat process is usually more focused and successful. The adolescent or young adult is more aware of his or her specific needs, the occupational therapy practitioner can assess strengths and limitations with greater accuracy, and the experience of the entire team generally makes the process more efficient and productive.

Chapter Summary

Chapter 7 provided an overview of adolescents and young adults with special needs who face unique challenges as they transition to adulthood. In the past few decades, society has begun to view the young person with special needs in a different light. The intrinsic value of the individual and the individual's ability to contribute in his or her own unique way are recognized. The enactment of new legislation combined with the understanding that children with special needs grow up to be adolescents who need vocational rehabilitation has led to a process focused on creating opportunities for young adults to achieve maximal participation. Laws and social policies have evolved to protect the individual and provide opportunities that in the past were not available, and occupational therapy services have advanced to provide social, cognitive, environmental, and work experience training and support throughout the life span. Identifying the unique needs of this population allows for the occupational therapy practitioner to provide the best services possible. The many theoretical models and evaluation tools can assist with developing effective strategies.

Despite the statistics indicating that employment rates for adolescents and young adults with special needs are lower than for the same age group without special needs, the literature suggests that when provided with appropriate support and training, these adolescents and young adults have better outcomes than those who do not receive intervention. Parents, family, caregivers, teachers, therapists, and employers are all important members of the team, and working together in concert helps to provide the optimal circumstances for achievement.

Case Resolution

Gail received transition services in a treatment setting that included a special education school and a vocational rehabilitation center. The intervention process lasted 3 years with an additional year of intermittent follow-up and guidance.

After Gail was integrated at the center, she chose to attend a workshop on the art of cooking. Subsequently, she participated in enrichment courses on community services, mobility, banking, and preparation for the workplace. Her functioning was affected greatly by her moods. Some of the moods were the result of fatigue caused by excessive effort at work or by comments she received from the staff. A behavioral program was created with Gail and her family to improve her ability to persevere in her tasks at the center. During therapeutic sessions in the occupational therapy department, a cognitive intervention was performed to improve Gail's functioning and to raise her awareness of her strengths, abilities, successes, and difficulties. The occupational therapist and Gail also sought to identify strategies designed to help her circumvent her difficulties and separate her functioning from her emotional state. Finally, Gail, her family, and the professional team defined the scope of work that would match her abilities and developed awareness of her strengths.

After the program was established, Gail's attendance at the center greatly improved, and she experienced increased success with the tasks assigned to her. After approximately a year and a half and many successful experiences, Gail applied to a cooking course conducted in cooperation with a participating hotel. At the beginning of the course, she regressed in perseverance and had difficulty with instructions, and her emotional states affected her work greatly. During this period, intervention included processing her difficulties with adaptation and using the tools she had acquired in earlier training. A few weeks later, she returned to her previous level of functioning. Only then was it possible to devote effort to acquiring the occupational skills that would enable her to function within the type of work she chose. She learned strategies for organizing the workspace and techniques for cooking tasks, such as selecting the right knife, holding it safely, and cutting, paring, or slicing proficiently. Gail also learned to seek help as needed, cope with criticism without a sense of failure, and work cooperatively with the supervisor to define the breaks she needed in order to continue to succeed.

At the end of the course, Gail was selected as an exceptional trainee. This commendation opened the possibility for her to obtain work at the hotel. Following a process of deliberation and clarification, Gail, her family, and the team decided that she would continue working in the kitchen and would work 3 days a week at the hotel. She learned to work with remote supervision and to seek assistance from her coworkers when necessary. Subsequently, she began working within the framework of supported employment with an adjusted minimum wage and was able to accept the authority of her supervisors and the rules of the workplace.

In parallel to the process at work, Gail became more independent in everyday living. She traveled independently using public transportation over long distances and initiated community services independently (social services, health services, banking, etc.). Gail helped daily with chores at her parents' home (cleaning, cooking, and laundry). In her leisure time, Gail met friends and shopped for herself.

References

Agran, M., Snow, K., & Swaner, J. (1999). A survey of secondary level teachers' opinions on community-based instruction and inclusive education. *Journal of the Association for Persons with Severe Handicaps, 24*(1), 58–62.

American Occupational Therapy Association (AOTA). (1998). *Standards of Practice for Occupational Therapists.* Bethesda, MD: AOTA Press. Permission to reprint for nonprofit, educational use only.

American Occupational Therapy Association (AOTA). (2008a). Occupational therapy practice framework: Domain and process, 2nd ed. *American Journal of Occupational Therapy, 62*, 625–683.

American Occupational Therapy Association (AOTA). (2008b). Transitions for children and youth: How occupational therapy can help. Retrieved from www.aota.org/Consumers/FactSheets/Children/Transitions.aspx.

American Psychiatric Association. (2000). *Diagnostic and Statistical Manual of Mental Disorders, 4th ed, Text Revision (DSM-IV-TRTM).* Washington, DC: American Psychiatric Association.

Baum, C. M., & Edwards, D. (1993). Cognitive performance in senile dementia of the Alzheimer's type: The kitchen task assessment. *American Journal of Occupational Therapy, 47*(5), 431–436.

Baum, C., Morrison, T., Hahn, M., & Edwards, D. (2007). *Executive Function Performance Test: Test Protocol Booklet.* St. Louis, MO: Program in Occupational Therapy, Washington University School of Medicine.

Bellini, J., & Royce-Davis, J. (1999). Order of selection in vocational rehabilitation: Implications for the transition from school to adult outcomes for youth with learning disabilities. *Work, 13*(1), 3–11.

Betz, C. L., & Nehring, W. M. (eds.). (2007). *Promoting Health Care Transitions for Adolescents with Special Health Care Needs and Disabilities.* Baltimore: Paul H Brookes Publishing.

Biernacki, S. D. (1993). Reliability of the Worker Role Interview. *American Journal of Occupational Therapy, 47*(9), 797–803.

Blomquist, K. B. (2006). Health, education, work, and independence of young adults with disabilities. *Orthopedic Nursing, 25*(3), 168–187.

Bollingmo, G. (1997). Survey of employment services and vocational outcomes for individuals with mental retardation in Norway. *Journal of Vocational Rehabilitation 8*(3), 269–283.

Braveman, B., Robson, M., Velozo, C., Kielhofner, G., Fisher, G. S., Forsyth, K., et al. (2005). *The Worker Role Interview (Version 10).* Chicago: Model of Human Occupation Clearinghouse: Department of Occupational Therapy.

Brown, C., Hamera, E., & Long, C. (1996). The Daily Activities Checklist: A functional assessment for consumers with mental illness living in the community. *Occupational Therapy in Health Care, 10*(3), 33–34.

Brown, B. V., Moore, K. A., & Bzostek, S. (2004). *A Statistical Portrait of Well-being in Early Adulthood.* Child Trends DataBank CrossCurrents Brief, Issue 2, #2004-18.

Canadian Association of Occupational Therapy (CAOT). (1997). *Enabling Occupation: An Occupational Therapy Perspective.* Toronto: CAOT Publications.

Carpenter, L., Baker, G. A., & Tyldesley, B. (2001). The use of the Canadian Occupational Performance Measure as an outcome of a pain management program. *Canadian Journal of Occupational Therapy, 68*(1), 16–22.

Chadsey-Rusch, J., & Heal, L. (1995). Building consensus from transition experts on social integration outcomes and interventions. *Except Child, 62*, 165–187.

Council of the European Union. (2000). Implementing the principle of equal treatment between persons irrespective of racial or ethnic origin, Council Directive 2000/43/EC. Retrieved from http://eur-lex.europa.eu/LexUriServ/LexUriServ.do?uri=OJ:L:2000:180:0022:0026:EN:PDF.

Cresswell, M. K., & Rugg, S. A. (2003). The Canadian Occupational Performance Measure: Its use with clients with schizophrenia. *International Journal of Therapy and Rehabilitation, 10*(12), 544–551.

Devine, M. A., & Koch, L. C. (2003). Recreational planning: An important component of career counseling for people with disabilities. *Work, 21*(1), 83–88.

Egan, M., Dubouloz, C. J., Vallerand, J., & Robichaud, L. (2008). Exploring the impact of a new translation process on the performance of French form writers of the Canadian Certification exam. *Canadian Journal of Occupational Therapy, 75*(3), 191–192.

Ekbladh, E., Haglund, L., & Thorell, L. (2004). The Worker Role Interview: Preliminary data on the predictive validity of return to work of clients after an insurance medicine investigation. *Journal of Occupational Rehabilitation, 14*(2), 131–141.

Evans, G. W. (2006). Child development and the physical environment. *Annual Review of Psychology, 57*, 423–451.

Evans, J. J., Chua, S. E., McKenna, P. J., & Wilson, B. A. (1997). Assessment of the dysexecutive syndrome in schizophrenia. *Psychological Medicine, 27*(3), 1–12.

Falvey, M., Forest, M., Pearpoint, J., & Rosenberg, R. (2003). *All My Life's a Circle—Using the Tools: Circles, MAPS, & PATHS.* Toronto: Inclusion Press.

Felce, D., & Perry, J. (1997). A PASS 3 evaluation of community residences in Wales. *Mental Retardation 35*(3), 170–176.

Forsyth, K., Braveman, B., Kielhofner, G., Ekbladh, E., Haglund, L., Fenga, K., & Keller, J. (2006). Psychometric properties of the worker role interview. *Work, 27*(3), 313–318.

Groce, N. E. (1999). Disability in cross-cultural perspective: Rethinking disability. *Lancet, 354*(9180), 756–757.

Hagner, D., & Sande, J. V. (1998). School-sponsored work experience and vocational instruction. In F. R. Rusch & J. G. Chadsey (eds.), *Beyond High School: Transition from School to Work.* Belmont, CA: Wadsworth.

Holland, J., Fritzsche, B., & Powell, A. (1994). *Self-Directed Search: Technical Manual.* Odessa, FL: Psychological Assessment Resources.

Holland, J., Powell, A., & Fritzsche, B. (1994). *Self-Directed Search: Professional User's Guide.* Odessa, FL: Psychological Assessment Resources.

Hughes, C. (2001). Transition to adulthood: Supporting young adults to access social, employment, and civic pursuits. *Mental Retardation & Developmental Disabilities Research Reviews, 7*(2), 84–90.

Hughes, C., & Carter, E. W. (2000). *The Transition Handbook: Strategies High School Teachers Use That Work!* Baltimore, MD: Paul H. Brookes.

Hughes, C., Eisenman, L. T., Hwang, B., Kim, J., Scott, S. V., & Killian, D. J. (1997a). Transition from secondary special education to adult life: A review and analysis of empirical measures. *Education and Training in Mental Retardation and Developmental Disabilities, 32*(2), 85–104.

Hughes, C., Hwang, B., Kim, J., Killian, D. J., & Harmer, M. L. (1997b). A preliminary validation of strategies that support the transition from school to adult life. *Career Development for Exceptional Individuals, 20*(1), 1–14.

Hughes, C., Kim, J., Bogseon, H., Killian, D. J., Fischer, G. M., Brock, M. G., Godshall, J. C., & Houser, B. (1997c).

Practitioner-validated secondary transition support strategies. *Education and Training in Mental Retardation and Developmental Disabilities, 32*(3), 201–212.

Hughes, C., Rung, L. L., Wehmeyer, M. L., Agran, M., Copeland, S. R., & Hwang, B. (2000). Self-prompted communication book use to increase social interaction among high school students. *Journal of the Association for Persons with Severe Handicaps, 25*(3), 153–166.

Individuals with Disabilities Education Improvement Act of 2004. Pub.L. 108-446, 20 U.S.C. § 1400 et seq.

Jahoda, A., Kemp, J., Riddell, S., & Banks, P. (2008). Feelings about work: A review of socio-emotional impact of supported employment on people with intellectual disabilities. *Journal of Applied Research in Intellectual Disabilities, 21*(1), 1–18.

Jett, A. M., & Cleary, P. D. (1987). Functional disability assessment. *Journal of Physical Therapy, 67*(12), 1854–1859.

Johnson, R., & Rosen, L. (2000). Sports behavior of ADHD children. *Journal of Attention Disorders, 4*(3), 150–160.

Kardos, M., & White, B. P. (2005). The role of the school-based occupational therapist in secondary education transition planning: A pilot survey. *American Journal of Occupational Therapy, 59*(2), 173–180.

Kardos, M., & White, B. (2006). Evaluation options for secondary transition planning. *American Journal of Occupational Therapy, 60*(3), 333–339.

Kaye, H. S. (1997). *Disability Watch: The Status of People with Disabilities in the United States.* Oakland, CA: Volcano Press.

Kemmis, B., & Dunn, W. (1996). Collaborative consultation: The efficacy of remedial and compensatory interventions in school contexts. *American Journal of Occupation Therapy, 50*(9), 709–717.

Kielhofner, G. E. (ed.). (2008). *A Model of Human Occupation: Theory and Application,* 4th ed. Baltimore: Williams & Wilkins.

Kielhofner, G., & Henry, A. (1988). Development and investigation of the Occupational Performance History Interview. *American Journal of Occupational Therapy, 42*(8), 489–498.

Kielhofner, G., Mallinson, T., Crawford, C., Nowak, M., Rigby, M., Henry, A., & Walens, D. (2004). The Occupational Performance History Interview (Version 2.1) OPHI-II. Chicago: Model of Human Occupation Clearinghouse.

Kielhofner, G., Mallinson, T., Forsyth, K., & Lai, J. S. (2001). Psychometric properties of the second version of the Occupational Performance History Interview (OPHI-II). *American Journal of Occupational Therapy, 55*(3), 260–267.

Kiernan, R., Mueller, J., Langston, W., & Van Dyke, C. (1995). *Cognistat: The Neurobehavioral Cognitive Status Examination.* Fairfax, CA: Northern California Neurobehavioral Group.

Kiernan, W. (2000). Where we are now: Perspectives on employment for persons with mental retardation. *Focus on Autism and Other Developmental Disabilities, 15*(2), 90–96.

King, G., Baldwin, P., Currie, M., & Evans, J. (2005). Planning successful transitions from school to adult roles for youths with disabilities. *Children's Health Care, 34*(6), 195–216.

Kjeken, I., Slatkowsky-Christensen, B., Kvien, T. K., & Uhlig, T. (2004). Norwegian version of the Canadian Occupational Performance Measure in patients with hand osteoarthritis: Validity, responsiveness, and feasibility. *Arthritis and Rheumatism, 51*(5), 709–715.

Kohler, P., & Field, S. (2003). Transition-focused education: Foundation for the future. *Journal of Special Education, 37*(3), 174–183.

Koller, J. R. (1994). Improving transition outcomes for persons with specific learning disabilities. *American Rehabilitation, 20*(2), 37–42.

Korpel, M. H. T. (1996). Supported employment behind the Netherland's dikes: Trends in vocational rehabilitation for person with psychiatric disabilities. *Journal of Vocational Rehabilitation, 6*(1), 97–106.

Law, M., Baptiste, S., Carswell, A., McColl, M. A., Polatajko, H., & Pollock, N. (1998). *The Canadian Occupational Performance Measure* (3rd ed.). Toronto: CAOT.

Law, M., & Dunn, W, (1993). Perspectives on understanding and changing the environments of children with disabilities. *Physical and Occupational Therapy in Pediatrics, 13*(3), 1–17.

Lawton, M. P., & Brody, E. M. (1969). Assessment of older people: Self-maintaining and instrumental activities of daily living. *Gerontologist, 9*(3), 179–186.

Levin, M., Kielhofner, G., Braveman, B., & Fogg, L. (2007). Narrative slope as a predictor of work and other occupational participation. *Scandinavian Journal of Occupational Therapy, 14*(4), 258–264.

Matheson, L., Ogden, L., Violette, K., & Schultz, K. (1985). Work hardening: Occupational therapy in industrial rehabilitation. *American Journal of Occupational Therapy, 39*(5), 314–321.

McColl, M., & Pollock, N. (2001). Measuring occupational performance using a client-centered perspective. In M. Law, C. Baum, & W. Dunn (eds.), *Measuring Occupational Performance: A Guide to Best Practice.* Thorofare, NJ: Slack.

McGlashing-Johnson, J., Agran, M., Sitlington, P., Cavin, M., & Wehmeyer, M. (2003). Enhancing the job performance of youth with moderate to severe cognitive disabilities using the self-determined learning model of instruction. *Research & Practice for Persons with Severe Disabilities, 28*(4), 194–204.

McManus, M. A., Newacheck, P., & Greaney, A. M. (1990). Young adults with special health care needs: Prevalence, severity, and access to health services. *Pediatrics, 86*(5), 674–682.

Michaels, C., & Orentlicher, M. (2004). The role of occupational therapy in providing person-centered transition services: Implications for school-based practice. *Occupational Therapy International, 11*(4), 209–228.

National Organization on Disability (NOD). (2004). Harris Surveys of Americans with Disabilities. New York: Harris Interactive, Study No. 20835.

Norris, G., & Tate, R. L. (2000). The behavioural assessment of the dysexecutive syndrome (BADS): Ecological, concurrent and construct validity. *Neuropsychological Rehabilitation, 10*(1), 33–45.

Office of Disability and Employment Policy (ODEP). (2001). Workforce Investment Act of 1998: Its application to people with disabilities. Retrieved from www.dol.gov/odep/pubs/ek01/act.htm.

Ohtake, Y., & Chadsey, J. G. (2001). Continuing to describe the natural support process. *Journal of the Association for Persons with Severe Handicaps, 26*(2), 87–95.

Orentlicher, M. (2007). Transition from school to adult life. In L. Jackson (Ed.), *Occupational Therapy Services for Children and Youth under IDEA,* 3rd ed. Bethesda, MD: AOTA Press.

Phelps, A., & Hanley-Maxwell, C. (1997). School-to-work transition for youth with disabilities: A review of outcomes and practices. *Review of Educational Research, 67*(2), 197–226.

Piek, J. P., & Dyck, M. J. (2004). Sensory-motor deficits in children with developmental coordination disorder, attention deficit hyperactivity disorder and autistic disorder. *Human Movement Science, 23*(3–4), 475–488.

Prellwitz, M., & Tham, M. (2000). How children with restricted mobility perceive their school environment. *Scandinavian Journal of Occupational Therapy, 7*(4), 165–173.

Ratzon, N., Ornoy, A., Greenbaum, C., Peritz, E., & Dulitzky, M. (1996). Developmental evaluation of school age children who were born to diabetic mothers, in comparison to children who were born to nondiabetic mothers. *Teratology, 53*, 93–94.

Reimer, B., D'Ambrosio, L. A., Coughlin, J. F., Fried, R., & Biederman, J. (2007). Task-induced fatigue and collisions in adult drivers with attention deficit hyperactivity disorder. *Journal of Traffic Injury Prevention, 8*(3), 290–299.

Rutkowski, S., Daston, M., Van Kuiken, D., & Riehle, E. (2006). Project SEARCH: A demand-side model of high school transition. *Journal of Vocational Rehabilitation, 25*(2), 85–96.

Schalock, R. L., Stark, J. A., Snell, M. E., Coulter, D. L., Polloway, E. A., Luckasson, R., Reiss, S., & Spitalnik, D. M. (1994). The changing conception of mental retardation: Implications for the field. *Mental Retardation, 32*(3), 181–193.

Sewell, L., Singh, S. J., Williams, J. E., Collier, R., & Morgan, M. D. (2005). Can individualized rehabilitation improve functional independence in elderly patients with COPD? *Chest, 128*(3), 1194–1200.

Spencer, K., & O'Daniel, S. (eds.). (2005). Transition services: From school to adult life. In J. Case-Smith (ed.), *Occupational Therapy for Children,* 5th ed. St. Louis: Elsevier.

Stapleton, D. C., & Burkhauser, V. B. (ed.). (2003). *The decline in Employment of People with Disabilities.* Kalamazoo, MI: W.E. Upjohn Institute for Employment Research.

Staub, D., Spaulding, M., Peck, C. A., Gallucci, C., & Schwartz, I. S. (1996). Using nondisabled peers to support the inclusion of students with disabilities at the junior high school level. *Journal of the Association for Persons with Severe Handicaps, 21*(4), 194–205.

Stewart, D. A., Law, M. C., Rosenbaum, P., & Willms, D. G. (2001). A qualitative study of the transition to adulthood for youth with physical disabilities. *Physical & Occupational Therapy in Pediatrics, 21*(4), 3–21.

Tiffin, J. (1987). *Purdue Pegboard Examiner's Manual.* Chicago: Science Research Associates.

Toglia, J. P. (1991). Generalization of treatment: A multicontext approach to cognitive perceptual impairment in adults with brain injury. *American Journal of Occupational Therapy, 45*(6), 505–516.

Toglia, J. P. (1994). *Dynamic Assessment of Categorization Skills: The Toglia Category Assessment.* Pequannock, NJ: Maddak.

Toglia, J. P. (2003). Lesson 4: Attention and memory. In C. B. Royeen (ed.), *AOTA Self-Study Series: Cognitive Rehabilitation.* Rockville, MD: American Occupational Therapy Association.

Toglia, J. P. (2005). A dynamic interactional approach to cognitive rehabilitation. In N. Katz (ed.), *Cognition and Occupation across the Life Span: Models for Intervention in Occupational Therapy,* 2nd ed. Baltimore: American Occupational Therapy Association.

Tuckwell, N. L., Straker, L., & Barrett, T. E. (2002). Test-retest reliability on nine tasks of the physical work performance evaluation. *Work, 19*(3), 243–253.

U.S. Department of Education, Institute of Education Sciences, National Center for Special Education Research. (2005). National Longitudinal Transition Study-2 (NLTS2), 2005; and National Longitudinal Survey of Youth (NLSY), 2001. (Youth surveys, responses for youth ages 17–21.) Fact sheet available at http://www.nlts2.org/fact_sheets/nlts2_fact_sheet_2005_11.pdf.

U.S. Department of Labor, Office of Disability Employment Policy (ODEP). (1993). Supported employment. Retrieved from www.dol.gov/odep/archives/fact/supportd.htm.

U.S. Equal Employment Opportunity Commission (EEOC). (2008). Americans with Disabilities Act: Questions and answers. Retrieved from www.ada.gov/q%26aeng02.htm.

Van Naarden Braun, K., Yeargin-Allsopp, M., & Lollar, D. (2006). A multi-dimensional approach to the transition of children with developmental disabilities into young adulthood: The acquisition of adult social roles. *Disabilities and Rehabilitation, 28*(15), 915–928.

Van Naarden Braun, K., Yeargin-Allsopp, M., & Lollar, D. (2009). Activity limitations among young adults with developmental disabilities: A population-based follow-up study. *Research in Developmental Disabilities, 30*(1), 179–191.

Vandercook, T., York, J., & Forest, M. (1989). The McGill Action Planning System (MAPS): A strategy for building the vision. *Journal of the Association for Persons with Severe Handicaps, 14*(3), 205–215.

Varga-Toth, J. (2006). *Meeting the needs of children and adolescents with special needs in rural and northern Canada: Summary report of a roundtable for Canadian policy-makers.* Canadian Policy Research Networks Inc. Retrieved from www.coespecialneeds.ca/PDF/meetingtheneeds.pdf.

Velozo, C. A., Kielhofner, G., Gern, A., Lin, F. L., Azhar, F., Lai, J. S., & Fisher, G. (1999). Worker Role Interview: Validation of a psychosocial work-related measure. *Journal of Occupational Rehabilitation, 9*(3), 153–168.

Verkerk, G. J., Wolf, M. J., Louwers, A. M., Meester-Delver, A., & Nollet, F. (2006). The reproducibility and validity of the Canadian Occupational Performance Measure in parents of children with disabilities. *Clinical Rehabilitation, 20*(11), 980–988.

Wagner, M. (1995). *Transition from high school to employment and post secondary education: Interdisciplinary implications for youths with mental retardation.* Paper presented at the 119th annual meeting of the American Association on Mental Retardation, San Francisco.

Walker, P. (1999). From community presence to sense of place: Community experiences of adults with developmental disabilities. *Journal of the Association for Persons with Severe Handicaps, 24*(1), 23–32.

Walsh, P. N., & Linehan, C. (1997). Factors influencing the integration of Irish employees with disabilities in the workplace. *Journal of Vocational Rehabilitation 8*, 55–64.

Wehmann, P. (2000). Foreword. In C. Hughes & E. W. Carter (eds.). *The Transition Handbook: Strategies High School Teachers Use That Work!* Baltimore: Paul H. Brookes.

Wehmeyer, M. L., & Bolding, N. (1999). Self-determination across living and working environments: A matched-samples study of adults with mental retardation. *Mental Retardation, 37*(5), 353–363.

Whetstone, M., & Browning, P. (2002). Transition: A frame of reference. *AFCEC Online Journal,* Special Issue, October, 1–9. Retrieved from www.afcec.org/pubs/journal/vol1/02F_definition1.pdf.

White, J., & Weiner, J. (2004). Influence of least restrictive environment and community based training on integrated employment outcomes for transitioning students with severe disabilities. *Journal of Vocational Rehabilitation, 21*(3), 149–156.

Wilson, B. A., Alderman, N., Burgess, P. W., Emslie, H., & Evans, J. J. (1996). *Behavioural Assessment of the Dysexecutive Syndrome.* Bury St. Edmunds, England: Thames Valley Test Company.

World Health Organization (WHO). (2008). International Classification of Fuctioning, Disability and Health. Retrieved from www.who.int/classifications/icf/site/icftemplate.cfm.

Glossary

Children with special needs are children who require supportive services to make the transition into the typical roles and occupations of adolescence and young adulthood.

Context encompasses a variety of interrelated conditions within and surrounding the client.

Physical environment encompasses the natural (geographic terrain, sensory qualities of environment, plants and animals) and built nonhuman settings (buildings) and the objects in them (furniture, tools, devices).

The **social environment** is constructed by the presence, relationships, and expectations of the persons, groups, and organizations with which the person has contact. The social environment includes the availability and expectations of significant individuals such as spouse, friends, and caregivers; relationships with individuals, groups, or organizations; and relationships with systems that are influential in establishing norms, role expectations, and social routines.

Social inclusion means "fully participating in the interactions that occur within an environment to the same extent as other people do who are a part of that setting" and a situation in which "individual differences are accepted and individual competencies are maximized and supported" (Hughes and Carter, 2000; Hughes, et al., 1997c).

Transition services are a collection of services designed to facilitate each student's transition from school to adult life through an individualized plan.

Resources

Individuals with Disabilities Education Act (IDEA)

http://idea.ed.gov

Americans with Disabilities Act

www.ada.gov

United States Equal Opportunity Commission

www.eeoc.gov

National Secondary Transition Technical Assistance Center (U.S.)

www.nsttac.org

Wrightslaw.Com

www.wrightslaw.com

A website for parents, educators, advocates, and attorneys for children with disabilities.

8

Older Workers
Maintaining a Worker Role and Returning to the Workplace

Jyothi Gupta and Dory Sabata

Key Concepts

The following are key concepts addressed in this chapter:

- The number of older workers is expected to increase significantly, and a majority of older Americans anticipate they will work, at least part time, past retirement age or will transition into retirement.
- Numerous factors, including financial pressures, extended life expectancy, and a limited pool of trained employees to replace the experienced older worker, result in older adults remaining in the workforce.
- Changes in organizational structure, globalization, and technology are just three drivers of change that have affected the modern-day workplace, the meaning of work, and opportunities for the older worker.
- Retirement impacts many aspects of a person's life, including identity, sense of purpose, aspirations, social networks, self-image, material wealth, habits, and routines of daily living.
- Discriminatory beliefs and pervasive myths about aging and older workers lead to discriminatory practices that affect the self-image of older workers and may in some instances become a self-fulfilling prophecy.
- While age-related changes to physical, sensory, and cognitive capabilities occur, these changes cannot be generalized to all older workers and do not always correlate with decline in skilled performance and/or overall poor job performance.

Case Introduction

Bev is a 64-year-old elementary school teacher in a public school. While she enjoys her work and plans to work for a few more years, she is beginning to think about retirement. Recently she has begun to think that she may need to work longer due to financial concerns. However, she is unsure about meeting the demands of her work as she gets older. She has worked as an elementary school teacher for nearly 40 years. In that time, she has adapted to changes in class sizes, teaching methods, curriculum, student evaluation techniques, and diversity of the student body. She has worked in the current school district for more than 20 years and has a good understanding of the community. Bev enjoys learning as well as teaching and has pursued advanced education and certificate courses to help her excel at her job. Bev has been committed to working in her field for decades and has an extensive history in the school where she currently works.

Bev derives meaning from her work as a teacher in several ways. She has meaningful relationships with her coworkers. She desires financial security from her job. She enjoys working with children and growing as a professional in her field. She feels competent at meeting many of the demands of her work. She is an effective problem-solver who is able to demonstrate student outcomes that result from her teaching. She has strong social networks with her team and collaborates efficiently and effectively with other teachers in her school.

Bev has many strengths that make her a successful teacher. Yet she has experienced some changes with aging that affect her performance, including the need to wear bifocals for reading. For the past few years, she has noticed difficulty getting up and down from the floor during activities with her class. She admits she is overweight and her knees "just don't work like they used to." She also does not enjoy playground duty because it sometimes requires running to the scene of an accident or injury. Bev is still working on finding ways to adapt to the changes in vision and mobility that are part of the natural aging process.

Not only has Bev experienced changes with aging, but also her work environment is rapidly transforming. Over the years, she has developed strategies for managing the stress and meeting necessary challenges. However, Bev is concerned about keeping up with the increasing demands of her work. Bev has experienced changes in the diversity of her students in terms of greater inclusion of children with disabilities and students who speak English as a second language. This has required her to be more aware and sensitive to the educational needs of a diverse student body. Technology has also affected education and Bev's role as a teacher. For instance, a significant amount of communication between administration and teachers occurs via email now, and grades and performance measures are tracked in systemwide databases. Additionally, she has needed ongoing training to keep up with advancements in education-related technologies as well as the continual revisions to software programs.

Introduction

The rapidly aging workforce in most industrialized countries is an issue of grave concern to workers, employers, and policymakers alike. In the United States, baby boomers (individuals born between 1946 and 1964) make up 40 percent of the workforce (Groeneman, 2008), and their retirement has the potential to impact the nation's economy at multiple levels. The "baby bust" cohort that followed the boomers into the work world is 16 percent smaller, and this discrepancy is bound to create severe job vacancies in the U.S. economy (Cappelli, 2003). With advances in health care and high standards of living, life expectancy has improved greatly, people are remaining active longer, and many choose to work beyond the expected social retirement age. Under the right circumstances, retaining older workers is a mutually beneficial arrangement for workers, employers, work environments, and society.

Under the right circumstances, retaining older workers is a mutually beneficial arrangement for workers, employers, work environments, and society

Who Is the Older Worker?

There is a great deal of variability in defining the *older worker,* and this appears to be both contextual and policy driven. Part of the problem is that the same metrics are not used by employers, researchers, academics, policymakers, and older adults themselves (Pitt-Catsouphes and Smyer, 2006). The one thing that is certain is that the older worker definition is not based solely on chronological age. Survey results on public perceptions of who is "old" showed that it depends on the age of the person being asked the question. Individuals in their 30s felt that 61 to 70 years is old, while those 50 to 64 years felt over 70 is old. Interestingly, no one over 65 thinks that 41 to 50 is old (MetLife, 2006). The Age Discrimination in Employment Act of 1967 (ADEA) uses age 40 for legal purposes. The ADEA has a broad agenda of age-related workplace discrimination and is not restricted to retirement issues alone. While this age may appear as too young for an individual to be categorized as an older worker, the U.S. Equal Employment Opportunity Commission (EEOC) has noted that discriminatory attitudes and practices in workplaces, in terms of the worth of the worker as human capital, appear to start around 45 years of age (EEOC, 1992, 2009). For example, workers may be denied advancement, training, and other opportunities for career growth. The U.S. Government Accounting Office (GAO), whose policy focus is on early retirement, uses 55 years and older as the cutoff, while the research literature on aging uses the normative 65 years and older as the lower limit.

The nature and demands of the work also influence how aging is defined in the context of work. For instance, many professional athletes and dancers may be "old" in their 20s and 30s, whereas scientists and academicians may be viewed as productive well into their 80s. In the former occupations, physical prowess is the defining attribute, which declines as one grows older. In the latter case, knowledge accrued over a lifetime is the valued attribute.

Older Workers' Patterns of Employment

The aging workforce is expected to impact society at many levels and in all sectors of the workforce. The number of Americans 65 years and older is expected to double and reach 89 million by 2030 (U.S. Department of Commerce, 2009). Since the mid- to late 1980s, the labor force participation rate for those ages 55 to 64 has steadily increased. The employment rate of persons ages 55 or older was about 29 percent in 1993 and has steadily increased to peak at 40.4 percent in May 2009. Despite the economic recession that began in December 2007, the employment rate of older workers has held at 40 percent, and interestingly, the jobless rate of older workers is lower than that of younger workers (Sok, 2010). Recent trends in employment indicate, for persons ages 55 to 61, a steady state for men at 71 percent and a slight increase for women at 61 percent being employed in 2003. At 62 to 64 years, about 47 percent of men and 37 percent of women are employed. Between 2006 and 2016, the number of workers in the labor force age 75 and older is expected to increase by 84.3 percent, and the percentage of workers ages 55 to 64 is expected to increase by 36.5 percent. At the same time, workers ages 25 to 54 are expected to increase by only 2.5 percent (Bureau of Labor Statistics, 2008). Given that a rapid rise in the number of dependent children is also expected during this period, the imbalance in the numbers of working-age adults to dependent children and older adults will place an enormous burden on this group (Johnson, 2004).

Employment rate is influenced by rate of economic growth, eligibility for benefits, and types of employer-sponsored pension plans (Purcell, 2007). A majority of older Americans anticipate they will work, at least part time, past retirement age or will transition into retirement (Cahill, Giandrea, and Quinn, 2006; Groeneman, 2008). There has been a steady increase in the percentage of workers who expect to retire after age 65: 11 percent in 1991 to 14 percent in 1995, 19 percent in 2000, 24 percent in 2005, and 33 percent in 2010 (Helman, Greenwald, Copeland, and VanDerhei, 2010). Today people are living longer and have to contend with high cost of living and health-care expenditures; this means that individuals need to finance more years of retirement. With the imbalance between the numbers of working adults and older workers exiting the workforce, there is grave concern about financing retirement benefits (Johnson, 2004). It is also evident that Social Security, Medicare, and Medicaid, in their present form, are not sustainable (U.S. General Accounting Office, 2003).

Social Security and Medicare are entitlements for seniors that are funded in a pay-as-you-go manner, and projections indicate that claims will exceed revenues by 2011 for Medicare and 2018 for Social Security. These projections were estimated prior to the 2009 financial collapse. Unless there is a dramatic change in work patterns of both working adults and older workers, this trend is bound to lower the standard of living, reduce per capita output, and place enormous burden on the working adult population (John and Levine, 2009). Besides Social Security and Medicare, American workers receive their retirement and health benefits through their employment. Traditionally, retirement was financed by an employment-based pension or a defined benefit plan. Pensions are, however, becoming a thing of the past, and nearly 50 percent of U.S. workers today do not have a pension plan (Pitt-Catsouphes and Smyer, 2005a). Instead, saving for retirement has dramatically shifted, especially in the private sector, to a defined contribution plan. In this case, the worker sets aside a pretax amount in a retirement account, and the employer may contribute a portion of or match employee contributions. With the shift from defined benefits to defined contributions, the responsibility has shifted from employers to workers to make not only voluntary contributions but also wise investment choices. Levels of participation in retirement plans vary across public and private sectors, with the former having higher levels of participation. However, overall rates of participation are dismal at about 42 percent (Employee Benefit Research Institute, 2007). Moreover, many workers report being clueless in estimating retirement expenses and have no or minimal savings and investments (Helman, Greenwald, Copeland, and VanDerhei, 2010). It is no wonder that the primary reason older workers give for wanting to work past their retirement age is for financial security (Pitt-Catsouphes and Smyer, 2005a).

When the Social Security Act was passed in 1935, the average life expectancy was 61 years. Today, life expectancy for American males is 75.78 years and for females is 80.81 years (CIA World Factbook, 2009). The retirement age had been decreasing in the past century but appears to have leveled somewhat. However, according to the National Council for Retirement Policy (NCRP, 1998), 60 percent of near retirees intend to retire as planned at 60 to 65, and many Americans who retire early may well spend a third of their life in retirement. The Social Security pension system typically penalizes those who leave the workforce early. This has been one strategy to ensure solvency of the system, and additional changes, such as reduced benefits, further delaying age of retirement, or privatization of social security, are bound to occur. For now, the eligibility for Social Security benefits has been raised from 65 years to 67 years for those born after 1959, and there is discussion whether this needs to change quickly to 70 years instead of 67 years (NCRP, 1998). This decision to increase the age of retirement translates to benefit cuts regardless of whether the older worker retires at 65 or remains on the job. For the worker who continues participating in the workforce, it will mean fewer years of benefits. Retirees will be penalized two ways. First, their benefits will decrease, and second, many will be subject to increased taxation of benefits. The argument to increase the age of retirement is also unfair on the grounds of racial disparity in life expectancy. Typically, African American males live nearly 7 years less than Caucasian males, and females are likely to live 4.5 years less than Caucasian females (Administration on Aging, 2010). Additionally, Social Security benefits will decrease as Medicare costs increase and claim a larger chunk out of social security (Munnell, 2007a). One way of decreasing the number of benefit claimants is by increasing labor-force participation by older workers. This will also help alleviate the labor shortage.

If the baby boomers who make up 40 percent of the U.S. labor force retire at 65 or earlier, businesses will find it hard to find equally qualified workers. In the past, the solution to labor shortages was increasing human capital by hiring immigrants. This approach is not as feasible today as in the past for a variety of reasons. First, after the 9/11 attacks, immigration laws have tightened, and it is increasingly difficult to procure visas to gain entry into the United States. Second, with growing opportunities in their native homeland, the number of individuals who come to the United States for advanced training and education has dropped considerably. Of those who do come for higher education, many are opting to return home to work after training. There has also been a small wave of first-generation immigrants who have acquired American citizenship and permanent residency returning to their country of origin. A second approach to increase labor capital that has been suggested is for employers to hire more women. This is feasible but may require employers to provide higher wages, child care options for women with children, flexible and/or part-time work, telecommuting options, and other incentives. Finally, businesses also have the option to relocate to developing economies of trained younger workers who demand lower wages. It has been projected that even if all these three approaches are implemented, it will still not meet the demands of the U.S. labor market. Any viable solution to the issue of labor shortage must therefore include retaining or hiring older workers.

Munnell (2007b) concludes that it is good public policy to encourage older workers to remain working longer, which will benefit all stakeholders. Employers will have access to experienced workers, the benefit system will not be overly burdened, and most important, healthy workers will not be spending long years in retirement. Occupational groups that are physically demanding, such as police, firefighters, miners, and construction workers, and that have a pension plan tend to promote early retirement. Workers feel entitled to cash in their benefits after working for the system, and they also want time for leisure. Many may return to some form of paid work after an initial period of full retirement either to use their time productively or for financial reasons.

To be considered retired, the individual should not participate in paid labor and must be a recipient of income from pension, Social Security, or retirement plans. However, in reality, some older workers have retired from one job and picked up another—so not everyone who receives a pension is retired. McDaniel (2003) argues that people do not smoothly transition out of work into retirement. Instead, they move in and out of jobs, and therefore multiple transitions occur before they fully disengage from paid work. According to Choi (2002), a vast majority of individuals, in particular women, do not completely withdraw from labor force but rather are in partial retirement. Benefits associated with this arrangement are continued activity and daily structure, less work and stress than full-time jobs, and guiding/mentoring the next generation (Raskin and Gettas, 2011). Productive activities, in general, positively impact psychological well-being of older adults, and furthermore this benefit is augmented by combining full-time work with some minimal degree of volunteering (Hao, 2008). For the enjoyment of working and the sense of well-being they experience through work, many older adults are willing to compromise and take low-paying jobs.

Meaning of Work

The fact that work and working are fundamental to one's life is supported empirically across nations and is agreed upon by researchers from diverse disciplines (Baker, Jacobs, and Tickle-Degnen, 2003; England and Harpaz, 1990; Harpaz and Fu, 2002). The centrality of paid work in the everyday lives and in the values and belief system of Americans is evident in the common query "What do you do?" when meeting a person for the first time. The typical response to this question is a title or description of one's job. Although the occupational therapy profession views work as one area of human occupation, "work" is what the term *occupation* means to most laypersons and is the most visible and "publically recognized occupation" (Davis and Polatajko, 2004, p. 164). Occupational therapy's categorization of productive occupations includes both paid employment and unpaid work, such as volunteer occupations (AOTA, 2008). For the purpose of this chapter, work is used in the context of paid employment unless otherwise stated.

Given the critical role of work in any society, it might appear that a uniform and accepted definition of work exists. In reality, defining work is a complex endeavor that is influenced by contexts, demography, and cultural values and beliefs (England and Harpaz, 1990). Often the different definitions of work address some or more of its attributes. The *Oxford English Dictionary* devotes nine pages to the definition of work, and *The American College Dictionary* provides 46 definitions of work (Drenth, 1991). In its broadest sense, work is the opposite of rest. Many studies have looked at work definition in the context of unemployment or job loss, and hence work is defined primarily in economic terms and is perceived as a means to meet basic needs or family responsibilities.

An empirically derived definition of work has emerged from a large cross-national study of employed workers from six countries, including the United States (England and Harpaz, 1990). Workers in all countries defined work in both economic and personal terms, although the economic rationale for working is the predominant work attribute identified. Table 8.1 adapts and summarizes the six patterns of work from the workers' perspectives (England and Harpaz, 1990). The authors have synthesized the older worker work pattern preferences from the literature and shown them in italics.

Table 8.1 Patterns and Attributes of Work Preferred by Older Workers

Pattern	Characteristics of Pattern
Pattern A: Low frequency (10.7% of workers)	Workers exchange largely *mental* effort and accountability for income Activity not directed by others Performance does not have negative impact on affect
Pattern B: High frequency; most professional definition of work (27.6% of workers) *Most favored by older workers*	Workers contribute to society and in exchange gain economic and affective benefits Compared to pattern A, relatively less directed Performance positively impacts affect, particularly identity
Pattern C (17.6% of workers)	Workers exchange effort that generates profit for others and income for self Physically strenuous activity Activity directed in a limited way
Pattern D: Second high frequency pattern (21.7% of workers) *Not favored by older workers*	Workers exchange effort for income Physically demanding activity Work is controlled and directed by others No positive impact on affect
Pattern E (10.6% of workers)	Physically and mentally demanding activity Relatively unpleasant activity No positive impact on affect Most self-oriented pattern
Pattern F (11.8% of workers)	Basic exchange of time for income Activity that takes place at specified times Not mentally strenuous No positive affect through performance Activity not profiting to others

Adapted from England and Harpaz, 1990.

People are proud of what they do and like to talk to others about their productive life experiences. The advantages to paid employment are many and are no different for the older worker than for any other paid worker. The most obvious is having an income with which to meet daily living expenses, such as for housing, transportation, food, and clothing, and that allows for some discretionary spending as well. As such, work can be viewed as a basic human right. With financial independence, people also experience a sense of competency and have freedom to make choices in their lives, which gives them a sense of personal control. Some people may choose to work solely for the income and gain satisfaction from having the money to meet their needs and to belong to a particular economic class for the social status it confers. For others, work also generates intangible benefits and diverse outcomes that impact a worker more deeply and intrinsically. Work enables individuals to be productive contributors to their communities and society; utilizes an individual's knowledge, skills, and abilities; and provides opportunities to experience self-efficacy, achieve goals, and, for the fortunate few, achieve self-actualization. Additionally, work organizes the day into work and nonwork (or personal) time, imposes daily routines and habits, and provides opportunities to cultivate relationships (Christiansen and Townsend, 2010). Many studies conclude that individuals' feelings of basic worth and sense of belonging is influenced by their employment status (Huang, Shaw, and Chen, 2004; Randolph, 2004). Hence, the activity of working and its outcomes are instrumental to the health and well-being of all individuals, including older adults, and society as a whole.

> *The activity of working and its outcomes are instrumental to the health and well-being of all individuals, including older adults, and society as a whole.*

It is a basic societal norm that all adults, particularly men, participate in work, and as such being a worker is an important social role and identity. McDaniel's (2003) study on the impact of loss of work on midlife men supports the integral role of work on self-perceptions of masculinity, identity, self-esteem, and sense of self that is intractably tied to the worker role, a successful career, and job status. Retirement detracts from this expectation and therefore impacts older men in a significant way.

The meaning of work shifts and is reinvented over the life span and develops and changes in relation to many social factors. For instance, women and men juggle many social responsibilities in various stages of their lives. Accordingly, they participate in education, training, work, and leisure at different times and life stages. Women, juggling motherhood and career, enter work later and may opt to work part time or pursue a slower career track. They may also withdraw from the workforce if they have to pick up the caregiver role in later life for aging parents. More women in the workplace, balancing their work and life roles and responsibilities, has changed the work culture and brought more fluidity into entering and leaving the workforce. Besides gender, age-based difference in attitude to time spent at work exists. For younger workers, career goals influence the perception of time spent at work, while for older workers, the focus shifts to how much time remains. This shift most likely happens as the worker becomes more aware of age-related changes to their physical capacities, cognitive abilities, emotional functioning, and social roles (Hedge, Borman, and Lammlein, 2006). For many older workers today, this awareness of age-related changes comes at a time when the very nature of work and workplace is undergoing massive transformation.

Changing Role of the Older Adult in the Modern-Day Workplace

The drivers that have changed the nature of work and the workplace include organizational structure, globalization, and technology. Organizational structures are increasingly less hierarchical, represented in models by flattened and overlapping circles, with project-oriented teams and work performed by a mix of associates, contingent workers, and others (O'Connell, McNeely, and Hall, 2008). Globalization has forced corporations to compete in the global arena and become more aware and accepting of diversity and different cultural norms and work behaviors. It has also heralded in novel terms such as *downsizing, rightsizing,* and *outsourcing.* The hardest hit has been the manufacturing sector, where en-masse shifting of manufacturing plants overseas to areas where costs of production are cheaper has displaced many workers who suddenly find their skills are obsolete and do not fit jobs in the local economy. Millions have lost jobs due to plant shutdowns, and older workers who counted on their jobs lasting until they retired are not immune to this type of job loss. In fact, their seniority is a liability because they end up leaving later and hence lose out on new employment opportunities (Root and Park, 2009). Older workers remain unemployed longer and unlikely to find new employment; if they do, they usually have to settle for lower wages. The residual manufacturing jobs that remain in the United States rely more on technology and less on skilled labor, and older workers' skills may not be easily transferable. Hispanic workers report greater difficulty adapting to technology compared to their Caucasian counterparts (Groeneman, 2008). Older blue-collar workers, in jobs that tend to be physically demanding, lose "the core of their existence" (p. 4), their worker identity, their status, along with workmates they have known over their work lives, and many are not willing to relocate (Root and Park, 2009). The decline in manufacturing-related jobs is associated with an increase in demand for white-collar employees or knowledge workers.

The nature of job demands in the new economy has shifted from jobs with physical demands to jobs that place greater cognitive and affective demands on the workers. Workers are required to engage in ongoing acquisition of new skills and knowledge, adapt quickly to workplace and work task changes, and be able to multitask capably while meeting higher productivity demands. These changes appear to have made work more stressful, time consuming, and accompanied by greater blurring of work/life boundaries (NIOSH, 1999).

Technology has changed dramatically how and where work gets done. Any information that can be digitized can be processed and distributed anywhere in the world. Employees are no longer bound to their offices, and many telecommute to work. Team meetings can be held in cyberspace, which calls for new skill sets in technology use and communication. Restructuring of the workplace includes more emphasis on teamwork, less supervision, growth of contingent workforces, and increased job flexibility. The rise in the number of contingent workers to roughly one-third of the labor force has changed the nature of social and professional relationships at the workplace (Cummings and Kreiss, 2008)

What have these workplace trends meant for the older worker? The reduction in physical demands of the job is actually beneficial for the workers because they can delay retirement and can work longer. However, older workers in jobs that are not physically demanding report having intense cognitive and affective demands placed on them. Examples cited are work tasks that require intense concentration, good eyesight, and increased teamwork that make work more difficult and stressful (Johnson, 2004).

Faced with changes to the workplace and subsequent stressors at work and home, why would older workers want to work? Finances continue to be a major motivator to remain in paid employment, both for meeting present living expenses for saving for anticipated retirement expenses (Groeneman, 2008). Many workers anticipate that Medicare benefits will be inadequate, and retirement income is insufficient to afford supplemental health insurance. In the United States, health insurance is linked to employment, so many older workers may have to continue to work to retain their health benefits. A close second reason for wanting to work longer is the chance to use perceived skills and talent. This most likely contributes to feelings of self-efficacy and self-esteem. By the year 2016, African Americans will account for more than 12 percent and Latinos for more than16 percent of the workforce (Johnson and Soto, 2009; Toossi, 2007). Older workers in these two racial/ethnic groups, when compared to their Caucasian counterparts, value work particularly for self esteem (Groeneman, 2008). Workplace social interactions are also valued by older workers who may have established long-term relationships with colleagues. The desire to work is linked to jobs that include friendly respectful relationships, satisfying work, and opportunities for growth and development.

Some researchers have devised taxonomic groupings of older workers based on the meaning of work: those who have to work, those who want to work, and those who work for both reasons (Pitts-Catsouphes and Smyer, 2006). Those who have to work do so for pragmatic reasons, such as income generation and/or health insurance; the second group wants to work for psychosocial benefits such as social networks or to apply their knowledge and skill; the last group derives more of a holistic work satisfaction. The American Association of Retired Persons (AARP) has four categories of workers: sustainers, providers, connectors, and contributors. For the sustainers, money is the main reason for working; providers work to meet obligations to others who are their dependents. Connectors have worked the longest with their employers and are linked to their workplace by the health and pension benefits. Finally, contributors live to work and perceive their work as contributing not just to self but to society (Montenegro, Fisher, and Remez, 2002).

Honig (1996) identified a bias in that the retirement literature reflects the attitudes and behaviors primarily of Caucasian men and found systematic differences in retirement expectations when gender, race, and ethnicity were factored in the analysis. For example, health status of Caucasian men, on average, is worse than for women and is a key deciding factor for continued work. Only Hispanic women ranked health status as an important factor, and their health status tends to be worse than that of Hispanic men. Honig found that, unlike men, married women may either not enter the labor market or else withdraw from it sooner if their health status is poor, and hence they are not represented in many reported studies. Participation of women in the labor force has steadily increased in the past decades and is, according to the Census Bureau, expected to reach 61 percent by 2012 (Munnell and Jivan, 2005).

It is evident that retirement is no longer tied to an arbitrary age when an individual is entitled to collect Social Security benefits. It is a matter of personal choice, and in the absence of a health crisis, the most common impetus is having a sense of financial freedom (Ameriprise Financial, 2006). According to these authors, it appears that retirement is perceived as a process with five distinct stages that commences nearly 15 years before the actual event: (1) imagination, (2) anticipation, (3) liberation, (4) reorientation, and (5) reconciliation. Typically, 15 to 6 years before retirement, workers begin to imagine retirement and focus their planning to financial retirement goals and needs. The anticipation stage lasts up to 5 years when workers now turn their attention to postretirement occupational planning, including leisure and second careers. Their financial planning is secure, and they look forward to retirement with hope and excitement. The first year postretirement is the liberation stage, which is the time retirees experience the most elation and freedom from the daily grind of work. However, this is a short-lived period, and then retirees spend the next 2 to 15 years trying to reorient themselves to their postwork lives. A majority who struggle during this phase are those who have not planned for their retirement, both financially and in terms of their daily occupations. While some feel content about their decisions, others may feel ambivalent or may try new occupations such as volunteering or hobbies. Nearly 16 years' postretirement, older adults have come to terms with their retired status. These stages, identified by Ameriprise Financial, suggest the attachment people have to their work and retirement appears to trigger emotions associated with loss akin to the grieving process. The question, then, is how does the absence of paid work impact the health and well-being of the worker?

Impact of Retirement on Health and Well-Being

The United States is a work-oriented society, and given the centrality of paid work to identity, individuals exiting the labor force may experience stress and decreased well-being (Ameriprise Financial, 2006). Work is central to a person's physical and mental health, and in fact, second to financial reasons, older workers want to work to remain healthy and active. It is therefore important that older workers be given equal access to opportunity for employment (Pitt-Catsouphes and Smyer, 2005a). Job satisfaction contributes to well-being as a whole, and it follows that all workers at least experience moderate levels of satisfaction at work. If people enjoy what they do, if their career reaffirms their values and beliefs, and if the income provides for their welfare, then they are more likely to experience a sense of well-being. Rebeiro (2001) concluded that job satisfaction is important in order to have a successful engagement in occupation and sense of overall well-being. A positive work environment is essential to job satisfaction, which in turn contributes to well-being. The organizational culture, interpersonal aspects of employer and coworkers, physical setting, and nature of job duties collectively contribute to a positive work environment. The way an employee is treated at work is critical to job satisfaction. Rebeiro points out that a focus on the employee's abilities rather than disabilities is conducive to acceptance and optimal performance. When a person is accepted and performing well at work, this can be directly related to his or her feelings of well-being.

Whether to retire outright or to phase into retirement is a decision for an older adult that is influenced by factors such as work environment, employer attitudes, and health issues. Intrinsic factors that keep workers committed to working and impact their job satisfaction appear to influence older workers similarly. These intrinsic factors in turn depend on work contextual factors such as those discussed in Chapter 15 (Shea and Hassan, 2006; Pitts-Catsouphes and Smyer 2006). Lim and Feldman (2003) hypothesized that the loss of productive role and time usage will lead to retirement anxiety and induce older workers to delay decisions to terminate work or to consider working part time. They showed that regardless of anxiety over retirement, workers will delay their retirement and expect life satisfaction to decline after retirement. Ageism, a systemic discrimination and stereotyping on the basis of age, is prevalent in many sectors of our society, including the workplace (Dennis and Thomas, 2007). Older workers who are attuned to age-related changes, their impact on perceived performance at work, and societal attitudes about aging may be particularly vigilant about coworkers' behaviors toward them. Some workers mention age discrimination and their own perceptions of having limited skills as barriers to work. Perceived discrimination and prejudice is likely to become self-fulfilling and discourages the worker from staying on the job. Powell (2010) draws attention to the dearth of research on workplace ageism and abuse and urges scholars to examine the intersection of ageism and abuse so that fair and equitable policies can be instituted to create safe workplaces for all workers.

Retirement impacts many aspects of a person's life, including identity, sense of purpose, aspirations, social networks, self-image, and material wealth, in a manner that takes some aspects away from the person. The hardest issues to deal with emotionally and financially are tied to health and health insurance, followed by loss of social networks (Ameriprise Financial, 2006). The best gainful feature of retirement is having control over time. Retirees and older workers transitioning out of work must recalibrate their daily routine and identify new ways to occupy time that once was dedicated to work. Leisure and life satisfaction, which are influenced by employment status, are also effected (Randolph, 2004). For many, this is also a time to think of new ways to generate income to supplement Social Security income and savings. Leaving the workplace also means individuals have to find alternative means to feel productive, experience self-competency, utilize the knowledge and skills gained over a lifetime of experience, and socialize. Unanticipated events that force an individual to take early retirement may make the adaptation process more difficult. If, on the other hand, the individual values time away from work, receives health insurance after retirement, has sufficient pension wealth, has no health problems, finds work mundane and repetitive, and has a retired spouse, then there is overall congruence in retirement expectations and behaviors (Honig, 1996).

Men who were satisfied with their retirement were those who were not career driven, had planned for their retirement, had enjoyed work prior to retirement, and had cultivated interests outside of work (Raskin and Gettas, 2011). Women's satisfaction with retirement was dependent on having sufficient financial support. Many retirees volunteer, and this productive use of their time is a benefit to both the community and the retirees. It helps the retirees structure the day, maintain venues for socialization, apply their experience in different ways, and remain actively engaged, positively impacting their well-being. Volunteerism is discussed in more depth in Chapter 10.

Earlier studies that reported either negative impact on health due to the stress of retirement or improvement of health due to leisure time are now losing support and have been criticized because the data was derived from self-reports rather than objective health measurements (Neuman, 2008, 2007). In fact, numerous studies over the last two decades have alluded to the fact that retirement is not a risk factor for poor health. However, a person who is unable to participate in work may not experience optimal health and may in fact sustain long-term negative impact on well-being. Involuntary job loss is detrimental to physical and mental health of older workers (Gallo, Bradley, Siegel, and Kasl, 2001; Gallo, et al., 2004; Tesch-Romer, 2009). It appears that retirement's impact on health, however, depends on the perception of retirement as either a loss, a gain, or of no consequence to health (Tesch-Romer, 2009). Individuals who have planned ahead for postwork life and ensured means to maintain the lifestyle they are accustomed to experience a greater sense of control and view retirement as a stage to indulge in occupations of choice. Finally, if a person accepts retirement as an epiphenomenon or a secondary consequence of aging, then inability to work is not viewed negatively. In general, if retirement occurs at a socially accepted age, it appears not to have any negative impact on health. On the other hand, forced retirement, regardless of cause, be it medical condition or restructuring, seems to be a high mortality risk factor and negatively impacts physical, mental, and subjective health in both the short and long term. So it is not retirement per se that impacts health but rather the circumstances in which one makes this life transition.

Retirement, whether voluntary or forced, can have both positive and negative consequences for the individual. Moen (1996) uses a life-course perspective and characterizes the outcomes of the retirement–well-being relationship as dynamic, embedded, and influenced by the interactions of the person and his or her social environment. A worker's past work experiences, choice, and control over timing of retirement and both personal and societal imperatives on the decision of leaving paid work have a bearing on well-being. McDaniel (2003) also emphasizes that patterns of work in late life are complex, dynamic, and gendered and are not captured adequately by policy and life-course theory. This view is congruent with theoretical models of occupational therapy that conceptualize occupations and their significance as changing over the life span and influenced greatly by the environment (Law, et al., 1996).

The decision to retire is not a simple matter of individual choice but a result of complex interplay among workers, work, context, and larger social influences. Some researchers see exit from the paid workforce as a "pull" phenomenon whereby individuals are drawn to pursue and engage in work that really matters, follow their dream, and so on. So their move away from the labor market is not really a retirement but a choice to pursue an alternative career path. Others take a different view with workers, particularly older workers, being "pushed" out of the labor market owing to socioeconomic restructuring brought on largely by globalization and technology (Root and Park, 2009).

> *The decision to retire is not a simple matter of individual choice but a result of complex interplay among workers, work, context, and larger social influences.*

Personal factors that lead workers to retire may include health status of self and/or family member, attitude toward work and leisure, financial status, and social support. The most common reasons workers retire are health problems and layoffs. Other common life challenges that older workers face include death, illness, divorce, empty-nest phenomenon, and marriage. Nearly 52 percent have to care for someone, usually a spouse, and about 14 percent of baby boomers take care of both an adult and a child. The burden of care is heavier for African Americans and Hispanics, who report caregiving responsibilities for spouses, children, and grandchildren. Nearly 15 percent of boomers identify themselves as the "sandwich" generation, juggling work with caregiving for children and aging parents. Sometimes, owing to caregiving responsibilities, workers may defer retirement to retain health benefits (Szinovacz, DeViney, and Davey, 2001). The average older worker experiences at least three life stressors during their pre-retirement years (Groeneman, 2008).

Systemic factors that influence the decision to leave the workforce are societal norms, policies at work, legislation, and economic conditions. In a "culture of retirement," workers are encouraged to leave work as early as possible and collect retirement benefits. For example, since the Social Security Act, the normative age for retirement is 65 years despite Social Security eligibility at 62 years of age. The choice of 65 years appears to be more of a sociocultural influence, with a large supply of young workers to meet the demands of employers, rather than medical reasons or any age-related issues. In the recent past, when jobs were physically demanding, many workers opted to retire as their physical strength and stamina declined with aging. Since the number of such jobs has declined dramatically and workers in general enjoy better health, older workers can opt to work longer. However, a deterrent for those workers who have started to collect benefits at 62 and may wish to return to work is increased taxation.

For the many couples who are a dual-income family, retirement decisions are made jointly with considerations being given to the health, work history, and pension wealth of both income earners. Pienta and Hayward (2002) studied the retirement decisions of married couples and the gendered expectations of retirement. The retirement expectations of husbands in this study are similar to those reported in other studies: based on pension wealth, health, and work environment. Women's expectations are not as clear and inequities exist. For instance, women's pension wealth was one-third the value of their husband's, and husband's characteristics and resources were more influential on joint retirement decisions. Although their own health did not influence early retirement decisions, the ill health or disability of a husband did cause exiting the workforce prematurely.

While health and family take precedence over productive occupations, nearly 30 percent of pre- and postretirees reported they value engaging in "more meaningful or satisfying work in retirement" (Ameriprise Financial, 2006, p. 8). However, there are many obstacles to hiring and keeping older workers. Many employers perceive the cost of hiring older workers is high and that costs outweigh the benefits. The rising costs of health insurance, training, and higher wages deter employers from hiring older workers. The same approach drives them to hire less expensive albeit inexperienced younger workers who are perceived as quick learners, more productive, and more adaptable. Employers also say the changing nature of the job and workplace may hinder some older workers from seeking employment and/or being hired.

However, with millions of skilled baby boomers exiting the workforce, *phased retirement* is an option employers use to induce older workers to remain employed while transitioning from full-time work to full-time retirement. Strategies for phased retirement, used by employers, include job-sharing, reduced or part-time work schedules, and temporary work. A deterrent in the past was pension laws, which disallowed accessing retirement funds until workers completely severed ties with their employer. However, after the enactment of the Pension Protection Act of 2006 (PPA, P.L. 109-280), pension funds can be paid out to workers who continue to maintain ties with their employers in a manner other than full-time contractual employment. The employers feel that phased retirement will be attractive to the older worker if pension funds can be available at early ages, between 55 and 62 years (Purcell, 2007).

Addressing issues regarding retirement income alone is insufficient to motivate older workers to remain in the labor market. Of equal importance are hiring practices of employers and workplace attitudes toward the older worker.

Ageism, Stereotyping, and Discrimination at the Workplace

Nearly three of five older workers believe that workplace age discrimination exists (Groeneman, 2008). All of us are impacted by pervasive cultural attitudes that see aging as a disease and that hold that all older adults are alike—that they tend to be orientated to the past; are critical, complaining, and inflexible; avoid challenges; have different job needs; and must retire and make room for younger workers. Such assumptions and beliefs lead to discriminatory practices that affect the self-image of older workers and may in some instances become a self-fulfilling prophecy (Shea and Haasen, 2006). Older workers are often viewed as lacking motivation and being less creative and less productive than their younger counterparts. As a result, they are often overlooked when it comes to promotions or new training.

More so than any other group, older workers tend to get grouped, and stereotypes abound. According to Shea and Haasen (2006), eight of the most commonly held (mis)beliefs are that older workers

1. must retire and make way for younger workers.
2. are all alike.
3. have specific job needs that are different from other younger workers.
4. focus on the past.
5. cannot change to meet changing demands at the workplace.
6. shy away from challenges.
7. are critical and complaining.
8. want calm and stability.

Such attitudes create a self-fulfilling prophecy and manifest as age discrimination that impacts the older workers' self-image and motivation to remain on the job. Gender-based discrimination results in women being underemployed in work that is not commensurate with their education level relative to men. Many are dissatisfied with their employment, do not wish to prolong their tenure at work, and retire early if they can afford to do so (Munnell and Jivan, 2006). Employer and employee perceptions of older worker productivity are more similar than one would think. Hard skills such as cognitive and physical capabilities tied to job performance are valued over soft, interpersonal skills by both groups. Moreover, productivity perceptions are biased by the age group of the workers as well as their position in the organizational hierarchy (van Dalen, Henkens, and Schippers, 2009).

A survey of 1,400 U.S. employed adults on older workers revealed the divergent perceptions held by older and younger workers. While 75 percent of older workers say they relate well to their younger colleagues, only 54 percent of the younger workers reciprocate these attitudes. Generally, lower numbers of younger workers than older workers said that their company values older workers, that they felt energized by older workers, or that they sought the advice of older workers. The only area where this trend differed was with learning from older workers: 64 percent of younger workers claim they learn from older workers, while 43 percent of older workers said they learn from younger workers (Randstad USA, 2006).

Individuals born in different cohorts are exposed to different social changes, and this influences the attitudes they bring to the job: their views on work itself, employers, peers, leaders, and subordinates (Moen, 1996). There are indeed differences in loyalty, teamwork, methods of communication, organizational structuring, and so on. While these differences may be perceived as an issue of age or ageism, they represent a deeper difference in core values. Given the transient nature of work today, younger workers are less likely to envision long-term relationships with or view any allegiance to their employers. They are also less favorable to hierarchy, function better in more egalitarian environments, and wish to participate in organizational decision-making. Additionally, they are at ease in using technology to communicate, and the use of language has evolved into cyberspeak with its own conventions.

Bennis and Thomas (2002) studied cohort differences on leadership skills and report the three significant generational differences between the digital age workers ("geeks") under 35 years of age and the analog group ("geezers") over 70 years of age. The digital group was more ambitious, more committed to achieving work/life balance, and far less likely to be influenced by images of successful leaders or larger-than-life heroes. Their ambition was both for personal gains and for their accomplishments having far-reaching and global impact. The older cohort viewed work primarily for making a steady income, gaining financial security, and influencing their social identity. Their leadership skills were influenced by and attributed to leadership heroes.

The managing director of operations and human resources for Randstad USA (2006) says that everyone benefits from a multigenerational workforce by leveraging the "synergy of ideas and insight that younger and older workers jointly bring to the table" and suggests that generation gaps can be bridged by not making assumptions, by being open-minded about diversity of ideas and talents, and by creating environments where all workers have opportunities to contribute.

As a group, older workers fare well in terms of their work performance. Countering ageist beliefs, empirical evidence shows that older workers have less absenteeism, less workplace aggression, less substance abuse, and fewer workplace injuries; that they are more dependable than younger workers; and that age is not linked to job performance. In addition, older workers are credited with a strong work ethic, valuable experience, and leadership. These days, older workers, particularly in white-collar occupations, are increasingly more comparable to younger workers in terms of education. There is not much difference in education level between workers age 55 or older and younger workers, as is the case for those 65 or older and younger workers. In fact, the bulk of the aging male baby boomer workers are better educated than younger males. The same trend holds true for women. Older workers bring a great deal of diverse experience gained with multiple employers. This has prepared them to adapt quickly, work efficiently, and be mobile. They are also healthier than in the past.

> *Countering ageist beliefs, empirical evidence shows that older workers have less absenteeism, less workplace aggression, less substance abuse, and fewer workplace injuries; that they are more dependable than younger workers; and that age is not linked to job performance.*

Age-Related Changes to the Worker

The body is susceptible to innate age-related changes at the cellular, tissue, and systems levels, and these changes impact occupational performance. Physical attributes are a product of genetics, environment, and lifestyle, so a great deal of variation exists in age-related physical decline. Some of the changes to the musculoskeletal system include decrease in the numbers, diameter, and types of muscle fibers; decreased number of motor units; increased amount of connective tissue; decreased oxidative capacity; increased contraction and relaxation time; and decreased bone density. These tissue-level changes lead to a decrease in range of motion, strength, power, endurance, speed, dexterity, and coordination. Examples of functional limitations are increased fatigue and difficulty with walking, lifting, maintaining postural balance, and recovering from impending falls. Exercise and aerobic training can reverse some of these changes and improve physical performance (Robnett and Murray, 2010).

The process of aging is multifaceted and complex. Originally proposed by Busse (1969, as cited in Stankov and Lord, 1993), aging entails aspects that are innate and hence beyond one's control and secondary aspects that are influenced by environmental and lifestyle choices. While age-related changes to physical and cognitive capabilities occur, these changes cannot be generalized to all older workers, and moreover, the changes do not always correlate with decline in skilled performance and/or overall poor job performance (Lee and Lee, 1999). The literature indicates that among older workers there are significant differences in the way individuals age and in their abilities, aptitude, and capacity to adjust and perform. While it is common to attribute cognitive decline to aging, often disuse and disease play a major role (Robnett, 2010). It is also important to keep in mind that cognitive attributes such as orientation, memory, and intelligence are interrelated, do not maintain distinct boundaries, and collectively influence occupational performance. Generally, older workers tend to adapt well and compensate for any changes they experience. Prior experiences enable older workers to use "anticipatory processing" to compensate for certain age-related changes and thereby preserve their ability to perform complex, real-world tasks (Salthouse, 1993). Table 8.2 identifies some workplace accommodation interventions for addressing needed performance skills in the workplace that may be affected by changes in body functions.

Williams, Sabata, and Zolna (2006) identified some of the most common motor, sensory, and mental limitations of older workers. Some of the most common difficulties reported included standing, sitting, changing positions, moving around the environment, and manipulating objects. Cognitive challenges included difficulty attending to tasks, remembering, and perceiving space and time. Nearly half of the respondents ages 55 to 64 reported

Table 8.2 Sample Work Outcomes, Person Factors, and Intervention Options

Sample Outcomes	Client Factors: Body Functions	Performance Skills	Interventions/ Adaptations
Occupational performance: Sufficient speed and accuracy in job tasks	Neuromusculo-skeletal system • Decreased speed of information processing by the nervous system • Decreased range of motion, strength, endurance • Loss of postural stability	Motor/praxis • Maintaining or changing positions: standing, sitting • Moving around the environment • Manipulating objects • Processing information • Reacting at a pace needed for productivity	• Special tools and furnishings • Communication devices • Modifications to entrance and bathrooms • Job restructuring • Redesign of workstation • Develop safety program • Allow more time for task
Adaptation: Adapt to changing roles in the workplace	Cardiovascular, hematological, immunological, and respiratory systems function • Decreased cardiac output • Shortness of breath		• Task simplification/ energy conservation • Use of equipment and assistive devices • Breaks during workday • Stress management sessions
Health and wellness: Older adults remaining healthy through engagement in work	Voice/speech • Volume, speech production	Communication and social • Speaking • Presenting • Developing relationships	• Communication devices • Assistive technology (e.g., voice amplification)
Quality of life: Engaging in work throughout the life span	Genitourinary and reproductive functions	Sensory, motor/praxis, and emotional regulation • Detecting urge to urinate • Accessing the bathroom in a timely manner • Responding appro-priately to hormonal changes	• Schedule • Bathroom modifications
Self-advocacy: Individuals advocating for what they need to do their job Organization developing supportive workplace policies	Digestive, metabolic, and endocrine sys-tems function • Longer to estab-lish homeostasis • Elevated cortisol response to stress may exacerbate health conditions		• Avoid extreme work temperatures • Preventative health-care education sessions • Strategies for managing changes in emotions and thermoregulation

(table continues on page 188)

Table 8.2 Sample Work Outcomes, Person Factors, and Intervention Options—cont'd

Sample Outcomes	Client Factors: Body Functions	Performance Skills	Interventions/ Adaptations
Occupational justice: People with disabilities in the workplace receiving same opportunities for advancement as others without disabilities	Sensory systems • Hearing loss • Vision changes • Decrease in sensory input ○ balance ○ proprioception ○ vestibular input ○ kinesthesia ○ tactile discrimination ○ stereognosis	Sensory skills • Accessing workstation • Using tools and equipment • Learning new skills through work training • Leading teams • Presenting	• Assistive technology • Flexible work hours • Lighting • Contrasts • Visual/auditory cues • Information in alternative formats
Participation: Engaging in the workplace as a member	Mental functions	Cognitive skills • Remembering • Initiating • Sequencing • Organizing	• Visual/auditory cueing • Equipment/assistive technology • Alarms/reminders
Prevention: Reducing injury; increasing safety in workplace	Skin and related structure functions	Sensory skills • Detecting sharp objects • Recognizing and responding to temperature	• Modify task to rely on alternative sensory skills (e.g., hearing, vision) • Assistive technology • Establish workplace policies that support safety

Based on research findings of Sabata, Williams, Milchus, Baker, and Sanford, 2008; Williams, Sabata, and Zolna, 2006; Zolna, Sanford, Sabata, and Goldthwaite, 2007; and language from the OTPF (AOTA, 2008).

visual impairments, while 57 percent of those 65 and older had some visual deficits. In terms of workplace accommodations used to address functional deficits, the older workers often reported having no accommodations. Some of the more commonly identified accommodations used by older workers included checklists and reminder devices for cognitive difficulties, custom lighting to address visual deficits, and written communication to compensate for hearing loss (Williams, et al., 2006).

Barriers to Work for the Older Worker

Although older workers are willing, able, and committed to work, research shows that employers do not view them in a favorable light in comparison to younger workers (Kite, Stockdale, Whitley, and Johnson, 2005). There are many barriers and obstacles to hiring and keeping older workers. Evidence shows that employers treat older workers differently, particularly when it comes to hiring practices. Many employers perceive that the cost of hiring older workers is high and that costs outweigh the benefits. Research is still not conclusive as to why employers prefer younger workers, although reasons for differential hiring are varied and include their belief that older workers are less energetic, have higher absenteeism due to health issues, possess obsolete knowledge and skills, lack flexibility, and block career paths for younger workers. From an investment perspective, employers feel that the career trajectory for the older worker is short and the salary expectation is higher; they also fear discrimination suits and increased costs of health insurance and pension (Lahey, 2005). The same attitude drives them to hire less expensive albeit inexperienced younger workers who are perceived as quick learners and as more productive and adaptable. Employers also cite that the changing nature of the job and workplace may hinder some older workers from seeking employment and/or being hired.

Strategies for Retaining Older workers

Telecommuting, or telework, is an increasingly popular alternative form of work arrangement that does not restrict the worker to working at the traditional "office"—a fixed place of employment—but allows flexibility and freedom to work from any place (Sharit, et al., 2004). This characteristic appeals to some workers because it increases flexibility, reduces travel costs and time, and allows balancing work and family duties (Bailey and Kurland, 2002). Benefits to the employer include heightened productivity and reduction in absenteeism (Di Martino and Wirth, 1990; Illegems and Verbeke, 2004). All these attributes of telecommuting are valued by older workers and are especially important for those who have restricted community mobility (Illegems and Verbeke, 2004). Opportunities for development, schedule input, job fit, flexibility, and perceived fairness were the drivers for engagement of older workers (James, Swanberg, and McKechnie, 2007). In general, most workers between 45 and 55 years of age want to have autonomy and experience self-efficacy at work. In the case of second careers, they are prepared to consult or be self-employed to gain more flexibility, pleasure, a sense of purpose, and have less stress (Brown, 2003).

To better understand aging workers in today's workplace and illustrate how current trends related to aging and employment may affect an aging worker, we return to our case example. Through Bev's experience, the decisions facing older workers regarding whether to stay in the workplace, retire, or return to work are considered. Examples of strengths of aging workers and factors that affect their capacity to work are explored. Strategies for supporting older workers are identified with particular focus on how organizations can support an aging workforce.

Can Occupational Therapy Help Older Adults Fully Participate in Employment and/or Retirement?

Bev, in our case study, is an example of a typical aging adult in the workforce today. She is faced with planning for retirement, identifying her own strengths and limitations in the workplace, and adapting as best as she can to perform her work. Like most aging people in the workplace, Bev may not be aware of strategies and environmental supports that can help her successfully perform her job.

Bev has seen many changes in her current workplace. She is faced again with the changing role of the older adult in today's workplace. Her role as an elementary school teacher is requiring greater cognitive and affective demands. The expectations for student learning and academic performance, the ever-changing technology used in instruction, and the diversity of her classroom are all contributing to her changing role.

Bev wants to continue to work for financial reasons as well as to keep social connections and contribute to her community. Like many older workers, job satisfaction is important to her continued employment as a teacher. Also, she may be interested in an alternative work schedule. She knows some coworkers who have retired and continue to teach as tutors, substitute teachers, and educational consultants. For now, she can work full time and enjoys her summers and weekends off. She wants to continue to have that flexibility in her work.

Bev knows changes have occurred with aging that can contribute to the challenge of her job. Her vision changes require her to wear bifocals. Sometimes she experiences eye strain and aches from excessive computer use. Additionally, she has some arthritis in her hands that can affect her ability to type or manipulate small objects used for teaching. New learning is also a challenge for Bev. She sometimes feels self-conscious in technology training sessions that seem rapid. She feels she cannot understand the use of these instructional technologies as rapidly as younger teachers who are familiar with similar technology and software. She often needs additional training time to master the new classroom technologies.

However, Bev's years of experience as a teacher help her to manage student behaviors, work effectively in teams, and adapt to new curriculum. Where younger teachers may lack the experience in managing students and the classroom, Bev is an excellent resource. Bev has learned to share with a team of teachers who draw from each other's strengths. When she needs technology assistance, she finds a younger teacher who can help. In turn, they come to Bev when they are faced with unfamiliar student situations. Bev's experience as a teacher is valued in the workplace.

Aging workers such as Bev can benefit from a range of workplace accommodations such as those presented in Table 8.2. However, older workers, perhaps who have experienced functional limitations gradually with aging, are underutilizing available workplace accommodations (Williams, et al., 2006). Bev has indicated that she needs more time for learning new technologies. Extra time for training is one example of a workplace accommodation. Occupational therapists apply a process to identify client needs, determine workplace accommodations, and facilitate effective work performance.

Applying the Occupation Therapy Process

The Occupational Therapy Practice Framework: Domain and Process (OTPF) outlines the occupational therapy process as having three main parts: evaluation, intervention, and outcomes (AOTA, 2008). Bev's case exemplifies how the occupational therapy process can be applied to determining workplace accommodation. The process can be applied to a client at the level of an individual, organization, or population (AOTA, 2008). For instance, considering the case presented, an aging schoolteacher is an individual client; an elementary public school system, including administration and teachers, is an organization; and aging schoolteachers in the United States are a population. Any of these could be a client of occupational therapy services. Bev's case is explored at the level of the individual (Bev) and the organization (the school).

Evaluation

During evaluation, occupational therapy practitioners are interested in understanding the meaning the client associates with a particular occupation and analyzing a client's performance of a particular occupation (AOTA, 2008). Insight into meaning is gathered by developing an occupational profile of the client. Analysis of performance can be understood through methods such as observation, interviews, and formal assessment.

Occupational therapy practitioners create an occupational profile of the client to understand the past, present, and future of the occupation. For an individual who is concerned about engaging in work, the occupational therapist should first understand the meaning the person associates with that activity or occupation. That occupational profile summarizes past work patterns and activities, the current work situation, and plans for the future.

An occupational profile of an organization looks somewhat different from that of an individual. Consider the school system (organization) as the client. This client's occupation is to manage the workforce that educates students in the school system. The workforce includes older workers. Historically, older teachers have retired. This organization values the commitment and experience of teachers who are seasoned educators and mentors to new teachers. Additionally, the organization wants, in its school system, new educators with new ideas and advanced technological skills. The organization recognizes a demand for qualified and competent professionals to teach a growing number of students and a diverse student body. The organization feels unprepared to meet the demand for educators if many of its current veteran teachers decide to retire. The school organization additionally finds meaning in building a workforce that contributes to the school system's educational outcomes and produces competent graduates.

Intervention

The OTPF (AOTA, 2008) identifies five intervention approaches (create/promote, establish/restore, maintain, modify, and prevent), most of which are drawn from the ecology of human performance model (Dunn, Brown, and McGuigan, 1994). The create/promote approach is focused on creating opportunities for engagement in occupation regardless of disability. When the focus of intervention is on building skills of the client, the approach is called establish/restore. Maintaining current functioning can involve any of the other approach techniques. Modifying addresses ways to change the environment or task. The final intervention approach takes into account ways to prevent disease, disability, or functional decline. Each approach can be applied to support older workers in the workplace. Examples are presented in Table 8.3 to illustrate how these approaches may be applied to an individual worker, such as Bev, as well as through an employer organization such as the school administration.

Table 8.3 Occupational Therapy Intervention Approaches and Workplace Examples

Intervention Approach	Workplace Intervention	Example for Individual Client	Example for Organizational Client
Create/promote	Universal design	Classroom designed to meet the needs of teacher and students	Basic accessibility software features for all computer systems in the organization (e.g., Ease of Access features in Windows)
Establish/ restore	Skill building Training	Tutorial on new instructional technology	Group training sessions on new teaching methods, technology
Maintain	Any intervention from other approaches	Larger computer monitor	Policies that allow older workers sufficient time for completing complex tasks
Modify	Workplace accommodations Assistive technology	Personal assistance services Alternative mouse/ keyboard	Provide critical information in alternative formats (e.g., large print or e-versions of memos)
Prevent	Ergonomics/injury prevention	Supportive seating and positioning	Energy conservation and task simplification techniques

In a survey of workplace accommodations, mobility accommodations, particularly changes that benefit multiple people such as ramps and bathroom modifications, were the most commonly reported type of accommodations (Williams, et al., 2006). While some individuals in the workplace may need specific, individualized accommodations, there may also be workplace accommodations that employers could implement to meet the needs of a larger aging workforce.

Mobility-related workplace accommodations are likely to be in place due to policies that require public facilities to be accessible. Their frequent use suggests that multiple workers are also benefiting from these accessibility accommodations. Employers may be more supportive of preventative workplace accommodations when they perceive that multiple workers' productivity can be maximized by them.

Public Policies and the Workplace

The workplace is influenced by public policies that address equal opportunity for employment, protection of civil rights, and retirement entitlement programs. The Equal Employment Opportunity Commission is charged with ensuring that workers, including those who are aging and/or have a disability, are provided an equal opportunity to work. Specifically, workers ages 40 and older are protected under the Age Discrimination in Employment Act (ADEA) of 1967, and the Americans with Disabilities Act of 1990 protects workers with a disability (ADA 1990; ADEA, 1967). Programs such as Social Security also effect the decisions workers make in terms of retirement or continuing to work.

Retired adults can begin to receive Social Security benefits at age 65. Consequently, this is a common age for retirement. The age for Social Security eligibility will increase to 67 in 2022. Historically, the mid-60s marked the beginning of retirement, but we now must reconsider this age range as a new era of older workers continue their jobs and careers (Montenegro, et al., 2002).

Role of Occupational Therapy

Occupational therapy practitioners have many opportunities to support aging workers in the workplace. Individuals will continue to have disabilities that increase the demands of the workplace and affect their ability to work. Occupational therapy practitioners can work one on one with individuals to identify and advocate for needed workplace accommodations. Organizations that comply with federal policies have already made workplace accommodations that may meet some of the needs of their workers. However, occupational therapy practitioners can work with employers and organizations to identify preventive measures and workplace accommodations that can be used not only to hire qualified workers with disabilities but also to meet the changing needs of the aging workforce. They can also engage with employers to institute health promotion and wellness programs at the workplace. The occupational therapy process outlined in this chapter can be applied and used by occupational therapists to help identify possible accommodations to maximize work performance and productivity of workplaces.

Chapter Summary

Employers have the opportunity to hire and retain qualified workers who are older and bring valued experiences to the workplace. The working population is aging just as society is aging. Individual workers may experience age-related changes. Workplace expectations, demands, and the use of advancing technologies are constantly evolving. Now is the time for occupational therapy to come forth and assist employers and workers to prepare for meeting the needs of an aging workforce.

Occupational therapy practitioners can work with both employers and aging workers to help identify workplace accommodations that will maximize performance of both the workers and the company. Occupational therapy has several approaches to interventions, such as establishing or restoring skills of workers, modifying or adapting the workplace or tasks, promoting and creating opportunities for all workers to be productive, and instituting prevention methods to reduce the risk of injury and illness in the workplace. Changing policies that neglect the needs of aging workers, meeting ADA accessibility guidelines, and modifying workstations to meet users' needs are all examples of workplace accommodations that may facilitate work participation and performance. Occupational therapy practitioners are also prepared to review the desired occupational outcomes of the individual or workplace organization once intervention has been implemented.

Case Resolution

Bev faced challenges that are common among older workers today. Skills and body functions change with aging. The workplace and job demands also change over time. Workplace accommodations are available to facilitate engagement in work by older workers such as Bev.

Bev has some strengths as well as declining skills that affected her participation in work activities. For instance, she has years of experience in the school system and understands the workplace and its demands. She also enjoys her work. However, Bev's vision changes and mobility limitations were affecting her work. Her vision was corrected with bifocals, but mobility was more problematic for her because her painful knees limited some of her interactions with the children.

Bev's job entails some consistent demands, such as playground monitoring duty, and some changing demands, such as keeping abreast of new technologies and applying them in her classroom. With her mobility limitations, playground duty had become increasingly difficult, and Bev also had difficulty lowering herself to the floor— and getting back up again—when necessary, for instance, during story time and other student–teacher interactions. Additionally, the technology training offered by the school was conducted at a rapid pace that made it difficult for Bev to follow and retain the information for application in her classroom.

An occupational therapy practitioner provided several options for Bev and her employer to address the workplace demands, including the interventions and examples outlined in Table 8.3. The occupational therapist also drew on the *prevent, modify,* and *establish* approaches to suggest other workplace accommodations.

Prevention is one approach the occupational therapist recommended to avoid pain or injury to Bev's knees. The intervention needed to reduce the physical demands made on Bev in the classroom and on the playground. After exploring options, the school administrators instituted a policy requiring teachers on the playground to work in pairs. As a team, the more agile teacher could respond quickly to students at a distance while the other teacher could resolve social conflicts that often occur among children at play. This solution maximized Bev's strengths as an experienced teacher and minimized the physical demands that exceeded her capacity.

To enhance Bev's skills in using instructional technology, the occupational therapist suggested the school provide training paced to fit Bev's learning style and opportunities for Bev to practice her new Internet skills at her own pace. Through this intervention, Bev was able to master new technologies and maximize their use in the classroom.

continued

Modifications are another approach to intervention. The therapist saw that the environment could be modified with simple accommodations such as rearranging the room and changing the level at which student–teacher interaction occurred. Instead of getting down on the floor to interact with students, Bev brought the students up to her level by placing chairs in a circle to facilitate interaction in close proximity.

The occupational therapy practitioner, using a tool similar to Table 8.2, worked with Bev to determine if the interventions were helping her to achieve her desired occupational outcomes. Although Bev's physical limitations interfered with her playground responsibilities, she was still able to participate in playground monitoring by emotionally and cognitively responding to students in conflict on the playground. This is an example of job restructuring. In the classroom, Bev created a space to interact with children seated in chairs rather than on the floor. This is an example of redesigning the workstation. These types of interventions led to her better achieving her occupational outcomes of caring for children on the playground and interactive learning with students in the classroom.

The occupational therapy profession has a process for identifying needs and implementing interventions such as workplace accommodations. Bev was probably aware of occupational therapy practitioners who worked with students in the school system. However, she and the school administrators may not have recognized the role of occupational therapy in maximizing work performance of aging workers. Regardless of the work setting, occupational therapy has an increasing opportunity to meet the needs of aging workers by building relationships with employers and employees.

References

Administration on Aging, Department on Health and Human Services. (2010). A statistical profile of black older Americans aged 65+. Retrieved from www.aoa.gov/aoaroot/aging_statistics/minority_aging/Facts-on-Black-Elderly-plain_format.aspx.

Age Discrimination in Employment Act of 1967, 29 U.S.C. 14 (1967).

Ameriprise Financial. (2006). The retirement mindscape: A groundbreaking, comprehensive study of the retirement journey. Retrieved from www.harrisinteractive.com/services/pubs/Ameriprise_Financial_New_Retirement_Mindscape.pdf.

Americans with Disabilities Act of 1990, Pub.L. 101-336, 104 Stat. 327 (1990).

American Occupational Therapy Association (AOTA). (2008). Occupational therapy practice framework: Domain and process, 2nd ed. *American Journal of Occupational Therapy, 62,* 625–683.

Bailey, D. E., & Kurland, N. B. (2002). A review of telework research: Findings, new directions, and lessons for the study of modern work. *Journal of Organizational Behavior, 23*(4), 383–400.

Baker, N. A., Jacobs, K., & Tickle-Degnen, L. (2003). A methodology for developing evidence about meaning in occupation: Exploring the meaning of working. *OTJR: Occupation, Participation and Health, 23*(2), 57–66.

Bennis, W. G., & Thomas, R. J. (2002). *Geeks and Geezers.* Boston: Harvard Business School Press.

Brown, K. S. (2003). Staying ahead of the curve 2003: The AARP working in retirement study. Retrieved from http://assets.aarp.org/rgcenter/econ/multiwork_2003.pdf.

Bureau of Labor Statistics. (2008). Older workers: Are there more older people in the workplace? (BLS Spotlight on Statistics). Retrieved from www.bls.gov/spotlight/2008/older_workers/.

Cahill, K. E., Giandrea, M. D., & Quinn, J. F. (2006). Added retirement patterns from career employment. *Gerontologist, 46*(4), 514-523.

Cappelli, P. (2003). Will there really be a labor shortage? *Organizational Dynamics, 32*(3), 221–233.

Central Intelligence Agency. (2009). *The World Factbook.* Washington, DC: Potomac, Poole. Retrieved from https://www.cia.gov/library/publications/the-world-factbook/geos/us.html.

Choi, N. G. (2002). Self-defined retirement status and engagement in paid work among older working-age women: Comparison between childless women and mothers. *Sociological Inquiry, 72*(1), 43–71.

Christiansen, C., & Townsend, E. (2010). An introduction to occupation. In C. Christiansen & E. Townsend (eds.), *Introduction to Occupation: The Art of Science and Living,* 2nd ed. (chap. 1). Upper Saddle River, NJ: Prentice Hall.

Cummings, K. J., & Kreiss, K. (2008). Contingent workers and contingent health: Risks of a modern economy. *Journal of the American Medical Association, 299*(4), 448–450.

Davis, J. A., & Polatajko, H. J. (2004). Occupational development. In C. Christiansen & E. Townsend (eds.), *Introduction to Occupation: The Art and Science of Living* (chap. 5). Upper Saddle River, NJ: Prentice Hall.

Dennis, H., & Thomas, K. (2007). Ageism in the workplace. *Generation, 31*(1), 84–89.

Di Martino, V., & Wirth, L. (1990). Telework: A new way of working and living. *International Labour Review 129*(5), 529.

Drenth, P. (1991). Work meanings: A conceptual, semantic and developmental approach. *European Work and Organizational Psychologist, 1*(2/3), 125–133.

Dunn, W., Brown, C., & McGuigan, A. (1994). The ecology of human performance: A framework for considering the effect of context. *American Journal of Occupational Therapy, 48*(7), 595–607.

Employee Benefit Research Institute. (2007). Facts from EBRI: Retirement trends in the United States over the past quarter-century. Retrieved from www.ebri.org/pdf/publications/facts/0607fact.pdf.

England, G. W., & Harpaz, I. (1990). How working is defined: National contexts and demographic and organizational role influences. *Journal of Organizational Behavior, 11,* 253–355.

Equal Employment Opportunity Commission (EEOC). (1992). *Employment Provisions (Title I) Technical Assistance Manual.* Washington, DC: Equal Employment Opportunity Commission.

Gallo, W. T., Bradley, E. H., Falba, T. A., Dubin, J. A., Cramer, L. D., & Kasl, S. V. (2004). Involuntary job loss as a risk factor for subsequent myocardial infarction and stroke: Findings from the Health and Retirement Survey. *American Journal of Industrial Medicine, 45*(5), 408–416.

Gallo, W. T., Bradley, E. H., Siegel, M., & Kasl, S. V. (2001). The impact of involuntary job loss on subsequent alcohol consumption by older workers: Findings from the Health and Retirement Survey. *Journals of Gerontology, 56*(1), S3–S9.

Groeneman, S. (2008). Staying ahead of the curve 2007: The AARP work and career study. Washington, DC: AARP. Retrieved from http://assets.aarp.org/rgcenter/econ/work_career_08.pdf.

Hao, Y. (2008). Productive activities and psychological well-being among older adults. *Journals of Gerontology, 63*(2), S64–S72.

Harpaz, I., & Fu, X. (2002). The structure and meaning of work: A relative stability amidst change. *Human Relations 55*(6), 639–667.

Hedge, J. W., Borman, W. C., & Lammlein, S. E. (2006). *The Aging Workforce: Realities, Myths, and Implications for Organizations.* Washington, DC: American Psychological Association.

Helman, R., Greenwald, M., Copeland, C., & VanDerhei, J. (2010). The 2010 retirement confidence survey: Confidence stabilizing, but preparations continue to erode. *EBRI Issue Brief/Employee Benefit Research Institute, 340,* 1–43.

Honig, M. (1996). Retirement expectations: Differences by race, ethnicity and gender. *Gerontologist, 36*(30), 373–382.

Huang Y., Shaw W., & Chen, P. (2004). Worker perceptions of organizational support and return-to-work policy: Associations with post-injury job satisfaction. *Work, 23*(3), 225–232.

Illegems, V., & Verbeke, A. (2004). Telework: What does it mean for management? *Long Range Planning, 37*(4), 319–334.

James, J. B., Swanberg, J. E., & McKechnie, S. P. (2007). Responsive workplaces for older workers: Job quality, flexibility and employee engagement. Retrieved from http://agingandwork.bc.edu/documents/IB11_Responsive Workplace.pdf.

John, D. C., & Levine, R. (2009). National retirement savings systems in Australia, Chile, New Zealand and the United Kingdom: Lessons for the United States. Retrieved from www.brookings.edu/papers/2009/07_retirement_savings_john.aspx.

Johnson, R. W. (2004). Trends in job demands among older workers, 1992–2002. *Monthly Labor Review, 127*(7), 48–56.

Johnson, R. W., & Soto, M. (2009). 50+ Hispanic workers: A growing segment of the U.S. workforce. Retrieved from http://assets.aarp.org/rgcenter/econ/hispanic_workers_09.pdf.

Kite, M. E., Stockdale, G. D., Whitley, B. E., Jr., & Johnson, B. T. (2005). Attitudes toward younger and older adults: An updated meta-analytic review. *Journal of Social Issues, 61*(2), 241–266.

Lahey, J. N. (2005). Do older workers face discrimination? Retrieved from http://thecenekreport.squarespace.com/storage/do%20older%20workers%20face%20age%20discrimination.pdf.

Law, M., Cooper, B. A., Strong, S., Stewart, D., Rigby, P. M., & Letts, L. (1996). The person-environment-occupation model: A transactive approach to occupational performance. *Canadian Journal of Occupational Therapy, 63*(1), 9–23.

Lee, J. W., & Lee, G. H. (1999). Effects of aging on pilot performance. In G.C.H. Lee (ed.), *Advances in Occupational Ergonomics and Safety* (pp. 385–394). Burke, VA: IOS Press.

Lim, V. K. G., & Feldman, D. (2003). The impact of time structure and time usage on willingness to retire and accept bridge employment. *International Journal of Human Resource Management 14*(7), 1178–1191.

McDaniel, S. A. (2003). Hidden in the household: Now it's men in mid-life. *Ageing International, 28*(4), 326–344.

MetLife, Inc. (2006). Living longer, working longer: The changing landscape of the aging workforce—A MetLife study. Retrieved from www.metlife.com/assets/cao/mmi/publications/studies/mmi-studies-living-longer.pdf.

Moen, P. (1996). A life course perspective on retirement, gender, and well-being. *Journal of Occupational Health Psychology, 1*(2), 131–144.

Montenegro, X., Fisher, L., & Remez, S. (2002). *Staying Ahead of the Curve: The AARP Work and Career Study.* A national survey conducted for AARP by RoperASW. Washington, DC: AARP.

Munnell, A. H. (2007a). Medicare costs and retirement security. Center for Retirement Research at Boston College, October 2007, Number 7-14. Retrieved from http://crr.bc.edu/images/stories/Briefs/ib_7-14.pdf?phpMyAdmin=43ac483c4de9t51d9eb41.

Munnell, A. H. (2007b). Working longer: A potential win-win proposition. In T. Ghilarducci & J. Turner (eds.), *Work Options for Older Americans* (pp. 11–43). Notre Dame: IN: University of Notre Dame Press.

Munnell, A. H., & Jivan, N. (2005). What makes older women work? Center for Retirement Research at Boston College, Series 1, Sept. 2005. Retrieved from http://crr.bc.edu/images/stories/Briefs/wob_1.pdf?phpMyAdmin=43ac483c4de9t51d9eb41.

Munnell, A. H., & Jivan, N. (2006). Earnings and women's retirement security. Center for Retirement Research at Boston College, Work Options for Older Americans Series, Working Paper #3. Retrieved from http://crr.bc.edu/images/stories/Working_Papers/wp_2006-12.pdf?phpMyAdmin=43ac483c4de9t51d9eb41.

National Council on Retirement Policy. (1998). Can America afford to retire? The retirement facing you and the nation. Retrieved from http://digitalcommons.ilr.cornell.edu/cgi/viewcontent.cgi?article=1005&context=institutes.

National Institute for Occupational Safety and Health (NIOSH). (1999). Stress at work. (NIOSH Publication No. 99-101). Retrieved from www.cdc.gov/niosh/docs/99-101/pdfs/99-101.pdf.

Neuman, K. (2007). Comments on "Continued labor force participation: Individual differences." In T. Ghilarducci & J. Turner (eds.), *Work Options for Older Americans* (pp. 83–90). Notre Dame, IN: University of Notre Dame Press.

Neuman, K. (2008). Quit your job and get healthier? The effect of retirement on health. *Journal of Labor Research, 29*(2), 177–201.

O'Connell, D. J., McNeely, E., & Hall, D. T. (2008). Unpacking personal adaptability at work. *Journal of Leadership and Organizational Studies,13*(3), 248–259.

Pienta, A. M., & Hayward, M. D. (2002). Who expects to continue working after age 62? The retirement plans of couples. *Journals of Gerontology, 57*(4), S199–S208.

Pitt-Catsouphes, M., & Smyer, M. A. (2005a). Older workers: What keeps them working? Retrieved from http://agingandwork.bc.edu/documents/IB01_OlderWrkrs.pdf.

Pitt-Catsouphes, M., & Smyer, M. A. (2005b). Businesses: How are they preparing for the aging workforce? Retrieved from http://agingandwork.bc.edu/documents/IB02_BusinessPreparing.pdf.

Pitt-Catsouphes, M., & Smyer, M. A. (2006). How old are today's older workers? Retrieved from http://agingandwork.bc.edu/documents/IB04_HowOldAreWrkrs.pdf.

Powell, M. (2010). Ageism and abuse in the workplace. *Journal of Gerontological Social Work, 53*(7), 654–658.

Purcell, P. (2007). Older workers: Employment and retirement trends. In T. Ghilarducci & J. Turner (eds.), *Work Options for Older Americans* (pp. 49–64). Notre Dame, IN: University of Notre Dame Press.

Randolph, D. S. (2004). Predicting the effect of disability on employment status and income. *Work, 23*(3), 257–266.

Randstad USA. (2006). Older workers underappreciated in workplace, says survey. Retirement News. Retrieved from http://seniorjournal.com/NEWS/Retirement/6-04-26-OlderWorkersUnderappreciated.htm.

Raskin, P. M., & Gettes, G. (2011). Continued labor force participation: Individual differences. In T. Ghilarducci & J. Turner (eds.), *Work Options for Older Americans* (pp. 65–82). Notre Dame, IN: University of Notre Dame Press.

Rebeiro, K. L. (2001). Enabling occupation: The importance of an affirming environment. *Canadian Journal of Occupational Therapy, 68*(2), 80–89.

Robnett, R. H. (2010). The cognitive and psychological changes associated with aging. In R. H. Robnett & W. C. Chop (eds.), *Gerontology for the Health Care Professional* (pp. 115–154). Sudbury, MA: Jones & Bartlett.

Robnett, R. H., & Murray, J. (2010). Functional performance in later life: Basic sensory, perceptual and physical changes associated with aging. In R. H. Robnett & W. C. Chop (eds.), *Gerontology for the Health Care professional* (pp. 155–178). Sudbury, MA: Jones & Bartlett.

Root, K. A., & Park, R. J. (2009). *Forced Out: Older Workers Confront Job Losses.* Boulder, CO: First Forum Press.

Sabata, D., Williams, M., Milchus, K., Baker, P., & Sanford, J. A. (2008). A retrospective analysis of workplace accommodations: Recommendations for addressing functional limitations. *Assistive Technology, 20*(1), 28–35.

Salthouse, T. A. (1993). Speed and knowledge as determinants of adult age differences in verbal tasks. *Journals of Gerontology, 48*(1), 29–36.

Sharit, J., Czaja, S. J., Hernandez, M., Yang, Y., Perdomo, D., Lewis, J. L., Lee, C. C., & Nair, S. (2004). An evaluation of performance by older persons on a simulated telecommuting task. *Journals of Gerontology, 59*(6), 305–316.

Shea, G. F., & Hassan, A. (2006). *The Older Worker Advantage: Making the Most of Our Aging Workforce.* Westport, CT: Praeger.

Sok, E. (2010). Record unemployment among older workers does not keep them out of the job market. Retrieved from www.bls.gov/opub/ils/summary_10_04/older_workers.htm.

Stankov, A. K., & Lord, S. (1993). Primary aging, secondary aging and intelligence. *Psychological Aging, 8*(4), 562–570.

Szinovacz, M. E., DeViney, S., & Davey, A. (2001). Influences of family obligations and relationships on retirement: Variations by gender, race, and marital status. *Journals of Gerontology, 56*(1), S20–S27.

Tesch-Romer, C. (2009). Health consequences of early retirement. *AARP International.* Retrieved from www.aarpinternational.org/resourcelibrary/resourcelibrary_show.htm?doc_id=918896.

Toossi, M. (2007). Labor force projections to 2016: More workers in their golden years. *Monthly Labor Review, 130*(11), 33–52.

U.S. Department of Commerce. (2009). Census bureau reports world's older population projected to triple by 2050. Retrieved from www.census.gov/Press-Release/www/releases/archives/international_population/013882.html.

U.S. Equal Employment Opportunity Commission (EEOC). (2009). Fact sheet: Age discrimination. Retrieved from www.eeoc.gov/eeoc/publications/upload/age.pdf.

U.S. General Accounting Office. (2003). Major management challenges and program risks. Department of Labor. Performance and Accountability Series. Retrieved from www.gao.gov/pas/2003/d03106.pdf.

U.S. Technology-Related Assistance for Individuals with Disabilities Act of 1988, Section 3.1. Pub.L. No. 100-407, 29 U.S.C. § 2202(2).

Van Dalen, H. P., Henkens, K., & Schippers, J. (2009). Unraveling the age-productivity nexus: Confronting perceptions of employers and employees. Retrieved from http://arno.uvt.nl/show.cgi?fid=90310.

Williams, M., Sabata, D., & Zolna, J. (2006). User needs evaluation of workplace accommodations. *Work, 27*(4), 355–370.

Williams, M., Sabata, D., & Zolna, J. (2008). Accommodating aging workers who have a disability In A. Mihailidis, J. Boger, H. Kautz, & L. Normie (eds.), *Assistive Technology Research Series, Volume 21, Technology and Aging: Selected Papers from the 2007 International Conference on Technology and Aging* (pp. 51–55). Fairfax, VA: ISO Press.

Zolna, J. S., Sanford, J., Sabata, D., & Goldthwaite, J. (2007). Review of accommodation strategies in the workplace for persons with mobility and dexterity impairments: Application to criteria for universal design. *Technology and Disability, 19*(4), 189–198.

Glossary

Accommodations in the job or workplace are changes in the work environment or the way in which work tasks are accomplished that enable a person with differing abilities to enjoy equal employment opportunities.

An **aging worker** is a person age 55 or older who is actively employed or seeking employment.

Alternative formats are various ways, other than standard oral or written, of presenting materials and information (e.g., large print materials, Braille, electronic format).

Assistive technology (AT) is "any item, piece of equipment, or product system, whether acquired commercially off the shelf, modified, or customized, that is used to increase, maintain, or improve functional capabilities of individuals with disabilities. AT service is directly assisting an individual with a disability in the selection, acquisition, or use of an assistive technology device" (U.S. Technology-Related Assistance for Individuals with Disabilities Act of 1988).

Cues (visual and auditory) are signals in the environment used to prompt or serve as a reminder.

Energy conservation encompasses strategies used to minimize effort required to complete a task.

Ergonomics is the science of designing equipment and workplaces to maximize the fit between the user and work tools and environment. A goal of ergonomics is to enhance safety and efficiency at the workplace while minimizing work-related injury.

Job restructuring entails modifying the essential job functions and redistributing or reallocating nonessential job functions to enable a worker with disabilities to continue to work. Job restructuring may involve changing the way the work gets done by modifying the environment and/or providing assistive technology.

Social Security is a social insurance program sponsored by the U.S. government that is funded by mandatory payments by employers and employees. In the context of this chapter, Social Security refers to payments for retired persons 62 and older who become eligible once they retire. Social Security also covers persons with disability and survivors.

Retirement is a transition point in work when an employee exits the paid workforce and stops working.

Phased retirement encompasses broad range of formal and/or informal employment arrangements that workers approaching retirement enter into with their employer to continue to work on a part-time basis and gradually transition into full-time retirement.

Contingent work is alternative or nontraditional temporary work arrangements involve no implicit or explicit contract for ongoing employment. This type of work typically does not provide employee benefits.

Telecommute, also called *telework,* is a work option whereby work is done offsite, typically from home rather than in the traditional workplace, with the help of telecommunications technology such as high-speed Internet, computers, fax, and telephone.

Resources

AARP

www.aarp.org

Staying ahead of the curve: AARP Work and Career Study

American Occupational Therapy Association

www.aota.org

AOTA tip sheets on workplace

Burton Blatt Institute, Syracuse University

http://bbi.syr.edu

Center for Retirement Research

http://crr.bc.edu

Disability and Business Technical Assistance Centers

www.adata.org/network/index.html

Employment and Disability Institute, Cornell University

www.ilr.cornell.edu/edi/

Job Accommodations Network (JAN)

www.jan.org

Meaning of Work (MOW) International Research Program

http://users.ugent.be/~rclaes/MOW/index.html

Office of Disability Employment Policy (ODEP)

www.dol.gov/odep/pubs/ek97/process.htm

Rehabilitation Engineering Research Center on Workplace Accommodations (WorkRERC)

www.workrerc.org

9

Mental Health and Work

Rachel Eisfelder and Rebecca Gewurtz

Key Concepts

The following are key concepts addressed in this chapter:

- The population of persons with mental illness who receive services from occupational therapists in mental health settings is described.
- Stigma and how it affects the employment process for those with mental illness is explored.
- The supported employment (SE) and the individual placement and support (IPS) models are described.
- Examples of work-related interventions for persons with mental illness are provided.

Case Introduction

Tammy is a 32-year-old African American female who is engaged to be married. She has completed a bachelor of science degree as well as a certificate program in a related field. At this time, she is working in a field unrelated to her degree; however, she has decided to continue searching for employment in her field while improving her work-related skills. She has recently started a job through an agency that hires individuals as custodians for local businesses. Individuals are typically responsible for emptying and taking out garbage, sweeping or vacuuming, cleaning restrooms, and other such tasks. Tammy reports she is very motivated to "keep this new job." She has a moderately good support system. She and her twin sister are very close and provide support to each other, and she is also supported by extended family and her fiancé. However, Tammy has reported on occasion that she can get frustrated with her fiancé because he telephones her frequently and is "needy" at times.

Tammy was diagnosed with schizoaffective disorder 10 years ago and has been followed by an interdisciplinary team, including a physician, a vocational rehabilitation specialist, a case manager, and an occupational therapist, through programs in a community mental health center. Tammy has been highly engaged with her team, has maintained good therapeutic relationships, and seeks support when needed. In addition to experiencing periods of profound depression alternating with periods of elevated or irritable mood, Tammy experiences auditory and visual hallucinations, which increase isolation and paranoia. Tammy's level of functioning becomes limited when she experiences hallucinations, as observed by a lack of home management tasks as well as increased disorganization. Tammy tends to experience bouts of depression more frequently than manic episodes, and her auditory and visual hallucinations seem to increase when she is feeling depressed. She reports increased depression when her stress level increases and she feels overwhelmed. Tammy has poor self-esteem and passive communication skills. She becomes increasingly stressed when confronted with conflict; however, when conflict occurs, she tends to ignore it and to personalize the other person's behavior. In conjunction with her psychosocial needs, Tammy has hypoglycemia, which requires her to maintain a balanced diet. Her employment specialist notes the hypoglycemia as a barrier because, during a job assessment, Tammy became lightheaded as a result of low blood sugar, and the employment specialist had to intervene.

Tammy expresses anxiety about her new job and is concerned that she may not be able to complete her job requirements in the time allotted. Tammy is currently working with an employment specialist through a nonprofit community mental health center and with her vocational rehabilitation counselor through the state. She also works closely with her psychiatrist and has been evaluated by the occupational therapist.

Introduction

In Chapter 1, you were introduced to the development of the occupational therapy profession and its long history of involvement in work-related occupations. In this chapter, we focus on the development of the profession's involvement in supporting people living with mental illness in their work-related occupations. Our understanding of how productive occupation, including work or employment, benefits people living with mental illness began primarily in the Progressive Era mental hygiene movement in the United States. During the first 30 years of the occupational therapy profession, most practitioners worked in mental health or psychiatric settings (Pitts, 2009). Individuals who were institutionalized during the 19th century, in the moral treatment era, began to be treated more humanely as the paradigm for treatment of psychiatric disorders shifted toward utilizing work and daily activity.

In the 1940s and 1950s, occupational therapy experienced a divergence in practice due to an increased focus on reductionism and the psychodynamic perspective. Grounded in the medical model, the perspective viewed people as representing states of homeostasis or disease, which contrasted with the ideas of holism and balance purported by earlier occupational therapy theorists (Kielhofner and Burke, 1977). Due to this paradigm shift, occupational therapy moved from working within vocational rehabilitation to focusing on how activity affects mental health and mental illness (Pitts, 2009). As a result of this shift and the limitations of the medical model, the 1960s and 1970s posed a difficult time for occupational therapy in mental health (Kielhofner and Burke, 1977).

As deinstitutionalization began to take hold, some occupational therapy practitioners became involved in various community-based models of service delivery in order to address the needs of their clients in the community; services included transitional employment programs (Beard, Schmidt, and Smith, 1963), psychosocial rehabilitation centers (Glasscote, Cumming, Rutman, Sussex, and Glassman, 1971), halfway houses (Glasscote, Gudeman, and Elpers, 1971), and assertive community treatment (ACT) teams (Stein and Test, 1985). Occupational therapy practitioners working within these models worked alongside other mental health professionals, often taking on generalist roles. During the late 1970s and 1980s, occupational therapy practice in mental health began to grow, and practice shifted back to an occupational perspective (Kielhofner and Burke, 1977). Occupational therapy practitioners in mental health began to explore their connection in psychosocial and psychiatric rehabilitation through occupation (Pitts, 2009). Practitioners working on interdisciplinary teams began to reclaim their occupational perspective and apply it to their work with individuals, clients, and communities (Krupa, Radloff-Gabriel, Whippey, and Kirsh, 2002)

Program models in psychiatric rehabilitation continued to flourish throughout the next several decades, and recovery began to emerge as a guiding conceptual framework in mental health practice (Blank and Hayward 2009; Slade and Hayward, 2007). Influenced by research suggesting that the deteriorating course of mental illness is not evitable (Harding, Brooks, Ashikaga, Strauss, and Breier, 1987) and the experiences of persons with mental illness (Deegan, 1988, 2001), recovery has been defined as "a way of living a satisfying, hopeful and contributing life, even with the limitations caused by the illness" (Anthony, 1993, p. 16). Recovery involves the development of meaning and purpose in one's life and transcending the experience of mental illness despite the ongoing, intermittent, or continuous presence of symptoms (Davidson, et al., 2001; Jacobson and Greenley, 2001). Recovery-oriented services focus on fostering hope for the future, empowering individuals to make real choices, building a system of support and companionship, and creating opportunities for engagement in meaningful occupation and community participation (Brown, 2001; Stoffel, 2011). Accordingly, occupational therapy practitioners are well suited to work within a recovery-oriented system of care. Promoting engagement in occupation for mental health and well-being and helping individuals who live with mental illness build a meaningful life are consistent with a recovery-oriented focus (Blank and Hayward 2009; Krupa and Clark, 2004; Rebeiro, 2005).

Recovery continues to be a key goal of mental health services (Farkas, Gagne, Anthony, and Chamberlin, 2005; Frese, Stanley, Dress, and Vogel-Scibilia, 2001; Ralph, Lambert, and Kidder, 2002). Target outcomes of service delivery increasingly include occupational and psychosocial outcomes that capture the complexity of recovery with a focus on social participation and inclusion (Krupa, et al., 2002). Consistent with a recovery-oriented focus, employment is a priority of mental health services as a means of helping individuals move beyond their experience of mental illness, recognize their capabilities, and develop ideas about their potential (Gewurtz and Kirsh, 2007; Provencher, Gregg, Mead, and Mueser, 2002; Strong, 1998). Employment is now a key indicator of recovery (O'Day and Killeen, 2002), and assisting individuals to find and keep jobs and advance their careers is a key focus of recovery-oriented mental health services.

> *Consistent with a recovery-oriented focus, employment is a priority of mental health services as a means of helping individuals move beyond their experience of mental illness, recognize their capabilities, and develop ideas about their potential.*

Despite progress in the field, unemployment continues to be a significant problem for individuals living with mental illness, and the provision of work-related services and supports is a key focus for occupational therapy in the mental health sector. According to Secker, Grove, and Seebohm (2001), 70 to 90 percent of people with mental health problems would like to have a job; however, employment rates among this population are as low as 10 to 30 percent across several developed countries, including the United States (Garske and Stewart, 1999; Noble, Honberg, Hall, and Flynn, 1999), the United Kingdom (Harvey, Henderson, Lelliot, and Hotopf, 2009; Marwaha and Johnson, 2004), Australia (Waghorn, Chant, and Whiteford, 2002), and Canada (Centre for Addiction and Mental Health, 2004). These staggering employment rates are particularly troubling in light of the growing evidence that employment is associated with multiple benefits for individuals living with mental illness and can contribute to an individual's recovery (Burns, et al., 2007; Crowther, Marshall, Bond, and Huxley, 2001).

The remainder of Chapter 9 reviews work-related occupational therapy practice with persons living with mental illness, including a description of the settings in which these services are provided as well as typical intervention strategies.

Description of the Population

Individuals with the lived experience of mental illness form a diverse and heterogeneous population that is typically defined in terms of level of disability, duration and severity, and diagnosis (Ontario Ministry of Health and Long-Term Care, 2000). *Disability* refers to difficulties that interfere with an individual's capacity to function in major life activities such as employment. *Duration and severity* are the acute, continuous, and intermittent experience of mental illness. *Diagnoses* typically include mood disorders, schizophrenia, and other types of psychoses. However, individuals living with mental illness often have concurrent conditions such as intellectual impairments, substance abuse or dependence, and physical health problems (Makikyro, et al., 1998; Mitchell and Malone, 2006; Regier, et al., 1990).

Work-related rehabilitation and occupational therapy services vary according to the individual's preexisting relationship to the workplace (Krupa, 2007; O'Halloran and Innes, 2005). Individuals with jobs who are either experiencing problems in the workplace or are on leave as a result of mental health problems or mental illness might encounter an occupational therapy practitioner through their employer or insurance company to help them maintain employment or return to work following a leave. These individuals might return to their previous job or a modified position, or they might return to another job within the same organization. However, their preexisting and ongoing relationship with an employer is critical and is often an asset in their work rehabilitation (Saint-Arnaud, Saint-Jean, and Damasse, 2006). Under these conditions, occupational therapy practitioners work in collaboration with disability management coordinators, case managers, and other health-care professionals, including occupational health physicians and nurses who can offer a range of assessment and interventions to facilitate the return-to-work process and negotiate reasonable accommodations (Krupa, 2007).

Individuals with no existing relationship with an employer who are either entering the workplace for the first time or returning to work after a long absence as the result of experiencing mental illness might encounter an occupational therapy practitioner through an employment or vocational program. These programs are usually government funded and may be government operated or operated by private for-profit or nonprofit community-based organizations. The focus is on helping individuals find and keep a job in the mainstream labor market. Unlike individuals with established relationships with employers, this group has to find jobs that meet their needs in the labor market (Krupa, 2007). Occupational therapy practitioners often work in collaboration with vocational rehabilitation specialists or counselors through publicly funded community mental health or vocational rehabilitation services to form connections with local employers to fill vacant positions that are suited to the skills, competencies, and strengths of the individual (Fig. 9.1).

Beyond their relationships with employers, these two groups often differ along social and diagnostic criteria. Individuals who have preexisting relationships with employers usually have recent work histories and sometimes have well-established careers. Therefore, they often have a worker identity (Gewurtz, Kirsh, Jacobson, and Rappolt, 2006) and the necessary skills, habits, and routines to maintain employment. They usually have access to financial resources through employment insurance or disability benefits, which can provide some protection from the impact of unemployment (Krupa, 2007). Furthermore, the onset of their illness or mental health problems might have occurred later in life, following the completion of their job training and education.

Conversely, those without these established connections could be young adults entering the workplace for the first time. Many experienced the onset of their illness during late adolescence or early adulthood while completing their education or job training, thereby interrupting their career trajectory (Gewurtz, et al., 2006; Krupa, 2007). Thus, many individuals in this group rely on government-administered income and may have incomplete education and job credentials. Living in a state of poverty and social marginalization can further complicate their transition to employment by restricting their opportunities and access to basic resources (Cook, 2006).

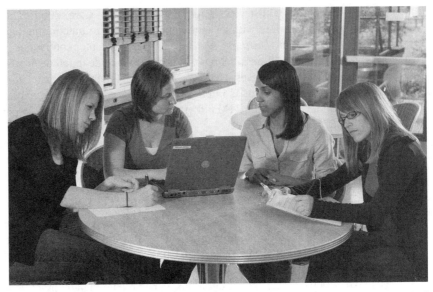

Figure 9.1 Occupational therapists and occupational therapy assistants often work as part of a multidisciplinary team to create connections with local employers.

Among both groups, employers and coworkers are particularly important in terms of negotiating accommodations in the workplace. Individuals with mental illness often benefit from accommodations that involve scheduling changes, changes to communication procedures and social interactions, and task modifications (MacDonald-Wilson, Rogers, Massaro, Lyass, and Crean, 2002). Despite their low costs, such accommodations are frequently challenging to implement because they can threaten established workplace rules and procedures (Harlan and Robert, 1998). Furthermore, the legitimacy of their illness, and therefore the need for accommodations, may be questioned because mental illness is often largely invisible and episodic, alternating between periods of illness and health (Gewurtz and Kirsh, 2009; Krupa, Kirsh, Cockburn, and Gewurtz, 2009). Open communication, education, and problem-solving are required to negotiate arrangements that meet the needs of the worker, the employer/manager, and the coworkers.

> *Individuals with mental illness often benefit from accommodations that involve scheduling changes, changes to communication procedures and social interactions, and task modifications. Despite their low costs, such accommodations are frequently challenging to implement because they can threaten established workplace rules and procedures.*

Stigma and Discrimination

Stigma and discrimination toward people living with mental illness are prevalent concerns for individuals returning to work or entering a new job and can complicate the decision to disclose a mental illness to an employer or coworker. Krupa and colleagues (2009) define stigma as "a social phenomenon, grounded in both the intolerance of human differences and the inability to meaningfully capitalize on human diversity" (p. 414). Discrimination is the behavioral expression of stigma: it involves treating people differently, negatively, or adversely because of their connection to a group. Both stigma and discrimination are detrimental to individuals living with mental illness in the workplace.

There are widespread assumptions that mental illness is associated with incompetency and that individuals with mental illness make unreliable and unpredictable employees (Krupa, et al., 2009). Stigma can create situations in which expectations and opportunities are restricted for individuals with mental illness, so individuals often actively conceal their condition at work and cover up their limitations even though disclosure could lead to helpful accommodations (Gewurtz and Kirsh, 2009). Without disclosure, employees with mental illness can miss their potential to be role models for others, to demonstrate their strengths, to create supported peer relationships, and to advocate for their rights (Krupa, et al., 2009). Furthermore, without disclosure and a culture of open communication, occupational therapists might be limited in their role in the workplace.

Efforts to better understand the attitudes and beliefs that foster stigma toward persons with mental illness are ongoing (Corrigan and Lam, 2007; Corrigan, Markowitz, and Watson, 2004; Feldman and Crandall, 2007). Krupa and colleagues (2009) suggest that antistigma campaigns targeting the workplace may educate employers, coworkers, and human resource professionals about mental illness and requirements to accommodate employees with disabilities, and may foster more positive attitudes toward persons with mental illness. Success in competitive employment can counter stigma linked to poverty and reliance on social assistance (Mickelson and Williams, 2008) and may counteract assumptions of incompetence in the workplace (Krupa, et al., 2009).

Stigma can create situations in which expectations and opportunities are restricted for individuals with mental illness.

Despite ongoing efforts to address stigma toward persons with mental illness in the workplace, it continues to hinder individuals with mental illness. Assumptions about mental illness are likely to fuel negative labeling and discrimination (Corrigan and Lam, 2007; Link and Phelan, 2006). To advance the development of theory related to the stigma associated with mental illness in the context of employment, Krupa and colleagues (2009) conducted a study using constructivist-grounded theory methodology of over 500 Canadian documents from a range of sources and perspectives and 19 informant interviews. Their findings suggest several key components of stigma in the context of work, including five assumptions that underlie the expressions of stigma toward persons with mental illness. For persons with mental illness, these assumptions (summarized in Box 9.1) can have several negative consequences that can hinder their opportunities in the workplace;

Box 9.1 Negative Assumptions About Persons With Mental Illness

1. People with mental illness lack the competence to meet the considerable task requirements and social demands of work.
2. People with mental illness are dangerous or unpredictable in the workplace.
3. Mental illness is not a legitimate illness.
4. Working is not healthy for people with mental illness.
5. Providing employment for people with mental illness is an act of charity.

(Krupa, et al., 2009)

for example, employers may hesitate to hire individuals with past or present mental illness because they are believed to be incapable of meeting the job demands.

Research examining employer perspectives on persons with mental illness confirms that stigma can impact hiring practices. For example, Shankar and Collyer (2004) found that employers were apprehensive about hiring people living with mental illness regardless of their qualifications because they did not feel comfortable providing constructive feedback about their work performance and were concerned about how to support an employee with a mental illness. They were also uneasy about the possibility of a future crisis in the workplace and uncertain about their responsibilities and obligations to the employee and coworkers. Similar findings were reported by Hand and Tryssenaar (2006) in their survey of small business employers and their hiring practices; they found that employers were particularly concerned with the social competency of potential employees with known mental illnesses.

Traditional strategies to entice employers to hire persons with mental illness, such as wage subsidies, can further perpetuate the assumption that persons with mental illness are deficient as workers. However, supported employment (SE) programs that place individuals directly into competitive employment positions with the provision of ongoing on-the-job support can counteract these assumptions by creating opportunities for individuals to be successful at work (Bond, Drake, and Becker, 2008).

The manner in which mental illness presents at work can perpetuate stigma toward people living with mental illness. Presenteeism refers to employees who are at work despite the presence of illness but are functioning at less than their full capacity (Dewa, Lesage, Goering, and Caveen, 2004). Presenteeism due to mental illness has significant productivity and economic costs for businesses. For example, Stewart, Ricci, Chee, Hahn, and Morganstein (2003) estimate that among U.S. workers, presenteeism productivity loss as a result of depression is about 4 hours per week, or $36 billion. Persistent presenteeism often burdens coworkers who must provide coverage. Furthermore, individuals often choose not to disclose their illness until their performance is in question following a crisis at work (Gewurtz and Kirsh, 2009). Such circumstances can raise further questions about the legitimacy of the condition. Box 9.2 provides an example of the impact of presenteeism in the workplace.

Box 9.2 Return-to-Work Case

Don is 40 years old and has been a high school math teacher for 15 years. He has always maintained good relationships with his coworkers and supervisors and is well liked among his students. Approximately 1 year ago, coworkers and students began to notice a change in Don. He became less sociable and more withdrawn, and he was less animated and enthusiastic in his classes. He began showing up late for his classes and appeared distracted. Nobody inquired about what was happening. Instead, coworkers covered for him, eventually becoming resentful.

After several months of noticeable behavioral changes and subpar performance, Don reportedly lost the final exams of several students. The school administration intervened and discussed disciplinary action with Don and his union representative. When confronted, Don disclosed that he had been experiencing stress, difficulty concentrating, and disruptions in his sleep. He requested a medical leave. After consulting with a psychiatrist, he was diagnosed with depression. His diagnosis was disclosed to his insurer, and he was deemed eligible for disability benefits.

Eight months later, Don was referred to an occupational therapist through his long-term disability provider, and they began developing a return-to-work plan. He is currently taking medication and reports an improvement in his symptoms and his ability to function at home and in his community. However, he is anxious about returning to the demands of teaching high school. He feels that he might be able to handle a gradual return to his full-time teaching responsibilities; however, he has ongoing difficulties with concentration and fatigue and concerns about coping with the pressures of his job, including planning his classes, marking exams, and attending to student and parent needs

Box 9.2   Return-to-Work Case—cont'd

and expectations. He is attending a mindfulness-based stress-reduction group to learn strategies for managing his mood, anxiety, and other symptoms.

His colleagues are also uncertain about Don's return. Although Don did not disclose his mental illness to them, some assume the behavioral changes they witnessed prior to his leave were the result of a "nervous breakdown." They are frustrated by the extra work they have taken on and worry that he will not be able to meet the demands of his job. Some have commented that everyone goes through rough times, and they wonder why Don has received "special treatment."

Connecting Individuals to the Workplace

Supported Employment and the Individual Placement and Support Models

The SE model of practice focuses on helping individuals with disabilities find and keep jobs in the mainstream labor market. It involves rapid placement of individuals into jobs that are well matched to their preferences and strengths, followed by ongoing support and skills training (Bond, 1998; Bond, et al., 2001; Drake, Becker, Clark, and Mueser, 1999). It marks a significant shift from traditional vocational programs that focused on preemployment services designed to help individuals develop skills necessary to succeed in the workplace.

In the mental health field, a group of clinical researchers developed the individual placement and support (IPS) approach as a standardized way of providing SE services to unemployed individuals with mental illness (Bond, 1998; Bond, Drake, Mueser, and Becker, 1997). Based on the SE and ACT models, IPS consists of integrating the employment specialists directly on comprehensive mental health treatment teams. The premise of this approach is that employment should be considered as part of the treatment plan for every individual interested in working (Drake, et al., 1999) and that individuals with mental illness require support in finding and keeping jobs.

To date, SE and IPS are considered the most widely studied models of service delivery for people with mental illness (Bond, et al., 2008; Bond, et al., 1997; Drake, et al., 1999). There is overall agreement that SE and IPS are best-practice approaches in community mental health and are associated with improved employment outcomes (Bond, et al., 2001; Bond, et al., 2008; Crowther, et al., 2001; Drake, et al., 2001; Rinaldi and Perkins, 2007). Randomized controlled trials have reported significant gains in competitive employment rates for individuals enrolled in SE programs compared with those in traditional vocational rehabilitation programs without any negative changes in nonvocational outcomes (Bond, et al., 2008; Crowther, et al., 2001; Lehman, et al., 2002). Specifically, in a review of 11 randomized control trials of the IPS model, Bond and colleagues (2008) found that 61 percent of individuals who received evidence-based SE secured competitive employment compared to 23 percent of individuals who received other vocational services.

Despite the positive outcomes associated with SE, some findings are disappointing. A significant proportion of individuals enrolled in SE programs remain unemployed (Bond, et al., 2008). In a randomized controlled trial of IPS in Montreal, Canada, Latimer and colleagues (2006) reported that only 13 percent of participants were able to average at least 5 hours of work per week over the 1-year follow-up period. Thus, even with improved employment outcomes, few individuals with mental illness are able to earn sufficient income through SE, and many remain dependent on social assistance (Becker, Whitley, Bailey, and Drake, 2007; Salyers, Becker, Drake, Torrey, and Wyzik, 2004). Although employment outcomes improve, the focus tends to be on part-time and entry-level work (Baron, 2000;

Bond, et al., 2001; Marrone, Foley, and Selleck, 2005), which does little to improve the economic circumstances of clients.

Clubhouse Model

The clubhouse model, which originated in New York City with Fountain House, is found around the world. The model supports individuals living with mental illness in their social, vocational, financial, and educational goals. It provides a community space for members to meet and participate in the operations of the clubhouse and offers services and supports grounded in the principles of psychiatric rehabilitation (International Center for Clubhouse Development [ICCD], 2008). Most clubhouses provide prevocational training, transitional employment, and/or SE programs. In the prevocational domain, clubhouses provide opportunities for members to participate in the operation and management of the clubhouse by working with staff in various work units. Typical work units include clerical, food services, maintenance, and membership services. When members express an interest in pursuing competitive employment, they might be provided with opportunities through transitional or SE programs offered within the clubhouse. As with SE, transitional employment provides clients paid employment opportunities in the labor market (Henry, Barreira, Banks, Brown, and McKay, 2001; Kirsh, Krupa, Cockburn, and Gewurtz, 2006). However, in transitional employment, the placements are temporary and "owned" by the program rather than the individual; the program secures the placements and guarantees coverage to the employer in the case of absenteeism (ICCD, 2008; Henry, et al., 2001; Kirsh, et al., 2006; Schonebaum, Boyd, and Dudek, 2006). Once the time limit is reached, another clubhouse member is offered the job (Henry, et al., 2001).

Recent research sheds light on the effectiveness of the clubhouse model in helping members connect to the workplace. Henry and colleagues (2001) conducted a retrospective study at a medium-sized clubhouse in an urban center. These authors found that 30.4 percent of members obtained competitive employment 1 year following their last recorded transitional employment placement. The jobs obtained by members tended to be part-time and entry-level positions. In a randomized controlled trial of 63 ACT and 58 clubhouse participants, Macias and colleagues (2006) found that employment outcomes across both programs met or exceeded published outcomes associated with SE. Although there were no significant differences in the employment rates (ACT, 64%; clubhouse, 47%), the clubhouse participants worked significantly longer, worked more total hours, and earned more money. Subgroup analysis based on the type and level of disability revealed that ACT was particularly effective for participants with co-occurring physical health problems or severe substance use, while the clubhouse was more effective for participants without these co-occurring conditions. Schonebaum and colleagues (2006) followed a group of 170 individuals with mental illness who were randomly assigned to either a clubhouse program ($N = 86$) or an ACT program ($N = 84$). After 30 months, 74 percent of ACT participants and 60 percent of clubhouse participants had been placed in at least one job. As with the study by Macias and colleagues, clubhouse participants earned significantly higher wages and lasted longer in each job than did ACT participants. Together, these findings suggest that clubhouses are effective at connecting people living with mental illness to the workplace.

Occupational therapy practitioners provide services within the clubhouse model in a number of capacities. Practitioners can assist with the work units, focusing on psychosocial aspects of employment such as wellness, communication skills, problem-solving skills, and stress management skills. Occupational therapy consultation with clubhouse members who seek competitive employment may improve their long-term success. Practitioners can provide their expertise with task analysis and options for adapting environment or task as well as assist members in exploring employment preferences through transitional and SE programs offered by the clubhouse.

Alternative Businesses

Alternative, consumer-run, affirmative, and agency-sponsored businesses are flourishing in some parts of the world (Kirsh, et al., 2006; Warner and Mandiberg, 2006). Although each of these business structures differ in terms of ownership and control, they share a common focus on economic and community development by addressing unemployment among individuals with mental illness (Kirsh, et al., 2006). These businesses provide goods and services to the public (much like any other business) but are staffed by individuals who have lived experience of mental illness. Employees are paid a competitive wage and receive eligible employment benefits. Such businesses are seen as an important means of creating jobs and opportunities for individuals with mental illness to develop work-related skills and leadership capacity in a supportive work environment (Kirsh, et al., 2006; Strong, 1998). Further advantages of alternative businesses include opportunities for empowerment, community development, and social support (Strong, 1998; Warner and Mandiberg, 2006). However, questions have been raised about opportunities for career development and advancement within alternative businesses, as many jobs tend to be entry level and employees rarely transition from such businesses to other competitive employment opportunities (Seyfried and Ziomas, 2005). Occupational therapy practitioners might be involved in referring individuals to local businesses in order to pursue employment opportunities or assisting businesses to create healthy work environments and accommodate the needs of their employees (Fig. 9.2) (Krupa, 1998).

Persons With Established Connections to the Workplace

The Return-to-Work Process

Important trends have occurred in return-to-work processes and the provision of employment supports for individuals who are on leave from work due to a mental illness. Most

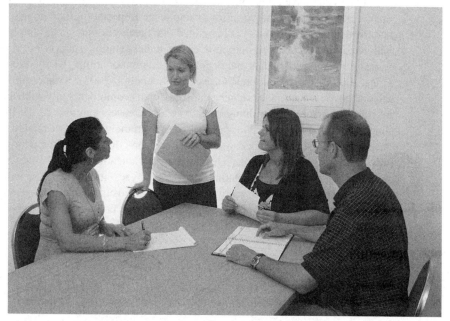

Figure 9.2 An alternative business manager and consumers consult with an occupational therapy practitioner on strategies for supporting consumer trainees and employees.

notably, recent evidence highlights the benefits of instituting early and gradual return-to-work plans (Canadian Psychiatric Research Foundation, 2007). Such plans can help maintain the individual's ongoing connection to the workplace and facilitate communication among the multiple stakeholders involved in the return-to-work process, including the employer, the worker, union representatives, disability management coordinators, and various health-care professionals.

However, there are several potential challenges to implementing early and gradual return-to-work plans. In a qualitative study examining the factors involved in the return-to-work process of employees on leave from work due to mental health problems, Saint-Arnaud and colleagues (2006) found that a gradual return-to-work plan can be contradictory to the goal of maximizing workplace productivity. As a result, individuals can be pressured to cut short this process. These authors state: "Gradual return to work can be effective only if the work context is favorable" (p. 310). Furthermore, Gewurtz and Kirsh (2009) conducted a qualitative metasynthesis on the experiences of persons with disabilities in the workplace and found that conditions such as mental illness that are largely invisible and poorly understood can evoke a sense of disbelief among coworkers and supervisors. This disbelief can pose further challenges to individuals trying to reintegrate and readapt to the demands and responsibilities of the workplace and can threaten the success of the return-to-work process. According to these authors, individuals often struggle to convince others about the significance of the limitations caused by their illness without compromising their reputation as a reliable and dependable worker. The episodic nature of many mental illnesses invites further disbelief and ambiguity. Gewurtz and Kirsh found that under such conditions, workplace accommodations are often perceived as special treatment, and individuals with mental illness are viewed as troublemakers. These findings highlight the complexity of negotiating workplace accommodations for persons with mental illness.

Creating Healthy Workplaces

Increasing evidence highlights the positive impact that healthy, supportive, and flexible workplaces can have on the mental health of employees (Kirsh, 2000; Strong, 1998). Tolerance and acceptance at work, for example, are important to individuals with disabilities and impact the way disability is integrated into the day-to-day operations at work (Gewurtz and Kirsh, 2009). Having supportive and understanding supervisors and coworkers is critical for job maintenance and negotiating accommodations (Kirsh, 2000; Saint-Arnaud, et al., 2006; Secker, Membrey, Grove, and Seebohm, 2003). Krupa (2007) further elaborated about how workplaces can be constructed to promote mental health and prevent mental illness. Specifically, training initiatives to increase awareness of the impact of mental illness at work and reasonable accommodations in the workplace can help improve acceptance and understanding. Occupational therapy practitioners can be involved in assessing and intervening at the workplace level to help organizations adopt healthy workplace practices that are more accommodating for all employees, including those with mental health problems. This type of intervention might include ensuring that managers are equipped to support their employees and modifying workplace policies and procedures to be more flexible and accommodating.

Occupational therapy practitioners can be involved in assessing and intervening at the workplace level to help organizations adopt healthy workplace practices that are more accommodating for all employees, including those with mental health problems.

Policy Issues

Policy developments such as the Americans with Disabilities Act (ADA) in the United States and comparable disability and human rights legislation in other developed countries have the potential to improve opportunities for individuals with disabilities at work (see Chapters 16 and 17). However, mounting evidence suggests that disabilities resulting from mental illness are particularly challenging to address through legislative means and that legislation alone is insufficient to effectively improve the integration of individuals with mental illness in the workplace (Gewurtz and Kirsh, 2009). For example, 7 years after the ADA was passed in the United States, the Office of Technology Assessment (OTA) conducted an evaluation of efforts under the ADA in the area of psychiatric disabilities and employment with the goal of improving future implementation efforts (Behney, Hall, and Keller, 1997). The findings from this evaluation highlight how persons with mental illness are particularly disadvantaged under the ADA because of an inadequate understanding of the relationship between mental illness and work. Identifying, removing, and preventing barriers to employment for individuals who have experienced mental illness can be difficult because the barriers are often less concrete and less visible than those associated with most physical disabilities.

Further policy issues concern those governing the administration of benefit systems. Many individuals with mental illness rely on income from various benefit systems. Each system has rules governing participation in employment and the treatment of earnings from employment. Efforts to assist individuals with mental illness to obtain paid employment are undermined by caps on earnings and recipients' fears about losing medication and drug coverage (Baron, 2000; Henry and Lucca, 2004; O'Day and Killeen, 2002). People living with mental illness face particular challenges in this regard due to the fluctuating and episodic course of many mental illnesses. Obtaining paid employment during a time of health and stability might lead to a financial crisis in the case of a relapse if income benefits and medication coverage are discontinued. Even during times of health and stability, many people living with mental illness rely on medication to manage symptoms to maintain their ability to participate in the workforce. Although prescription drug coverage could shift from the public to private spheres as individuals enter the workforce, many jobs obtained by people living with mental illness are low-paying and entry-level positions without adequate employee benefits (Baron, 2000; Bond, et al., 2001; Marrone, et al., 2005).

Research examining the impact of income support substantiates these concerns. Warner (2001) notes that employment among people living with mental illness is highest in jurisdictions that have less severe disincentives to work in their disability pension programs. Using a narrative approach, Estroff, Patrick, Zimmer, and Lachicotte (1997) conducted a 32-month prospective cohort study to describe how people living with mental illness apply for and receive disability income benefits. The findings suggest that the arduous process of applying for and being approved for benefits, coupled with fear of losing medical and drug coverage, can discourage individuals from pursuing employment opportunities. These findings highlight the significant impact that benefit systems can have on employment pursuits of recipients. Many recipients limit their employment participation or choose not to work at all for fear of losing their eligibility for income support.

To address these fears, many jurisdictions have attempted to remove disincentives to work within their benefit systems. For example, some jurisdictions have increased benefits available to recipients who start work, developed provisions for recipients to keep their health and dental benefits if equivalent benefits are not provided by their employer, and instituted rapid reinstatement processes in the case of job loss or relapse. However, the fear of losing benefits is deeply rooted, and efforts to remove disincentives are often met with apprehension and disbelief (Baron, 2000; Lawand and Kloosterman, 2006). This fear can be a strong deterrent to pursuing employment and must be acknowledged and addressed within employment supports for persons living with mental illness. Occupational therapy practitioners working in this area should be aware of the benefits available to individuals with mental illnesses who pursue employment in their jurisdiction and provide individualized benefits counseling to their clients so clients can make informed decisions about their employment.

Where Are Work-Related Services Provided to Persons With Mental Illness?

Work-related services are often provided to persons experiencing mental health problems in the workplace through SE services or job coaching. SE programs can be found in community mental health centers or psychosocial rehabilitation agencies where housing supports, skills training, and other preemployment supports may also be available. SE services may also be found in psychiatric hospitals and in freestanding employment programs (Bond, et al., 2002).

Return-to-work services for individuals with established connections to the workplace, by contrast, are often delivered through private insurance companies or disability management organizations. In some cases, these agencies have more contact with employers and the workplace and may be involved in negotiating return-to-work plans and reasonable accommodations. However, in many cases, individuals must negotiate these arrangements on their own. Given the lack of awareness and understanding associated with mental illness, such circumstances can pose challenges and lead to ongoing problems. As a result, efforts are ongoing in Canada and elsewhere to develop educational materials for employers to assist them in meeting their obligations and providing appropriate accommodations to their employees (Canadian Psychiatric Research Foundation, 2007). Box 9.3 provides an example of how an occupational therapist can work with individuals to support their successful return to work following a leave due to mental illness.

Work-Related Intervention in Mental Health

A wide variety of practice models are utilized by occupational therapy practitioners in planning and providing work-related intervention for persons living with mental illness.

Box 9.3 Return-to-Work Case Resolution

The occupational therapist and Don discussed what he felt he needed to successfully return to work. In order to regain confidence in his skills and to assess his ability to concentrate and interact appropriately, the occupational therapist facilitated permission from his long-term disability provider for Don to do occasional work as a tutor through a private tutoring agency. When he felt confident he could reenter the classroom, they agreed he would benefit from a gradual return to work, starting with one class per day and eventually returning to a full-time schedule. The occupational therapist and Don considered his options regarding the class he should begin with in light of the multiple pressures and demands involved. In developing their plan, they engaged multiple stakeholders, including the long-term disability provider, the union representative, the board of education disability manager, and the school principal. Don will continue to be followed by his psychiatrist throughout the return-to-work process.

Box 9.3   Return-to-Work Case Resolution—cont'd

Don felt it was important to speak to some of his colleagues about the challenges he experienced and to acknowledge the extra work they were doing. Although he did not wish to disclose the specifics of his mental illness, he decided to explain that he has been experiencing some difficulty with his concentration and sleeping pattern, which is why he decided to take a medical leave and why he was now returning to his position on a part-time basis. While a few colleagues appeared uncomfortable by this disclosure, some teachers approached Don privately and told him that they too had experienced "difficult" times in their lives. One math teacher specifically told Don that she would be happy to help him out during her spare period if he needed any assistance with his classes. It took a few months for Don to resume his full course load, and he found each addition to his work schedule challenging. Don experienced increases in his anxiety at times of heavier workload (e.g., marking exams and completing report cards); however, with ongoing support, he utilized the strategies he had learned to assist him in managing these predictable stressors.

A number of these are discussed in depth in Chapter 4 and other chapters of this book. Table 9.1 lists common conceptual practice models and other models used in mental health work-related services and briefly identifies their contribution to service planning and delivery.

In combination with the occupational therapy conceptual practice models are a number of interventions that may be used when working with individuals with mental illness. Such interventions are often used by occupational therapists working across different employment and vocational programs for individuals with established connections to the workplace and individuals trying to enter the workplace and find a suitable job.

Table 9.1   Common Models and Their Contributions to Service Planning and Delivery

Model	Contributions
Model of human occupation	Focuses on occupation, prioritizes the needs of clients, provides a holistic and client-centered approach
Canadian model of occupational performance and engagement	Focuses assessment and intervention on clients' performance and satisfaction with their occupations; works to improve transactions between person, occupation, and environment through enablement
Person-environment-occupation performance framework	Assesses areas of fit or lack of fit in interactions between the person, environment, and occupation
Allen model of cognitive disability	Assesses functional cognition to determine individuals' cognitive abilities and the activity context that produces observable performance
Transtheoretical stages of change	Involves progress through six stages of change; explores individuals' readiness for change and how to assist in making changes in behavior
Cognitive-behavioral therapy	Focuses on clients' goals and educating client's on the skills necessary to manage thoughts that create unhealthy emotion and behavior responses
Social model of disability	Focuses on how environmental factors such as cultural expectations, physical structures, and stigmatizing/discriminatory attitudes restrict opportunities for persons with disabilities in their communities

(table continues on page 212)

Table 9.1 Common Models and Their Contributions to Service Planning and Delivery—cont'd

Model	Contributions
Psychiatric rehabilitation	Focuses on restoring community functioning and well-being of individuals by teaching skills and effecting change in individuals' environment and the way they manage their environmental resources
Recovery and wellness	Encourages individuals to gain insight into their illness and the associated symptoms and to collaborate with mental health professionals to improve their coping strategies

The *Wellness Recovery Action Plan* (WRAP) was developed to assist individuals in taking control over their illness and moving forward with their lives by identifying strategies or responses that will help them relieve symptoms and/or enhance their wellness (Copeland, 2001). Occupational therapy practitioners can assist in exploring an individual's symptoms and assisting in identifying ways to manage those symptoms with a structured plan. Both the recovery and wellness models assist in focusing treatment on a more active life for the individual. The WRAP tool is useful for occupational therapy practitioners to assist individuals in planning for times when they may become unwell. It provides structure to help individuals develop a daily maintenance plan, deal with triggers and early warning signs and symptoms, and develop a crisis plan (Copeland 2002). The WRAP is a beneficial tool to provide a planned course of action as well as an opportunity to rehearse before a person experiences symptoms that will hinder performance in employment (Waghorn, Lloyd, and Clune, 2009).

In addition to the above-mentioned frames of reference, occupational therapists have been part of traditional mental health vocational rehabilitation services, typically utilizing a "train-then-place" approach (Waghorn, et al., 2009). This model assumes that individuals require a long period of preparation (preemployment training) before being "placed" or entering into competitive employment (Crowther, et al., 2001). This approach differs from the SE model, which focuses on a rapid job search and placing individuals into competitive employment positions that are well matched to their preferences and skills, with the provision of ongoing postemployment support (Crowther, et al., 2001).

The Role of Occupational Therapy in Work-Related Services for Persons With Mental Illness

Occupational therapy practitioners are utilized in a number of ways in the provision of employment supports for individuals with mental illness. Traditionally, occupational therapy practitioners focused on prevocational skills training with the idea that an individual must be fully trained prior to being placed in employment. However, the role of the occupational therapy practitioner in the vocational arena is changing, and there is a wide range of tasks and opportunities for practitioners within the SE and IPS models. Specifically, occupational therapy practitioners have expertise that can help match individuals to appropriate job placements by considering the worker skills, competencies, and limitations; the workplace; and the demands of the work (Cockburn, Kirsh, Krupa, and Gewurtz, 2004). Often, this information can be ascertained by exploring patterns from their work history, both the successes they have experienced and the challenges they have encountered. Occupational therapy practitioners are also involved in providing ongoing support to individuals. Examples of occupational therapy interventions include cognitive training, work-related social skills interventions, assessment of work performance, financial and benefits counseling, managing personal information, improving work-related self-efficacy, establishing a work/life balance, and preparing clients for possible relapses of their mental illness by teaching them to recognize early warning signs (Waghorn, et al., 2009).

> *However, the role of the occupational therapy practitioner in the vocational arena is changing, and there is a wide range of tasks and opportunities for occupational therapists within the SE and IPS models.*

Cognitive training has been found to help individuals develop problem-solving strategies (Waghorn, et al., 2009). Such training can be focused generally or on a particular task. Research with individuals with schizophrenia has found that deficits in problem-solving can include attempting to identify a problem when it occurs, defining a problem, understanding the problem, generating alternative solutions, evaluating and choosing the best alternative, and evaluating the efficacy of the problem-solving effort (Malouff, Thorsteinsson, and Schute, 2007; Stalberg, Lichtenstein, Sandin, and Hultman, 2008). Focusing on cognitive training after employment has been established is useful for resolving problems as they arise in the workplace (Waghorn, et al., 2009).

Training in social skills continues to be an important component of the employment support process. SE participants often have difficulty in social situations at work, and training is often specifically focused on interactions with coworkers and customers and on learning to accept feedback from supervisors (Mueser, et al., 2005). The ability to apply these skills has been found to be most useful after employment is established, as the skills can then be learned in context (Cheung and Tsang, 2005).

Assessing work performance by targeting work-related occupations such as social interaction, concentration, time management, emotional regulation, behavior management, and physical work demands can be beneficial for job retention (Behney, et al., 2005; MacDonald-Wilson, Rogers, and Anthony, 2001). Occupational therapy practitioners can assess performance in work-related occupations and suggest modifications, skill training, or reasonable accommodations in order to improve performance. For example, an occupational therapy practitioner could provide on-the-job training to assist an individual with stress management strategies appropriate for the workplace and could explore ways to communicate more assertively with the individual's employer or coworkers if conflicts arise. Environmental modification may also help improve work performance. Changing the physical environment by utilizing reminders, making lists, or organizing tools and materials are examples of simple modifications or accommodations (Brown, 2009).

Individuals participating in SE programs who are reliant on social assistance often require guidance in developing a financial plan that takes into account the rules and regulations associated with how earnings from employment are treated by various income support programs (Bond, 2004). Occupational therapy practitioners often help clients with weekly budgets and with meeting income support notification standards in order to maintain eligibility. Paperwork and processes associated with government-administered income support programs can be complicated and difficult for clients to complete on their own. Financial planning may be useful for all SE service users (Auerbach and Jeong, 2005).

Occupational therapy practitioners may also help individuals improve their self-efficacy in the workplace, especially when focusing on the specific tasks of their job (Waghorn, et al., 2005). With the use of self-report measures such as the Career Self-Efficacy Scale (McDonald, 1999; Solberg, et al., 1994), the Work Limitations Questionnaire

(Lerner, 2000), and the Work Behavior Inventory (Bryson, Bell, Lysaker, and Zito, 1997), occupational therapy practitioners can assess how much assistance an individual may require with certain tasks within their job descriptions (Waghorn, Chant, and King, 2005). Occupational therapists can also help individuals make use of supports available within their workplace, such as human resource personnel, coworkers, and supervisors.

Occupational therapy practitioners can assist individuals with establishing a healthy work/life balance. Finlay (2004) defines work/life balance as the relationship between a person, his or her occupations, and his or her environments. There has been little research to explore the lack of occupational balance and its relation to poor employment outcomes. According to Crist, Davis, and Coffin (2000), individuals who are unemployed tend to put more emphasis on self-care and play/leisure. Thus, individuals entering the workplace for the first time or after a long absence may require support to manage their multiple responsibilities and the necessary changes in their routines and habits. Neglecting self-care and home management needs could have negative implications on their work performance and job retention.

Group Interventions

Occupational therapy practitioners use a wide range of group interventions focused on psychosocial skills that are important for individuals as they explore vocational options and after they acquire employment. Examples of such groups are listed in Box 9.4.

Group intervention sessions are typically held on a daily or weekly basis and within specific programming. Job clubs or employment groups commonly focus on the skills needed to find and keep employment. Many topics focus on the psychosocial aspects of how to maintain employment once the individual has obtained a job. Group members may also need to explore hygiene and grooming along with proper attire and etiquette in order to present in an interview. Group intervention allows participants to practice these newly acquired skills. Preparation for increased social interaction in the workplace becomes necessary for many individuals with mental illness. Basic social skills, such as initiating and terminating a conversation, knowing what information to share with others and how to do so in an assertive and socially appropriate manner, setting boundaries with self and others, managing anger, and advocating for oneself in an appropriate way, can often be addressed effectively in a group setting. However, it is important to assess individuals prior to including them in a therapeutic group to ensure that they will benefit from the group and that group members will be able to work together.

Individual Intervention

When occupational therapy practitioners provide individual intervention, the focus may also include psychosocial aspects needed for employment and/or the daily living skills that affect a person's employment success. Daily living skills may include, for example, meal planning and preparation and teaching the importance of balanced meals and snacks in maintaining energy and focus while working.

Box 9.4   Examples of Occupational Therapy Group Interventions

- Anger management
- Assertive communication skills
- Time management
- Stress management/coping skills
- Anxiety management
- Wellness

New employees may require assistance with community mobility. They may need to learn about public transportation schedules and routes in order to get to and from work safely and on time. Observing a client in this public space allows the therapist to assess the individual's anxiety level, identify any problems with sequencing or problem-solving, and assess the individual's ability to provide correct change.

New employees may also require assistance with financial management. If an individual is losing benefits due to newfound employment, the occupational therapist may need to assess the client's ability to develop and follow a budget as well as to read and pay bills. Individuals may need to budget for new expenses that arise with employment, such as a monthly bus pass, increased gasoline expenses, and increased clothing costs if uniforms are not provided by the employer. They must sometimes learn to manage an increase in income without over-spending. Individuals may also require assistance with self-care and grooming, as they now have to dress according to the standards of their workplace, perhaps requiring a uniform. This may lead to education on laundry tasks as well as basic organizational skills and time management skills in order to be prepared for work shifts.

Chapter Summary

We briefly explored the history of occupational therapy in mental health from the moral treatment era to recovery and the challenges faced by people with mental illness in relation to work and employment. Occupational therapy practitioners work in many capacities and provide many options for individuals in this population. Problems with employment often coincide with mental illness and difficulties with day-to-day functioning. Despite efforts to provide services through transitional employment, IPS, and SE programs, the rate of employment among persons living with mental illness continues to be low.

Stigma toward persons with mental illness continues to pose challenges; however, there has been improvement. Occupational therapy practitioners have been involved in advocacy efforts for individuals with mental illness in the workplace. Occupational therapy can provide assessment and assist in negotiating appropriate workplace accommodations. Through occupational therapy intervention, individuals with mental illness can focus on improving psychosocial and life skills that can enable them to meet the demands of the workplace.

Case Resolution

After Tammy's evaluation with her occupational therapist, it was determined that she would benefit from exploring stress management strategies, symptom management strategies, and assertive communication skills. Tammy also identified a need to become more organized at home and to work on meal planning and preparation in order to manage her hypoglycemia. Tammy also requested assistance in identifying strategies to improve her time management skills in order to complete all the tasks required of her in the time allotted.

Tammy met with her occupational therapist once a week in her home to work on the areas identified in the site-specific evaluation. With the interventions provided, Tammy was able to develop multiple strategies to manage her stress and symptoms when feeling overwhelmed or experiencing an increase in her symptoms of depression or hallucinations. After Tammy's case manager requested she take an online assertiveness quiz, Tammy was able to measure her level of assertiveness. She then developed specific skills with her occupational therapist to improve communication. Role-play was especially effective for Tammy because she was able to practice assertive communication in a safe environment. After 6 months of services, Tammy was encouraged to retake the online assertiveness quiz. She reported she had improved by 40 percent and felt proud of her accomplishment. With the occupational therapist's assistance, Tammy developed a schedule for meals and snacks in order to manage her symptoms of hypoglycemia.

Tammy did not feel it was necessary for the occupational therapist to come to her workplace to work on time management. She felt that by discussing it during the sessions in her home, she could implement those skills independently at work. Tammy was also encouraged to talk with her supervisor for suggestions on how to improve her use of time and productivity.

Tammy continues to meet with her occupational therapist once a month primarily for support with employment. She has improved her time management and stress management skills. She sometimes experiences depression and hallucinations, but she has learned strategies to manage them and utilizes her support system as needed. She recently got married and requested occupational therapy services to continue working on assertive communication and organizational skills, as she feels she could still benefit from services in these areas.

References

Anthony, W. A. (1993). Recovery from mental illness: The guiding vision of the mental health service system in the 1990s. *Psychosocial Rehabilitation Journal, 16*(4), 11–23.

Auerbach, E. S., and Jeong, G. (2005). Vocational programming. In E. Cara & A. MacRae (eds). *Psychosocial Occupational Therapy,* 2nd ed. (pp. 591–619). Clifton Park, NY: Thomson Delmar Learning.

Baron, R. (2000). Employment policy: Financial support versus promoting economic independence. *International Journal of Law and Psychiatry, 23*(3–4), 375–391.

Beard, J. H., Schmidt, J. R., & Smith, M. M. (1963). The use of transitional employment in the rehabilitation of the psychiatric patient. *Journal of Nervous and Mental Disease, 136*(5), 507.

Becker, D., Whitley, R., Bailey, E., & Drake, R. E. (2007). Long-term employment trajectories among participants with severe mental illness in supported employment. *Psychiatric Services, 58*(7), 922–928.

Behney, C., Hall, L. L., & Keller, J. T. (1997). *Psychiatric disabilities, employment, and the Americans with Disabilities Act background paper.* U.S. Office of Technology and Assessment. Retrieved from http://earthops.org/ada_ota.html.

Blank, A., & Hayward, M., (2009). The role of work in recovery. *British Journal of Occupational Therapy, 72*(7), 324–326.

Bond, G. (1998). A brief history of the individual placement and support model. *Psychiatric Rehabilitation Journal, 22*(1), 3–7.

Bond, G. (2004). Supported employment: Evidence for an evidence-based practice. *Psychiatric Rehabilitation Journal, 27*(4), 345–359.

Bond, G., Becker, D. R., Drake, R. E., Rapp, C. A., Meisler, N., Lehman, A. F., et al. (2001). Implementing supported employment as an evidence-based practice. *Psychiatric Services, 52*(3), 313–322.

Bond, G., Campbell, K., Evans, L. J., Gervey, R., Pascaris, A., Tice, S., et al. (2002). A scale to measure quality of supported employment for persons with severe mental illness. *Journal of Vocational Rehabilitation, 17*(4), 239–250.

Bond, G., Drake, R. E., & Becker, D. (2008). An update on randomized controlled trials of evidence-based supported employment. *Psychiatric Rehabilitation Journal, 31*(4), 280–290.

Bond, G., Drake, R. E., Mueser, K. T., & Becker, D. R. (1997). An update on supported employment for people with severe mental illness. *Psychiatric Services, 48*(3), 335–346.

Brown, C. (2001). Introduction: Recovery and wellness: Models of hope and empowerment for people with mental illness. *Occupational Therapy in Mental Health, 17*(3/4), 1–3

Brown, C. (2009). Functional assessment and intervention in occupational therapy. *Psychiatric Rehabilitation Journal, 32*(3), 162–170.

Bryson, G., Bell, M., Lysaker, P., & Zito, W. (1997).The work behavior inventory: A scale for the assessment of work behavior for clients with severe mental illness. *Psychiatric Rehabilitation Journal, 20*(4), 47–55.

Burns, G., Catty, J., Becker, T., Drake, R., Fioritti, A., Knapp, M., et al. (2007). The effectiveness of supported employment for people with severe mental illness: A randomised control trial. *Lancet, 370* (9593), 1146–1152.

Canadian Psychiatric Research Foundation. (2007). *When Something's Wrong: Strategies for the Workplace.* Toronto, ON: Author.

Centre for Addiction and Mental Health, Canadian Mental Health Association, Ontario Division, Ontario Mental Health Foundation, & Government of Ontario. (2004). Making a difference: Community mental health evaluation initiative. Retrieved from www.ontario.cmha.ca/cmhei/making_a_difference.asp.

Cheung, L. C. C., & Tsang, H. W. H. (2005). Factor structure of essential social skills to be salespersons in retail markets: Implications for psychiatric rehabilitation. *Journal of Behaviour Therapy and Experimental Psychiatry, 36*(4), 265–280.

Cockburn, L., Kirsh, B., Krupa, T., & Gewurtz, R. (2004). Mental health and mental illness in the workplace: Occupational therapy solutions for complex problems. *Occupational Therapy NOW, 6*(5), 7–14.

Cook, J. A. (2006). Employment barriers for persons with psychiatric disabilities: Update of a report for the president's commission. *Psychiatric Services, 57,* 1391–1405.

Copeland, M. E. (2001). Wellness recovery action plan: A system for monitoring, reducing and eliminating uncomfortable or dangerous physical symptoms and emotional feelings. *Occupational Therapy in Mental Health,* *17*(3/4), 127–50.

Copeland, M. E. (2002). *Wellness Recovery Action Plan.* West Dummerston, VT: Peach Press.

Corrigan, P. W., & Lam, C., (2007). Challenging the structural discrimination of psychiatric disabilities: Lessons learned from the American disabilities community. *Rehabilitation Education 21*(1), 53–58.

Corrigan, P. W., Markowitz, F. E., & Watson, A. C. (2004). Structural levels of mental illness stigma and discrimination. *Schizophrenia Bulletin, 30*, 481–491.

Crist, P. H., Davis, C., & Coffin, P. S. (2000). The effects of employment and mental health status on the balance of work, play/leisure, self-care, and rest. *Occupational Therapy in Mental Health, 15*(1), 27–42.

Crowther, R., Marshall, M., Bond, G., & Huxley, P. (2001). Helping people with severe mental illness to obtain work: Systematic review. *British Medical Journal, 322*(7280), 204–208.

Davidson, L., Stayner, D. A., Nickou, C., Styron, T. H., Rowe, M., & Chinman, M. L. (2001). "Simply to be let in": Inclusion as a basis for recovery. *Psychiatric Rehabilitation Journal, 24*(4), 375–388.

Deegan, P. (1988). Recovery: The lived experience of rehabilitation. *Psychosocial Rehabilitation Journal, 11*(4), 11–19.

Deegan, P. (2001). Recovery as a self-directed process of healing and transformation. *Occupational Therapy in Mental Health, 17*(3), 5–21.

Dewa, C., Lesage, A., Goering, P., & Caveen, M. (2004). Nature and prevalence of mental illness in the workplace. *Healthcare Papers, 5*(2), 12–25.

Drake, R. E., Becker, D. R., Clark, R. E., & Mueser, K. T. (1999). Research on the individual placement and support model of supported employment. *Psychiatric Quarterly, 70*(4), 289–301.

Drake, R. E., Goldman, H. H., Leff, S. H., Lehman, A. F., Dixon, L., Mueser, K. T., et al. (2001). Implementing evidence-based practices in routine mental health services. *Psychiatric Services, 52*(2), 179–182.

Estroff, S. E., Patrick, D. L., Zimmer, C. R., & Lachicotte, W. S., Jr. (1997). Pathways to disability income among persons with severe, persistent psychiatric disorders. *Milbank Quarterly, 75*(4), 495–532.

Farkas, M., Gagne, C., Anthony, W., & Chamberlin, J. (2005). Implementing recovery oriented evidence-based programs: Identifying the critical dimensions. *Community Mental Health Journal, 41*(2), 141–158.

Feldman, D. B., & Crandall, S. C. (2007). Dimensions of mental illness stigma: What about mental illness causes social rejection? *Journal of Social and Clinical Psychology, 26*(2),137–154.

Finlay, L. (2004). *The Practice of Psychosocial Occupational Therapy,* 3rd ed. Cheltenham: Nelson Thornes.

Frese, F., Stanley, J., Dress, K., & Vogel-Scibilia, S. (2001). Integrating evidence-based practices and the recovery model. *Psychiatric Services, 52*(11), 1462–1468.

Garske, G. G., & Stewart, J. R. (1999). Stigmatic and mythical thinking: Barriers to vocational rehabilitation services for persons with severe mental illness. *Journal of Rehabilitation, 65*(4), 4–8.

Gewurtz, R., & Kirsh, B. (2007). How consumers of community mental health services come to understand their potential for work: Doing and becoming revisited. *Canadian Journal of Occupational Therapy, 74*(3), 173–185.

Gewurtz, R., & Kirsh, B. (2009). Disruption, disbelief, and resistance: A meta-synthesis of disability in the workplace. *Work, 34*(1), 33–44.

Gewurtz, R., Kirsh, B., Jacobson, N., & Rappolt, S. (2006). The influence of mental illnesses on work potential and career development. *Canadian Journal of Community Mental Health, 25*(2), 207–220.

Glasscote, R. M., Cumming, E., Rutman, I. D., Sussez, J. N., & Glassman, S. M. (1971). *Rehabilitating the Mentally Ill in the Community: A Study of Psychosocial Rehabilitation Centers.* Washington, DC: American Psychiatric Association and the National Association of Mental Health.

Glasscote, R. M., Gudeman, J. E., & Elpers, J. R. (1971). *Halfway Houses for the Mentally Ill: A Study of Programs and Problems.* Washington, DC: American Psychiatric Association and the National Mental Health Association.

Hand, C., & Tryssenaar, J. (2006). Small business employers' views on hiring individuals with mental illnesses. *Psychiatric Rehabilitation Journal, 29*(3), 166–173.

Harding, C. M., Brooks, G. W., Ashikaga, T., Strauss, T. S., & Breier, A. (1987). The Vermont longitudinal study of persons with severe mental illness: II. Long-term outcome of subjects who retrospectively met DSM-II criteria for schizophrenia. *American Journal of Psychiatry, 144*(6), 727–735.

Harlan, S., & Robert, P. (1998). The social construction of disability in organizations: Why employers resist reasonable accommodation. *Work and Occupations, 25*(4), 397–435.

Harvey, S. B., Henderson, M., Lelliot, P., & Hotopf, M. (2009). Mental health and employment: Much work still to be done. *British Journal of Psychiatry, 194*(3), 201–203.

Henry, A. D., Barreira, P., Banks, S., Brown, J.-M., & McKay, C. (2001). A retrospective study of clubhouse-based transitional employment. *Psychiatric Rehabilitation Journal, 24*(4), 344–354.

Henry, A. D., & Lucca, A. M. (2004). Facilitators and barriers to employment: The perspectives of people with psychiatric disabilities and employment service providers. *Work, 22*(3), 169–182.

International Center for Clubhouse Development. (2008). International standards for clubhouse programs. Retrieved from http://iccd.org/quality.htmlp.

Jacobson, N., & Greenley, D. (2001). What is recovery? A conceptual model and explication. *Psychiatric Services, 52*(4), 482–485.

Kielhofner, G., & Burke, J. (1977). Occupational therapy after 60 years: An account of changing identity and knowledge. *American Journal of Occupational Therapy, 31*(10), 675–689.

Kirsh, B. (2000). Work, workers, and workplaces: A qualitative analysis of narratives of mental health consumers. *Journal of Rehabilitation, 66*(4), 24–30.

Kirsh, B., Krupa, T., Cockburn, L., & Gewurtz, R. (2006). Work initiatives in Canada: A decade of development. *Canadian Journal of Community Mental Health, 25*(2), 173–191.

Krupa, T. (1998). The consumer-run business: People with psychiatric disabilities as entrepreneurs. *Work, 11*(1), 3–10.

Krupa, T. (2007). Interventions to improve employment outcomes for workers who experience mental illness. *Canadian Journal of Psychiatry, 52*(6), 339–345.

Krupa, T., & Clark, C. (2004). Occupational therapy in the field of mental health: Promoting occupational perspectives on health and well-being. *Canadian Journal of Occupational Therapy, 71*(2), 69–74.

Krupa, T., Kirsh, B., Cockburn, L., & Gewurtz, R. (2009). Understanding the stigma of mental illness in employment. *Work, 33*(4), 413–425.

Krupa, T., Radloff-Gabriel, D., Whippey, E., & Kirsh, B. (2002). Occupational therapy and assertive community treatment. *Canadian Journal of Occupational Therapy, 69*(3), 153–157.

Latimer, E., Lecomte, T., Becker, D. R., Drake, R. E., Duclos, I., Piat, M., et al. (2006). Generalisability of the individual placement and support model of supported employment for people with severe mental illness: Results of a Canadian randomised controlled trial. *British Journal of Psychiatry, 189*(1), 65–73.

Lawand, N., & Kloosterman, R. (2006). The Canada Pension Plan Disability Program: Building a solid foundation. In M. A. McColl & L. Jongbloed (eds.), *Disability and Social Policy* (pp. 267–283). Concord, ON: Captus Press.

Lehman, A. F., Goldberg, R. W., Dixon, L. B., McNary, S. W., Postrado, L., Hackman, A., et al. (2002). Improving employment outcomes for persons with severe mental illness. *Archives of General Psychiatry, 59*, 165–172.

Lerner, D. (2000). *The Work Limitations Questionnaire.* Boston: New England Medical Center, Tufts University School of Medicine.

Link, B., & Phelan, J.C. (2006). Stigma and its public health implications. *Lancet, 367*(9509), 528–529.

MacDonald-Wilson, K. L., Rogers, E. S., & Anthony, W. (2001). Unique issues in assessing work function among individuals with psychiatric disabilities. *Journal of Occupational Rehabilitation, 11*(3), 217–232.

MacDonald-Wilson, K. L., Rogers, E. S., Massaro, J. M., Lyass, A., & Crean, T. (2002). An investigation of reasonable workplace accommodations for people with psychiatric disabilities: Quantitative findings from a multi-site study. *Community Mental Health Journal, 38*(1), 35–50.

Macias, C., Rodican, C. F., Hargreaves, W. A., Jones, D. R., Barreira, P. J., & Wang, Q. (2006). Supported employment outcomes of a randomized controlled trial of ACT and clubhouse models. *Psychiatric Services, 57*(10), 1406–1415.

Makikyro, T., Karvonen, J. T., Hakko, H., Nieminen, P., Joukamaa, M., Isohanni, M., et al. (1998). Comorbidity of hospital-treated psychiatric and physical disorders with special reference to schizophrenia: A 28-year follow-up of the 1966 Northern Finland general population birth cohort. *Public Health, 112*(4), 221–228.

Malouff, J. M., Thorsteinsson, E. B., & Schute, N. S. (2007). The efficacy of problem solving therapy in reducing mental and physical health problems: A meta-analysis. *Clinical Psychology Review, 27*(1), 46–57.

Marrone, J., Foley, S., & Selleck, V. (2005). How mental health and welfare to work interact: The role of hope, sanctions, engagement, and support. *American Journal of Psychiatric Rehabilitation, 8*(1), 81–101.

Marwaha, S., & Johnson, S. (2004). Schizophrenia and employment. *Social Psychiatry & Psychiatric Epidemiology, 39*(5), 337–347.

McDonald, R. (1999). Career self-efficacy in people who have psychiatric disabilities. *Australian Journal of Career Development, 8*(3), 31–37.

Mickelson, K. D., & Williams, S. D. (2008). Perceived stigma of poverty and depression: Examinations of interpersonal and intrapersonal mediators. *Journal of Social and Clinical Psychology, 27*(9), 903–930.

Mitchell, A. J., & Malone, D. (2006). Physical health and schizophrenia. *Current Opinion in Psychiatry, 19*(4), 432–437.

Mueser, K. T., Aalto, S., Becker, D. R., Ogden, J. S., Wolfe, R. S., Schiavo, D., et al. (2005). The effectiveness of

skills training for improving outcomes in supported employment. *Psychiatric Services, 56*(10), 1254–1260.

Noble, J. H., Honberg, R. S., Hall, L. L., & Flynn, L. M. (1999). NAMI executive summary. *Journal of Disability Policy Studies, 10*(1), 10–17.

O'Day, B. L., & Killeen, M. B. (2002). Does U.S. federal policy support employment and recovery for people with psychiatric disabilities? *Behavioral Sciences and the Law, 20*(6), 559–583.

O'Halloran, D., & Innes, E. (2005). Understanding work in society. In G. Whiteford & V. Wright-St Clair (eds.), *Occupation and Practice in Context* (pp. 299–316). Marrickville: Elsevier Australia.

Ontario Ministry of Health and Long-Term Care. (2000). *Making it work: Policy framework for employment supports for people with serious mental illness.* Retrieved from www.health.gov.on.ca/english/public/pub/mental/pfes.html.

Pitts, D. B. (2009). Introduction to special section on occupational therapy. *Psychiatric Rehabilitation Journal, 32*(3), 151–154.

Provencher, H. L., Gregg, R., Mead, S., & Mueser, K. T. (2002). The role of work in the recovery of persons with psychiatric disabilities. *Psychiatric Rehabilitation Journal, 26*(2), 132–149.

Ralph, R., Lambert, D., & Kidder, K. (2002). *The recovery perspective and evidence-based practice for people with serious mental illness.* Illinois Department of Mental Health.

Rebeiro, K. (2005). The recovery paradigm: Should occupational therapists be interested? *Canadian Journal of Occupational Therapy, 72*(2), 96–102.

Regier, D. A., Farmer, M. E., Rae, D. S., Locke, B. Z., Keith, S. J., Judd, L. L., et al. (1990). Comorbidity of mental disorders with alcohol and other drug abuse: Results from the Epidemiologic Catchment Area (ECA) study. *Journal of the American Medical Association, 264*(19), 2511–2518.

Rinaldi, M., & Perkins, R. (2007). Comparing employment outcomes for two vocational services: Individual Placement and Support and non-integrated pre-vocational services in the UK. *Journal of Vocational Rehabilitation, 27*(1), 21–27.

Saint-Arnaud, L., Saint-Jean, M., & Damasse, J. (2006). Towards an enhanced understanding of factors involved in the return-to-work process of employees absent due to mental health problems. *Canadian Journal of Community Mental Health, 25*(2), 303–315.

Salyers, M. P., Becker, D., Drake, R. E., Torrey, W. C., & Wyzik, P. F. (2004). A ten-year follow-up of a supported employment program. *Psychiatric Services, 55*(3), 302–308.

Schonebaum, A. D., Boyd, J. K., & Dudek, K. J. (2006). A comparison of competitive employment outcomes for the clubhouse and PACT Models. *Psychiatric Services, 57*(10), 1416–1420.

Secker, J., Grove, B., & Seebohm, P. (2001). Challenging barriers to employment, training and education for mental health service users: The service user's perspective. *Journal of Mental Health, 10*(4), 395.

Secker, J., Membrey, H., Grove, B., & Seebohm, P. (2003). The how and why of workplace adjustments: Contextualizing the evidence. *Psychiatric Rehabilitation Journal, 27*(1), 3–9.

Seyfried, E., & Ziomas, D. (2005). *The Establishment of Social co-operatives in Greece: Pathways to Social Integration for People with Mental Health Problems: A*

Synthesis Report on the Peer Review Held in Athens, 6–6 October 2005. Brussels, Belgium: European Commission DG Employment, Social Affairs and Equal Opportunities. Retrieved from www.peer-review-social-inclusion.net.

Shankar, J., & Collyer, F. (2004). Welfare reform and its impact on the employment prospects of individuals with psychiatric disabilities. *Journal of Social Work in Disability and Rehabilitation, 3*(4), 19–44.

Slade, M., & Hayward, M. (2007). Recovery, psychosis and psychiatry: Research is better than rhetoric. *Acta Psychiatrica Scandinavica, 116*(2), 81–83.

Solberg, V. S., Scott, V., Good, G. E., Nord, D., Holm, C, Hohner, R., et al. (1994). Assessing career search expectations: Development and validation of the Career Search Efficacy Scale, *Journal of Career Assessment, 2*(2), 111–123.

Stalberg, G., Lichtenstein, P., Sandin, S., & Hultman, C. M. (2008). Video-based assessment of interpersonal problem solving skills in patients with schizophrenia, their siblings and non-psychotic controls. *Scandinavian Journal of Psychology, 49*(1), 77–82.

Stein, L., & Test, M. (1985). The evolution of the training in community living model. *New Directions for Mental Health Services, 26,* 7– 16.

Stewart, W. F., Ricci, J. A., Chee, E., Hahn, S. R., & Morganstein, D. (2003). Cost of lost productive work time among US workers with depression. *Journal of the American Medical Association, 289*(23), 3135–3144.

Stoffel, V. C. (2011). Recovery. In V. C. Stoffel & C. Brown (eds.), *Occupational Therapy in Mental Health: A Vision for Participation* (pp. 3–16). Philadelphia: F.A. Davis.

Strong, S. (1998). Meaningful work in supportive environments: Experiences with the recovery process. *American Journal of Occupational Therapy, 52*(1), 31–38.

Waghorn, G., Chant, D., & King, R. (2005). Work-related self-efficacy among community residents with psychiatric disabilities. *Psychiatric Rehabilitation Journal, 29*(2), 105–113.

Waghorn, G., Chant, D., & Whiteford, H. (2002). Clinical and non-clinical predictors of vocational recovery for Australians with psychotic disorders. *Journal of Rehabilitation, 68*(4), 40–51.

Waghorn, G., Lloyd, C., & Clune, A. (2009). Reviewing the theory and practice of occupational therapy in mental health rehabilitation. *British Journal of Occupational Therapy, 72*(7), 314–323.

Warner, R. (2001). Work disincentives in US disability pension. *Journal of Mental Health, 10*(4), 405–409.

Warner, R. & Mandiberg, J. M. (2006). An update on affirmative businesses or social firms for people with mental illness. *Psychiatric Services, 57*(10), 1488–1492.

Glossary

Recovery is a personal process of actively engaging in community life despite the ongoing presence of mental illness (Krupa and Clark, 2004).

Supported employment (SE) is a model of practice focused on helping individuals with disabilities find and keep jobs in the mainstream labor market. It involves rapid placement of individuals into jobs that are well matched to their preferences and strengths, followed by the provision of support and skill training.

Assertive community treatment is a model of service delivery that draws on the expertise of a multidisciplinary team to provide ongoing treatment, rehabilitation, and support to individuals diagnosed with a serious mental illness and who have high service needs (Krupa, et al., 2002). ACT teams typically operate 24 hours a day, 7 days a week, in the client's community environment to address crisis situations, and support community living.

Individual placement and support (IPS) is based on the SE and ACT models; IPS consists of integrating the employment specialists directly on comprehensive mental health treatment teams.

The **clubhouse model** originated in New York City with Fountain House in the 1940s. It is designed to support individuals living with mental illness in their social, vocational, financial, and educational goals. It provides a community space for members to meet and participate in the operations of the clubhouse and also offers services and supports grounded in the principles of psychiatric rehabilitation (ICCD, 2008). Most clubhouses provide prevocational training through the work-ordered day and integrated work experiences in the community through transitional employment and/or supported employment programs.

Transitional employment is a model of vocational programming that provides time-limited job placements (usually 6–9 months) within the mainstream labor market.

Stigma is a disposition, attitude, or orientation toward social exclusion of groups of individuals (Krupa, et al., 2009).

Discrimination is the behavioral expression of stigma. Discrimination involves treating people differently, negatively, or adversely because of their connection to a group.

The purpose of a **halfway house,** also called a recovery house or sober house, is generally to allow people to begin the process of reintegration with society while still receiving monitoring and support; this is generally believed to reduce the risk of recidivism or relapse when compared to a release directly into society. Some halfway houses are meant solely for reintegration of persons who have been recently released from prison or jail, others are meant for people with chronic mental health disorders, and most others are for people with substance abuse issues. These sober halfway houses are often voluntary places of residence, and many of the residents may have no criminal record whatsoever. There is often opposition from neighborhoods where halfway houses attempt to locate.

Psychosocial rehabilitation centers are agencies that provide a range of social, educational, occupational, behavioral, and cognitive interventions for increasing the functioning of persons with serious and persistent mental illness and enhancing their recovery.

Resources

Mental Health Works

www.mentalhealthworks.ca

An initiative of the Canadian Mental Health Association, Ontario, Mental Health Works began in 2001 as a partnership research project involving the voluntary sector, government, and business. In 2004, Mental Health Works began selling products and services to the business community. It provides resources for employers and employees with mental illness.

When Something's Wrong: Strategies for the Workplace

http://healthymindscanada.ca

This handbook by the Canadian Psychiatric Research Foundation is a useful tool to help employers, managers, human resource personnel, occupational health and safety personnel, disability management providers, union representatives, and employees address mental health problems in the workplace.

Workplace Strategies for Mental Health

www.gwlcentreformentalhealth.com/index.asp

This website is dedicated to helping all Canadian employers who wish to address mental health issues in the workplace. An initiative of Great-West Life Centre for Mental Health in the Workplace, the website is a freely available public resource providing strategies, tools, and support for research and initiatives aimed at improving workplace mental health for all Canadians. The Centre was established by the The Great-West Life Assurance Company.

Living Well With a Psychiatric Disability in Work and School

www.bu.edu/cpr/jobschool/index.html

The Center for Psychiatric Rehabilitation, Boston University, maintains this interactive and informative website for people with a psychiatric condition; it addresses issues and reasonable accommodations related to work and school.

Reasonable Accommodations: An Online Resource for Employers and Educators

www.bu.edu/cpr/reasaccom/employ-read-macdon.html

On this site is a helpful 1994 report: "Reasonable Workplace Accommodations for People with Psychiatric Disabilities" by Kim MacDonald-Wilson, M.S., Reasonable Accommodations Project Director, Center for Psychiatric Rehabilitation, Boston University.

Mental Health Commission of Canada

www.mentalhealthcommission.ca/english/pages/default.aspx

A nonprofit organization funded by the government of Canada, the Mental Health Commission of Canada was created to focus national attention on mental health issues and to work to improve the health and social outcomes of people living with mental illness.

Dartmouth IPS Supported Employment Center

www.dartmouth.edu/~ips/

This organization studies and develops resources about evidence-based supported employment.

Center on Mental Health Services Research and Policy, Employment Intervention Demonstration Program (EIDP)

www.psych.uic.edu/eidp/

The EIDP is a multisite research study of innovative programs that combine vocational rehabilitation with clinical services and supports for mental health consumers. This website offers several tools for accommodations and workplace culture and provides evidence about employment for individuals living with mental illness.

U.S. Substance Abuse and Mental Health Services Administration

www.samhsa.gov

The SAMHSA site is dedicated to providing therapeutic interventions for individuals with substance abuse and mental health needs. It also has a toolkit on evidence-based supported employment (http://store.samhsa.gov/product/SMA08-4365).

10

Volunteerism and Play
Alternative Paths to Work Participation

Brent Braveman

Key Concepts

The following are key concepts addressed in this chapter:

- Volunteerism plays a key role in both industrialized and developing countries by providing communities with critical support that would not otherwise be afforded by federal, state, or local governments or private organizations.
- Approximately 77 million Americans were born between 1946 and 1964, and the first of these "baby boomers" reach age 65 in 2011. Volunteering can provide aging adults with opportunities to remain active and engaged while contributing their experience and skills.
- Volunteer and leisure occupations can be used as occupation-as-means with adults who are not yet ready or are not appropriate for exploration of paid employment or return-to-work to promote participation.

Case Introduction

Jerry is a 46-year-old Latino client in a return-to-work program for persons living with HIV/AIDS in Chicago operated by a local nonprofit agency. He has been HIV-positive for over 20 years. He is unemployed and has received private disability payments and health insurance for the past 4 years. Jerry lives in a small condominium, which he and his partner bought together. Jerry paid off the remainder of his mortgage using the life insurance benefits he received when his partner died of AIDS 8 years ago.

Jerry had a stable work history as an information technology (IT) expert for a large local company until his partner died. He worked full time for the same employer for 14 years and enjoyed his work. Jerry's depression after the death of his partner began to impact his job performance, and he began to miss work. He reported that several symptoms related to his AIDS and its treatment became markedly worse during his last few years of work. These symptoms included significant fatigue and severe lower extremity neuropathy. The symptoms persist currently and interfere with many daily activities.

Jerry left work 4 years ago when his doctor suggested that he consider applying for disability benefits. Jerry decided to apply and was approved and classified as disabled due to his health condition. He reports that since being on disability, he spends most of his time in his condominium and only leaves to visit the doctor, to walk his dog in front of his building a few times a day, or to go out with his family when they visit. His family lives 3 hours away, and they visit him every other month. Jerry reports that walking long distances or standing for long periods of time aggravates his neuropathy symptoms (e.g., severe burning and tingling in his feet and legs), so he stays off his feet as much as possible. He has groceries delivered and barters with other residents in his building to get other needs met. For example, he recently spent 2 days installing software on new computers for a woman who owns a cleaning service. In return, she sent people to clean Jerry's apartment. He entered the return-to-work program to explore opportunities for working, although he expresses pessimism given his neuropathy and fatigue.

Introduction

Most of this book focuses on paid employment and strategies to assess the potential for entry or return to paid work roles and to support competitive employment. However, some people may not be ready for paid or competitive employment, and some experience disincentives to entering or returning to paid work. For example, a client who is receiving public or private disability payments may worry that obtaining paid employment could result in a decrease or loss of those disability payments as well as the associated health insurance that accompanies these benefits. Other clients may not be interested in paid work but may be interested in adding or returning to *worklike* occupations in their daily lives. People that have retired from paid employment may experience some sense of loss after they end their worker role and may miss the rewards, social interaction, and sense of satisfaction and achievement they received when working.

Chapter 10 discusses the benefits of volunteerism and leisure occupations and how they may be used to explore and promote paid employment. Volunteer and leisure roles as an alternative to paid employment are also discussed. Strategies for using volunteer and leisure occupations to assess client factors, explore interests, develop skills, and safely test capacity for work are presented and applied using case examples. Opportunities for occupational therapy practitioners to address volunteerism and leisure with individual clients, client groups, and populations are presented. While volunteerism is prevalent in both industrialized and developing countries around the globe, a description of volunteerism in America is provided next as a background for the remainder of the chapter.

Volunteerism in America

According to the Corporation for National and Community Service (CNCS; 2008), in the United States 60.8 million volunteers serve nationwide, and the national volunteer rate is 26.2 percent. Volunteers provided an estimated 8.1 billion hours of service in 2008. The CNCS also reported that the annual number of hours provided by many volunteers has increased, with over a third of volunteers (34%) providing more than 100 hours a year. After a large drop-off in volunteering among the members of generation X (born between 1965 and 1976), the millennials (born between 1980 and 1995) are embracing public service in numbers not seen since the baby boomers who were born between 1946 and 1964.

According to the Corporation for National and Community Service (CNCS; 2008), in the United States 60.8 million volunteers serve nationwide, and the national volunteer rate is 26.2 percent. Volunteers provided an estimated 8.1 billion hours of service in 2008.

The visibility of volunteerism in America and other countries increases or decreases over time, and trends in volunteerism are often couched in terms of corresponding upturns or downturns in economic conditions (CNCS, 2008). Regardless of the decade, however, a steady feature of American society is the act of volunteering time, skill, and energy to give to others. The prevalence of organizations such as the American Red Cross, the Peace Corps, and countless community organizations are built on the enduring values of altruism, caring, and giving to others. Our federal, state, and local governments also have a long history of organizing and relying on volunteers to improve daily life in our communities.

Government Support of Volunteerism

Federal, state, and local governments are heavily involved in supporting volunteerism. For example, in 1993, President Bill Clinton signed the National and Community Service Trust Act, which established the CNCS. This act created *AmeriCorps,* a network of national service programs that engage Americans in intensive service to meet the nation's critical needs in education, public safety, health, and the environment. The newly created AmeriCorps incorporated two existing national service programs: the longstanding VISTA (Volunteers in Service to America) program, created by President Lyndon Johnson in 1964, and the National Civilian Community Corps (NCCC) (AmeriCorps, 2009).

When the CNCS was created, Congress also charged individual states with a critical role in managing volunteer and service resources on a national basis through the creation of governor-appointed state service commissions. The CNCS website provides the following description of these commissions: "In addition to setting national service funding priorities and making and monitoring AmeriCorps grants, these commissions typically serve as the lead statewide agency to mobilize volunteers and promote community service within their respective states. Every year, governors and State Service Commissions distribute more than $250 million dollars from federal national service funds, which in turn leverage more than $100 million in local funding to support citizen service and volunteering in America" (CNCS, 2009). Volunteers also save governments money. Volunteers in America represent the equivalent of 9 million full-time workers at a value of $239 billion (Young, 2004).

Many local governments also have organized efforts to promote volunteerism and to get their citizens involved in a wide range of community service. These networks are great opportunities for occupational therapy practitioners to connect their clients with a variety of volunteer experiences. For example, Chicago has a *volunteer network* that can be accessed via its website (www.CityofChicago.org). Opportunities range from volunteering in the public schools, links to programs such as *Big Brothers* and *Big Sisters*, animal foster care programs, and involvement in city cultural events (City of Chicago, 2009).

Long-Distance Volunteering and Volunteer "Vacations"

A relatively new phenomenon in volunteering is *long-distance volunteering,* including *volunteer vacations,* or organized trips to volunteer for a week to several weeks in a distant location. For example, since the hurricanes in the southern United States in 2005, many volunteers from all around the country have traveled to help with cleanup efforts. In 2007, about 3.7 million people volunteered at a long-distance site and traveled at least 120 miles to work with an organization located in the United States but outside their communities (CNCS, 2008).

Organizations such as the *Sierra Club* (www.sierraclub.org) run programs in which participants may volunteer for a week to several weeks working on national service projects. According to the Sierra Club website, "Service trips range from helping with research projects at whale calving grounds in Maui to assisting with archaeological site restoration in New Mexico. Usually, service trip participants team up with forest service rangers or park service personnel to restore wilderness areas, maintain trails, clean up trash and campsites, and remove non-native plants" (Sierra Club, 2009).

International volunteering has benefits beyond the services that are directly provided and may help occupational therapy practitioners to become effectively *globally connected.* David Caprara (2009), director of the International Volunteering and Service Initiative at the Brookings Institution in Washington, D.C, testified before the U.S. House Committee on Education and Labor: "Our nations' volunteers have also made great headway in promoting global solutions. Freedom from Terror polls have noted a marked drop in support for violent terrorism and a dramatic increase in positive views toward the United States in populous Muslim nations like Indonesia, Bangladesh, and Pakistan following our national and volunteer responses after the tsunami and earthquake disasters that were sustained beyond the initial period of aid." International volunteering is also a great way for occupational therapy practitioners to contribute on a global level. An example of such volunteer efforts by an occupational therapy practitioner, Paula Jo Belice, is described in Box 10.1.

Box 10.1 International Volunteerism in Occupational Therapy: Global Contributions by Paula Jo Belice, an Occupational Therapy Practitioner

---

The Belize Service Project is an interdisciplinary, international immersion experience offered to students enrolled at a small Midwestern health-care university. The first Belize project was organized in 1999 as an initiative of the student nursing organization. I joined the project in 2000 as a faculty advisor. Little did I know at the time how a simple volunteer experience would alter my path in the field of occupational therapy.

Journal entry 2000:

I return home with a renewed soul enriched by the people I met here. The toothless grins, but grins nonetheless, the smells, the stench, and the poverty. Although many live in squalor, their lives are richer than those who live in fancy homes, because they have the love of their people and their God. Sister Mary B. said it is important to realize many have family who love them and they are happy.

The project's aim is to engage in community and social outreach programs for the schools and local health agencies in Belize City, Belize, Central America. The volunteer work helps to serve immediate needs of a community lacking the basic necessities of life. The first week, participants are assigned to a variety of service agencies in Belize City. Speech therapy and occupational therapy professions do not exist in Belize. This is an excellent opportunity for the participants from the health-care disciplines to screen and identify therapy needs and provide services for the children, parents, and teachers. The second week of the trip, the participants are engaged in the Building for Change program. A small (16' × 16') home is constructed for the poorest of the poor. Home recipients are offered life skills classes on topics such as hygiene, personal finances, and parenting. As part of the experience, the project participants conduct one of these classes focused on a health-related topic.

The Belize Service Project provides the participant with an opportunity for a hands-on experience to work in a developing country and learn about the world and themselves. To encounter a region rich in culture and kindness, yet in the grip of social injustice, is something not provided in a textbook or classroom. The interdisciplinary nature of the trip allows the participant to develop an appreciation for the health-care team as they rely on the knowledge of the collective. Multicultural awareness and social concerns are cultivated as participants are removed from their familiar world and come face to face with poverty and health-care disparities.

I am fortunate to see the Belizean people through an occupational lens. My years of occupational therapy training provide me with the capacity to listen to their stories, identify the meaning in their lives, and offer my partnership to work toward their goal of leading a dignified life. Building a home with a family provides a basic necessity and allows them to engage in meaningful occupations to improve their circumstances.

My role as an occupational therapist is to promote independence and participation in life and society. In a developing country where conditions and resources can limit engagement, this presents a challenge. The adage "doing more with less" applies when working to provide adaptations for disabilities. At times overwhelmed, I called upon my training and experience as an occupational therapist to guide me. In these challenges, however, rewards are often found. Service can have a sustainable impact on the lives of many. There are personal rewards to be sure, but most important is the developed capacity in those who receive the services delivered in the project. With the Building for Change program, the recipients acquire more than a house. They cross a threshold to a better and more hopeful life.

Someone once said, "You will leave here and return to your daily life. You may even forget your experience. But what you have done remains here. You have made a difference." Living your life is a daily experience, but engaging in service is a reminder of our responsibility beyond our profession to the lives of others. Through 10 years of volunteering in Belize, I discovered a natural symbiotic relationship between my passion for occupational therapy and my passion for service.

Benefits of Volunteering

Volunteering is not an isolated activity driven solely by a desire to contribute to the social good, although such a desire indeed motivates many people to volunteer. Instead, as noted by Fried, et al. (2004), "Volunteering is a reflection of an underlying quality of social connectedness that may manifest itself in many ways: through work or social life, formal community service or informal helping, secular civic engagement or faith-based good works. Social connectedness is also strongly associated with the health and welfare of the individuals in a community, which is a necessary precondition for engaging in community service."

> *Volunteering is a reflection of an underlying quality of social connectedness that may manifest itself in many ways: through work or social life, formal community service or informal helping, secular civic engagement or faith-based good works. Social connectedness is also strongly associated with the health and welfare of the individuals in a community, which is a necessary precondition for engaging in community service.*

The benefits of volunteerism to our communities are considerable. One study reported that greater than 50 percent of managers in the public sector believe that volunteers provide substantial cost savings and productivity gains to organizational endeavors, including improved feelings of goodwill among the community. The *Independent Sector* (www.independentsector.org), a prestigious coalition of philanthropic and charitable organizations, reported that volunteering—among many other things—adds value to services, promotes social harmony, and creates public trust (Young, 2004).

Volunteerism is recognized as an effective way to combine public participation with nonprofit organization or governmental operations. This involvement can improve not only decision-making but also the outcomes of services. Volunteers can interject skills and knowledge through their various voluntary experiences that might not otherwise be accessed. As a result, public interests and needs are met. Young (2004) reported, "The literature, in many cases, suggests that volunteers 'improve citizenship' and serve as an effective conduit 'to educate' individuals outside philanthropic and governmental circles as to the merits of public service. In one study of local governments, it was found that 91% of volunteer supervisors felt that volunteers permitted local governments to do considerably more without expense or undue cost."

Brundy (1995) identified other benefits commonly associated with the use of volunteers in the public sector:

- Volunteers add to the quality and capacity of programmatic services.
- Volunteers provide enthusiasm, extra resources, and many times, much needed skills.
- Volunteers supplement the normal workforce during times of crisis and especially when workload demands peak.
- Volunteers who are trained and experienced provide a ready pool of applicants for employment.
- Volunteers often provide services outside the normal purview of government employees, such as fundraising and advocacy.

Older Volunteers

Approximately 77 million Americans were born between 1946 and 1964. These adults are now commonly called the baby boomers. In 2011, the oldest of these persons begin turning 65, and, on average, they can expect to live to 83. Many of the baby boom generation will live well into their 90s, and these older Americans can make invaluable contributions to society through volunteerism (Harvard School of Public Health and Metropolitan Life Foundation, 2004).

It is sometimes thought that as people enter retirement, their involvement in volunteer efforts increases because they "have more time on their hands," but this is only partially correct (Harvard School of Public Health and Metropolitan Life Foundation, 2004). As a general rule, the percentage of people who volunteer reaches a peak in midlife—not in retirement—and then gradually declines as people age. You may have heard it said, "If you want to get something done, ask a busy person," and this may be true in regard to volunteering. The peak in volunteering at middle age is associated with having more, rather than fewer, obligations and commitments. However, it is also true that individuals who volunteer during their early years of retirement do so with greater frequency than midlife volunteers.

The Harvard report also challenges traditional thinking about some of the common words we use and the imagery and assumptions they foster. The report notes, "Words like *work, retirement, volunteer* and all of the language related to aging (e.g., 'seniors') oversimplify a complex reality and may serve as barriers to change. To combat the negative image of the frail, dependent elder that underpins a grim view of the future, society may have too willingly embraced the contrasting image of the 'active senior'—indefatigable, healthy, usually wealthy, and eternally young. Both images have limitations. New language, imagery, and stories are needed to help boomers and the general public re-envision the role and value of elders and the meaning and purpose of one's later years."

There are organized programs focused on tapping the resources and skills of older adult volunteers. *Senior Corps* is a network of programs including the *Retired and Senior Volunteer Program (RSVP),* the *Foster Grandparent Program (FGP),* and the *Senior Companion Program (SCP).* These programs take advantage of the experience, skills, and talents of more than 500,000 volunteers age 55 and older to meet community needs. Senior Corps volunteers serve in more than 65,000 local nonprofits, public agencies, and faith-based and other community organizations through the three Senior Corps programs (Corporation for National and Community Service, 2006).

Leisure and Play in Adulthood

Leisure and Occupation

Leisure is defined in the Occupational Therapy Practice Framework: Domain and Process (OTPF; AOTA, 2008) as "a nonobligatory activity that is intrinsically motivated and engaged in during discretionary time, that is, time not committed to obligatory occupations such as work, self-care, or sleep" (Parham and Fazio, 1997, p. 250). The OTPF further delineates *leisure exploration* and *leisure participation.* Leisure exploration includes occupations and processes related to identifying interests, skills, opportunities, and appropriate leisure activities. Leisure participation includes occupations and processes related to planning and participating in appropriate leisure activities; maintaining a balance of leisure activities with other areas of occupation; and obtaining, using, and maintaining equipment and supplies as appropriate.

Numerous perspectives exist on how leisure fits into persons' daily lives, and some perspectives classify leisure pursuits in some ways. For example, Primeau (2009) notes that definitions of leisure tend to converge into four categories: (1) leisure as discretionary time, (2) leisure as context, (3) leisure as activity or observable behavior, and (4) leisure as disposition or experience. For some persons, and for each of us at some times, having time to just do whatever we want or to do nothing and just relax is experienced as leisure. Conceptualizations of leisure as context focus on contexts that are friendly, safe, and comfortable with a variety of materials, objects, people, and activities (p. 634). Conceptualizations of leisure as activity or behavior are those with which we may be most familiar. Everyday leisure occupations and games such as golf, cards, bowling, baseball, and swimming are just a few examples. Finally, leisure as disposition or experience has to do with our state of mind as we experience participation in leisure. Leisure may include the qualities of experiencing freedom from obligation and everyday duties, freedom of choice, relaxation, suspension of reality, and fun.

The perception that a dichotomy must exist between leisure and other areas of occupation such as work or instrumental activities of daily living (IADL) has also been the topic of discussion in the literature. While earlier conceptualizations were more likely to draw clear lines between work and leisure, more recent theorists describe interrelationships that allow for more variability and interconnection. Zuzanek (2010) notes that conceptualizations of the relationship between work and leisure have included the spillover, compensation, and compartmentalization hypotheses in which leisure is viewed either as something that relates to work (spillover), fills needs not met by work (compensations), or has no relationship to work at all (compartmentalization).

Primeau (2005) shared a similar observation regarding what may be a false dichotomy between involvement in leisure occupations and parenting. She reported that parents, even when involved in tasks often perceived as unpleasant such as laundry, vacuuming, cooking, and doing the dishes, seemed to be enjoying themselves. She further noted, "Later, during intensive interviews, when asked to reflect back to the times when they were observed to embed play with their children within their work, many of the parents stated that they were having fun. All the parents said that they were working, but four mothers specifically stated that they were both working and playing. They described the experience of embedding play with their children within their household work as work that was fun or as a blending of work and play. For many parents, play with their children within the context of household work is a continuous experience combining elements from both work and leisure. Thus, work and leisure occupations may not always be experienced as separate and dichotomous phenomena within daily life" (p. 575).

It is important as occupational therapy practitioners that we avoid the assumption of clear divisions and necessary dichotomies in the occupational participation of our clients. Remaining client centered and using a variety of assessment approaches can help assure that we obtain the client's perspective when developing the occupational profile as the first step in the occupational therapy process. Regardless of how individuals fit leisure pursuits into their lives, the benefits of leisure are many and commonly identified.

The Benefits of Leisure

The National Center on Physical Activity and Disability at the University of Illinois at Chicago (2009) identified the following benefits of leisure:

- Leisure allows for the development of skills not only for a particular activity but also for those useful in other aspects of life.
- Leisure facilitates personal independence and growth.
- Leisure experiences help to develop a sense of competence because they provide individuals with freedom of choice.
- Leisure allows for the discovery of who we truly are and what we can become free of others labels and stigmas.
- Leisure experiences positively influence one's self-perceptions.
- Leisure empowers people to clarify their values and determine what is worth doing.

Additional benefits, listed by the University of Alberta's Academy of Leisure Sciences (2001) in a white paper on leisure, include a perceived sense of freedom, independence, and autonomy; enhanced self-competence, improved sense of self-worth/esteem, self-reliance, and self-confidence; improved leadership skills; better ability to relate to others; increased cognitive efficiency, including better problem-solving ability; greater adaptability and resiliency; and reduced personal sense of social alienation.

> *Additional benefits of leisure include a perceived sense of freedom, independence, and autonomy; enhanced self-competence, improved sense of self-worth/esteem, self-reliance, and self-confidence; improved leadership skills; better ability to relate to others; increased cognitive efficiency, including better problem-solving ability; greater adaptability and resiliency; and reduced personal sense of social alienation.*

In many cases, occupational therapy practitioners are concerned with leisure occupations as ends. In other words, assisting clients with the performance of the leisure occupations themselves is sometimes an end goal of occupational therapy intervention. In other cases, occupations, particularly leisure occupations, may be used as means. Trombly (1995) explained the use of occupation as means in her 1995 Eleanor Clarke Slagle lecture: "Occupation-as-means refers to occupation acting as the therapeutic change agent to remediate impaired abilities or capacities." This, of course, is how occupation is often used in the occupational therapy process in general and how leisure occupations may be used not only for the promotion of leisure but toward promoting other functional activity. Both volunteer and leisure occupations and opportunities may be used as *occupation-as-means* to assist with the exploration of entry to or return to competitive employment. Through such use of occupation, we may help to remediate impaired abilities or capacities or to alter task demands or the environment to facilitate performance.

Using Volunteerism and Leisure With Adolescents and Adults to Promote Participation

Volunteer and leisure occupations can provide opportunities to explore and develop work and career interests and options and to gain practical experience and develop skills to support employment. They can also help individuals to develop general skills such as effective interpersonal communication or basic work habits that contribute to being a more effective worker. Volunteering can also lead to specific opportunities for paid employment in the same or related settings.

Involvement in volunteer activities provides an opportunity for the occupational therapy practitioner and the client to explore, assess, and collaborate to develop an accurate knowledge of capacity. Such involvement also may contribute to an increase in self-confidence, skills, and the sense of occupational identity and competence as a worker. For example, in a study in England of 215 young people aged 11 to 25 (57% female, 43% male; 20% from black and minority ethnic communities; and just over 10% with some kind of disability), the following results were reported (National Youth Agency, 2007):

- Young people identify for themselves a wide range of personal and social skills developed through volunteering, but opportunities to reflect on and articulate this learning are often underdeveloped.

- Findings clearly support the evidence that young people can and do increase their self-confidence and self-esteem, develop a range of communication skills, and improve their ability to work with other people through volunteering.
- Volunteering can act as a catalyst for young people to engage more effectively with other learning, or in some cases re-engage with formal learning or training, putting them in a position where they can develop skills and potentially gain qualifications.
- Many young people also develop practical skills related to their specific experiences of volunteering.

Of course, these same outcomes can be found with people of all ages.

The following section briefly outlines ways in which volunteering and leisure opportunities can be used with clients to explore entry or return to employment. Brief examples are provided to highlight each part of the process. Following this section, we return to Jerry, who was introduced at the start of the chapter, for an in-depth application.

Assessing Capacity and Efficacy

To be successful at work, clients must accurately be able to assess both task (job) demands and their capacities to meet those demands. As noted by Kielhofner, Braveman, Levin, and Fogg (2008, p. 39), "Achieving an accurate view of one's capabilities and efficacy is not always easy. Persons with newly acquired impairments have not yet discovered what their capacities will be. Similarly, persons with progressive conditions or those who have exacerbations and remission cannot anticipate what abilities they will have in the future." For persons who have been removed from the challenges associated with typical occupational performance (either by choice or due to illness or disability), both the accuracy of self-assessment of capacity and the belief that they can bring about what they want (self-efficacy) may be decreased.

Volunteer and leisure occupations can be used by an occupational therapy practitioner in collaboration with his or her client to assess both capacity and self-efficacy. For example:

- Volunteering with a set schedule allowed Ellen to assess her ability to complete activities of daily living and manage transportation to arrive at work on time.
- Gradually increasing time spent volunteering or in steady participation in leisure helped Christopher assess his tolerance and ability to persist in an activity and to effectively manage fatigue.
- Volunteer roles with multiple demands and games or leisure occupations with more complex rules can help a client and the occupational therapy practitioner assess attention, memory, sequencing, problem-solving, and other cognitive and perceptual skills. Shelly found that playing board games regularly helped her assess just how much of a problem her short-term memory might be.
- Rita's occupational therapist assessed her social, communication, and interaction skills and her capacity for working as a member of a team while she was answering phones and helping out in her senator's campaign office.

Exploring Interests

Clients often identify a specific type of job they wish to pursue or are interested in returning to a prior workplace or career. Other clients are unable to envision a particular work path either because of a spotty or nonexistent work history or because they cannot return to their previous work. For example, clients who had physically demanding jobs but who have conditions that challenge their strength or level of endurance may need to consider changing to less taxing employment. Taking on a volunteer role or starting a new leisure pursuit is a simple and low-risk way for clients to explore and develop new interests. For example:

- Kristy volunteered at a travel agency to learn if customer service or sales were a good match for her and to take advantage of her interest in learning about life in other countries.
- Martin volunteered at a local health clinic, answering phones, and began training to answer calls on a suicide hotline to explore a possible interest in enrolling in a health professions program.
- Angelique joined a community gardening program to gain knowledge and skills to help her learn if a job in the landscaping business would be a good fit.
- After cutting his time at work by 50 percent to accommodate his more frequent symptoms, Russell found that he had too much unstructured time. Because he was not sure how he wanted to fill his days, he joined an online community that publicized local social activities and events, and he committed to trying one new thing each week until he found his leisure "passion."

Developing Habits and Routines

The ability to arrive at work on time and to organize and maintain the daily routines that are required by a workplace or are part of the established workplace culture is critical to work success. As previously identified, habits are the automatic behaviors integrated within routines or the patterns associated with specific occupations that support performance. All jobs involve routines at some level, although the demands and the requirements to flexibly respond to alternative routines can vary greatly. In addition to assessing capacity, volunteer works and regularly scheduled participation in leisure events such as clubs, team activities, or social groups can aid in establishing productive routines and the habits to support them. For example:

- Juan was struggling with getting to work on time and found that by joining a social bowling league with scheduled weekly practice and games, he became more skilled at planning his day.
- Chandra was easily distracted and had struggled in jobs where she could not isolate herself from noise and interaction. At the suggestion of her occupational therapy assistant, she began volunteering at the little league hotdog stand and focused on developing habits and self-cues to return to tasks after interruptions.
- Ellen volunteered for her church soup kitchen each morning to support her goal of getting a job in a restaurant. She intentionally chose a site where she would have to use public transportation. Under the guidance of her occupational therapist, she developed checklists and cue cards to guide her evening and early morning routine.

Developing Work Skills

Obtaining and maintaining competitive employment rests on the development of the basic skills required to meet the task demands of the job. In instances where occupational therapy services are focused on assisting workers to return to existing positions, practitioners may focus more on adaptation of the environment, remediation of physical performance, or identifying accommodations. In these situations, the occupational therapy practitioner may not need to attend as much to basic work skills.

However, when intervention is more focused on *work readiness,* the practitioner may help clients identify opportunities to develop basic vocational skills such as using a computer, answering phones, or other varied tasks. In earlier chapters, you read about various types of formal settings where such skill development might be fostered. Unfortunately, not everyone has access to or may qualify for formal vocational preparation programs.

Others may not be ready for the rigors of such programs but may still benefit from opportunities to develop skills that will help prepare them for employment. For example:

- Amy became better at regulating her emotions and controlling her frustration by volunteering to work a cash register at a local secondhand shop.
- In exchange for stocking shelves and cleaning aisles for a small, family-owned grocery store, the owner agreed to spend an hour three times a week training Roger to learn basic Internet skills.
- Crystal became more confident in speaking to and interacting with others by joining a local games group that met twice a week to provide an opportunity for socialization and networking.
- Shivan developed the basic computer skills she needed to apply for part-time work as a receptionist at a local dentist's office by volunteering as a note-taker for a student with a disability.

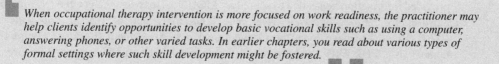

When occupational therapy intervention is more focused on work readiness, the practitioner may help clients identify opportunities to develop basic vocational skills such as using a computer, answering phones, or other varied tasks. In earlier chapters, you read about various types of formal settings where such skill development might be fostered.

Reestablishing Social Connections

One function that work serves for many of us is to provide a source of social interaction and connectedness. Persons experiencing work disability often report decreased socialization and increased feelings of isolation and loneliness. This can result because of the decrease of everyday interaction that comes with loss of the worker role and of work-associated social events and interactions. Volunteering and leisure activities are simple ways to create opportunities for social interaction, and these experiences can prevent depression, provide outlets for social energy, and allow clients to develop and maintain their social skills. For example:

- Booker reported increasing depression since he had left his job due to a chronic illness. He hoped to return to work at some point but agreed to follow the recommendation of his occupational therapy practitioner to volunteer to hand out water at a local marathon. He reported feeling more upbeat at their next session and agreed to discuss other volunteer opportunities.
- Omar worried about how coworkers and others would react to his physical appearance after an accident in which his face was burned. He had spent most of his time alone since the accident. To help overcome his fears, he joined a running club so that he could begin to meet others who shared a similar interest.
- Rachel retired 14 months ago. At first, she enjoyed her newfound free time, but recently she began feeling lonely and isolated. Her friend Joan, an occupational therapy aid, suggested she volunteer a few mornings a week at the local hospital. Rachel followed the suggestion and soon noticed that she not only enjoyed her time at the hospital but also began to enjoy her free time and time alone more.

At the start of the chapter, you met Jerry, who enrolled in a return-to-work program for people living with HIV/AIDS. The next section discusses the occupational therapy assessment and intervention process used with Jerry and highlights how volunteerism and leisure pursuits can help clients explore competitive employment.

Using Volunteerism and Leisure with Jerry

Assessment

Jerry's occupational therapist, Brent, first met Jerry when he enrolled in the Employment Options Program operated through a nonprofit agency serving persons living with HIV/AIDS. Occupational therapy practitioners have developed several programs for this population, and detailed descriptions of the programs are available in the occupational therapy literature (Braveman, 2005; Kielhofner, et al., 2008; Kielhofner, et al., 2004). The Employment Options Program included group psychoeducational sessions on topics common to all participants, such as résumé preparation, interviewing, and the Americans with Disabilities Act of 1990 (ADA), combined with individualized occupational therapy assessment and intervention. The theoretical basis for the program was the model of human occupation (MOHO).

In the first individual session with Jerry, Brent completed a narrative interview that provided information he needed to score two MOHO-based assessments, the *Occupational Performance History Interview, version 2.1 (OPHI-II)* and the *Worker Role Interview (WRI)*. Brent also gave Jerry the Occupational Self-Assessment (OSA) to complete at home. (The OPHI, WRI, and OSA are discussed in Chapter 4.) They arranged for Brent to visit Jerry at his home to complete a functional assessment of Jerry's level of endurance and performance in IADL (i.e., cleaning, meal preparation, laundry). Finally, Brent and Jerry discussed strategies for assessing his readiness for return to work and the process of seeking employment, including review of his résumé, his interview skills, and his level of competency in work tasks specific to his field of IT.

Table 10.1 summarizes the focus and purpose of each assessment and the findings.

OPHI-II

Each of the three subscales of the OPHI-II was scored, and Jerry and Brent constructed a narrative slope that provided a visual representation of the major events in Jerry's life and their trajectory. The OPHI-II summary is shown in Figure 10.1, and Jerry's narrative slope is shown in Figure 10.2. The OPHI-II revealed that Jerry had maintained a solid sense of identity as a worker despite his extended period of unemployment and so scored as having appropriate occupational functioning on all items of the occupational identity subscale. He scored lower on some items on the occupational competence subscale as evidenced by some level of occupational dysfunction in the areas of (1) participation in interests; (2) organizing his time despite the lower level of occupational demand; (3) not meeting his own standards for performance, especially regarding upkeep of his home; (4) limited progress toward his goals, such as not following through with enrolling in courses to improve his skills; (5) not fulfilling his expectations as a worker, homemaker, family member, and friend; and 6) overall reporting that he did not find his lifestyle satisfying.

Regarding occupational behavior settings, Jerry's biggest problems were in performance related to lack of leisure pursuits and his major occupational roles of worker and home maintainer. Most significant were the development and discussion of Jerry's narrative slope. Jerry and Brent agreed to describe the slope as stable (neither getting better or worse) but noted that Jerry felt negative events were becoming more common and his outlook on life was becoming more pessimistic. He shared that he saw taking the "leap of faith" to give up his disability benefits on merely the assumption that he would be successful in return was a major obstacle. He also described increasing feelings of loneliness and isolation that added to his pessimism.

Table 10.1 Assessments Used With Jerry

Assessment	Focus and Purpose	Findings: What We Learned About Jerry
Occupational Performance History Interview, version 2.1 (OPHI-II)	Includes three subscales: • Occupational Identity • Occupational Competence • Occupational Behavior Settings Provides an opportunity to develop and validate a narrative slope, or a visual representation, of major life events and fosters discussion of the direction clients feel their lives are taking.	Jerry has maintained a reasonably strong identity as a worker despite his 4-year period of unemployment and has appropriate occupational functioning on all items related to identity. In the area of competence and occupational settings, he has numerous areas of occupational dysfunction. Despite being able to identify interests, goals, and a desired lifestyle, he is not currently pursuing these areas and states he is unable to make progress toward his goals. Through the life history narrative, Jerry shared his story, and the occupational therapist learned that Jerry still is optimistic about the future.
Worker Role Interview (WRI)	Measures the construct of psychosocial potential for return to work. Can be combined with the OPHI-II and scored after asking additional work-specific questions.	Jerry has a number of strengths in regard to his psychosocial potential for return to work. He enjoys work and is committed to attempting to return to work if he can overcome his obstacles. However, numerous factors interfere with and detract from his potential to return to work. He is worried about stigma associated with his condition and interacting with a boss and coworkers. His daily routine has deteriorated, and he has little activity and does not pursue interests. Because of his fear of aggravating his symptoms with too much activity, Jerry's role of home maintainer interferes in some ways with involvement in work-related pursuits.
Occupational Self-Assessment (OSA)	Designed to capture clients' perceptions of their own occupational competence or their occupational adaptation. From a list of everyday occupations, clients assess their level of ability when participating in the occupation and their value for that occupation.	Despite concerns over coworkers' reactions to his condition, Jerry notes that interpersonal relationships with others are strengths, as are expressing himself and solving problems. He noted some difficulty with most items related to habituation, routines, and performance. He most values developing a satisfying routine and making progress toward his goals among other items ranked as highly important.

WRI

By asking a few additional questions specific to work during the administration of the OPHI-II, Brent was able to score the WRI using the format suggested for persons with longstanding disability. The negatives or disadvantages related to return to work were

Client: Jerry   Age: 46   Diagnosis: HIV/AIDS   Date of Assessment: 9/1/2009

Therapist: Brent   Therapist Signature: *Brent Bravern*

Ratings Key: 4 = Exceptionally competent occupational functioning, 3 = Appropriate, satisfactory occupational functioning, 2 = Some occupational functioning problems, 1 = Extreme occupational functioning problems

Occupational Identity Scale	1	2	3	4
Has personal goals and projects			X	
Identifies a desired lifestyle			X	
Expects success			X	
Accepts responsibility			X	
Appraises abilities and limitations			X	
Has commitment and values			X	
Recognizes identity and obligations			X	
Has interests			X	
Felt effective (past)			X	
Found meaning and satisfaction in lifestyle (past)			X	
Made occupational choices (past)			X	

Occupational Identity Scale
OPHI-II Key form results
Client Measure: 60
Standard Error: 5

Occupational Competence Scale	1	2	3	4
Maintains satisfying lifestyle		X		
Fulfills role expectations		X		
Works toward goals		X		
Meets personal performance standards		X		
Organizes time for responsibilities		X		
Participates in interests		X		
Fulfilled roles (past)			X	
Maintained habits (past)			X	
Achieved satisfaction (past)			X	

Occupational Competence Scale
OPHI-II Key form results
Client Measure: 46
Standard Error: 4

Occupational Settings (Environmental) Scale	1	2	3	4
Home-life occupational forms	X			
Major productive role occupational forms	X			
Leisure occupational forms	X			
Home-life social group	X			
Major productive social group	X			
Leisure social group	X			
Home-life physical spaces, objects, and resources			X	
Major productive role physical spaces, objects, and resources			X	
Leisure physical spaces, objects, and resources			X	

Occupational Settings (Environmental) Scale
OPHI-II Key form results
Client Measure: 42
Standard Error: 4

Analysis/Plan: Since Jerry has maintained a relatively strong sense of identity in all of his roles, including worker, despite his unemployment and disability, occupational therapy intervention will focus on increasing his participation in a full repertoire of roles and associated occupations. Through discussion, Jerry has acknowledged that he does not have a full understanding of his physical capacity and is limiting involvement in occupations due to the fear that activity will make his neuropathy and fatigue unmanageable. Jerry has agreed to explore options for increasing his involvement and participation, including volunteer and leisure pursuits, in addition to participation in the Employment Options Program.

Figure 10.1 OPHI-II Clinical Summary Report Form.

Client: ____Jerry_____

Therapist: _Brent_____

Date: _____9/1/2009_____

Narrative Slope

Draw slope including major life events and how the client's life got better or worse from these events. Angle of slope indicates severity or changes in events.

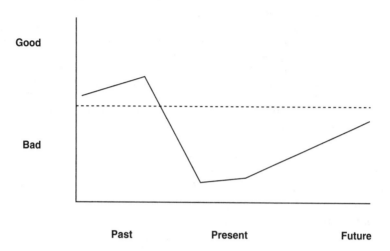

Meaning/Implication of the life story: Jerry describes his current life narrative as most closely resembling an unfinished "tragedy" with hopes for a happy ending. He describes a childhood that was "normal and happy" and that as a young man he was filled with hope for a bright future. He describes the best time of his life as living happily with his partner in their first home, before his partner became ill. He balances this point with the lowest point in his life which is when his partner died 8 years ago. Since that time he has struggled with depression and the symptoms associated with his own HIV became worse. He eventually left work and since has been in a "holding pattern." He currently describes being at a low point in his life, but states that he remains optimistic for the future and hopes that he can overcome his current challenges and return to living "a normal, pleasant and functional life."

Life History Narrative

Illustrating the slope drawn above, describe the client's life history. Where possible, make appropriate reference to the five thematic areas (Activity/Occupational Choices, Critical Life Events, Daily Routine, Occupational Roles, and Occupational Settings [Environment])

Jerry is a 46-year-old black male living alone in a small condominium. He is ADL and I/ADL independent but has difficulties with symptoms secondary to HIV/AIDS including significant lower extremity neuropathy and significant fatigue. He has been unemployed for 4 years but prior to that he had a long-term stable work history with a single employer as an information technologist. Despite his unemployment he includes the worker role in his self-description and notes he would like to return to work but does not think it is likely.

He describes a childhood and college years that are positive and "just like any typical kid" with good family support and friends. Just out of college Jerry met his life partner and they moved in together. Jerry reports living with his partner as the best time of his life. Jerry and his partner both learned they were HIV positive over 20 years ago and his partner became ill and died of AIDS-related

Figure 10.2 Life History Narrative Form.

complications 8 years ago. Jerry notes that time as the hardest time in his life. Since that time Jerry has lived alone and 4 years ago he filed for private disability benefits and left work.

Jerry has become socially isolated and while he can identify interests, he pursues few of them. He worries that standing or walking for extended periods of time can cause an exacerbation of pain and tingling in his feet but is unable to state how long he can walk or stand without this happening. As a result he avoids most activities outside of the home. He reports that depression is becoming more of a problem and that he misses the socialization that came with going to work every day. He noted that he gets along well with most people and that interacting with others is a strength. He is aware of the ADA but is concerned about the reaction of coworkers if he were to disclose his condition and request reasonable accommodations.

Jerry expresses optimism for the future and has enrolled in a return-to-work program to explore options for reentering the field of information technology. While he describes his life story as a "Great American Tragedy" he is able to see that things could get better in the future and that there are ways he could overcome the current challenges facing him. He is open to participating in group educational sessions and to working individually in occupational therapy to explore options for increasing his involvement in social groups and the community and for exploring return to work as long as that does not jeopardize or can replace the health benefits he is currently receiving.

Figure 10.2—cont'd

perceived to outweigh the positives or advantages in the areas of personal causation (lowered knowledge of capacity resulted in difficulty assessing his capacities and limitations), values (lowered work goals), habits (poor or diminished habits, disrupted and insufficient routines, limited ability to adapt and change his routines), and the environment (worries over reaction of and relationships with coworkers and boss, worries requesting reasonable accommodations, and being perceived as a "weak link").

Based on the combined results of the OPHI-II and the WRI, Jerry and Brent identified the challenges Jerry faced in attempting the transition back to work. They concluded that entering directly into paid employment was not a realistic option for Jerry because beginning to receive a salary could have a negative impact on receiving his disability payments and health insurance. Additionally, Jerry's true capacity for work-related activity was in question. The summary of the WRI is shown in Figure 10.3.

OSA

The OSA Jerry completed at home revealed that he had some difficulty with all of the volition items (doing activities I like, working toward my goals, making decisions based on what I think is important, accomplishing what I set out to do, and effectively using my abilities). It also showed Jerry had some difficulty with all of the habituation items (i.e., relaxing and enjoying myself; getting done what I need to do; having a satisfying routine; handling my responsibilities; being involved as a student, worker, volunteer, and/or family member).

Jerry identified some difficulty with three of the skill and performance items but also identified strengths in this area. He noted some difficulty with physically doing what he needs to do, taking care of his condo, and getting to where he needed to go. However, he felt that he concentrated on tasks and managed his finances well and that he took care of himself, managed his basic needs, expressed himself to others, got along with others, and identified and solved problems very well. Jerry marked "taking care of others" as not applicable. An important part of the discussion between Jerry and Brent focused on Jerry's increasing feelings of awkwardness when talking with others in social situations—a skill that had previously been a strength. Jerry explained that conversations often turned to work, and he never knew how to respond to the question, "What do you do?" Jerry experienced these interactions as very negative; he felt they led to his increasing tendency to isolate himself from social situations and were the primary reason he abandoned most of his leisure pursuits. The summary of the OSA is shown in Figure 10.4.

Name of Client: _____ Jerry _____ Client date of birth: _____ 3/1/1963 _____ Client condition/diagnosis: _____ HIV/AIDS _____

Name of Therapist: _____ Brent _____ Purpose of evaluation: Initial Evaluation Discharge Evaluation Date of assessment: _____ 9/1/2009 _____

☐ Client is rated relative to his/her previous job ☒ Client is rated relative to return to work in general

Strongly Supports SS Strongly supports client returning to previous employment or finding and keeping work in general	Supports S Supports the client returning to previous employment or finding and keeping work in general	Interferes I Interferes with the client returning to previous employment or finding and keeping work in general	Strongly Interferes SI Strongly interferes with the client returning to previous employment or finding and keeping work in general	Non-Applicable N/A Not applicable or not enough information to rate
1. Assesses abilities and limitations				
SS	S	I	(SI)	N/A
2. Expectations of job success				
SS	S	(I)	SI	N/A
3. Takes responsibility				
SS	(S)	I	SI	N/A
4. Commitment to work				
SS	(SS)	S	I	N/A
5. Work-related goals				
SS	(S)	I	SI	N/A
6. Enjoys work				
SS	(S)	I	SI	N/A
7. Pursues interests				
SS	S	I	(SI)	N/A
8. Appraises work expectations				
SS	(S)	I	SI	N/A
9. Influence of other roles				
SS	(S)	(I)	SI	N/A
10. Work habits				
SS	(S)	I	SI	N/A
11. Daily routines				
SS	S	I	(SI)	N/A
12. Adapts to minimize difficulties				
SS	S	(I)	SI	N/A
13. Perception of work setting				
SS	S	(I)	SI	N/A
14. Perception of family and peers				
SS	S	(I)	SI	N/A
15. Perception of boss				
SS	S	(I)	SI	N/A
16. Perception of coworkers				
SS	S	(I)	SI	N/A

Key Comments: Jerry's strengths include his continued identity as a worker and his commitment to working if possible. He is able to articulate clear work goals and accepts responsibilities for his actions. Major obstacles to returning to his work in information technology include a poor understanding of his physical capacity, the lack of a regular routine, and the large amount of time he spends alone. Jerry fears activity and has become socially isolated. He is very concerned about stigma and discrimination if coworkers find out he has AIDS.

Figure 10.3 Worker Role Interview Summary Form.

Client: ___Jerry___ DOB: ___3/1/65___ Diagnosis: ___HIV/AIDS___

Date Completed: ___9/8/09___

Myself	Competence				Values				Priority
	A Lot of Problems	Some Difficulty	Well	Extremely Well	Not So Important	Important	More Important	Most Important	
Concentrating on my tasks			X				X		
Physically doing what I set out to do		X				X			
Taking care of the place where I live		X				X			
Taking care of myself				X				X	
Taking care of others for whom I am responsible									
Getting where I need to go		X				X			
Managing my finances		X				X			
Managing my basic needs (food, medicine)				X		X			
Expressing myself to others				X	X				
Getting along with others				X			X		
Identifying and solving problems				X			X		
Relaxing and enjoying myself		X				X			
Getting done what I need to do		X						X	
Having a satisfying routine		X						X	
Handling my responsibilities		X						X	
Being involved as a student, worker, volunteer, and/or family member		X					X		
Doing activities I like		X				X			
Working toward my goals		X						X	
Making important decisions based on what I think is important		X					X		
Accomplishing what I set out to do		X						X	
Effectively using my abilities		X						X	

Competence Scale	Values Scale
OSA Key Form Results	OSA Key Form Results
Client Measure: 47	Client Measure: 56

Comments: Jerry identifies some difficulty in numerous areas related to volition, habituation, and performance. He also has strengths, most notably in social skills, although he currently is isolated. The biggest gap between competence and values relates to the lack of a satisfying routine and frustration over not making progress on work-related goals.

Figure 10.4 OSA Data Summary Sheet: Initial OSA Results.

Functional Assessment

Brent arranged to observe Jerry at his home to get a more objective perspective on the extent to which his neuropathy and fatigue interfered with Jerry's ADL. Brent watched Jerry prepare a small meal, perform some household tasks including vacuuming and putting a load of laundry in the washing machine, and walk his dog. There was no evidence of any difficulty with performance of the tasks, although Jerry noted that he typically would not have done much more without taking a significant rest period during which he would have watched television. Jerry explained that standing or walking for longer durations some-times resulted in flare-ups of pain and tingling in his feet or significant fatigue. When asked, "How much more would it take to cause these symptoms?" Jerry replied, "I'm not exactly sure. I have learned to stop way short of that." No cognitive or perceptual difficulties were reported or observed at any point of the assessment process.

Work Skills Assessment

Jerry began to attend group educational sessions on topics related to disability and employment as the process of completing the occupational therapy assessment continued. From a local volunteer group, Brent found someone who also worked in IT to meet with Jerry to discuss typical job demands, recent changes and advances in the field, the current job market, and strategies for updating his skills. Brent also arranged for Jerry to meet with a volunteer career counselor who reviewed his résumé and suggested strategies he could use to make himself more marketable. Through these processes, Jerry and Brent learned more about the potential gap in skills that developed while Jerry was unemployed, and they developed a shared understanding of the activity demands associated with the various work occupations that Jerry would be required to complete.

Intervention

Brent used MOHO to guide the intervention planning and to address Jerry's volition (personal causation, values, and interests), habituation (roles, performance patterns, habits), performance capacity and skills (physical capacity and work skills), and the environment (physical and social). Brent and Jerry collaborated to address the primary goal of simultaneously increasing the accuracy of Jerry's knowledge of his capacity and increasing his physical and psychological tolerance and his ability to persist in the performance of work, leisure, and IADL occupations.

Jerry had maintained a relatively strong identity as a worker despite his 4 years of unemployment. He expressed a strong work ethic that included feeling the responsibility to financially provide for himself—to get off disability, earn a regular income, and contribute to payment for his own health care. In planning occupational therapy intervention, Brent focused on this and other strengths that would help Jerry experience success and build his confidence.

Despite his strong occupational identity as a worker, Jerry had serious doubts about his capacity and his competence to reenter paid employment. His fears over the possibility of losing the steady income from his disability insurance and the associated health care essentially had paralyzed Jerry. Because of this and because of Jerry's poor understanding of his true tolerance for occupational involvement, Brent suggested that they begin by exploring volunteer and leisure occupations that Jerry could use to assess his capacity, improve his skills, and develop new social connections.

As homework, Brent suggested Jerry search the Internet and local newspapers for volunteer opportunities where he could use his IT skills and leisure opportunities that would help Jerry reestablish routines. Jerry was also asked to identify any leisure activities that he previously had enjoyed but had dropped for one reason or another. Jerry reported that he had enjoyed going to church, but had stopped, so he set a goal of attending church every week. He also reported that he used to belong to two different book clubs, so he invited several neighbors and a friend from one of his old book clubs to form a new club. At Brent's suggestion, Jerry established that the book club would alternate locations each week, which put additional demands on Jerry's schedule and was another opportunity to assure that Jerry would get out of the house. Finally, Jerry began going on outings arranged by a local volunteer group called Take-A-Hike. The Chicago-based organization arranges free nature trips to provide continuing education and promote activities conducive to improving the psychological and physical well-being of its members. These trips "serve to relieve the stress and anxiety associated with HIV/AIDS, allowing members an opportunity to reconnect with nature while learning about its intricacies." The outings also "give the opportunity to exercise and meet other people in a safe environment" (Take-A-Hike, 2009). Jerry perceived that the outings achieved all of their stated goals, and importantly, Jerry felt "safe" because, while his new activities were related to improving his likelihood of returning to work, he knew that his financial and health benefits were not yet in question.

Jerry found several volunteer opportunities that served multiple purposes: (1) updating his IT skills, (2) reestablishing daily routines and habits, (3) increasing his level of socialization, (4) creating current contacts who could act as references, and (5) providing a mechanism to accurately establish his tolerance level for sustained activity. Brent and Jerry developed a daily schedule that allowed sufficient rest and time for Jerry to take frequent breaks with the agreement that he would increase his time spent in productive activity each week. Jerry and Brent placed special emphasis on developing a schedule that balanced IADL, leisure, social activities, and activities related to work/productive activity.

Through discussions with several IT specialists arranged by the occupational therapist, Jerry identified specific skill areas where he was deficient and developed a strategy for updating those skills. He enrolled in a class at a local community college, which had the added benefits of requiring him to meet a schedule, providing opportunities for socializing, and requiring him to use public transportation more frequently. On days when he had class, Jerry kept his afternoons free to assure that he did not overdo it, and it allowed him to feel more confident in his ability to attend class regularly.

As Jerry began to increase his involvement in occupations outside of the home, he also used walking his dog as a method of assessing his capacity and building endurance for activity. IADL were scheduled for specific days and times of the week to promote a consistent routine and allow Jerry and his occupational therapist to closely monitor the rate at which he was increasing his activity level.

As more and more activities were added to Jerry's schedule, he noted that his tolerance for activity seemed to improve. His course was not without complications, and from time to time he would report that he had overdone it and that his neuropathy or his fatigue interfered. However, he also reported that his ability to accurately predict when he needed to take a break to avoid flare-ups of his neuropathy and to manage his fatigue had greatly improved.

Through his involvement in his volunteer position and his leisure pursuits, including his hikes and book club, Jerry's level of socialization had dramatically increased. After 8 months, Jerry reported that meeting new people and socializing with others was no longer an area of concern for him and that interacting with others was once again becoming a strength. While he still worried about negotiating reasonable accommodations with a boss, he felt more comfortable about how to interact with coworkers. His occupational therapist suggested that Jerry contact the Great Lakes ADA Center, which is one of 10 disability and technical assistance centers across the United States (Disability and Business Technical Assistance Centers, 2009). The Great Lakes ADA Center provided Jerry with some informal guidance through its toll-free information line, answered some of Jerry's questions, and provided additional resources to help him identify specific, reasonable accommodations that would be appropriate for him and the type of work he did. Getting this information was a significant boost to Jerry's confidence.

Chapter Summary

Chapter 10 has pointed out that not every client we come in contact with as occupational therapy practitioners is ready for preparation for competitive paid employment. For a variety of reasons, clients may want to explore volunteering as an initial alternative to paid work. For example, some clients need to develop skills before exploring paid work, and others want to explore working without risking loss of benefits.

Volunteerism and participation in leisure activities can be used as methods of developing basic skills and habits to support working and as an alternative to work for clients for whom competitive employment is not an option. The benefits of volunteerism and leisure participation are broad and varied, and both can be associated with improved quality of life.

Jerry's case highlights how volunteerism and leisure participation can be used with a client to assess capacity and improve skills and performance capacity and how occupational therapy assessments and intervention strategies can be used to help a client explore whether return to work is his or her best option.

Case Resolution

Jerry and Brent worked together for approximately 9 months. Because of Jerry's significant concerns over losing his private disability income and the associated health benefits, his concerns over abilities to socialize and interact with coworkers and a boss, and his limited understanding of his true capacities, involving Jerry immediately in work-related occupations did not seem the best course of action. Instead, Brent helped Jerry to identify first leisure and then volunteer opportunities that served multiple purposes. Jerry was able to assess and improve his tolerance for productive occupation in nonthreatening environments while at the same time establishing a productive routine, reestablishing habits to support involvement in work, and improving his confidence.

As Jerry gradually incorporated an increasing number of commitments to his schedule, his identity and sense of competence as a worker also gradually increased. Involvement in structured leisure activities helped Jerry to regain his sense of being an outgoing and sociable individual and forced him to manage his daily and weekly schedule in ways that also helped him learn to manage his neuropathy and fatigue. His volunteer position helping to manage the nonprofit agency's IT system and his coursework at the community college helped to update Jerry's skills, and the multiple resource agencies available locally, nationally, and on the Internet armed Jerry with all the information he needed to begin to make difficult decisions about the possibility of returning to work.

During one meeting to discuss next steps, Jerry reported that there would soon be an IT job fair at a local hotel. He did not think he was ready to begin interviewing for jobs but thought it might be a good opportunity to practice talking with recruiters and to get a sense of what else he needed to do to update his skills. Brent supported this idea, as Jerry had been working on his résumé, and Brent agreed that talking with recruiters would provide an opportunity for Jerry to get feedback on his skills, his résumé, and how he might come across in an interview.

Jerry attended the job fair and was surprised to find that a communications company was actively recruiting a large number of IT professionals to help with a planned expansion. Despite his worries, he found that they were willing to hire him and enroll him in a paid training program for 4 months that would allow Jerry to update his skills. Moreover, Jerry decided to take a risk and disclose to the recruiter that he was managing a chronic illness that might require some minor accommodations, and the recruiter was very supportive. The recruiter said he had hired a number of employees with disabilities in recent years, and the company was flexible and supportive in providing reasonable accommodations.

Through his involvement in the Employment Options Program and occupational therapy, Jerry had learned much about his true capacities for activity. He learned that he

(case study continues on page 242)

could use strategies effectively to manage his symptoms, allowing him to increase his participation in ADL, work, and leisure occupations. Jerry's sense of competence increased to match his identity as a worker, and he decided he was ready to take another risk. Jerry accepted the position in the paid training program and continued to work intermittently with Brent to learn additional strategies for managing his increasingly busy life.

References

Academy of Leisure Sciences, University of Alberta. (2001). White paper #7: The benefits of leisure. Retrieved from www.eas.ualberta.ca/elj/als/alswp7.html.

American Occupational Therapy Association. (2008). Occupational therapy practice framework: Domain and process, 2nd ed. *American Journal of Occupational Therapy, 62*, 625–683.

AmeriCorps. (2009). History, legislation, and budget. Retrieved from www.americorps.gov/pdf/PERFREP/ perfrep_acstate_full.pdf.

Braveman, B. (2005). Development of a community-based return to work program for people with AIDS. *Occupational Therapy in Health Care, 13*(3), 113–131.

Brundy, J. L. (1995). Preparing the organization for volunteers. In T. Connors (ed.), *Volunteer Management Handbook* (pp. 36–60). New York: Wiley.

Caprara, D. (2009). Renewing America through national service and vounteerism. The Brookings Institution. Retrieved from www.brookings.edu.

City of Chicago. (2009). Volunteer network. Retrieved from www.CityofChicago.org.

Corporation for National and Community Service (CNCS). (2006). AmeriCorps: State Commission performance report. Retrieved from www.americorps.gov/pdf/ PERFREP/ perfrep_acstate_full.pdf.

Corporation for National and Community Service (CNCS). (2008). Volunteering in America research highlights. Research brief. Retrieved from www.volunteeringinamerica .gov/index.cfm.

Corporation for National and Community Service (CNCS). (2009). Government support for volunteering. Retrieved from www.volunteeringinamerica.gov/search.cfm?q= Volunteering+in+America+Research+Highlights.

Disability and Business Technical Assistance Centers. (2009). The DBTAC Network. Retrieved from www.adata.org/Static/Home.aspx.

Fried, L. P., Carlson, M. C., Freedman, M., Frick, K. D., Glass, T. A., Hill, J., et al. (2004). A social model for health promotion for an aging population: Initial evidence on the Experience Corps model. *Journal of Urban Health: Bulletin of the New York Academy of Medicine, 81*(1), 64–78.

Harvard School of Public Health & Metropolitan Life Foundation. (2004). *Reinventing Aging: Baby Boomers and Civic Engagement.* Boston: Center for Health Communication, Harvard School of Public Health.

Kielhofner, G., Braveman, B., Finlayson, M., Paul-Ward, A., Goldbaum, L., & Goldstein, K. (2004). Outcomes of a vocational program for people with AIDS. *American Journal of Occupational Therapy, 58*(1), 64–72.

Kielhofner, G., Braveman, B., Levin, M., & Fogg, L. (2008). A contolled study of services to enhance productive participation among persons with HIV/AIDS. *American Journal of Occupational Therapy, 62*(1), 36–45.

National Center on Physical Activity and Disability. (2009). Benefits of leisure for individuals with and without disabilities. Retrieved from www.ncpad.org/get/ discoverleisure/leisure2.html.

National Youth Agency (Great Britain). (2007). *Young People's Volunteering and Skills Development.* Leicester, England: Department of Education and Skills.

Parham, L. D., & Fazia, L. S. (1997). *Play in Occupational Therapy.* St. Louis, MO: Mosby.

Primeau, L. A. (2005). Work and leisure: Transcending the dichotomy. *American Journal of Occupational Therapy, 50*(7), 569–577.

Primeau, L. A. (2009). Play and leisure. In E. B.Crepeau, E. S. Cohn, & B. A. Boyt Schell (eds.), *Willard and Spackman's Occupational Therapy,* 11th ed. (pp. 633–648). Philadelphia: Lippincott Williams & Wilkins.

Sierra Club. (2009). Get something back with a volunteer vacation. Retrieved from www.sierraclub.org.

Take-A-Hike. (2009). Welcome to Take-A-Hike. Retrieved from www.take-a-hike.org.

Trombly, C. A. (1995). Occupation: Purposefulness and meaningfulness as therapeutic mechanisms: 1995 Eleanor Clarke Slagle lecture. *American Journal of Occupational Therapy, 49*(10), 960–972.

Young, R. D. (2004). *Volunteerism: Benefits, incidence, Organizational Models, and Participation in the Public Sector.* Columbia: University of South Carolina Institute for Public Service and Policy Research.

Zuzanek, J. (2010). Work, occupation, and leisure. In C. H.Christiansen & E. A. Townsend (eds.), *Introduction to Occupation: The Art and Science of Living,* 2nd ed. (pp. 281–302). Upper Saddle River, NJ: Pearson Education.

Glossary

AmeriCorps is a network of national service programs that engage Americans in intensive service to meet the nation's critical needs in education, public safety, health, and the environment.

Baby boomers are Americans born between 1946 and 1964.

Leisure is any nonobligatory activity that is intrinsically motivated and engaged in during discretionary time, that is, time not committed to obligatory occupations such as work, self-care, or sleep.

Occupation-as-ends is occupation as it occurs in everyday life and not performed as part of occupational therapy intervention.

Occupation-as-means is occupation as a therapeutic change agent to remediate impaired abilities or capacities.

Volunteer vacations are run through organizations such as the Sierra Club, and volunteers pay to join a group and complete a volunteer service project while on vacation.

Resources

American Therapeutic Recreation Society

http://atra-online.com

Provides resources for recreation therapists and helpful hyperlinks and resources for all persons concerned with recreation and leisure.

National Center on Physical Activity and Disability

www.ncpad.org

An information center located at the University of Illinois at Chicago and concerned with physical activity and disability.

Sierra Club

www.sierraclub.org/outings/national/

A service organization that arranges volunteer vacations.

ServiceLeader.org

www.serviceleader.org

A project of the RGK Center for Philanthropy and Community Service at the Lyndon B. Johnson School of Public Affairs of the University of Texas at Austin, ServiceLeader.org provides information on all aspects of volunteerism.

U.S. Government Public Service and Volunteerism

www.usa.gov/Citizen/Topics/PublicService.shtml

Volunteer opportunities and information provided by the U.S. government.

Occupational Therapy Work-Related Assessment

Chapters 11, 12, and 13 focus on specific areas of occupational therapy assessment (psychosocial, physical, and cognitive) in relationship to work-related services. These chapters provide specific examples of assessments that occupational therapy practitioners can use, and they present important links between assessment and occupational therapy intervention. Chapters 14 and 15 discuss occupational therapy assessment specifically focused on ergonomics, environment, and workplace modifications to better meet the worker's abilities and needs. Because occupational therapy intervention in work-related practice includes intervention strategies that are used by occupational therapy practitioners in all settings (e.g., cognitive intervention strategies), this section focuses heavily on assessment; however, work-related occupational therapy intervention and outcomes are discussed throughout this section and the entire text.

11 Psychosocial Assessment of the Worker

Thomas Fisher

Key Concepts

The following are key concepts addressed in this chapter:

- The theoretical underpinnings, guiding rationales, and models of practice that support psychosocial assessment of the worker are presented.
- Specific psychosocial factors that influence work performance and return to work are identified.
- The chapter discusses psychosocial factors from an occupational therapy perspective, including:
  - Supervisor and coworker relationships.
  - Self-perceived identity and competence as a worker.
  - Influence of the family.
  - Influence of the environment, including the physical context, social context, and organizational climate.
- The Worker Role Interview (WRI) is introduced as an assessment of a client's psychosocial capacity for return to work.

Case Introduction

Corrine is a 47-year-old divorced white female who is the mother of three children ages 2, 5, and 9. She is 4 weeks postcervical laminectomy and has not worked since her surgery. While the symptoms she experienced prior to her surgery (e.g., pain, upper extremity numbness, and some lack of coordination) have improved, she continues to experience some difficulties. She is fearful of reinjury, is afraid to drive, and worries about the daily child-care activities she must perform, such as lifting her toddler on and off the commode and bathing him.

Corrine has been employed for 4 years at a construction firm as a clerical worker in the front office. She enjoys her work and has what she describes as a "generally positive" relationship with her boss and coworkers. However, she reports that she has not always felt supported at work as the sole caretaker for her children and that getting time off when her children are ill is stressful. There are few women at her workplace, and she perceives that requests for time away from work for illness or to tend to family needs are seen as "problems" and a "sign of weakness." Despite that her condition is not work-related and that she has adequate personal leave saved to cover a 6-week absence, she is worried that her relationship with her employer is becoming strained. She reports that her employer is involved in two contentious workers' compensation cases, and Corrine perceives that this is affecting how she is being treated. She is increasingly nervous about returning to work and is unsure of her ability to handle it along with her family responsibilities. She mentioned the possibility of exploring "temporary disability" to her physician, who referred Corrine to a work rehabilitation program. As part of that service, Corrine is evaluated by an interdisciplinary team, including an occupational therapy practitioner.

Introduction

Occupational therapy has been recognized as a health and rehabilitation profession since becoming formally organized as a profession in 1917 when the National Society for the Promotion of Occupational Therapy was formed. As members of a health and rehabilitation profession, occupational therapy practitioners provide services to a variety of clients, including individuals, groups, organizations, and populations. Occupational therapy practitioners have a long tradition of addressing the psychosocial concerns of these clients in a wide range of practice and intervention settings, including work-related services.

The influence of psychosocial factors on human performance, including work, is well documented in the profession's literature (Bond, et al., 2007; Fidler, 1957; Meyer, 1948/1921; Miller, 2004). In fact, some early occupational therapy clinical programs were centered on the construct of work (Olson, 1995). Unfortunately, psychosocial issues have not always received the same level of attention as other issues when examining worker performance, perhaps because of their complexity, the difficulty in studying these issues, or their influence in the current health environment. This chapter highlights concepts associated with *psychosocial assessment* of worker performance and the practice of occupational therapy within the context of work-related services.

Comprehensive assessment of the worker and work performance includes assessment of both physical factors and psychosocial factors (mental health, emotional health, self-perceptions, and functional abilities). Physical factors can be assessed by a variety of health-care providers, including physicians, nurses, physical therapists, and occupational therapy practitioners. Several health-care disciplines may also assess the psychosocial component of human performance despite the lack of reimbursement at times for assessment of these factors. Unfortunately, these factors are not consistently addressed as they relate to understanding worker performance. From an occupational therapy perspective, the psychosocial domain requires consideration of both occupational health and wellness. The domain includes "psychological demand, job control (decision latitude), social support and intrinsic and extrinsic rewards" (Bond, et al., 2007, p. 3).

Risk factors associated with the psychosocial domain may be observed when the human (i.e., person factors), job tasks (occupations), and environment intersect. Occupational therapy practitioners call this interaction *occupational performance*. Occupational performance in the worker role is a result of the interaction among the individual (psychological), work environment, business culture, and the employers' attitudes toward its employees (social) (Keough and Fisher, 2001; Miller, 2004; Woodside, 1971). The work environment includes not only the physical context but also the attitudinal culture in the workplace. For example, is the environment supportive of workers, punitive, or inconsistent? The nature and quality of worker interactions and relationships with coworkers and supervisors should be considered when fostering a productive work environment. Effective communication is critical and cannot be neglected or ignored; it must include all stakeholders in the process. Employers and service providers such as occupational therapy practitioners who support a return-to-work philosophy after injury, illness, or disease will address the psychosocial factors because they value their importance and recognize the influence of these factors on the return-to-work process.

Occupational therapy is well suited to address the psychosocial domain because of its documented roots in humanism, including the psychosocial influence, and occupational therapy practitioners can play a significant role with injured workers. Returning or facilitating productivity is a basic tenet of occupational therapy (Dunton, 1915; Fidler, 1957; Law, 2002; Meyer, 1948/1921; Moyers and Dale, 2007; Reilly, 1966; Woodside, 1971).

Occupational therapy is well suited to address the psychosocial domain because of its documented roots in humanism, including the psychosocial influence, and occupational therapy practitioners can play a significant role with injured workers.

The occupational therapy profession's history is important to understand when exploring its role in work-related services, especially in the context of psychosocial factors. Occupational therapists have always assessed clients and provided interventions, whether for physical or psychosocial issues, to promote participation and productivity in the clients' chosen occupations. Promoting participation and productivity is a core belief of the profession. Recently, however, occupational therapists and occupational therapy assistants have reemphasized the profession's commitment to occupation, embracing the cognitive, emotional, psychological, and social dimensions as well (AOTA, 2008; Moyers and Dale, 2007). The history and philosophy of occupational therapy, as well as the industrial rehabilitation movement, support the human need to work, rest, be productive, and engage in activities of daily living (ADL). Occupational therapy practitioners understand and promote the human drive to be productive; they refer to this drive as *volition* (Kielhofner, 2009).

According to the Occupational Therapy Practice Framework: Domain and Process (OTPF), work includes both paid employment and volunteer activities (AOTA, 1992, 2008; Moyers and Dale, 2007). For example, some persons who manage their homes or care for others but are not paid for these activities may consider these activities as work. Volunteerism as "work" is discussed in more depth in Chapter 10. It is not surprising that occupational therapy practitioners, researchers, and scientists recognize the complexity of work. They understand that job performance is dependent on physical, cognitive, perceptual, psychological, social, and environmental demands. The education of occupational therapy practitioners supports the required knowledge, skills, attitudes, and clinical reasoning to address these demands.

The education of occupational therapy practitioners in contemporary curricula, including a rich fieldwork preparation, provides students with an ideal opportunity for learning how to assess the psychosocial dimension of persons who have had injury, disease, or illness that impact their ability to return to work. Occupational therapy practitioners, in their professional preparation, are exposed to a complement of the biological, psychological, and social sciences (Moyer and Dale, 2007). Occupational therapy practitioners understand the person–activity–environment interaction and occupational performance, and through this understanding and expertise, they are well suited to influence human performance (AOTA, 2008; Baum and Christiansen, 2005; Moyer and Dale, 2007).

Occupational therapy practitioners are concerned with individuals, populations, and groups in *doing* or *performing* meaningful occupations. They provide direct services to assist with individuals' successful performance in the role of worker. In addition, they provide a wide range of services to employers, including (1) recommending work accommodations (individual and workstation) or modifications to work practices, (2) making job tasks safer, (3) preventing injuries, (4) promoting health and wellness, (5) supporting workers' return to work after injury, and (6) providing education and training about risk factors for musculoskeletal or psychosocial injuries to prevent workplace injuries.

Returning injured workers to the worksite and maintaining workers on the job are major concerns of employers. Occupational therapy practitioners have a significant role in the rehabilitation process for individuals injured on the job or who have had an injury, illness, or disease that has taken them away from the work environment for a period of time.

Overview of Psychosocial Aspects of Work Performance

To most effectively help workers with impairment or disability return to work, it is necessary to understand the factors that influence the return-to-work process, such as (1) administrative policy, (2) payment, (3) physical factors such as strength or mobility, (4) cognitive and perceptual factors, (5) social factors including working relationships, and (6) environmental factors. In successful outcomes-driven, evidence-based, best practice approaches, all of these factors must be addressed. Other chapters in this book specifically address the physical factors, cognitive factors, policies, and environment and their impact on worker performance. This chapter explores the psychosocial factors that affect work performance and describes how occupational therapy practitioners assess these factors. The factors to be discussed include:

• Self-perceived identity and competence of the worker.
• Environmental influences.
• Family influences.
• Supervisor and coworker relationships.

Not all workers who have sustained an injury or disability and are pursuing return to work have psychosocial problems related to their reemployment. However, screening all injured workers and conducting an in-depth assessment when appropriate is beneficial because it informs providers about this dimension. Typically, if there is a formal psychological diagnosis, providers know to examine the psychosocial factors. Unfortunately, in the absence of such a diagnosis, this examination does not always occur. Regardless of the nature of the injury and issues the client faces, assessing these factors provides the team additional information about the client and how to meet all of his or her needs.

The American Psychiatric Association includes the psychosocial domain with environment in the *Diagnostic and Statistical Manual of Mental Disorders, Fourth Edition, Text-Revision* (DSM-IV-TR) (2000). The DSM-IV-TR Axis IV reports psychosocial and environmental problems that may affect the diagnosis, treatment, and progression of mental disorders (Axes I and II). It identifies psychosocial problems as including problems related to (1) the primary support group, (2) the social environment, (3) education, (4) occupation, (5) housing, (6) finances, (7) access to health services, and (8) the legal system. These factors from the DSM-IV-TR demonstrate the cohesion between occupational therapy and medicine in terms of the psychosocial construct. Employers, health-care providers, and others should consider these problems when engaged with workers returning after injury, illness, or disease. In addition, unemployment, job dissatisfaction, threat of job loss, and coworker relationships are problems in the industry and must be considered when assessing psychosocial functioning.

Because the psychosocial domain encompasses many factors, addressing each factor effectively requires attention from and involvement of all stakeholders (e.g., employers, workers, health-care providers, third-party payers). Many professionals may participate in addressing the various psychosocial dimensions of the worker (Fig. 11.1), and their roles may vary depending on the setting in which services are provided: the makeup of a "team" is not the same in all settings. For example, social workers often address financial and community resources, while psychologists address psychological health and functioning. However, social workers and psychologists are not present in every work rehabilitation program or setting and are not always involved in intervention with every client. The role of occupational therapy practitioners can also vary, and the range of factors they address can be broad. It is important to recognize that, in some settings, occupational

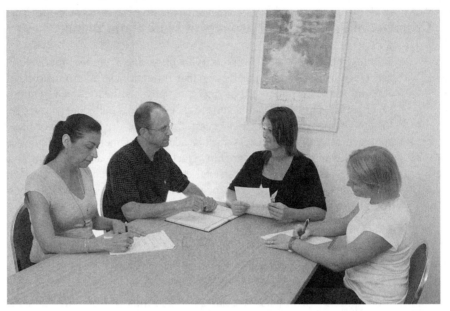

Figure 11.1 Members of the team in work-related services can include occupational therapists, physical therapists, social workers, vocational rehabilitation counselors, psychologists, and others.

therapy practitioners may be the only professionals to consider the psychosocial domain in the context of the worker's environment. This may be the case when working with some workers' compensation clients; working with clients with specific types of injuries, such as hand injuries; or, in private practice, providing onsite services and direct training and education of employees.

According to Miller (2004), understanding psychosocial issues and utilizing the resources available can be the difference between return to work and no return to work. Miller recognized the need for occupational therapy practitioners to assess strength, movement, agility, coordination, and endurance of the worker but, more important, the need to address the psychosocial aspects of the worker that may be interfering in occupational performance. Addressing these psychosocial issues provides a critical contribution to the process of predicting outcomes of intervention designed to aid workers to return to work. Predicting outcomes for populations is a complex process that must consider the full range of factors in addition to psychosocial variables.

The biomechanical theoretical framework (discussed in Chapter 4) is useful when assessing the physical components of performance in the worker role. Biomechanical components lend themselves to objective measures, which are well documented in the literature (Bettencourt, Carlstrom, Brown, Lindar, and Long, 1986; Caruso, Chan, and Chan, 1997; Isernhagen, 2000; Kornblau and Jacobs, 2000; Matheson, Ogden, Violette, and Schultz, 1985). However, the biomechanical framework is limited in depth and breadth and does not provide all of the information needed for comprehensive intervention. Therefore, practitioners must use additional theoretical models, such as the model of human occupation (MOHO; Kielhofner, 2009) and the readiness for return to work model (Franche and Krause, 2002). Using these two models as the theoretical underpinning for this chapter reflects the occupational therapy profession and return to work from a holistic and global perspective. These two models are compatible, as they recognize the influence that occupational performance and disability have on the industry of occupational medicine and industrial rehabilitation.

Theoretical Models of Practice

The MOHO is a theoretical approach or framework to understand human occupation (Kielhofner, 2008). Occupations are those everyday activities in which an individual engages. The person, as viewed through the MOHO, is understood through three sets of issues: volition, habituation, and skills (Kielhofner, 2008). *Volition* includes an individual's values, beliefs, attitude toward work, interests, personal causation, and participation. *Habituation* is the patterns and routines of behavior to which an individual is accustomed and that he or she follows at work, at home, and in other roles. Components of habituation are roles, habits, and routines of the person. The importance of habituation for human development and performance is supported by the MOHO framework. *Skills* consist of motor, cognitive/process, and communication/interaction components.

The readiness to return to work theory focuses on the interpersonal context of the worker. When applying this theory, the worker is referred to as a *work-disabled employee*. It recognizes the worker's interactions at the workplace and considers the insurance system as including the health and rehabilitation component. This model supports the worker's need to understand change and its three dimensions: decisional balance, self-efficacy, and change processes. It also considers individual variation to account for an individual's readiness to return to work and addresses the individual-level (which precedes a broader group-level) framework. It has its roots in assessment of psychosocial function.

Franche and Krause (2002) propose that return to work after injury or illness is a "behavior influenced by physical, psychological, and social factors" (p. 233). Their model of readiness for return to work is based on the readiness for change model and phase model of disability (Linton, 2001; Prochaska, Velicer, DiClemente, and Fava, 1988, 1992; Sinclair, et.al., 1998). Both of these theoretical models are compatible and support the assessment identified for use.

Psychosocial Factors Assessed by Occupational Therapists

Occupational therapy practitioners view the role of worker as multidimensional and human beings as interacting in a variety of environments with the need to perform numerous roles (MOHO views people as dynamic systems). This perspective makes occupational therapy practitioners well suited to address psychosocial factors when working in industrial rehabilitation programs and other work-related services. Practitioners recognize that establishing support for workers is critical and necessary. Developing collaborative relationships with clients injured on the job is important and is supported by the therapeutic use of self: the occupational therapy practitioner must address the workers' interests, abilities, concerns, and limitations. Whether the focus of intervention is on returning to previous work, seeking alternative work, or seeking other means of productivity, the practitioner must address, at a minimum, the client's supervisor and coworker relationships, self-perceived identity as a worker, competence as a worker, influence of family support, and environment or organizational climate.

> *Occupational therapy practitioners view the role of worker as multidimensional and human beings as interacting in a variety of environments with the need to also perform numerous other roles.*

Self-Perceived Identity and Worker Competence

Chapter 2 introduced the concept of *occupational identity* as "a composite sense of who one is and wishes to become as an occupational being generated from one's history of occupational participation" (Kielhofner, 2008, p. 106). Caplow (1954) explained that all societies, even the simplest, must maintain themselves through functional skills transmitted from each generation to the next. He suggested that in any society there is a human need to be employed and to work. Work offers a sense of mastery, and as workers, individuals can contribute to their needs. Because work occupies the majority of time for adults, many adults define themselves by their work. One of the first questions asked by people meeting for the first time is "What do you do for a living?" Therefore, developing an identity as a worker has become a social norm in industrialized countries. In order to have an income and survive, people need to work, and in down economies, the worker role can become even more important to the individual (Isernhagen, 2000; Siporin and Lysack, 2004).

Many issues play into the selection of and participation in the role of worker. For example, over time, the role of worker for women has changed, especially in the United States. During the 20th century, more women began to work outside the home, which has contributed to employers' acceptance of women as workers and a change in attitude by American society toward women and the contributions they bring to the workplace. Women's presence in the workforce is sometimes driven by need for personal fulfillment or other career rewards but is often most driven by financial need. Women's reasons for working influence their commitment and work performance (Johnson, 2005; Mortimer, 2003).

Zvonkovic, Schmiege, and Hall (1994) reported that women commonly identified family issues and associated demands as a factor that influences their participation at work, commitment to the job, and job satisfaction. Employers must pay attention to this issue, especially if they have a large workforce of women. The authors pointed out that while work–family decisions in the past were primarily based on the husband's work situation, such decisions today are more often collaborative because of the number of families in which both the husband and wife work. Hanson (1995) suggested that employers who recognize the value of workers and are flexible with both their benefits and working hours have more success with employee satisfaction. Over time, employee satisfaction has become even more important when attempting to implement an organizational change.

Chapter 2 also discussed *occupation competence,* defined as "the degree to which one sustains a pattern of occupational participation that reflects one's occupational identity" (Kielhofner, 2008, p. 107). Employees who feel competent at the workplace are often also satisfied employees, which contributes to job retention. However, it is important for both employers and health professionals to understand what the employee identifies as the intrinsic and extrinsic rewards for working. Practitioners cannot assume that because a worker has been with an employer for some time, he or she is satisfied. Many employees remain in their jobs because of the compensation, benefits, or lack of other employment opportunities. Employees' worth to an organization must be acknowledged in order for them to form the identity of a valued and competent employee. Without validation of their worth, employees may feel devalued and dissatisfied, not wishing to return to work after injury, illness, or disease.

Family Influences

The importance of family and its influences on workers and work performance is well documented (Hill, Hawkins, Ferris, and Weitzman, 2001; Johnson, 2005; Zvonkovic, et al., 2001). Employers who demonstrate flexibility and acknowledge the importance of family–work balance are predicted to have more satisfied and committed employees. Increasing demands at work without recognizing the demands employees have at home can be a serious error for employers to make. It may cause frustration for and lack of commitment by the employee. This issue may be even more important for employees preparing to return to work after a job-related injury. Johnson (2005) found that it is important for employers to assess whether intrinsic rewards or extrinsic rewards contribute to individual employees' work ethic. Her research suggests fathers place greater importance on extrinsic rewards than do men who are not parents. Extrinsic rewards are obtained from the job but are external to the job tasks and include pay, security, and prestige. Intrinsic rewards of work are obtained from the job tasks and include responsibility and challenge. These issues can influence workers' performance when they return to work after an injury, illness, or disease.

Hochschild (1997) reported that the stress of home life can drive workers to invest more in their jobs. Therefore, family life can affect job performance, and vice versa. Being a parent or a spouse influences people's values, increasing their sense of responsibility because their actions now affect other lives. Exploring family–work interrelations with workers provides additional information to providers for consideration when assessing psychosocial factors (Hill, et al., 2001; Johnson, 2005).

Environment

The environment (discussed in depth in Chapter 15) is widely recognized as an important component of assessment of psychosocial factors in the workplace (American Psychiatric Association, 2000; Fisher, 2000, 2003; Fisher and Gibson, 2008; Pejtersen, Allermann, Kristensen, and Poulsen, 2006; Snow, 2002). Negative environmental factors encountered by workers can cause emotional stress and physical discomfort. Most employers recognize that noise, temperature, dust, debris, and poor equipment can result in decreased employee performance. Therefore, such physical aspects of the environment are important for employers to consider.

Pejtersen and colleagues (2006) found that the design of the environment is important for employers to consider and to influence when they have the opportunity. In a survey of 2,000 office employees, they found that employees with open-plan offices are more likely than those in cellular offices to perceive thermal discomfort, poor air quality, and noise. They also may complain more frequently about central nervous system (CNS) and mucous membrane symptoms. The researchers also recognized that open-plan offices are not suitable for all job types: because open-plan workspace supports a social relations approach, workers tend to talk and interact with fellow employees more than they would in a cellular office. The noise and distraction of constant talking is likely to interfere with worker productivity.

Space, air quality, thermal comfort, and lighting are important, and the occupational therapy practitioner should assess such factors through direct observation when possible. It is also important to listen to the employee's perception of the environment, particularly when the practitioner cannot physically visit the workplace. Different employees have different preferences and sensitivities. Some workers identify crowded spaces, poor ventilation, or smells as problems, while to other workers, the same environmental factors are not problematic.

In assessing the environment, occupational therapy practitioners must consider the work climate, or *organizational climate* (Fuller, Barnett, Hester, and Relyea, 2003; Schiff, 2009; Snow, 2002; Stokols, Clitheroe, and Zmuidzinzs, 2002), which includes factors such as the beliefs, values, and attitudes of management. In the OTPF, these concepts are included as part of the social context. Organizational climates can send various messages, which, depending on the message, can have positive or negative influences on employees. Through discussions with the employee during the assessment process, the occupational therapy practitioner learns about the organization through the eyes of the worker.

Snow (2002) identified six dimensions of an organizational climate. She found that climate accounts for up to 30 percent of variance in performance of nurses on hospital units. She reported climate influences employee motivation: a positive climate promotes a level of comfort and satisfaction at work. The six dimensions of climate are (1) flexibility, (2) responsibility, (3) standards, (4) rewards, (5) clarity, and (6) team commitment. Problems with any of these six dimensions can be revealed during the occupational therapy assessment process.

Supervisor and Coworker Relationships

A number of relationships exist in the workplace, including relationships among workers, among workers and supervisors, and among supervisors and other management staff. The most critical is between employee and supervisor. Fuller and colleagues (2003) revisited the literature supporting that perceived organizational support from management is positively related to commitment by employees. Landry and Vandenberghe (2009) explored the role of commitment to supervisors. They surveyed over 200 employees and examined relationships between supervisors and employees. Turnover was one of the outcomes cited. If workers do not feel a commitment from supervisors, they are likely to leave and pursue employment elsewhere. Conflict with supervisors is one of the consistent examples identified in the literature around supervisor–employee relationships. Landry and Vandenberghe concluded that employers may want to assess this relationship because of its impact on employees' feelings of self-worth. Occupational therapists, as well, must assess the supervisor and coworker relationships.

Hung, Chi, and Lu (2009) explored the notion of coworker loafing and counterproductive work behaviors. They collected data from 184 supervisor–employee pairs from multiple sources. Participants self-rated, and supervisors of employees rated their perceptions of coworkers engaged in productive work and unproductive work (loafing). The researchers concluded that when employees perceive that coworkers are loafing, there is an increase in counterproductive behaviors toward both the organization and the coworkers. In the context of a person returning to work after an injury, coworkers and supervisors may believe that the employee is not really hurt and therefore may perceive the worker's modified duty as a means of loafing. The returning employee is then resented, and a revenge motive can emerge. Exploring these concerns during the assessment is important.

Assessment of Psychosocial Factors

For successful return-to-work outcomes, the assessment of psychosocial factors must address the role of workers, measure human performance, and evaluate workers' ability to meet job requirements. Understanding and supporting worker motivation, performance capacity, and environmental considerations requires a comprehensive assessment. The MOHO considers all these factors. The *Worker Role Interview (WRI)* is an assessment based on MOHO and used by occupational therapy practitioners in the United States and other countries (Fig. 11.2). A growing body of evidence supports the use of this assessment.

The WRI is a semistructured interview designed to identify the psychosocial and environmental factors that may influence a person's ability to return to work. It is used in conjunction with the observations made through the typical physical and behavioral assessments such as a functional capacity evaluation or assessment of ADL or activities and instrumental activities of daily living (IADL).

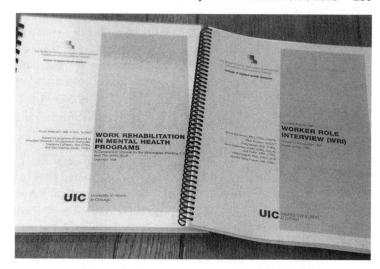

Figure 11.2 The Worker Role Interview (WRI) and other assessments and literature based on the model of human occupation can be obtained from the Model of Human Occupation Clearinghouse listed under "Resources" at the end of the chapter.

A number of studies demonstrate the validity and reliability of the WRI. In a study of 30 adults with work-related upper extremity injuries, Biernacki (1993) found high test–retest reliability and high total interrater reliability. Velozo (1999) found preliminary evidence from 62 workers with low back pain that 15 of the 17 items of the original version of the WRI constituted a unidimensional construct, thereby suggesting that the instrument should not be separated into different content areas for analysis. Haglund, Karlsson, Kielhofner, and Lai (1997) examined the construct validity of the Swedish WRI (WRI-S) in a psychiatric population. The results indicated that the WRI is a psychometrically sound assessment, since all but two environment-related items (perception of boss, perception of coworkers) assessed psychosocial work ability. The WRI is now used extensively in Sweden and is mandated as part of a comprehensive assessment of workers with all forms of disability.

Velozo (1999) reported three studies on the WRI. Two of them examined the construct validity, and the third examined the predictive validity of the WRI in returning to work. The findings showed that the WRI items, except some in the environment area, constitute a unidimensional construct for assessing psychosocial work ability and that neither the WRI items nor other variables, such as chronicity, diagnosis, number of surgeries, attorney involvement, or age, were useful in predicting return to work. Following these studies, the environment-related items were modified to reflect the person's perception of the environment. The aim of this change was to improve the fit of environment items with the rest of the scale. Ekbladh, Haglund, and Thorell (2004) investigated the predictive validity of the WRI for return to work at a 2-year followup of clients who attended an insurance medicine investigation center in Sweden. Five of the 17 items in the WRI had a tentative predictive validity of return to work. All three items related to the personal causation concept in MOHO, and the items appraising work expectations and perceptions of work setting were found to be predictive for returning to work.

Recently, an Icelandic translation of the WRI was found to replicate the item hierarchy of the English and Swedish versions (Fenger and Kramer, 2007). Similarly to other WRI studies, two environment items, perception of family and peers and perception of work setting, did not fit the construct of psychosocial ability to return to work. The remainder of the items validly and reliably measured return to work. Forsyth and colleagues (2006) examined the psychometric properties of the WRI rating scale. Data were collected from 21 raters on 440 participants from the United States, Sweden, and Iceland. A multifaceted Rasch model was used to analyze the data. Most items of the scale worked effectively to measure the underlying construct for which the WRI was designed. The scale validly measured 90.23 percent of the participants, who varied by nationality, culture, age, and diagnostic status. The scale's items distinguished participants into approximately three strata and were appropriately targeted to the participants. Seventeen of the 21 raters used the scale in a valid manner. This study demonstrated that the WRI scale and items are valid across ages, diagnoses, and culture and effectively measure a wide range of persons.

The WRI interview covers various aspects of the employee's life and job setting associated with his or her past work experience. The most recent version of the WRI includes 16 items and suggested interview formats for both workers with a recent injury and workers with longstanding disability or chronic illness (Braveman, et al., 2005). The WRI manual provides suggested questions associated with the underlying theoretical principals assessed by the tool. The associated principal from MOHO is in parentheses after each question. For example, "Do you think you were good at your job before your injury? (PC)" relates to personal causation, an underlying principal of the volitional subsystem. Samples of the suggested questions for injured workers are provided in Box 11.1, and sample questions for persons with longstanding disability or chronic illness are provided in Box 11.2.

The WRI may be utilized as part of the initial evaluation and may be repeated at the conclusion of intervention so the worker's initial and discharge responses can be compared. The questions are designed to solicit information relevant to rating the 16 items included on the WRI scale. The content areas of the assessment are based on the constructs of the MOHO:

- *Personal causation,* or the beliefs of what is expected for the worker to be effective at the workplace.
- *Values,* or what the worker sees as good or important in his or her job and about himself or herself as a worker.
- *Interests,* or the enjoyment the worker finds inside and outside employment.
- *Roles,* or how the individual sees himself or herself as a worker, student, son or daughter, and so on, and the obligations accompanying each role.
- *Habits,* or the routines and use of time both at and away from the workplace.
- *Environment,* or the objects, persons, and events with which the worker interacts during his or her daily routines.

Box 11.1   WRI Format 1: The Injured Worker

Questions from Section IV. Present Job

Let's talk about what work was like before your injury.

1. Tell me about this job: what did you do? (R)
2. Do you like your work? What do you like or dislike about it? (R)
3. How did you choose your present job? (V)
4. Did other family members have similar jobs or influence you in choosing your job?
5. Do you think you were good at your job before your injury? (PC)
6. What exactly do you feel you did especially well or better than others? (PC)
7. What are you most proud of in terms of your work? (V)
8. Do you have high standards for your work? (V)
9. Did you set goals for yourself at work (e.g., advances, promotions, productivity targets)? (V)
10. Have you had promotions or other recognitions with regard to your work? (V)
11. Describe what a typical workday was like. Start from when you arrived at the job to when you came home. (H)
12. When you think about your workday, tell me about your good work habits. (H)
13. How about work habits that aren't so good or habits that you would like to change? (H)

H, habits; PC, personal causation; R, roles; V, values.

Box 11.2   WRI Format II: Chronic Illness or Disability

Questions from Section II, Present Roles and Routines

1. Describe a typical day now. Describe a typical week. For example, are you working, attending any type of job training or therapy? (H)
2. What responsibilities have you got at the moment? (R)
3. Are you able to structure your days to meet your current responsibilities? (H)
4. How did your routine change when you got sick? (H)
5. Have you been able to make adjustments in your routines or in your responsibilities (or things you needed to do) while you have been sick? (H/R)
6. What aspects of your routine have you been successful in changing? (H)
7. Do you miss working? (V)
8. Is work the most important role for you at the moment? In the future? (V)
9. Do you feel that your current routine would support returning to work? (H)

H, habits; PC, personal causation; R, roles; V, values.

After the worker is assessed, the information obtained is used to score the 16 items that comprise the single scale reflecting psychosocial capacity for return to work. Each item is scored from 1 to 4. A score of 4 strongly supports the client's return to work; 1 indicates significant interference with the client's return to work. A score of 2 is associated with "interferes," and a score of 3 is associated with "supports." The rating scale and descriptions of each score are presented in Box 11.3. Full administration of the assessment, including scoring the 16 items, typically takes between 30 and 60 minutes for the experienced occupational therapy practitioner. An intervention plan is developed on the basis of information obtained through the WRI and other parts of a comprehensive evaluation. When the individual is being prepared for discharge, the occupational therapy practitioner again administers the WRI. The ratings at discharge reflect the impressions from the completed rehabilitation program in which the worker participated. The practitioner then can assess in which areas the worker improved, worsened, or stayed the same when the discharge ratings are compared to the initial scores.

A sample of a completed initial WRI assessment form for Corrine, introduced at the start of this chapter, is shown in Figure 11.3.

Box 11.3   Rating Scale for Items of the Worker Role Interview

Each subcontent area is scored according to a 4-point scale. The grading scale is based on the following four definitions:

4 = Strongly supports: Item strongly supports the client returning to previous employment or finding and keeping work in general. The outcome from this item yields good results for the client. It is highly probable that the positive aspects of this item will benefit the client in returning to previous employment.
3 = Supports: Item supports the client returning to previous employment or finding and keeping work in general. The positive aspects of this item outweigh the negative aspects, giving the client an advantage in returning to previous employment.
2 = Interferes: Item interferes with the client returning to previous employment or finding and keeping work in general. The negative aspects of this item outweigh the positive aspects, giving the client a disadvantage in returning to previous employment.
1 = Strongly interferes: Item strongly interferes with the client returning to previous employment or finding and keeping work in general. The outcome from this item yields negative results for the client. It is highly probable that the negative aspects of this item will interfere with the client returning to previous employment.
NA = Not applicable: Not enough information to rate the item or item does not apply to the client's particular employment situation.

Worker Role Interview Summary Scoring Sheet For Corrine				
Strongly Supports	Supports	Interferes	Strongly Interferes	Not Applicable
4	3	2	1	N/A
Strongly supports client returning to job	Positive qualities outweigh negative qualities: advantage for returning to job	Negative qualities outweigh positive qualities: disadvantage for returning to job	Strongly interferes with returning to job	Not applicable or not enough information to rate

	4	3	2	1	N/A
Personal Causation					
Assess abilities and limitations	I				
Expectations of job success		I			
Takes responsibility		I			
Values					
Commitment to work	I				
Work-related goals	I				
Interests					
Enjoys work		I			
Pursues interests		I			
Roles					
Identifies with being a worker	I				
Appraises work expectations		I			
Influence of other roles			I		
Habits					
Work habits	I				
Daily routines	I				
Adapts routine to minimize difficulties		I			
Environment					
Perception of work setting			I		
Perception of family and peers			I		
Perception of boss			I		
Perception of coworkers			I		
Use il's" for initial ratings and "D's" for discharge ratings. Connect the "I's" together and connect the "D's" together to create a graphic profile.					

Figure 11.3 Worker Role Interview Summary scoring sheet for Corrine.

Using the Worker Role Interview in Assessment and Intervention

Comprehensive assessment and intervention includes the full range of factors discussed in this and other chapters, including the client's personal factors, such as age, education, strength, and endurance. Both the physical and social contexts of environment must be considered, and as laid out in this chapter, assessment of the psychosocial factors influencing return to work is a critical element.

The WRI is intended for use as part of a comprehensive assessment of the worker, which may include assessment of basic ADL and IADL, other assessments of worker capacity such as a functional capacity evaluation, and a thorough assessment of the workplace. The results of all of these assessments are used together to identify a worker's strengths and weaknesses, both the factors that may support return to work and those that may make return to work less likely.

Failure to address the full picture can result in negative outcomes regardless of the level of motivation of the client. For example, a client may be making significant physical gains, and acceptable adaptations to the workplace may be identified, but if relations between the worker and his or her peers or supervisors are strained and are not addressed effectively in intervention, the success of other interventions may be compromised. Likewise, the influence of other roles, such as of a parent or spouse, on the return-to-work process must be recognized.

The complexity of intervention with injured workers or workers with longstanding disability must not be minimized. In order to simplify the process of learning about assessment and intervention in work-related services, the various components of the occupational therapy process are broken into different chapters throughout this text. However, you must remember to consider each component, such as the psychosocial assessment of the worker, in context and remain aware that such an assessment is just one piece of a complicated puzzle.

Chapter Summary

This chapter provided an overview of the psychosocial factors that affect individuals' perception of their worker role, their occupational performance, and at times the likelihood that they can return to work after the onset of illness or disability. With the MOHO and the readiness to work theory as a backdrop, several key categories of psychosocial factors were described: (1) supervisor and coworker relationships, (2) self-perceived identity and competence as a worker, (3) the influence of family roles, and (4) psychosocial environmental factors.

Assessing the influence of psychosocial factors on an individual's psychosocial capacity for work was described, and you were introduced to a commonly used occupational therapy assessment, the Worker Role Interview, or WRI. Assessment of psychosocial capacity for work and of the personal and environmental psychosocial factors described in this chapter are only part of the comprehensive evaluation of a client. Other chapters in this book describe assessment of additional key factors that influence work performance, such as cognition, physical capacity, and the environment.

Case Resolution

Corrine was evaluated by the interdisciplinary team in the work rehabilitation program. The evaluation process included a traditional functional capacity evaluation (FCE), the administration of the Worker Role Interview and a visit to Corrine's workplace and her home. The FCE validated that, although Corrine had continuing symptoms she was able to complete the required functions of her position and necessary IADL tasks at home. With additional training and education in body mechanics Corrine became more confident in her physical capacity to complete tasks at work and at home. Further, recommendations were made to make changes to her workstation and to pursue some simple accommodations at work such as taking more frequent breaks.

(case study continues on page 260)

Despite the initial progress that Corrine made, she continued to express worry over returning to work and if she would be supported by her employer and her coworkers. During the administration of the WRI the occupational therapist identified factors that appeared to support Corrine's return to work and factors that might interfere. Psychosocial factors that could be considered problems and potentially interfere with return to work included Corrine's perceptions of her boss and coworkers related to her worry that they would not support her. The occupational therapist also learned that Corrine's mother and siblings might be a negative influence on Corrine returning to work as they were encouraging pursuit of temporary disability status. The psychosocial factors that supported Corrine's return to work included her capacity to assess her abilities and limitations, her commitment to work, her strong identification as a worker, her work habits, and her ability to adapt her routines.

In collaboration with Corrine, the occupational therapist completed a worksite assessment that included consultation with Corrine's boss. During this consultation, the occupational therapist concluded that Corrine's boss valued her contributions highly and noted that her boss acknowledged that he did not express his appreciation to Corrine directly. Corrine's boss was open to all the suggestions regarding altering the workstation and providing reasonable accommodations to allow Corrine to return to work sooner. In their discussions, Corrine's boss even suggested that perhaps Corrine could return to work on "light duty" status and asked if there were actions he could take to better support her. When Corrine's occupational therapist shared this information with her, Corrine was quite surprised and realized that some of her worries might not be well founded. Corrine agreed that returning to work on light duty was a good option, and she and her occupational therapist scheduled a final visit to the worksite to make the recommended changes to her workstation. After 2 weeks of light duty, Corrine returned to full-time employment, needing to only occasionally take advantage of the accommodations provided to her. Her confidence increased, and she reported at discharge that she was completing all of her IADL at home, caring for her children independently, and making good use of proper body mechanics.

References

American Occupational Therapy Association. (1992). Occupational Therapy Services in Work Practice Statement. Commission on Practice. Approved by the Representative Assembly 3/92.

American Occupational Therapy Association (AOTA). (2008). Occupational therapy practice framework: Domain and process, 2nd ed. *American Journal of Occupational Therapy, 62,* 625–683.

American Psychiatric Association. (2000). *Diagnostic and Statistical Manual of Mental Disorders Fourth Edition, Text Revision.* Washington, DC: American Psychiatry Association.

Baum, C., & Christiansen, C. (2005). *Occupational Therapy: Enabling Function and Well-Being,* 3rd ed. Thorofare, NJ: Slack.

Bettencourt, C. M., Carlstrom, P., Brown, S. H., Lindar, K., & Long, C. M. (1986). Using work simulation to treat adults with low back injuries. *American Journal of Occupational Therapy, 40*(1), 12–18.

Biernacki, S. D. (1993). Reliability of the worker role interview. *American Journal of Occupational Therapy, 47*(9), 797–803.

Bond, M. A., Kalaja, A., Markkanen, P., Cageca, D., Daniel S., TsuriKova, L., & Punnett, L. (2007). *Expanding Our Understanding of Psychosocial Work Environment: A Compendium of Measures of Dissemination, Harassment and Work-Family Issues.* Department of Health and Human Services, Centers for Disease Control and Prevention, National Institute for Occupational Safety and Health.

Braveman, B., Robson, M., Velozo, C., Kielhofner, G., Fisher, G. S., Forsyth, K., et al. (2005). *The Worker Role Interview (Version 10).* Chicago: Model of Human Occupation Clearinghouse, Department of Occupational Therapy.

Caplow, T. (1954). *The Sociology of Work.* University of Minnesota: Minnesota Press.

Caruso, L. A., Chan, D. E., & Chan, A. (1987). The management of work-related back pain. *American Journal of Occupational Therapy, 41*(2), 112–117.

Dunton, W. R. (1917). History of occupational therapy. *Modern Hospital, 8*(6), 380–382.

Ekbladh, E., Haglund, L., & Thorell, L.-H. (2004). The worker role interview: Preliminary data on the predictive validity of return to work of clients after an insurance medicine investigation. *Journal of Occupational Rehabilitation, 14*(2), 131–141.

Fenger, K., & Kramer, J. M. (2007). Worker role interview: Testing the psychometric properties of the Icelandic version. *Scandinavian Journal of Occupational Therapy, 14*(3), 160–172.

Fidler, G. S. (1957). The role of occupational therapy in a multi-discipline approach to psychiatric illness. *American Journal of Occupational Therapy, 11*(1), 8–35.

Fisher, T. F. (2000). Perception differences among groups of employees in identifying the factors influencing a return to work after a work-related musculoskeletal injury. Unpublished dissertation. University of Michigan.

Fisher, T. F. (2003). Perception differences between groups of employees in identifying the factors influencing a return to work after a work-related musculoskeletal injury. *Work, 21*(3), 211–220.

Fisher, T. F., & Gibson, T. (2008). A measure of employees' exposure to risk factors for work-related musculoskeletal disorders in a university. *American Association of Occupational Health Nurse Journal, 56*(3), 1–15.

Forsyth, K., Braveman, B., Kielhofner, G., Ekbladh, E., Haglund L., Fenger, K., & Keller, J. (2006). Psychometric properties of the worker role interview. *Work, 27*(3), 313–318.

Franche, R.-L., & Krause, N. (2002). Readiness to work following injury or illness: Conceptualizing the interpersonal impact of health care, workplace, and insurance factors. *Journal of Occupational Rehabilitation, 12*(4), 233–256.

Fuller, J. B., Barnett, T., Hester, K., & Relyea, C. (2003). A social identity perspective on the relationship between perceived organizational support and organizational commitment. *Journal of Social Psychology, 143*(6), 789–791.

Haglund, L., Karlsson, G., Kielhofner, G., & Lai, J. S. (1997). Validity of the Swedish version of the worker role interview. *Scandinavian Journal of Occupational Therapy 4*(1–4), 23–29.

Hill, E. J., Hawkins, A. J., Ferris, M., & Weitzman, M. (2001). Finding an extra day a week: The positive influence of perceived job flexibility on work and family life balance. *Family Relations, 50*(1), 49–58.

Hochschild, A. (1997). *The Time Bind: When Work Becomes Home and Home Becomes Work.* New York: Metropolitan Books.

Hung, T.-K., Chi, N.-W., & Lu, W.-L. (2009). Exploring the relationships between perceived coworker loafing and counterproductive work behaviors: The mediating role of a revenge motive. *Journal of Business Psychology, 24*(2), 257–270.

Isernhagen, S. J. (2000). Matching the worker and work benefits to the worker: Benefits to the employer. *Work, 15*(2), 125–132.

Johnson, M. K. (2005). Family roles and work values: Process of selection and change. *Journal of Marriage and Family, 67*(3), 352–369.

Keough, J. L., & Fisher, T. F. (2001). Occupational-psychosocial perceptions influencing return to work and functional performance of injured workers. *Work, 16*(2), 101–110.

Kielhofner, G. (2008). *A Model of Human Occupation: Theory and Application,* 4th ed. Baltimore: Lippincott Williams & Wilkins.

Kielhofner, G. (2009). *Conceptual Foundations of Occupational Therapy Practice,* 4th ed. Philadelphia: F.A. Davis.

Kornblau, B., & Jacobs, K. (2000). *Work: Practice and Principles.* Bethesda, MD: AOTA Press.

Landry, G., & Vandenberghe, C. (2009). Role of commitment to the supervisor, leader–member exchange, and supervisor-based self-esteem in employee–supervisor conflicts. *Journal of Social Psychology, 149*(1), 5–27.

Law, M. (2002). Participation in the occupations of everyday life. *American Journal of Occupational Therapy, 56*(6), 640–649.

Linton, S. J. (2001). A review of psychological risk factors in back and neck pain. *Spine, 25*(9), 1148–1156.

Matheson, L. N., Ogden, L. D., Violette, K., & Schultz, K. (1985). Work hardening: Occupational therapy in industrial rehabilitation. *American Journal of Occupational Therapy, 39*(5), 314–321.

Meyer, A. (1948/1921). The contributions of psychiatry to the understanding of life problems: An address at the celebration of the 100th anniversary of Bloomingdale Hospital. In A. Lief (ed.), *The Commonsense Psychiatry of Dr. Adolf Meyer: Fifty-Two Selected Papers* (pp. 1–15). New York: McGraw Hill.

Miller, D. M. (2004). Psychosocial issues and the return-to-work process. *OT Practice, 9*(3), 16–20.

Mortimer, J. T. (2003). *Working and Growing Up in America.* Cambridge, MA: Harvard University Press.

Moyers, P. A., & Dale, L. M. (2007). *The Guide to Occupational Therapy Practice,* 2nd ed. Bethesda, MD: AOTA Press.

Olson, L. (1995). *Work Readiness: Day Treatment for the Chronically Disabled.* Chicago: Model of Human Occupation Clearinghouse, Department of Occupational Therapy.

Pejtersen, J., Allermann, L., Kristensen, T. S., & Poulsen, O. M. (2006). Indoor climate, psychosocial work environment and symptoms in open-plan offices. *Indoor Air, 16*(15), 392–401.

Prochaska, J. O., DiClemente, C. C., & Norcross, J. C. (1992). In search of how people change. Applications to addictive behaviors. *American Psychologist, 47*(9), 1102–1114.

Prochaska, J. O., Velicer, W. F., DiClemente, C. C., & Fava, J. (1988). Measuring processes of change: Applications to the cessation of smoking. *Journal Consulting Clinical Psychology, 56*(4), 520–528.

Reilly, M. (1966). A psychiatric occupational therapy program as a teaching model. *American Journal of Occupational Therapy, 20*(2), 61–67.

Schiff, J. W. (2009). A measure of organizational culture in mental health clinics. *Best Practice in Mental Health: An International Journal, 5*(2), 89–111.

Sinclair, S. J., Hogg-Johnson, S. H., Mondloch, M. V., & Shields, S. A. (1997). The effectiveness of an early active intervention program for workers with soft-tissue injuries. The Early Claimant Cohort Study, *Spine, 15*(22), 2919–2931.

Siporin, S., & Lysack, C. (2004). Quality of Life Supported Employment: A case study of three women with developmental disabilities. *American Journal of Occupational Therapy, 53*(4), 455–465.

Snow, J. (2002). Enhancing work climate to improve performance and retain valued employees. *Journal of Occupational Nursing, 32*(7/8), 393–397.

Stokols, D., Clitheroe, C., & Zmuidzinzs, M. (2002). Qualities of work environments that promote perceived support for creativity. *Creativity Research Journal, 14*(2), 137–147.

Velozo, C. (1999). Worker Role Interview: Toward validation of a psychosocial work-related measure. *Journal of Occupational Rehabilitation, 9*(3), 153–168.

Woodside, H. (1971). The development of occupational therapy, 1910–1929. *American Journal of Occupational Therapy, 25*(5), 226–230.

Zvonkovic, A. M., Schmiege, C. J., & Hall, L. D. (1994). Influence strategies used when couples make work-family decisions and their importance for marital satisfaction. *Family Relations, 43,* 182–188.

Glossary

Habits include work routines and routines outside the workplace as well as use of time.

Interests include the enjoyment the worker finds inside and outside employment.

Environment includes the objects, persons, and events with which the worker interacts during daily routines.

Occupational identity is "a composite sense of who one is and wishes to become as an occupational being generated from one's history of occupational participation" (Kielhofner, 2008, p. 106).

Occupational competence is "the degree to which one sustains a pattern of occupational participation that reflects one's occupational identity" (Kielhofner, 2008, p. 107).

Organizational climate includes factors such as the beliefs, values, and attitudes of management of an organization.

Personal causation is a list of beliefs of what is expected for the worker to be effective at the workplace.

Psychosocial domain includes "psychological demand, job control (decision latitude), social support, and intrinsic and extrinsic rewards" (Bond, et al., 2007, p. 3).

Roles encompass the individual's view of himself or herself as a worker, student, son or daughter, and so on, and the obligations associated with each identification.

Values are what the worker sees as good or important in his or her job and about himself or herself as a worker.

Work includes both paid employment and volunteer activities (AOTA, 2008).

Resources

Model of Human Occupation Clearinghouse

www.moho.uic.edu/

This website lists resources based on the Model of Human Occupation, including assessments such as the Worker Role Interview (WRI).

12 Physical Assessment of the Worker

Jill J. Page

Key Concepts

The following are key concepts addressed in this chapter:

- The components of conventional functional capacity evaluation are described.
- Modified functional capacity is described, and times when it is appropriate for use are explained.
- The basics of preemployment testing and the point in the process of hiring a new employee are explained.
- Opportunities for occupational therapy practitioners to provide onsite services for employers are described.
- The importance of job demands analysis in the return-to-work/stay-at-work process is explained.

Case Introduction

Jeff worked for 17 years as a maintenance worker at Acme Foundry. He liked his job and really felt that he was part of the team and took pride in doing a good job. Jeff is 45 years old and has always been physically active, both at work and in his leisure pursuits and family activities. Jeff experienced a sharp, pulling sensation that radiated from his neck down to his left upper arm while installing a heating element at work and sought medical help through his employer. He was diagnosed with a cervical strain. It was recommended that he take off work for 4 weeks and receive outpatient occupational therapy. Jeff was very concerned about returning to work and expressed this anxiety to his treating therapist during their initial meeting. The occupational therapist noted the concern and explained that treatment would be wide-ranging and address his physical abilities to ready him for return to work. The program would include an evaluation of his function as well as his description of his job and a job site visit that would help provide additional detail and prepare the occupational therapist to better provide a comprehensive treatment program.

Introduction

This chapter addresses the need for physical assessment of the worker and the challenges often encountered with such assessment. The history of occupational therapy in work assessment and the physical factors that influence work performance and return to work after the onset of illness or disability are discussed. Strategies for assessing physical factors are described, and types of work performance and work demands assessments are overviewed. The chapter discusses traditional strategies such as *functional capacity evaluation* in clinical settings and more recent strategies, including *modified functional capacity evaluation, preemployment testing, onsite services*, and *job demands analysis*. The current climate in medicine, occupational therapy, and other disciplines has increasingly focused on evidence-based clinical decision-making (Maddern, 1998). Using standardized assessments that provide reliable and valid data supply evidence-based information that substantiates the occupational therapy contribution to an interdisciplinary evaluation process and plan of care (Gutman, Mortera, Hinojosa, and Kramer, 2007). An occupational therapist simply cannot make the best recommendation possible regarding a client's work abilities or job requirements without sound data.

Evolution of Functional Assessment of the Worker

Occupational therapy has a rich history of utilizing work for therapeutic purposes (Harvey-Krefting, 1985). As noted in Chapter 1, the occupational therapy profession began with a strong foundation in mental health facilities. The use of work occupations as a treatment modality in work programs did not begin to focus on measuring the physical aspects of both work and the worker until after World War II (Cromwell, 1985). Lillian S. Wegg was honored with the Eleanor Clark Slagle Lecture in 1959 and expressed the need in occupational therapy work programs for an emphasis on testing the client, stating, "The purpose of the testing is to diagnose and evaluate the client's ability and capacity for work" (1960, p. 55). Wegg reported that her work evaluation team did not find work capacity information in the more traditional tests commonly associated with occupational therapy physical disability evaluations, such as range-of-motion and strength testing, and emphasized the need for work testing that utilized real work tasks or the work setting to assess work capacity.

In the 1970s and early 1980s, an industrial boom in the United States created opportunity for occupational therapy practitioners to interact in a more substantial fashion with workers in both industrial rehabilitation and work hardening (Jacobs and Baker, 2000). The increased industrial activity required improved control of rising injury rates (Darphin, 1995; King, 1998; Lechner, 1994; Ogden-Neimeyer and Jacobs, 1989). Industrial rehabilitation is an encompassing term that includes all aspects of treating and evaluating the injured worker (Ha, Page, and Wietlisbach, 2006). Work hardening is described as a structured, multidisciplinary approach to maximize the injured worker's functional abilities, and the term is typically attributed to Leonard Matheson (Darphin, 1995; King, 1998; Lechner, 1994; Matheson, Ogden, Violette, and Schulz, 1985; Ogden-Neimeyer and Jacobs, 1989). The physical assessment of the worker was included in work hardening programs as a key element in treatment planning, goal-setting, and discharge. usually identified as a functional capacity evaluation (FCE) (Darphin, 1995; King, 1998; Lechner, 1994).

In early 2006, the American Occupational Therapy Association (AOTA) officially adopted the Centennial Vision for the profession, with a principal goal of preparing occupational therapy to meet the changing and evolving needs of society (AOTA, 2007). One of the primary focus areas identified in the Centennial Vision was work and industry (AOTA, n.d.). AOTA has long recognized and promoted the skills of occupational therapists and occupational therapy assistants in the provision of work-related services. In its "Occupational Therapy Services in Facilitating Work Performance" (2000), occupational therapy's educational background, which includes both biological and behavioral sciences, is emphasized as central to the value that occupational therapy brings to the evaluation of work performance. The Occupational Therapy Practice Framework: Domain and Process (OTPF) was first published by AOTA in 2002, with latest revisions occurring in 2008. The purpose of the OTPF is to describe the "interrelated constructs that define and guide occupational therapy practice" (2008, p. 625) and provide documentation of how occupational therapy practitioners use a holistic view encompassing the individual, organization, and population levels. This provides a strong foundation for occupational therapy practitioners who are employed in the area of work. The OTPF identifies work as an area of occupation and specifically names job performance as a component of work.

Types of Assessments

Functional Capacity Evaluation

FCE is generally defined as an assessment of a client's ability to physically perform work related activity (Gibson and Strong, 2003; Lechner, Roth, and Stratton, 1991). FCE can be performed for a variety of reasons, including collaborating with clients to set treatment goals, making decisions about return to work, evaluating functional capacity remaining after an injury, deciding if an individual qualifies for disability, assisting in selecting an appropriate applicant during a hiring process, and closing cases for settlement purposes (Page, 2001). FCE is performed by professionals from a number of disciplines; occupational therapy is one of the primary disciplines to conduct these assessments. Occupational therapy practitioners, because of their educational background and their ability to observe task performance on multiple levels, are exceptionally qualified to assess the physical performance of the worker and the physical demands of the work (AOTA, 2000, 2008). Functional capacity falls within the OTPF definition of performance skills, which are described as the "abilities clients demonstrate in the actions they perform" (2008, p. 639).

> *Occupational therapy practitioners, because of their educational background and their ability to observe task performance on multiple levels, are exceptionally qualified to assess the physical performance of the worker and the physical demands of the work.*

FCE typically begins with a thorough review of the medical records, an interview with the client, brief musculoskeletal screening, assessment of physical capacities, and report generation including results and recommendations if indicated (King, Tuckwell, and Barrett, 1998). The medical record review must be as inclusive as possible because detailed information about previous interventions can greatly improve the recommendations developed at the conclusion of the FCE. The client interview ordinarily covers review of demographic information, the mechanism of injury and resulting treatment, the client's employment history, and any medications the client may be taking (Ha, et al., 2006). Subjective pain ratings are often collected at the beginning of the evaluation and throughout the FCE to monitor the correlation between functional activity and the client's pain level. It is important to note that pain response, or the client's perception of soreness or discomfort, following FCE can be expected and interpreted as a normal reaction to the administration of FCE (Soer, et al., 2008). Soer and colleagues (2008) found no apparent significant difference between the pain response to FCE of healthy workers and patients with chronic low back pain. This is likely the case because FCE is a test of an individual's maximum abilities and is physically demanding for both the injured and uninjured alike.

The musculoskeletal screening provides a baseline of range of motion (ROM) and strength abilities and limitations, which enables the therapist to be judicious with the functional assessment of physical ability (see Fig. 12.1) (King, et al., 1998). Red flags may be identified during the screening, such as limited cervical ROM that may impede the client's ability to work overhead on a ladder. Such red flags help to ensure client safety during the FCE (Lechner, 1998). The assessment of physical abilities addresses the client's ability to perform work-related activity, usually within the context of physical demands of various work occupations described by the U.S. Department of Labor's (1991a, 1991b) *Dictionary of Occupational Titles (DOT)* and *The Revised Handbook for Analyzing Jobs* (King, et al., 1998); see Table 12.1. These publications provide specific information about occupations and the physical demands that make up each occupation, and they provide standardized nomenclature for classifying physical demands (Ha, et al., 2006). The physical demands selected for testing can be broad in scope or focused to be job or injury specific, depending on the client's needs or the referral request. Full FCE usually is classified as either "any occupation," which tests all demands for any job; "own job," which tests for the demands of the client's job description, such as truck driver for ABC Trucking; or "own occupation," which tests demands for a generic job category, such as truck driver; see Box 12.1 (Ha, et al., 2006). If performing an "own job" FCE, a job description is assembled from either the employer or the client, sometimes from both for comparison's sake. The FCE focus could also be on a particular injury or body part; see Figure 12.2 (Ha, et al., 2006).

The client's physical abilities are evaluated in the areas of strength, static postures, and dynamic movements through the therapist's observation of biomechanical change and response during the task performance, according to the FCE's scoring criteria (Ha, et al., 2006). Strength tasks are evaluated in a graded fashion, starting the client at no weight or a very low weight and increasing the load incrementally, providing the occupational

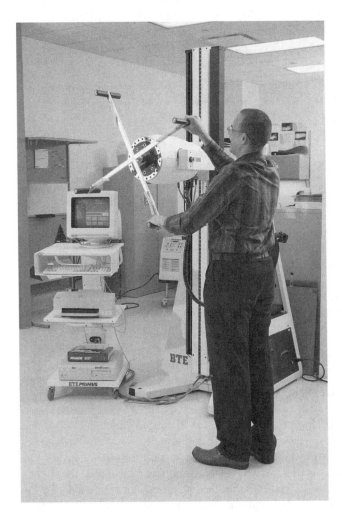

Figure 12.1 Evaluation of shoulder function using the BTE work simulator by BTE Technologies.

Table 12.1 Twenty Physical Demands of Work*

• Lifting	• Pushing	• Kneeling	• Fingering
• Standing	• Pulling	• Crouching	• Feeling
• Walking	• Climbing	• Crawling	• Talking
• Sitting	• Balancing	• Reaching	• Hearing
• Carrying	• Stooping	• Handling	• Seeing

*As defined by the *Dictionary of Occupational Titles* and *The Revised Handbook for Analyzing Jobs* (United States Department of Labor, 1991a, 1991b)

Box 12.1   Types of FCEs

Own Job—Testing to an individual's own job demands, such as for a cashier at John's Quick Stop
Own Occupation—Testing to an individual's own occupational demands, such as for "cashier" as described in the DOT
Any Job—Testing all physical demands to determine which, if any, jobs an individual may be able to perform

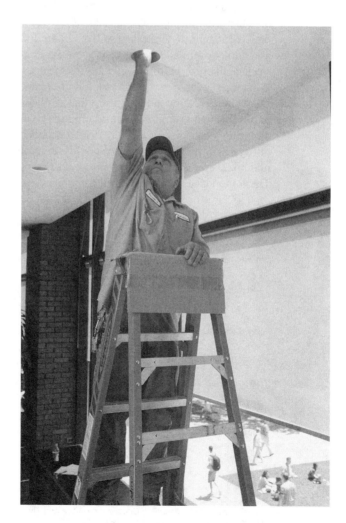

Figure 12.2 Evaluating the ability to sustain reach overhead while on a ladder would be important in a job-specific FCE.

therapy practitioner with the opportunity to see biomechanical changes over the course of progressive loading and allowing a safe maximum weight to be established with minimum risk to the client (Box 12.2). It is the therapist's responsibility not to push the client beyond his or her capability but to incorporate client feedback with objective examination into evaluating capacity (Ha, et al., 2006; Lechner, 1998). Vital statistics, including heart rate and blood pressure, are often monitored throughout the physical assessment to maintain cardiovascular safety. The client's abilities are usually reported in terms of the frequency that the physical demand can be performed during the course of the workday, using the DOT language or some derivative thereof (Table 12.2). The philosophy behind the assessment of a client's work-performance skills is described in the OTPF and incorporates a focus on the occupational performance of the client (AOTA, 2008). The report is formulated at the conclusion of the evaluation and may include information about the client's overall level of work ability, tolerance for a given level of work for the length of the workday, specific physical demand or task abilities, job demands match, information about the client's level of cooperation during the course of the FCE, and recommendations regarding possible interventions (King, et al., 1998; Lechner, 1998) (Table 12.3).

To be considered comprehensive, an FCE must include, at a minimum, the physical demands defined by the U.S. Department of Labor (Gibson and Strong, 1997; Ha, et al., 2006; U.S. Department of Labor, 1991a). Additional test items may be added to address specific questions that were included in the referral for the FCE. It is also important that the client find meaning in the tasks of the test so he or she will fully engage in the occupational nature of the tasks (AOTA, 2000, 2008). For example, if a dental hygienist is asked to perform a crawling task when she does not have to perform this task on her job, she is unlikely to perform well because she doesn't understand the reasoning behind it and is being asked to perform the task out of context (AOTA, 2008; Page, 2001).

Standardization in FCE means that the evaluation has structure, including a procedure manual, verbal task instructions, definitions, equipment and task setup requirements, and a scoring mechanism (Lechner, 1998; Lechner, et al., 1991; Page, 2001). The FCE needs this type of structure to ensure stability in the testing design and implementation and to minimize evaluator bias and ensure client safety (Ha, et al., 2006; Lechner; 1998). The importance of the verbal instructions cannot be overlooked. The tone of the entire

---

Box 12.2 Traits of a Well-Designed FCE

A well-designed FCE must be:

- Comprehensive   • Objective
- Standardized   • Reliable
- Practical   • Valid

(King, Tuckwell, and Barrett, 1998; Lechner, 1998; Rothstein and Echternach, 1993)

Table 12.2 Physical Demand Frequency Definitions*

Never	Activity or condition does not exist
Occasionally	Up to $\frac{1}{3}$ of the day
Frequently	$\frac{1}{3}$ to $\frac{2}{3}$ of the day
Constantly	$\frac{2}{3}$ to full day

*As defined by the *Dictionary of Occupational Titles* and *The Revised Handbook for Analyzing Jobs* (United States Department of Labor, 1991a, 1991b)

Table 12.3   Definitions for Overall Level of Work*

Sedentary	Exerting up to 10 pounds of force occasionally or a negligible amount of force frequently to lift, carry, push, pull, or otherwise move objects, including the human body. Sedentary work involves sitting most of the time but may involve walking or standing for brief periods of time. Jobs are sedentary if walking and standing are required only occasionally but all other sedentary criteria are met.
Light	Exerting up to 20 pounds of force occasionally or up to 10 pounds of force frequently or a negligible amount of force constantly to move objects. Physical demand requirements are in excess of those for sedentary work. Even though the weight lifted may be only a negligible amount, a job should be rated light work (1) when it requires walking or standing to a significant degree, (2) when it requires sitting most of the time but entails pushing or pulling of arm or leg controls, or (3) when the job requires working at a production-rate pace entailing the constant pushing or pulling of materials even though the weight of those materials is negligible. Note: The constant stress and strain of maintaining a production-rate pace, especially in an industrial setting, is physically demanding of a worker even though the amount of force exerted is negligible.
Medium	Exerting 20–50 pounds of force occasionally or 10–25 pounds of force frequently or greater than negligible up to 10 pounds of force constantly to move objects. Physical demand requirements are in excess of those for light work.
Heavy	Exerting 50–100 pounds of force occasionally or 25–50 pounds of force frequently or 10–20 pounds of force constantly to move objects. Physical demand requirements are in excess of those for medium work.
Very Heavy	Exerting force in excess of 100 pounds of force occasionally or in excess of 50 pounds of force frequently or in excess of 20 pounds of force constantly to move objects. Physical demand requirements are in excess of those for heavy work.

*As defined by the *Dictionary of Occupational Titles* and *The Revised Handbook for Analyzing Jobs* (United States Department of Labor, 1991a, 1991b)

evaluation process is set during the initial interview, and the establishment of rapport is critical to ensuring cooperation and maximum participation (Lechner, 1998).

The FCE needs to be practical in both time required to administer, score, and generate reports and in its space and equipment requirements. If purchased, the FCE system must be cost effective and be able to demonstrate a return on investment (Lechner, 1998; Page, 2001). A variety of FCE systems are commercially available (Table 12.4), but many

Table 12.4   Various Commercially Available FCE Systems

Arcon VerNova	Matheson
Blankenship	Medigraph
BTE Technologies	OccuCare
DSI	ProComp
ErgoScience	Valpar-Joule
Evaluwriter	WEST-EPIC
J-Tech	WorkHab
Key	WorkSteps
	WorkWell

therapists choose to perform an FCE of their own design (Cotton, Schonstein, and Adams, 2006). This choice seems to be influenced primarily by the cost of purchasing an FCE system and not by the lack of reliability and validity behind their approach.

The term *objectivity* in the context of FCE is often thought to mean units of measure expressed in pounds, inches, force pounds, and so on, but subjective observation can be expressed objectively through the use of operational definitions (Ha, et al., 2006). Operational definitions give precise descriptions of terms that could be interpreted differently by different people. For example, *kneeling* and *crouching* cannot be misconstrued if *kneeling* is defined as having both knees resting on the ground and *crouching* as having one knee on the ground and the other off the ground. Clear definitions enable evaluators to communicate and collaborate effectively. Decision-making processes, which include the clinical judgment of the therapist, must be free of observer bias (Rothstein and Echternach, 1993).

Reliability and validity are two of the most important aspects of FCE (Ha, et al., 2006; Innes and Straker, 1999a, 1999b; Pranksy and Dempsey, 2004). These characteristics assist referral sources such as physicians and workers' compensation insurers in understanding the value of FCE results (King, et al., 1998; Lechner, 1998; Lechner, et al., 1991). The literature suggests that interrater and intrarater reliability are are the two most important types of reliability in FCE (Chen, 2007; Innes and Straker, 1999a; Lechner, et al., 1991). Interrater reliability in FCE is the consistency of the measure (King, et al., 1998). In other words, if two occupational therapists give the same FCE to the same patient, it is essential that they get the same end result. Intrarater or test–retest reliability is the instrument's ability to react the same way when the therapist administers the test more than once (King, et al., 1998). If agreement cannot be reached between two therapists observing the same performance, it becomes difficult, if not impossible, to determine which result is correct (King, et al., 1998). Ascertaining reliability is the initial step in establishing validity in an evaluation (Rothstein and Echternach, 1993).

Validity in FCE is much more difficult to demonstrate. *Validity* is a scientific term meaning accuracy, or in terms of an FCE, whether the evaluation result truly represents the client's work ability (Lechner, 1998; Rothstein and Echternach, 1993). Content validity, criterion validity (both concurrent and predictive), and construct validity are all important in FCE (Kielhofner, 2006; King, et al., 1998; Lechner, 1998; Polgar, 2009). Content or face validity determines that the evaluation is testing what it is supposed to be testing. Content validity is described as being defined by a panel of experts, job demands analysis, or a document standard, such as the DOT (Lechner, 1998; Lechner, et al., 1991; Page, 2001). Criterion validity is often demonstrated by comparing an instrument against a "gold standard" or another tool that is proven reliable and valid and, in FCE, would show that clients can actually perform the work the evaluation concludes they can. This can be challenging because few FCE instruments have been studied in their entirety for reliability and validity, with the results published in peer-reviewed literature, to allow comparison against other instruments. Concurrent validity is an instrument's aptitude to determine existing ability, whereas predictive validity is its ability to detect future ability. Both have value in FCE, as concurrent validity determines whether or not a client can return to a given level of work, and predictive validity allows a therapist to determine who can return to work and expect to remain on the job without injury (King, et al., 1998; Lechner, 1998; Lechner, et al., 1991). Beware of language that describes client effort as "valid" or "invalid" based on level of client participation or perceived sincerity of effort, as this is a misuse of the word. Being able to demonstrate the FCE results are both reliable and valid support an evidence-based approach in occupational therapy.

FCE referrals come from a variety of sources and will depend on the local market. Physicians, insurance companies, case managers, attorneys, and employers are usual referral sources and are often approached by practitioners for referrals (Ha, et al., 2006).

Depending on facility, payer, and state regulations and requirements, a physician's prescription may be required for an occupational therapist to perform an FCE. Contacting a payer to determine if payment is approved (precertifying) before completing the FCE is recommended to ensure that reimbursement will be received. Compensation for FCE will vary according to local market and geography and is often governed by state workers' compensation fee schedules (Ha, et al., 2006).

The results of FCE are used to determine whether or not a client can return to work, whether the client qualifies for disability, or if a case should be settled or closed (Ha, et al., 2006). The decision reached with FCE has tremendous impact on the client's life, and this reality must be at the forefront of the therapist's mind when choosing an assessment and formulating conclusions (King, et al., 1998; Lechner, 1998).

Modified FCE

Studies suggest that modifying the FCE to suit the needs of the client and to be able to answer the referral question can be done with improved efficiency and accuracy. Modified FCE can be in the form of abbreviated FCE, postoffer employment screening, job or injury specific, and *return-to-work/fit-for-duty testing*. When compared to standard FCE administration, short-form FCE seems to reduce time to perform while not affecting recovery outcomes (Gross, Battié, and Asante, 2007). Frings-Dresen and Sluiter (2003) found that by developing a job-specific FCE protocol by utilizing job-site observation, it was possible to improve the external validity over the original, non-job-specific protocol, with the added benefit of having a test protocol that was one-fourth the length of the original protocol. Fit-for-duty testing is an assessment of readiness for return to work designed to ensure that the client can perform the tasks of the work without risk to self or others' safety (Saeki and Hachisuka, 2004).

Preemployment Testing

The intended benefit of preemployment testing is that by performing a test of physical abilities before an applicant is placed in a job, an employer has the opportunity to hire employees who are physically capable of performing the job, lessening the chances of the employee sustaining an on-the-job injury. Preemployment testing is often one piece of a company's comprehensive injury management program (Perry, 1998). When a company implements this type of testing, it is usually the result of a close examination of injury rates and costs, both direct and indirect. The employer must consider not only the medical cost related to an injury but also the costs related to the injured employee's benefit package, loss of production, hiring and training of replacement personnel, and potential overtime for workers who cover the added workload (Ha, et al., 2006).

A variety of approaches have been used in preemployment testing, ranging from isokinetic strength testing, generic fitness testing to job specific, and postoffer screening (POS). Although this type of testing can occur at many points throughout the course of hiring, the literature suggests that it occur after a conditional offer of employment has been extended to a potential employee, often called postoffer or preplacement testing (Harbin and Olson, 2005; Littleton, 2003; Pruitt, 1995; Ratzon, 2004; Scott, 2002). The Equal Employment Opportunity Commission (EEOC) describes processes related to employment testing *Uniform Guidelines on Employee Selection Procedures* (1978) and provides further clarification in the *Fact Sheet on Employee Testing and Selection Procedures* (2007), which covers the guidelines, the Americans with Disabilities Act (ADA; 1991), and the Age Discrimination in Employment Act (ADEA; 1967). The recommended steps in preemployment screening are (1) interview of the applicant, (2) conditional offer of employment, if decision is made to hire, with start date based on the individual successfully completing a drug screen, (3) physical examination, and (4) physical ability testing (see Fig. 12.3).

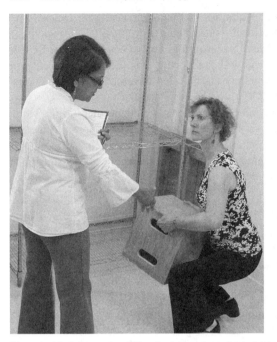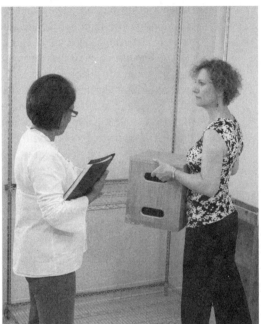

Figure 12.3 Assessing lifting from floor to waist height.

Both the *Uniform Guidelines on Employee Selection Procedures* and the ADA prohibit medical testing prior to the extension of an offer of employment (ADA, 1991; EEOC, 1978, 2007). If an occupational therapist is administering the test, the test could be considered medical because occupational therapy is a health-related profession. This also extends to the collection of physiological data, such as heart rate and blood pressure. Under the ADA, this information is deemed medical and prohibited in the preoffer stage of hiring. The EEOC (1978, 2007) maintains that any physical testing be job specific and consistent with business necessity or be representative of what the employer requires for the job to be performed. Preplacement screening must test only the essential functions of the job, address the need for reasonable accommodation if needed by the applicant, and extend a conditional offer of employment pending passing the POS as part of the employee selection process (Pruitt, 1995). Case law has supported this. The most prevalent reason for courts deciding against preemployment evaluation is the lack of job relatedness in measuring performance. Arbitrary requirements such as applicant height and weight requirements as a condition for employment have been found to be illegal because they are not job related (Jackson, 1994). For instance, assume that a job requires that the worker must lift 100 pounds from the floor to a counter 30 inches from the floor, and this task is part of the postoffer screen. If most of the female applicants do not pass the screen, the employer must be prepared to be able to prove that the 100-pound lift to 30 inches is part of the job and that the screen tested exactly the task as required on the job. Employers also have to be vigilant in the design of the testing to avoid adverse impact on the basis of age, race, sex, color, religion, or national origin or be able to demonstrate why adverse impact is occurring. Adverse impact occurs when a selection rate for any race, sex, or ethnic group is less than four-fifths (80%) of the rate for the group with the highest selection rate (EEOC, 1978, 2007); see Box 12.3. In *EEOC v. Dial* (2006), the U.S. Court of Appeals for the Eighth Circuit upheld a lower court's decision that Dial Corporation had discriminated against women during a hiring screen because the screen was more difficult than the job.

Box 12.3 Determining Adverse Impact

Suppose that 40 applicants participated in a POS and 24 were hired. The gender and ethnicity information for the 40 applicants was collected, and the results are listed in the following table. The four-fifths, or 80 percent, selection rule is applied, and the impact ratio is determined by dividing the selection rate of a given group by the selection rate of the highest selected group. In this example, the company must be prepared to explain the business necessity of the adverse impact on female applicants.

Applicants	Hired	Selection Rate	Impact Ratio	Adverse Impact
31 Male	20	20/31 = 0.67 = 67%	N/A	N/A
9 Female	4	4/9 = 0.44 = 44%	0.44/0.67 = 0.66 = 66%	Yes
20 Caucasian	10	10/20 = 0.50 = 50%	N/A	N/A
12 African American	8	8/12 = 0.67 = 67%	0.67/0.50 = 1.34 = 134%	No
8 Hispanic	6	6/8 = 0.75 = 75%	0.75/0.50 = 1.55 = 155%	No

Many studies have found limited or no value in strength testing alone in predicting work injury (Dueker, Ritchie, Knox, and Rose, 1994; Harbin and Olson, 2005). Mostandi, Noe, Kovacik, and Porterfield (1992) found that isokinetic low back–strength scores, previous history of injury, or reported pain are not positively correlated with future low back pain or injury in jobs where heavy loads are lifted and postures inconsistent. However, evidence supports the use of job-specific testing as part of an employer's hiring process (Box 12.4). Harbin and Olson (2005) found a strong correlation between an employee's physical abilities and the physical job demands. If an employee's physical abilities enabled him or her to perform the essential functions of the job, there was a much lower injury rate than among employees whose physical abilities were less than what the job required. In their study, the rate of low back injury for those who demonstrated the capacity to do the job was 3 percent; among those whose abilities were below the job requirements, the rate was 33 percent. Harbin and Olson found that application of

Box 12.4 Steps in Developing a POS

The following are steps in the development of a POS process:

1. The company decides which jobs will be selected for screening (usually jobs with high injury rates or in which injuries occur within the first 6 months of hire).
2. Perform job demands analysis on the selected jobs.
3. Develop a physical screen from the most difficult physical demands of the job.
4. In conjunction with human resources and legal input, develop policy and procedures for the screening process.
5. Select evaluators and ensure they have adequate training to administer the screen.
6. Validate the screen, preferably by evaluating incumbents and making any necessary modifications to the screen upon completion of this step.
7. Put the screening into operation and follow up to maintain good documentation and quality assurance.
8. Amend the screen as necessary because job demands may change over time.

(Ha, et al., 2006; Perry, 1998)

suitable postoffer, preplacement testing demonstrates a good return on investment by lowering the rate of work injuries. Others have found that through use of job-related strength testing, workers whose abilities met or exceeded the job demands were injured less often than those whose abilities did not meet the job demands (Keyserling, Herrin, Chaffin, Armstrong, and Foss, 1980).

Although the cost of developing a POS program can be considerable (Box 12.5), the long-term savings can outweigh the initial costs (Perry, 1998). Well-designed POS that includes job demands analysis, clear scoring criteria, and standardized tests with job-specific focus can dramatically diminish both the rate of injury and costs, according to Scott (2002). Littleton (2003) compared data collected 3 years before POS was implemented to data collected 3 years after it was introduced and found an 18 to 1 return on investment. This study also discovered a decline in the number of work-related injuries, total cost related to injury, and cost per case.

Ratzon (2004) discussed the potential uses for the results of POS and presented a case study in which an otherwise qualified applicant did not meet the physical demands of a job; remediation was offered, and the client was able to successfully perform the job. This is an excellent example for employers who are interested in choices for applicants beyond "pass/fail" in the POS process.

> *Littleton (2003) compared data collected 3 years before POS was implemented to data collected 3 years after it was introduced and found an 18 to 1 return on investment. This study also discovered a decline in the number of work-related injuries, total cost related to injury, and cost per case.*

The aim of POS is to accurately match the worker to job demands (Scott, 2002). Ongoing documentation and focus on job relatedness in the screening process are key elements in a successful POS program (Perry, 1998).

Onsite Services

In some instances, performing the FCE or even rehabilitation is best conducted at the job site. Some researchers contend that onsite role assessments have more face and content validity and are more effective methods for measuring the demands of the job (Innes and Straker, 1999b). Cheng and Hung (2007) found a higher return-to-work rate in onsite work rehabilitation programs than in clinic-based work rehabilitation. They also found a statistically significant lower rate of self-reported shoulder and functional work capability problems in the work-based group, providing evidence to support provision of onsite services. Others have reported that onsite intervention (including job-site assessment, work modification, and case management) can produce safe and more efficient return to work

---

Box 12.5 How to Use the Results of a POS

The results of postoffer employment testing can help determine:

- If an applicant meets the job demands and can begin work.
- If the applicant does not meet the job demands and has a disability, and if an accommodation is appropriate or reasonable.
- If the applicant does not meet the job demands and does not have a disability, and the conditional offer of employment should be rescinded.
- If the applicant does not meet the job demands and remediation is available to provide the applicant with an opportunity to improve deficiencies and retest.

than usual offsite care in a cost-effective fashion (Steenstra, et al., 2006). Lindström, Ohlund, and Nachemson (1994) suggested that an onsite visit by a therapist may benefit the rehabilitation process. It is critical to be aware of issues of safety and productivity for services provided at the workplace (Gibson and Strong, 2003).

Challenges in FCE

Impairment versus Disability

The differences between the medical model of disability and impairment is sometimes difficult to resolve (Chen, 2007). *Impairment* is described by the American Medical Association, in its *Guides to the Evaluation of Permanent Impairment,* as a change of a person's physical condition that has been assessed by medical means (Rondinelli, 2008). Please note, this definition does not take into account changes in the client's social, emotional, or vocational state, but the term *disability* does bridge this gap (Chen, 2007). Impairment is often seen as a measurement of strength or range or motion but supplies no functional information about the injury and the impact on occupational performance (Gibson and Strong, 2003). FCE is recognized as a primary tool used to determine impairment and disability (Taiwo and Cantley, 2008) and is important in clarifying the worker's abilities (Wyman, 1999). However, it is challenging to incorporate a client-centered approach to making return-to-work decisions, which the literature supports, including not only functional status but also subjective information like pain reports and affective status (Linn, Granger, Disler, and Yang, 2001).

Other perspectives on the concepts of impairment and disability are commonly used by occupational therapy practitioners. Most noted is the perspective provided by *The International Classification of Functioning, Disability and Health,* or ICF (World Health Organization, 2001). The ICF defines *impairments* as "problems in body function or structure such as a significant deviation or loss." The term *functioning* refers to "all body functions, activities, and participation," while *disability* is similarly "an umbrella term for impairments, activity limitations, and participation restrictions." This approach to conceptualizing impairment and disability is different than the medical model approach commonly used in FCE.

In an article exploring design flaws of commercially available FCE systems, Innes and Straker (1998) found an apparent common disconnect between the functional information obtained and the client's context and functional level. Gibson and Strong (2003) also found a frequent misunderstanding between occupational therapy practice and the theoretical basis of FCE. They developed a conceptual framework for FCE within the context of occupational therapy practice, utilizing the work of Mathiowetz, Moyers, and ICF. According to Gibson and Strong, "FCE is primarily an evaluation of activity and activity limitations . . . its content needs to be based on evaluation of activities rather than body function or body structure." Some studies found that the client's functional self-efficacy beliefs influence lift performance during FCE and suggested that strategies for addressing self-belief and how it affects functional performance should be investigated, lending support to Gibson and Strong's theory (Asante, Britnell, and Gross, 2007). The OTPF also uses the WHO ICF model in the description of client factors, linking the client's body function and body structures with their values, beliefs, and spirituality. Because of occupational therapy's holistic view of the client, it is important to consider all of the client factors and how they influence work performance. There are many functions behind each performance skill, not just the physical performance but also sensory, emotional, cognitive, communication, and social skills (AOTA, 2008). Not all components can or should be assessed during an FCE, but the occupational therapist should be aware of the client as a whole and be prepared to make appropriate recommendations regarding these components should the need arise. Physicians recognize that job satisfaction, psychosocial factors, and work-related elements are related to an injured worker's return-to-work success. Other physicians reported primary obstacles in return-to-work process were (1) the worker's lack of understanding and fears about their injury and (2) a nonsupportive work environment evidenced by the behavior of coworkers and supervisors (Guzman, Yassi, Cooper, and Khokhar, 2002). Barriers can also include lack of information about work demands and lack of workplace accommodation in either design or work tasks (Schweigert, McNeil, and Doupe, 2004). Further studies have found that communication with the workplace can be fraught with worry regarding confidentiality and partiality issues (Russell, Brown, and Stewart, 2005).

Pranksy and Dempsey (2004) found a current lack of meaningful data in the studies relating to FCE, especially linking FCE results to significant occupational results, and this lack of data presents difficulty in knowing when FCE is best administered in the health-care continuum. Others concur about the lack of reliability and validity in FCE literature (Innes and Straker, 1999a, 1999b; King, et al., 1998). This indicates an opportunity for occupational therapy to contribute to the body of evidence supporting these evaluations. The first FCE studied for reliability and validity was developed by occupational therapists and remains an important contribution to the literature (Smith, Cunningham, and Weinberg, 1986).

Job Demands Analysis

Job demands analysis (JDA) encompasses cognitive and physical demands, environmental conditions, tools and equipment used, and personal protective equipment (Schulze, Delclos, and Pinglay, 2001). Job demands closely parallel the OTPF's description of activity demands, which are "the specific features of an activity that influence the amount of effort required to perform the activity" (AOTA, 2008, p. 634). The evaluation of job demands provides a detailed documentation process that can serve as a foundation for written job descriptions, hazard identification and abatement, development of job-training materials, preplacement screening, suggestions for *transitional* and/or *modified duty,* rehabilitation goal-setting, and return-to-work documentation. While a JDA may set the stage for hazard identification and abatement, it does not serve the same purpose, and the distinction is important (Bohr, 1998). Hazard identification assesses the work practice and identifies risks that may be remedied and is addressed in more detail in Chapter 14. The objective information provided in JDA assists the treating therapist in developing specific goals in treatment and planning for graded work return by modifying the job tasks or physical demands. It is important to note that in making return-to-work decisions, physicians rely on FCE, the DOT job demands evaluations, subjective reports from the worker and work supervisor, and information from the medical staff at the client's place of work as important sources of data (Wyman, 1999).

Simonelli and Camarotto (2008) suggested a JDA model that includes interviews of the worker and supervisor, filming the job as it is being performed, analysis of the physical demands of the job, and the application of a checklist to detail the skills involved in the job tasks. The model discussed in their study was designed to assist in placing clients with disabilities into jobs, as they had discovered that attempting to place people with disabilities into jobs without sufficient evaluation of the worksite led to problems "of adaption, accidents and losses" that impact both the company and the disabled worker.

Methods for JDA include interview, self-administered questionnaires, review of the DOT, and informal inspection and structured assessment of the job (Bohr, 1998). Studies suggest that work sampling and activity monitoring are better methods for job analysis than self-report (Homan and Armstrong, 2003; Mikkelsen, et al., 2007). In Homan and Armstrong's study (2003), they discovered that the subjective report tended to be overestimated and more variable than the two other methods recommended. Mikkelsen and colleagues (2007) also found that self-report of job demands was inaccurate and was likely to be overestimated.

The DOT terminology used in FCE is also best utilized for the description of the physical demands of jobs to promote easier communication among disciplines involved in the return-to-work process (Ha, et al., 2006). The DOT was last revised in 1991, and the U.S. government determined that it would be more effective to develop a new taxonomy and descriptive technique than to modify the DOT again and awarded the redesign project to the American Institutes of Research (AIR) by way of the Utah Department of Social Security, which acted on behalf of the U.S. Department of Labor (Ha, et al., 2006).

AIR developed O*NET, which is an online searchable database for seeking occupational information. O*NET uses new terminology for describing occupations and provides an easier mechanism to keep the information updated. As described on O*NET's Online Question FAQ page, although the initial data was provided by experts, the ongoing data collection is intended to be from the "real world" of individuals who are actually performing the work they describe. O*NET does not utilize the language of the DOT, and the descriptions of strength, postural, and movement demands are difficult for a therapist to test against to determine a match. O*NET describes itself as a guide for "career exploration" and does not purport to take the place of JDA (O*NET, 2006). This has created opportunity for crosswalk systems, such as OccuBrowse, to enter the market (see Fig. 12.4 and Fig. 12.5). Software programs such as these allow users to take advantage of the combined benefit of the broad occupational descriptors of O*NET with the more concrete structure of the DOT (Field and Field, 1999).

DOT Code	DOT Title	Industry	SVP	Str	O*NET
900.683-010	Batch-Mixing-Truck Driver	Construction	3	M	53-3032.00
900.683-010	Concrete-Mixing-Truck Driver	Construction	3	M	53-3032.00
906.683-022	Crew-Truck Driver	Any Industry	3	M	53-3033.00
292.353-010	Delivery-Route Truck Driver	Retail Trade	3	M	53-3031.00
905.663-014	Delivery-Truck Driver, Heavy	Any Industry	4	M	53-3032.00
902.683-010	Dump-Truck Driver	Any Industry	2	M	53-3032.00
902.683-010	Dump-Truck Driver, Off-Highway	Any Industry	2	M	53-3032.00
902.683-010	Dust-Truck Driver	Any Industry	2	M	53-3032.00
903.683-010	Explosives-Truck Driver	Ordnance and Accessories	3	M	53-3032.00
905.663-014	Fire-Truck Driver	Petroleum and Natural Gas	4	M	53-3032.00
905.663-014	Hole-Digger-Truck Driver	Construction	4	M	53-3032.00
904.683-010	Log-Truck Driver	Logging	4	M	53-3032.00
292.463-010	Lunch-Truck Driver	Hotel and Restaurant	2	M	53-3031.00
906.683-022	Mail-Truck Driver	Any Industry	3	M	53-3033.00
904.383-010	Pole-Truck Driver	Construction	4	M	53-3032.00
903.683-014	Powder-Truck Driver	Ordnance and Accessories	3	M	53-3032.00
900.683-010	Ready-Mix-Truck Driver	Construction	3	M	53-3032.00
853.663-018	Road-Oiling-Truck Driver	Construction	5	L	47-2071.00
904.383-010	Semi-Truck Driver	Any Industry	4	M	53-3032.00
906.683-022	Sprinkler-Truck Driver	Any Industry	3	M	53-3033.00
903.683-018	Tank-Truck Driver	Petroleum Refining	3	M	53-3032.00
905.663-014	Tower-Truck Driver	Telephone and Telegraph	4	M	53-3032.00

Figure 12.4 Screenshot from Vertek, OccuBrowse.

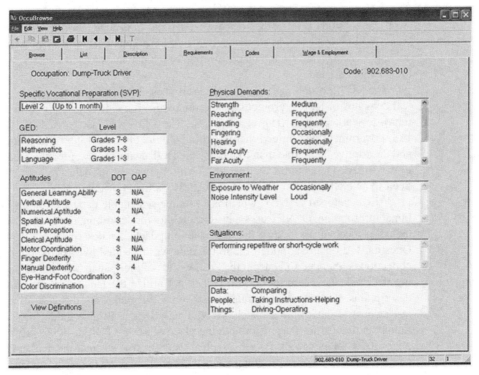

Figure 12.5 Screenshot from Vertek, OccuBrowse.

Because JDA often is used as a basis for developing POS, it is important to begin with a determination of the job's essential tasks so the evaluator knows what to evaluate. The ADA (1991) allows only for the preemployment testing of job tasks that are deemed essential, and it defines *essential tasks* as the basic tasks that an employee must be able to perform. In determining if a task is essential, it is helpful to find out if the job exists in order to perform the task, whether the task can be allocated to other employees, and what type of skill or proficiency is required to perform the task (ADA, 1991). This determination can be difficult because employers and employees are not accustomed to thinking about work in this fashion (Ha, et al., 2006). Being patient and thorough with a systematic question-and-answer process can make this initial step easier.

Before the onsite visit, preliminary information can be gathered by telephone, allowing the therapist to confirm tasks based on review of any previously written job descriptions or DOT descriptions, find out what personal protective equipment (PPE) is required, confirm work hours and shift information, and get directions (Ha, et al., 2006). Once the job task list is developed, the physical demands of each task can be analyzed (see Fig. 12.6). After analyzing each task, an aggregate of the physical demands frequency can be established, along with the maximum weights handled, forces applied, and distances both for ambulation and reaching (Bohr, 1998). It is vital for the therapist to represent a proportionate rate for the physical demands as they occur in the tasks and give appropriate emphasis to the tasks that occur for a greater length of time; see Box 12.6 (Ha, et al., 2006). For example, a data-entry clerk works an 8-hour shift. During the shift, he performs data entry for 6 hours and files documents for 2 hours. Therefore, two tasks make up the job of data-entry clerk. The physical demands of data entry include sitting, reaching, handling, fingering, and walking to and from the workstation. The physical demands that comprise document filing are walking, standing, reaching, handling, and fingering.

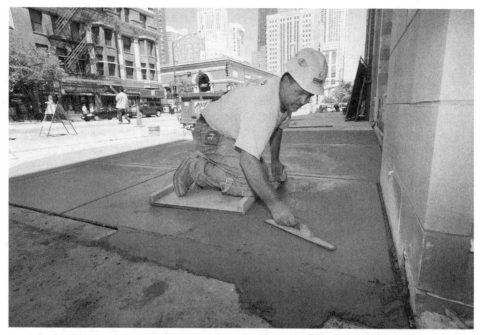

Figure 12.6 This job task requires crawling, reaching, and handling.

Box 12.6   JDA Checklist

The JDA report must include:

- List of essential tasks
- Overall level of work
- Physical demands that comprise the tasks
- Frequency of the physical demands
- Maximum weights handled

- Distances traveled and reached
- Work environment
- Equipment used
- Personal protective equipment required

Because the task of data entry is where the worker spends the bulk of his day, the physical demands that occur in this task occur more frequently than those that happen during the document filing task, which is the less frequently occurring task. The final report must reflect the actual physical demands in proportion to the task time allotment.

JDA products and educational courses are available to those who wish to pursue additional training in this area.

It is important to keep in mind that JDA is not a static process. It is dynamic because the reality of work is that jobs change. Physical plants make structural changes, processes become more efficient, and products evolve. The OTPF recognizes that a change in one aspect of an activity can have a ripple effect and may change other aspects or the activity as a whole (AOTA, 2008). Emphasize and encourage companies to develop a plan for reevaluation of the jobs in order to keep their information current.

JDA is not a static process. It is dynamic because the reality of work is that jobs change.

Chapter Summary

Jette (2006) suggests the WHO ICF model has the potential to become a standard language to address how people live with their circumstances to improve communication across disciplines and nations. The OTPF emphasizes using language that reflects existing and emerging areas of practice (AOTA, 2008). There are many opportunities in the area of work practice for occupational therapy practitioners to be involved and innovative in the care of workers. Occupational therapy practitioners have the unique skill set, background, and education to excel in the physical assessment of the worker and to assist in strengthening the links in the continuum of work-related services.

Case Resolution

The occupational therapist asked Jeff about the physical demands of his job. Jeff hesitated; he'd never thought about his work in this way. The occupational therapist began asking specific questions about the physical demands to help guide Jeff in his thinking. "Do you have to lift anything from the floor on your job?" "What is the heaviest thing that you have to lift?" "How often do you have to lift it?" The occupational therapist planned to perform a JDA, and the questions helped lay the groundwork for the onsite evaluation. To set appropriate treatment goals related to return to work, physical demands of the job needed to be identified, and this would allow the occupational therapist to evaluate Jeff's physical abilities and compare them to the actual demands of the job.

Jeff said, "Well, the heaviest thing I have to lift from the floor by myself is my tool box, and it weighs, gosh, I don't know, maybe 100 pounds?" The occupational therapist nodded and recorded this information. "Is that also the heaviest thing you would carry in one hand? How far would you have to carry it?" Jeff thought, "Probably about 50 feet on average." "How far is the greatest distance you'd have to carry it?" Jeff replied, "No more than 300 feet at any one time." "Great," the occupational therapist replied. "Okay, what is the heaviest thing to lift overhead?" and continued asking Jeff about the physical demands of his job. When she contacted the employer, she was able to ask questions related to the work and the equipment Jeff used. Once on site, the occupational therapist attempted to confirm the weights Jeff had reported and found that his tool box weighed 80 pounds, not the 100 pounds he had reported. This was helpful, as this was the heaviest weight Jeff had to handle, and would allow the occupational therapist to focus treatment goals around accurate job demands.

Back in the clinic, the occupational therapist conducted a job-specific FCE on Jeff to determine if he was physically able to go back to work or, if not, what areas needed to be addressed in treatment. Jeff was able to lift only 55 pounds with one hand and could carry the load only 50 feet before his mechanics deteriorated to an unsafe point. Among the rest of the tasks at which Jeff was deficient in his job demands, treatment goals were set. Jeff was eager to return to work, and his employer had expressed the desire for Jeff to return, indicating that his job was still available.

References

Age Discrimination in Employment Act of 1967 (ADEA), Pub.L. No. 90-202, §634, 81 Stat. 602 (1967).

American Occupational Therapy Association (AOTA). (2000). Occupational therapy services in facilitating work performance. *American Journal of Occupational Therapy, 54*(6), 626–628.

American Occupational Therapy Association (AOTA). (2007). AOTA's Centennial Vision and executive summary. *American Journal of Occupational Therapy, 61*(6), 613–614.

American Occupational Therapy Association (AOTA). (2008). Occupational therapy practice and framework: Domain and process. *American Journal of Occupational Therapy, 62*(6), 625–683.

American Occupational Therapy Association (AOTA). (n.d.). AOTA's Centennial Vision: What is it, why it is right. Bethesda, MD: AOTA Press. Retrieved from www.aota .org/nonmembers/area16/index.asp.

Americans with Disabilities Act of 1990 (ADA), Pub.L. No. 101-336, §2, 104 Stat. 328 (1991).

Asante, A. K., Britnell, E. S., & Gross, D. P. (2007). Functional self-efficacy beliefs influence functional capacity evaluation. *Journal of Occupational Rehabilitation, 17*(1), 73–82.

Bohr, P. C. (1998). Work analysis. In P. M. King (ed.), *Sourcebook of Occupational Rehabilitation* (pp. 229–245). New York: Plenum Press.

Chen, J. J. (2007). Functional capacity evaluation. *Iowa Orthopedic Journal, 27,* 121–127.

Cheng, A. S., & Hung, L. K. (2007). Randomized controlled trial of workplace-based rehabilitation for work-related rotator cuff disorder. *Journal of Occupational Rehabilitation, 17*(3), 487–503.

Cotton, A., Schonstein, E., & Adams, R. (2006). Use of functional capacity evaluation by rehabilitation providers in NSW. *Work, 26*(3), 287–295.

Cromwell, F. S. (1985). Work-related programming in occupational therapy: Its roots, course and prognosis. *Occupational Therapy in Healthcare, 2*(4), 9–25.

Darphin, L. E. (1995). Work-hardening and work-conditioning perspectives. In S. J. Isernhagen (ed.), *The Comprehensive Guide to Work Injury Management* (pp. 443–462). Gaithersburg, MD: Aspen Publishers.

Dueker, J. A., Ritchie, S. M., Knox, T. J., & Rose, S. J. (1994). Isokinetic trunk testing and employment. *Journal of Occupational Medicine, 36*(1), 42–48.

EEOC v. Dial Corporation. Case Nos. 05-4183 and 05-4311 (U.S. Court of Appeals for the Eighth Circuit).

Equal Employment Opportunity Commission (EEOC). (1978). *Uniform Guidelines on Employee Selection Procedures.* Washington, DC: Equal Employment Opportunity Commission.

Equal Employment Opportunity Commission (EEOC). (2007). Fact sheet on employment tests and selection procedures. Retrieved from www.eeoc.gov/policy/docs/factemployment_procedures.html.

Field, J. E., & Field, T. F. (1999). *COJ 2000 with an O*NET^TM* 98 Crosswalk.* Athens, GA: Elliot & Fitzpatrick.

Frings-Dresen, M. H, & Sluiter, J. K. (2003). Development of a job-specific FCE protocol: The work demands of hospital nurses as an example. *Journal of Occupational Rehabilitation, 13*(4), 233–248.

Gibson, L., & Strong, J. (1997). A review of functional capacity evaluation practice. *Work, 9*(1), 3–11.

Gibson, L., & Strong, J. (2003). A conceptual framework of functional capacity evaluation for occupational therapy in work rehabilitation. *Australian Occupational Therapy Journal, 50*(2), 64–71.

Gross, D. P., Battié, M. C., & Asante, A. K. (2007). Evaluation of a short-form functional capacity evaluation: Less may be best. *Journal of Occupational Rehabilitation, 17*(3), 422–435.

Gutman, S. A., Mortera, M. H., Hinojosa, J., & Kramer, P. (2007). Revision of the occupational therapy framework. *American Journal of Occupational Therapy, 61*(1), 119–126.

Guzman, J., Yassi, A., Cooper, J. E., & Khokhar, J. (2002). Return to work after occupational injury. Family physicians' perspectives on soft tissue injuries. *Canadian Family Physician, 48*(12), 1912–1919.

Ha, D. H., Page, J. J., & Wietlisbach, C. M. (2006). Work evaluation and work programs. In H. M. Pendleton & W. Schultz-Krohn (eds.), *Pedretti's Occupational Therapy Practice Skills for Physical Dysfunction,* 6th ed. (pp. 264–307). St. Louis, MO: Mosby.

Harbin, G., & Olson, J. (2005). Post-offer, pre-placement testing in industry. *American Journal of Industrial Medicine, 47*(4), 296–307.

Harvey-Krefting, L. (1985). The concept of work in occupational therapy: A historical review. *American Journal of Occupational Therapy, 39*(5), 301.

Homan, N. M., & Armstrong, T. J. (2003). Evaluation of three methodologies for assessing work activity during computer use. *American Industrial Hygiene Association Journal, 64*(1), 48–55.

Innes, E., & Straker, L. (1998). A clinician's guide to work-related assessments: 2—design problems. *Work, 11*(2), 191–206.

Innes, E., & Straker, L. (1999a). Reliability of work-related assessments. *Work, 13*(2), 107–124.

Innes, E., & Straker, L. (1999b). Validity of work-related assessments. *Work, 13*(2), 125–152.

Jackson, A. S. (1994). Preemployment physical evaluation. *Exercise and Sport Science Reviews, 22*(1), 53–90.

Jacobs, K., & Baker, N. A. (2000). The history of work-related therapy in occupational therapy. In B. L. Kornblau & K. Jacobs (eds.), *Work: Principles and Practice* (pp. 1–11). Bethesda, MD, AOTA Press.

Jette, A. M. (2006). Toward a common language for function, disability and health. *Physical Therapy, 85*(5), 726–734.

Keyserling, W. M., Herrin, G. D., Chaffin, D. B., Armstrong, T. J., & Foss, M. L. (1980). Establishing an industrial strength testing program. *American Industrial Hygiene Association Journal, 41*(10), 730–736.

Kielhofner, G. (2006). *Scholarship in Occupational Therapy: Methods of Inquiry for Enhancing Practice.* Philadelphia: F.A. Davis

King, P. M. (1998). Work hardening and work conditioning. In P. M. King (ed.), *Sourcebook of Occupational Rehabilitation* (pp. 209–227). New York: Plenum Press.

King, P. M., Tuckwell, N., & Barrett, T. E. (1998). A critical review of functional capacity evaluations. *Physical Therapy 78*(8), 852–866.

Lechner, D. E. (1994). Work hardening and work conditioning interventions: Do they affect disability? *Physical Therapy, 74*(5), 102–124.

Lechner, D. E. (1998). Functional capacity evaluation. In P. M. King (ed.). *Sourcebook of Occupational Rehabilitation* (pp. 209–227). New York: Plenum Press.

Lechner, D. E., Roth, D., & Stratton, K. (1991). Functional capacity evaluation on work disability. *Work, 1*(1), 37–47.

Lindström, I., Ohlund, C., & Nachemson, A. (1994). Validity of patient reporting and predictive value of industrial physical work demands. *Spine, 19*(8), 888–893.

Linn, R. T, Granger, C. V., Disler, P. B., & Yang, J. (2001). Applications of functional assessment to musculoskeletal disability evaluation. *Physical Medicine and Rehabilitation Clinics of North America, 12*(3), 529–541.

Littleton, M. (2003). Cost-effectiveness of prework screening program for the University of Illinois at Chicago physical plant. *Work, 21*(3), 243–250.

Maddern, G. A. (1998). Surgery and evidence-based medicine. *Medical Journal of Australia, 169*(7), 348–349.

Matheson, L. N., Ogden, L. D., Violette, K., & Schulz, K. (1985). Work hardening: Occupational therapy in industrial rehabilitation. *American Journal of Occupational Therapy, 39*(5), 314–321.

Mikkelsen, S., Vilstrup, I., Lassen, C. F., Kryger, A. I., Thomsen, J. F., & Andersen, J. H. (2007). Validity of questionnaire self-reports on computer, mouse and keyboard usage during a four-week period. *Occupational and Environmental Medicine, 64*(8), 541–547.

Mostandi, R. A., Noe, D. A., Kovacik, M. W., & Porterfield, J. A. (1992). Isokinetic lifting strength and occupational injury. A prospective study. *Spine, 17*(2), 189–193.

O*NET (2006). O*NET homepage. Retrieved from http://online.onetcenter.org.

Ogden-Niemeyer, L., & Jacobs, K. (1989). Definition and history of work hardening. In *Work Hardening State of the Art* (pp. 1–11). Thorofare, NJ: Slack.

Page, J. J. (2001). Functional capacity evaluation: Making the right decision. *RehabPro, 9*(4), 34–35.

Perry, L. L. (1998). Preemployment and preplacement testing. In P. M. King (ed.), *Sourcebook of Occupational Rehabilitation* (pp. 167–183). New York: Plenum Press.

Polgar, J. M. (2009). Critiquing assessments. In B. Crepeau, E. S. Cohn, & B. A. Boyt-Schell (eds.), *Willard & Spackman's Occupational Therapy,* 11th ed. (pp. 519–536). Philadelphia: Lippincott, Williams & Wilkins.

Pranksy, G. S., & Dempsey, P. G. (2004). Practical aspects of functional capacity evaluations. *Journal of Occupational Rehabilitation, 14*(3), 217–229.

Pruitt, R. H. (11995). Preplacement evaluation: Thriving within the ADA guidelines. *American Association of Occupational Health Journal, 43*(3), 124–130.

Ratzon, N. (2004). Functional capacity evaluations as a post-offer employment: A case study. *Work, 23*(1), 59–66.

Rondinelli, R. (ed.). (2009). *Guides to the Evaluation of Permanent Impairment,* 6th ed. Chicago: American Medical Association Press.

Rothstein, J., & Echternach, J. (1993). *Primer on Measurement: An Introductory Guide to Measurement Issues Featuring the APTA's Standards for Tests and Measurements in Physical Therapy Practice.* Alexandria, VA: American Physical Therapy Association.

Russell, G., Brown, J. B., & Stewart, M. (2005). Managing injured workers: Family physicians' experience. *Canadian Family Physician, 51*(1), 78–79.

Saeki, S., & Hachisuka, K. (2004). Medical fitness to return to work for disabled workers. *Journal of University of Occupational and Environmental Health, 26*(1), 41–50.

Schulze, L. J., Delclos, G. L., & Pinglay, N. (2001). Integrated job analysis: A technique to document job activities and identify occupational risk factors and modes of remediation and accommodation. *International Journal of Occupational and Environmental Health, 7*(3), 222–229.

Schweigert, M. R., McNeil, D., & Doupe, L. (2004). Treating physicians' perceptions of barriers to return to work of their patients in southern Ontario. *Occupational Medicine (Oxford, England), 54*(6), 425–429.

Scott, L. R. (2002). Post offer screening. *American Association of Occupational Health Nurses Journal, 50*(12), 559–563.

Simonelli, A. P., & Camarotto, J. A. (2008). Analysis of industrial tasks as a tool for the inclusion of people with disabilities in the work market. *Occupational Therapy International, 15*(3), 150–164.

Smith, S. L., Cunningham, S., & Weinberg, R. (1986). The predictive validity of the functional capacities evaluation. *American Journal of Occupational Therapy, 40*(8), 564–567.

Soer, R., Groothoof, J. W., Gerrtzen, J. H., van der Schans, C. P., Reesink, D. D., & Reneman, M. F. (2008). Pain response of healthy workers following a functional capacity evaluation and implications for clinical interpretation. *Journal of Occupational Rehabilitation, 18*(3), 290–298.

Steenstra, I. A., Anema, J. R., van Tulder, M. W., Bongers, P. M., de Vet, H. C., & van Mechelen, W. (2006). Economic evaluation of a multi-stage return to work program for workers on sick-leave due to low back pain. *Journal of Occupational Rehabilitation, 16*(4), 557–578.

Taiwo, O. A., & Cantley, L. (2008). Impairment and disability evaluation: The role of the family physician. *American Family Physician, 77*(12), 1689–1694.

U.S. Department of Labor, Employment and Training Administration. (1991a). *Revised Dictionary of Occupational Titles, Vol. I & II,* 4th ed. Washington, DC: US Government Printing Office.

U.S. Department of Labor, Employment and Training Administration. (1991b). *The Revised Handbook for Analyzing Jobs.* Indianapolis, IN: JIST Works.

Wegg, L. (1960). The Eleanor Clarke Slagle Lecture: The essentials of work evaluation. *American Journal of Occupational Therapy, 14,* 65–69.

World Health Organization. (2001). *International Classification of Functioning, Disability, and Health (ICF).* Geneva: Author.

Wyman, D. O. (1999). Evaluating patients for return to work. *American Family Physician, 59*(4), 844–848.

Glossary

Functional capacity evaluation (FCE) is an evaluation of an individual's physical ability to perform work. Most FCEs cover, at a minimum, the physical demands of work as described in the *Dictionary of Occupational Titles* (DOT).

Job demands analysis (JDA) is the evaluation of the physical demands that comprise a particular job. Also known as physical demands analysis (PDA) and job site analysis (JSA).

Preemployment testing is an evaluation of a prospective employee's ability to perform the physical demands of the job. Also known as preplacement screening (PPS), postoffer screening (POS), postoffer physicals (POP), and postoffer employment testing (POET).

Return-to-work/fitness-for-duty screening is usually an abbreviated FCE focusing on specific job demands.

Transitional duty/job modification is graded work entry in which changes are made to the job, shift, or work hours to assist an employee to begin or return to work.

Resources

"Vocational Assessments" by J. J. Page and R. L. Simon. In I. E. Asher (ed.), *Occupational Therapy Assessment Tools: An Annotated Index,* 3rd ed. (pp. 137–176) (Bethesda, MD: AOTA Press, 2007).

National Safety Council National and State Chapters

www.nsc.org

International Association of Rehabilitation Professionals (IARP) National and State Chapters

www.rehabpro.org

National Ergonomic Expo

www.ergoexpo.com/NECE

ErgoWeb

www.ergoweb.com

Equal Employment Opportunity Commission

www.eeoc.gov

Vertek, Inc. (or pricing information on OccuBrowse)

www.vertekinc.com

12835 Bel-Red Road, Suite 300
Bellevue, WA 98005
Phone: (800) 220-4409

13 Performance-Based Work Assessment
A Cognitive/Perceptual Approach

Timothy J. Wolf and Matthew B. Dodson

Key Concepts

The following are key concepts addressed in this chapter:

- The cognitive functional evaluation is presented as an approach for how occupational therapy practitioners should assess cognition and perception in the context of daily life—in this case, work.
- The process and usefulness of performance-based assessment in regard to cognition and function are described.
- Assessment of attention, memory, and higher-level cognitive functions is addressed.
- An assessment of the work environment and the demands of work tasks and their match or mismatch with a client's abilities and limitations is a critical component of a cognitive assessment, and this component is described.

Case Introduction

Stan is a 48-year-old male with a wife and two children. He holds an extremely well-paying job as a senior account manager at a leading communications and information systems company. As one of fewer than 10 senior account managers in the entire company who is recognized as a star performer, his client accounts are frequently measured in the hundreds of thousands and account for millions of dollars in profit for his company. His job requires him to sometimes work as much as 16 hours a day, and he has been working this schedule for 20 years to reach his current level of professional success. He takes great pride in his ability to fulfill the "provider" role in his family, and although he is frequently unable to attend to family matters (which he leaves in the hands of his wife), he has a high level of satisfaction with his life overall. Four months ago, Stan sustained a moderate traumatic brain injury in a car accident. He lost consciousness briefly at the scene of the accident and required a 3-day hospital stay because he suffered some disorientation and needed surgical repair of multiple facial fractures. After 3 days, he was released from the hospital with doctor's orders to stay at home 2 or 3 weeks until he felt better and the pain from his facial injuries had lessened. Stan returned to work 5 days after his discharge because he "felt fine" and was concerned about losing a lucrative performance-incentive bonus.

Unfortunately, Stan was unable to keep up with the demands of his job and was told by his manager to go home and relax until he could keep up. He was referred to occupational therapy to address his work-performance issues. Stan reported significant amounts of anxiety related to loss of his ability to work and apprehension about his future with his company. He wanted a clearly defined date when he would be "100 percent again." This chapter focuses on how occupational therapy practitioners assess the cognitive and perceptual deficits that will impact Stan's ability to return to do his work.

The Role of Occupational Therapy in Cognitive and Perceptual Assessment of Work

According to the Occupational Therapy Practice Framework: Domain and Process (OTPF), the domain of occupational therapy in general is to support health and participation in life through engagement in occupation (AOTA, 2008). For a large percentage of individuals, work is a primary occupation in which they engage on a daily basis. When a working individual, such as Stan, has an injury or illness that impacts his or her ability to return to work, occupational therapy practitioners have a clear and important role in helping the individual return to work. The OTPF states that assisting someone like Stan to return to work is accomplished by facilitating interactions among the client, the environments/contexts, and the activities or occupations to help the person reach the desired outcomes that will support his health and participation in work (AOTA, 2008). The focus on assessment and intervention with the complex interaction of person, environment, and occupation is unique to occupational therapy and transcends all aspects of its practice. The person, environment, and occupation constructs are further described in the OTPF as the aspects of the domains of occupational therapy. The client factors, or person factors, include mental (cognitive) factors (attention, memory, perception, higher-level cognitive processes). Cognitive factors are critical in supporting individuals to engage in work because work involves a series of integrated complex tasks that require judgment, organization, sequencing, and planning. While cognition is crucial to work, all aspects of occupational therapy are of equal value, and together they interact to influence the client's engagement in work (AOTA, 2008). While other professionals assess and intervene in some of these aspects, occupational therapy practice is based on examining how they all interact to impact participation and success at work. Therefore, discussing an assessment of cognition and perception as it relates to work has to be accomplished through a framework that examines not just cognition and perception in isolation but also the constructs in the context of how they interact with the environment and the individual's occupational goals. The cognitive functional evaluation (CFE; Hartman-Meier, Katz, and Baum, 2009) was chosen to frame this chapter on occupational therapy assessment of cognition and perception at work because the CFE was designed as an approach for how we as occupational therapy practitioners should assess cognition and perception in the context of daily life—in this case work.

Cognitive Functional Evaluation

Occupational therapy practitioners have a distinct role in assessing cognitive constructs in the performance of daily life and work (Katz and Hartman-Maeir, 2005). By assessing a person's cognition in the context of work activity, it is possible to determine the individual's cognitive capabilities and limitations as they relate to his or her chosen employment. The information from this assessment enables the occupational therapy practitioner to develop an individualized treatment plan to help remediate or compensate for cognitive loss and maximize the person's ability to participate in work-related activities. Cognitive assessment of this nature is not without challenges. First, individuals with cognitive loss are not always aware of their deficits; even if they are aware of their deficits, they may not be able to accurately identify how those deficits may affect their ability to work (Fleming, Strong, and Ashton, 1996; Katz and Hartman-Maeir, 2005; Prigatano, 2005). Second, the nature of work is complex and can include a wide variety of activities, tasks, roles, habits, and routines. It is essential for the occupational therapy practitioner to employ a client-centered approach that assesses cognitive deficits within the context of occupational performance. The CFE was designed as such a client-centered approach. It is a six-stage process of systematic evaluation of functional cognitive performance. For the purposes of work-specific evaluation, CFE framework was adapted to five stages and incorporates work-specific evaluation methods and assessments that can guide intervention (Table 13.1). Four key concepts of the CFE used to gather information on functional performance are (1) methods of direct observation of performance, (2) specific questioning pertaining to the manifestations of cognitive deficits in daily life, (3) information obtained from third parties, and (4) assessment of the environment (Hartman-Meier, et al., 2009).

Stage 1: Interview and Background Information Including an Occupational History

The purpose of the first stage of the assessment is to establish an occupational profile and a baseline of the individual's awareness of deficits (Hartman-Maeir, et al., 2009). The occupational history assists in establishing the individual's employment goals. To accomplish this first step, the occupational therapy practitioner employs interviews and questionnaires with the client and, when available, with a third party (e.g., spouse) to compare answers. The interviews and questionnaires can be used for comparison of actual task performance later in the process (Fleming, et al., 1996; Hartman-Maeir, et al., 2009; Katz and Hartman-Maeir, 2005; Lezak, Howieson, and Loring, 2004; Prigatano, 2005).

An established measure that can be used for this initial interview with the client is the Canadian Occupational Performance Measure (COPM; Law, et al., 1998). The COPM was designed as a structured interview to obtain a firsthand understanding of the client's goals related to the activities in which the client perceives challenges to occupational performance. The COPM covers multiple areas of occupation, including self-care, social, and work activities. Through an interview format, the client is asked to identify specific tasks and activities that he or she perceives as difficult and rate each task or activity using two different 10-point scales: performance and satisfaction. Performance ratings are based on how well the individual perceives that he or she can perform the activity (1, poor; 10, perfect) and satisfaction ratings are based on how satisfied the individual is with his or her reported performance rating (1, not at all satisfied; 10, completely satisfied). Therefore, the individual could report the ability to perform the activity as high (e.g., 8), but compared to the ability to perform the activity before injury or illness, the individual may not be satisfied with performance at the current level (e.g., 2). As a result, the individual would like to focus on this activity in treatment. The opposite could also occur: the individual may rate current performance as low (e.g., 3) but may be completely satisfied with current performance (e.g.,10) and therefore would not like to focus on that activity in intervention The occupational therapy practitioner then has to use this information as a starting point to develop client-centered goals. The balance must occur between the client's goals and the essential job functions the client must be able to perform at a certain level in order to return to work. Therefore, for the purpose of a work-related

Table 13.1 Five Stages in the Work-Specific Process of the Cognitive Functional Evaluation (CFE)

Stage 1	Interview and background information including an occupational history
Stage 2	Cognitive screening and baseline status tests
Stage 3	General measures of cognition in occupations
Stage 4	Cognitive tests for specific domains
Stage 5	Environmental assessment

Hartman-Meier, Katz, and Baum (2009)

assessment, the COPM should focus on the client's essential job functions in depth. The Job Performance Measure (JPM) was designed for just this purpose. Because work was only a small part of the COPM and there was not a method beyond self-report to discover the client's essential job functions, the JPM was developed as a work-focused assessment of the essential functions of the client's job and the client's perceived ability to perform these functions (Kaskutas and Seaton, 2008).

The JPM was developed with the understanding that clients sometimes have difficulty in recalling the essential functions of their job. Recalling this information appears to become increasingly difficult with the complexity of the job. If we use the case of Stan, his essential job functions were very difficult to identify because of the ever-changing environment in which he worked. To account for this difficulty, the therapist can employ one of two strategies: (1) seek permission to contact the client's employer to obtain a job description or (2) obtain the essential functions of the job from the Occupational Information Network (O*NET; http://online.onetcenter.org). The O*NET system was developed by the U.S. Department of Labor/Employment and Training Administration (USDOL/ETA) through a grant to the North Carolina Employment Security Commission and serves as the nation's primary source of occupational information, providing comprehensive information on key attributes and characteristics of workers and occupations (North Carolina Employment Security Commission, 2009). Rehabilitation professionals can search for the individual's reported job in the O*NET database and pull a list of essential job functions free of charge. The essential job functions are then discussed and rated as part of the JPM.

The results of the JPM are used later to set goals for intervention at the completion of all stages of the CFE. At this point, the information obtained is self-report only. Given the issues seen in awareness, it would be inappropriate to set treatment goals at this point in the process, but it would be appropriate to ask the client if you could ask a third person who knows the client well to rate how he or she feels the client would be able to perform the work activities on the JPM. The comparison of the first-person and third-person rating serves as a screen of the client's awareness. Discrepancies in the ratings may indicate an awareness issue on the part of the client, and these results have to then be verified later in assessment of the client's actual performance.

Stage 2: Cognitive and Perceptual Screening and Baseline Status Tests

The purpose of stage 2 is to develop a preliminary profile of clients' cognitive and perceptual abilities and deficits using standardized instruments (Hartman-Maeir, et al., 2009). In the context of work rehabilitation, this stage is important as an initial screen of cognition and perception; it serves as a baseline measure of overall cognitive status and screens for perceptual deficits that may not yet have been identified. The results of this screen are used to determine if the client is appropriate for work-oriented occupational therapy services or needs additional assessments from other health-care professionals such as speech-language pathology or neuropsychology. The following assessments were selected as a sample of possible assessments that can be used for stage 2 (Table 13.2). They were selected on the basis of easiest availability, minimal training required, and the most widely accepted.

Short Blessed Test
The Short Blessed Test (SBT) is a brief screening tool to evaluate general cognitive status (Katzman, et al., 1983). It includes questions regarding cognitive orientation, a short memory test, counting backward, and months of the year in reverse order. The SBT has scoring instructions listed on the assessment. Scores above 10 indicate significant cognitive impairment. In the context of work rehabilitation, a score of 10 or higher may indicate the

Table 13.2 Stage 2 Cognitive Screening and Baseline Status Tests

Cognitive or Perceptual Domain	Selected Measure
General cognitive status	Short Blessed Test
Neglect, visual field loss, aphasia	National Institutes of Health Stroke Scale (NIHSS)
Perceptual screen	Occupational Therapy-Adult Perceptual Screening Test (OT-APST)
Cognitive flexibility	Trail Making Test

inability to participate in work rehabilitation at this time and may suggest a need to refer to neuropsychology. The Short Blessed Test is publically available online: http://alzheimer.wustl.edu/About_Us/Forms.htm.

National Institutes of Health Stroke Scale (NIHSS)

The NIHSS is an assessment that quantifies neurological deficits following stroke (cerebrovascular accident [CVA]) and widely considered the gold-standard stroke scale (Brott, et al., 1989). The NIHSS was originally designed to evaluate persons with strokes in clinical trials; it is now widely used to evaluate acute stroke status, determine appropriate medical treatment and rehabilitation, and predict patient outcome. The NIHSS is a 15-item impairment scale that assesses level of consciousness, extraocular movements, visual fields, facial muscle function, extremity strength, sensory function, coordination, language, speech, and neglect. While the NIHSS was developed specifically for work with the stroke population, it covers cognitive and perceptual constructs that may be affected as a result of a wide variety of neurological impairments. For the purposes of a work assessment, the test for speech, language, visual fields, and neglect can be used as a screen for aphasia, neglect, and hemianopsia. Language deficits identified from the NIHSS may require a referral to a speech-language pathologist and also could identify areas of deficit that must be addressed as part of the treatment plan. The NIHSS is publically available through the National Institutes of Health, and the information related to the assessment and the information needed for training on the instrument are all publically available online: www.strokecenter.org/trials/scales/nihss.html.

Occupational Therapy–Adult Perceptual Screening Test (OT-APST)

The OT-APST is a standardized tool that enables occupational therapists to screen for perceptual deficits and includes subscales to measure agnosia, visuospatial relations (body scheme and neglect), constructional skills, apraxia, acalculia, and functional skills (Cooke, McKenna, and Fleming, 2005). The functional skills subscale includes observation of reading, writing, math, telling time, and manipulating objects. The OT-APST is a screening tool intended to be used in conjunction with functional task observation. Its reliability and validity has been established (Cooke, McKenna, Fleming, and Darnell, 2005; Cooke, McKenna, and Fleming, 2006a, 2006b). The OT-APST is available for purchase: www.functionforlife.com.au.

Trail Making Test

The Trail Making Test (TMT) was originally designed as part of a testing battery for the U.S. Army in 1944; over the course of its existence, it has been widely used as an assessment of scanning, divided attention, and cognitive flexibility (Lezak, et al., 2004). There are many different versions and editions of the TMT, and most are publically available and can be reproduced without permission. The TMT is given in two parts. In part A, the client is to connect consecutively numbered circles that are spread out across a page in a random fashion (Fig. 13.1). In part B, the client is to connect the circles in a similar manner;

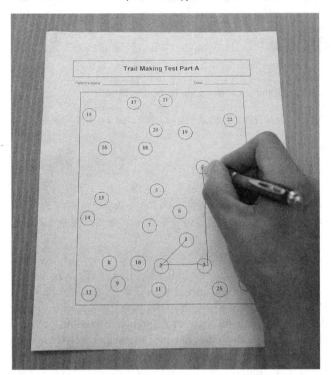

Figure 13.1 The Trail Making Test is freely available in different versions and can be reproduced without permission.

however, they have to alternate between connecting letters and numbers in consecutive order (e.g., A-1-B-2). The assessment is then scored on speed of completion and accuracy. Different versions can include multiple conditions; however, the commonalities between the versions are the parts A and B. For the purposes of work assessment, the TMT is used as a screening tool of cognitive flexibility. Deficits observed on the TMT could indicate a need to refer to neuropsychology for a full cognitive assessment. An example of a publically available TMT with instructions and scoring information is provided as a hyperlink in the resources section.

By this point in the assessment, the occupational therapy practitioner will have sufficient interview information and assessment data to determine the need for further testing by the practitioner or by other health-care professionals and whether or not the client is appropriate for work rehabilitation services at this time. The perceptual deficits identified in this stage of the assessment must be accounted for in treatment planning and may need to be addressed as part of a multidisciplinary effort with other health-care professionals. The next stages of the assessment are then completed if the person is going to be seen for treatment and will provide vital information related to the client's cognitive capabilities and limitations and how they may impact the client's ability to work.

Stage 3: General Measures of Cognition in Occupations

Stage 3 of the assessment process is focused on the functional impact of cognitive deficits and also examines *higher-level cognitive functions* (executive functions) in the context of activity (Hartman-Maeir, 2009). Traditional assessments of higher-order cognitive functions are usually short in duration, well-structured, and have clearly defined goals and outcomes, which all contradict defined components of higher-order cognitive functions (Adams, Parsons, Culbertson, and Nixon, 1996; Wolf, Morrison, and Matheson, 2008). For this reason, assessments that test higher-level cognitive functions within the context of everyday life have been developed and are used in conjunction with neuropsychological testing. This form of testing is *ecologically valid,* which means that the test is representative of real-world performance (Shallice and Burgess, 1991; Wolf, et al., 2008). In the context of work rehabilitation, ecologically valid assessment is of great importance because, while performance-based testing does not necessarily allow the clinician to identify specific cognitive and perceptual deficits that may exist, it does demonstrate how those deficits will impact the client's ability to perform complex work-related activities. The selected assessments have a self-assessment component that is compared to actual performance to evaluate awareness of deficits. For stage 3, only one assessment should be completed in the interest of time; however, two different assessments are presented here as options.

> *While performance-based testing does not necessarily allow the clinician to identify specific cognitive and perceptual deficits that may exist, it does demonstrate how those deficits will impact the client's ability to perform complex work-related activities.*

Executive Function Performance Test (EFPT)

The EFPT (Baum, et al., 2008) was developed as a measure of higher-level cognitive functions in the context of a performance-based assessment. The EFPT focuses on what the client can do and the level of support necessary for him or her to successfully perform a task. It uses a structured cueing and scoring system in order to cue the person to perform the activity correctly. The EFPT was validated most recently with a population of people following mild to moderate stroke (Baum, 2008).

The EFPT assesses four basic instrumental activities of daily living (IADL) tasks: simple cooking, telephone use, medication management, and bill payment. The task for simple cooking requires the participant to prepare oatmeal following written instructions; for telephone use, the participant must look up a grocery store number in the phone book (see Fig. 13.2), call the store, and ask if they deliver groceries; for medication management, a simulation is provided using fake medication in labeled prescription bottles; for bill payment, two bills and checks are provided in an envelope, and the client is required to get the bills, pay them, and balance the account. Before starting, the client is asked about familiarity with these tasks and whether he or she performs them usually relatively independently or with assistance. All the necessary materials are provided for the assessment. The participant is evaluated on ability to adhere to the following higher-level cognitive constructs: (1) initiation, (2) execution of a task (organization, sequencing, safety/judgment), and (3) completion of a task. The participant is cued to successfully complete the tasks, and the level of cueing necessary to support task performance is recorded. The levels of cueing are as follows: 0, no cue required; 1, verbal guidance; 2, gestured guidance; 3, direct verbal assistance; 4, physical assistance; 5, do for the participant. With this scoring system, a lower score indicates a higher level of independence with the activity.

Complex Task Performance Assessment (CTPA)

The CTPA was developed as a higher-level cognitive function performance assessment (Wolf, et al., 2008). The CTPA uses the same criteria as used in the development of multitasking assessments in neuropsychology established by Paul Burgess (Burgess, 2000). While the CTPA is still being validated, it is presented here because it is specifically focused on the assessment of work-related tasks that are similar to those found in many occupations. Two clerical-based work-simulation tasks are used in the CTPA: bookkeeping–current

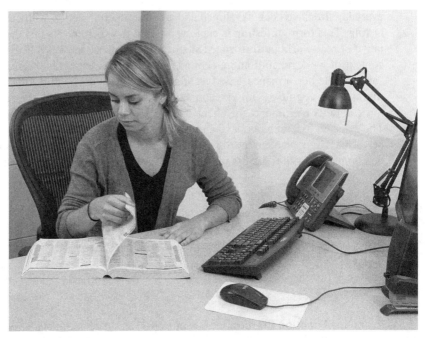

Figure 13.2 Telephone use is part of the Executive Function Performance Assessment (EFPT).

inventory control and telephone messaging activities from the Structured Work Activity Groups (SWAG; Matheson, Kaskutas, and Seaton, 2003). These tasks are administered simultaneously in order to meet the multitasking criteria. The bookkeeping–current inventory control SWAG work simulation requires the participant to calculate current fines and replacement costs for books and videos that are overdue (Wolf, et al., 2008). The client must determine from the information given if the library patron is likely to either pay the fine or pay to replace the item. Next, the information is used in the participant's calculations to complete an inventory control worksheet. The telephone messaging activity is a work simulation in which the participant listens to recorded telephone messages played on a CD player (Wolf, et al., 2008). The messages have multiple levels of difficulty that require different types of actions by the participant and that interact with the bookkeeping task. In addition, a set of rules is provided, and once the assessment begins, the client works independently until the assessment is complete. Performance is assessed by measuring the following constructs: accuracy of the inventory control activity, the number of tasks completed, the number of executive decisions made, the number of phone messages completed, and the inventory control percentage completed. A derived score, "performance efficiency," is generated on the basis of performance. This is the ratio of the sum of tasks completed added to the number of executive decisions made, divided by total time in minutes (TC + ED)/Time (Wolf, et al., 2008).

After stage 3, the occupational therapist must determine the next step in the assessment. If the therapist concludes that the client's performance on this stage of the assessment was poor given his or her occupational goals, it may be appropriate to refer to neuropsychology for a full cognitive profile, which will provide in-depth information about the client's cognitive capabilities and limitations. If the client has an evaluation by neuropsychology, the therapist may skip the fourth stage of the assessment and complete the environmental assessment. If the therapist determines that the client does not need a full neuropsychological evaluation, the following stage of the assessment can provide information about specific cognitive domains to help with treatment planning if needed.

Stage 4: Cognitive Tests for Specific Domains

The purpose of stage 4 is to see how specific cognitive domain deficits will affect occupation (Hartman-Maeir, et al., 2009). Stage 3 focused on overall performance in a cognitively demanding performance-based assessment. While that information is of high value to the occupational therapy practitioner, it does not point to the specific cognitive domains that may be impacted. This stage of the assessment is completed at the discretion of the occupational therapist depending on how much information is needed in regard to the specific cognitive domains.

The current understanding of cognitive domains is centered on the use of models. Cognitive models organize knowledge around the cognitive domain and drive the selection and interpretation of assessments. Each cognitive domain discussed here has been studied extensively in multiple disciplines and has many existing investigation and clinical models that are in use today. The models described for each construct are clinical models, and even though they were selected for the purposes of this description, there are many other models in the literature that would also be appropriate for this stage of the assessment.

Cognitive models organize knowledge around the cognitive domain and drive the selection and interpretation of assessments.

Attention

Attention is the ability to selectively focus on stimuli. This includes our ability to shift what we are focusing on and even at times divide our focus between different stimuli. Attention is essential to our ability to work, and it is considered to be supervisory over other cognitive domains (Norman and Shallice, 1986). If a person is unable to selectively focus on stimuli in his or her work environment, the individual will not be able to function at a high-level and will be easily distracted and frustrated by the inability to complete work-related tasks. To describe attention, the attention process training (APT) model is used (Sohlberg and Mateer, 2001). The APT model was developed from the clinical observations of clients with brain injury. It is a way to organize our knowledge of attention and provides a guide for assessment and treatment to remediate attentional deficits. The APT model includes five systems of attention organized in a hierarchical fashion: *focused attention, sustained attention, selective attention, alternating attention,* and *divided attention* (Sohlberg and Mateer, 2001). A description of each system and its importance in work is described in Table 13.3.

Assessment of attention is accomplished through a combination of structured observation and standardized assessment. Using the APT model as a guide, a simulated work task can be used to observe the attentional abilities of the client in the context of an activity. By starting at the base of the hierarchy, focused attention, and gradually adding attentional demands to the task, the occupational therapy practitioner can observe at what level the client is able to maintain his or her attention and then incorporate this information into treatment planning. For example, if the client is successfully working on a budgeting task without distraction but must pause to answer the phone once and is unable to return to the budgeting task, the occupational therapist would determine that the client can selectivity use his or her attention but cannot alternate attention. Treatment planning would include activities structured to progress through the hierarchy starting at alternating attention. To support the observations seen in the

Table 13.3 Five Hierarchical Systems of Attention and Their Relation to Work Tasks

Attention System	Definition	Relation to work
Focused attention	Ability to respond to an auditory, visual, or tactile stimulus: lowest level of attention	Phone rings, employee turns to the phone
Sustained attention	Ability to maintain behavioral response during activity	Ability to complete a budget task over a period of time
Selective attention	Capacity to maintain a behavior or focus in the face of competing stimuli	Ability to complete the budget task over time with people talking nearby
Alternating attention	Capacity to shift focus of attention and move between multiple tasks having different cognitive requirements	Ability to work on the budgeting task and also stop to answer the phone when it rings and then come back to the budgeting task
Divided attention	Highest level of attention: the ability to respond simultaneously to multiple tasks	Ability to talk on the phone while simultaneously working on the budgeting task

Sohlberg and Mateer (2000)

structured observation, a standardized assessment should also be included. We describe the Test of Everyday Attention (TEA), but many other assessments are available.

The TEA was designed to assess selective attention, sustained attention, alternating attention, and divided attention using eight subtests: map search, elevator counting, elevator counting with distraction, visual elevator, auditory elevator with reversal, telephone search, telephone search dual task, and lottery (Robertson, Ward, Ridgeway, and Nimmo-Smith, 1994). The TEA is widely accepted as a measure of attentional abilities and can be used with anyone aged 18 to 80, which encompasses the majority of the working population. The structured observation combined with the results of the TEA provide the therapist an in-depth understanding of the client's attentional abilities and deficits.

Memory

Memory is generally accepted as the process by which we encode, store, and then retrieve information (Tulving, 1991). Memory is essential to optimal work performance. If the client cannot remember instructions, what was said at a meeting, how to fill out a report, or even to go to work, the client's ability to be competitively employed is limited. Like other cognitive domains, memory is understood through the use of models. The classification of memory and the models used to describe it are highly debated in the literature. However, there is a high level of consensus on a few concepts of memory: the general model of memory, the Atkinson-Shiffrin model, and the further classification of long-term memory into subcomponents. This hybrid of concepts is the model of memory used to guide the assessment and treatment of memory in work rehabilitation.

The Atkinson-Shiffrin model involves a sequence of three stages: sensory register (store), short-term store, and long-term store (Atkinson and Shiffrin, 1968). This model proposed that sensory information can enter the sensory register for a very brief period of time. If the information in the sensory store needs to be retained, it can selectively pass to the short-term store where it can be retained long enough to be used in an activity (e.g., remembering a phone number long enough to dial the phone). If the information is

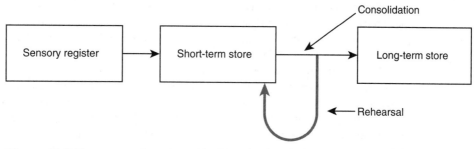

Figure 13.3 The process of memory consolidation model of memory (Atkinson and Shiffrin, 1968).

needed long term (e.g., remembering the number of a person you need to call numerous times), it can, through the process of rehearsal, pass into the long-term store where it can be retained for an extended period of time. This process of moving information from sensory store to long-term store through rehearsal is called *memory consolidation* (see Fig. 13.3). This basic understanding of memory has served as the basis for most models and research since the 1960s.

The criticism of the Atkinson-Shiffrin model is that it is an oversimplistic understanding of long-term memory. Since its development, long-term memory has been further classified (Cohen, 1984; Graf and Schacter, 1985; Tulving, 1991). Its classification into categories and systems has taken many different forms and is still an area of debate; however, the classification presented here is a representative composite of memory adapted from the description of Endel Tulving (Tulving, 1991); see Figure 13.4. One primary difference is the inclusion of prospective memory, which is a relatively new memory construct.

Memory is first classified as either *short-term memory* or *long-term memory*. Long-term memory is classified as either *declarative* (explicit) or *nondeclarative* (implicit). This classification is based on whether the information remembered is consciously recalled

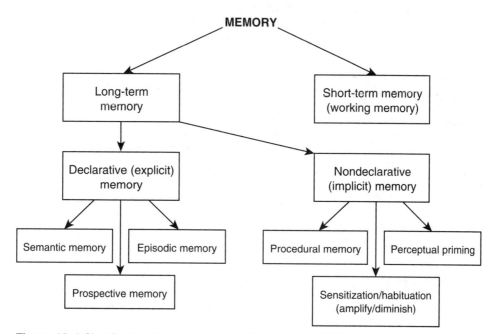

Figure 13.4 Classification of memory based on Endel Tulving's (1991) memory systems.

(e.g., fact, events) or was learned but cannot be consciously recalled (e.g., motor memory). Declarative memory is further classified as *semantic* (facts), *episodic* (events), and *prospective* (future events). Nondeclarative memory is classified as *procedural, perceptual priming,* and *sensitization/habituation* (Table 13.4).

Our understanding of the classification of memory is extremely important for work rehabilitation assessment and treatment for two primary reasons: (1) Because memory systems are controlled by distinct neuroanatomic systems, some memory systems will likely be affected by injury or illness while others will be relatively untouched. (2) Different essential job functions rely on different memory systems. Therefore, the assessment of memory is cross-referenced with a task analysis of the essential job functions to determine if the observed memory impairments are likely to impact specific essential job functions. For example, if the assessment yields that the individual has impaired prospective memory, the individual will likely have difficulty remembering to show up for meetings on time, so the occupational therapy practitioner will have to work with the client to compensate for this deficit. Different cognitive intervention models of memory use different memory systems, which allows the occupational therapist to select an approach best suited to the client's memory capabilities and limitations. Memory is assessed a little differently than attention. Memory assessment relies mainly on standardized instruments. We describe the Rivermead Behavioral Memory Test (RBMT; Wilson, Cockburn, and Baddeley, 1985), but many other assessments are available.

The RBMT was designed in 1985 with the following goals: (1) to predict everyday memory problems and (2) to monitor change over time (Wilson, et al., 1985). The RBMT includes the following subtests: (1) remembering an appointment; (2) remembering a short route: immediate and delayed; (3) remembering a belonging; (4) remembering to deliver a message; (5) picture recognition; (6) orientation story recall: immediate and delayed; (7) remembering a name; (8) face recognition; and the newest edition, RBMT-III, now includes (9) the novel test. The RBMT can yield a screening score and a profile score and can be used with anyone of working age. It is a widely accepted standardized memory assessment and provides a very good profile of the client's memory capabilities and limitations.

Higher-Level Cognitive Functions

Higher-level cognitive function is commonly called executive function. The difficulty in using the term *executive function* is that across disciplines and lines of research, executive

Table 13.4   Classification of Long-Term Memory

Long-term memory construct	Definition
Declarative (Explicit)	Memory that can be consciously recalled
Semantic	General knowledge and facts about the world
Episodic	Recollection of the personal past
Prospective	Memory for future events—appointments
Nondeclarative (Implicit)	Memory that cannot be consciously recalled
Procedural	Skills and motor learning
Perceptual Priming	Identification of objects
Sensitization/Habituation	Amplification or diminution of a behavioral response after repeated stimulus

Adapted from work of Endel Tulving (1991)

function has a different definition, which leads to a great deal of miscommunication. The World Health Organization's *International Classification of Functioning, Disability and Health* (ICF) was developed to eliminate confusion of terminology across disciplines and "establish a common language for describing health and health-related states in order to improve communication between health care workers, researchers, policy-makers and the public, including people with disabilities" (2001, p. 5). The ICF developed *higher-level cognitive functions* in lieu of executive functions and defines it as follows:

> Specific mental functions especially dependent on the frontal lobes of the brain, including complex goal-directed behaviors such as decision-making, abstract thinking, planning and carrying out plans, mental flexibility, and deciding which behaviors are appropriate under what circumstances; often called executive functions. (p. 57)

Essentially, higher-level cognitive processes refer to the "if" and "how" of performance. More specifically, higher-level cognitive processes refer to *if* a person will perform an action and *how* the person will perform that action. Compromised higher-level cognitive processing ability can have devastating effects on ability to function in complex, real-world environments like those encountered in the work world. A well-established model for describing higher-level cognitive functions is Norman and Shallice's automatic and willed control-to-action theory (Norman and Shallice, 1986).

The automatic and willed control-to-action theory breaks performance down into two primary categories: automatic behaviors and willed behaviors. Automatic behaviors consist of a series of routines and habits. Behavior is guided by *schemas* (automatic behavior patterns) that are automatically put into action by cues and prompts in the environment and also by internal motivations. For example, not a lot of effort needs to be expended to brush our teeth or wash our hands, and both of these activities can occur without our conscious awareness of it happening. Think about leaving the house in the morning and wondering, "Did I take my vitamin?" or "Did I grab my bag?" These types of behaviors are considered automatic in this model and are the simplest form of behavior. They occur outside of conscious effort and therefore are easily forgotten that they were completed. To further describe these behaviors, schemas that are selected are said to contend with each other and are selected automatically, which Norman and Shallice call *contention scheduling*. Schemas are selected to achieve the behavior, but sometimes the wrong schema can be selected—for example, you leave your house to go to the store but instead automatically take the route you take to work every day. Since the process is automatic and schemas are in contention, the wrong schema can be selected for the behavior. Willed behaviors are necessary to account for all other actions that are not routine and require a higher degree of cognitive involvement to organize and plan the behavior. Norman and Shallice propose that this is accomplished through the supervisory attentional system (SAS). When a nonroutine behavior is necessary, the SAS can organize, coordinate, and monitor (through the expenditure of cognitive effort) schemas to accomplish novel or complex behaviors. In essence, when working in an environment that is constantly changing, the SAS is necessary to organize behavioral patterns (schemas). When working in an environment that is relatively stable and involves tasks that are overlearned, the behavior can occur automatically and does not need the SAS or higher-level cognitive functions to be successful.

The automatic and willed control-to-action theory is extremely important when assessing higher-level cognitive functioning in relation to work. If the individual is attempting to return to work in a complex, dynamic work environment (e.g., restaurant server), he or she must have a high degree of higher-level cognitive ability. If the individual is returning to a fairly routine job where the environment is stable (e.g., factory work), the person may likely be successful even if he or she has a high degree of higher-level cognitive functioning impairment. The work environment and task demands are crucial to the interpretation of the results of the higher-level cognitive functioning assessment. The results have to be evaluated with the work demands in mind to determine if the occupational therapy practitioner will have to work with the client to develop the adaptive strategies necessary to accommodate for deficits. In addition, the occupational therapy practitioner may have to work with the client to accommodate the work environment in order for the client to be successful.

Assessment of higher-level cognitive functions in relation to work is best achieved using performance-based assessments. To best guide treatment planning, the results of the performance-based assessment completed in stage 3 can be used in conjunction with further assessment to reveal how higher-level cognitive functions are being disrupted. The assessment described here is the Behavioral Assessment of Dysexecutive Syndrome (BADS) battery of tests (Wilson, Evans, Emslie, Alderman, and Burgess, 1998). The battery targets a variety of higher-level cognitive function components such as alternating attention, planning different tasks, and temporal judgment (Katz and Hartman-Maeir, 2005). The Dysexecutive Questionnaire (DEX) is a 20-item self-report or caregiver-rating questionnaire used with the BADS; it is constructed to sample the range of behavioral problems commonly associated with higher-level cognitive function deficits (dysexecutive syndrome) (Wilson, et al., 1998). The DEX is used as part of the battery and includes both a self-rating form and a caregiver-rating form. The BADS has established high interrater reliability, construct validity, and high correlation of profile score and prediction to DEX rating by the caregiver (Katz and Hartman-Maeir, 2005).

At end stage 4 of the CFE, the occupational therapist should have one of two things: a full-cognitive profile completed by a neuropsychologist or the specific cognitive domain assessments needed to provide the necessary information to guide treatment planning. Regardless of how the information is obtained, the use of cognitive models is necessary to organize and interpret the assessment results and guide treatment. At this point, the assessment of the occupation, perceptual deficits, and cognitive status is complete. The remaining component is the environment. An assessment of the work environment is necessary to interpret how the other three components will affect work functioning.

Stage 5: Environmental Assessment

The final stage of the assessment focuses on providing information about the environment in which the client will have to participate given his or her cognitive and perceptual capabilities and limitations (Hartman-Maeir, et al., 2009). An environmental assessment is critical to the assessment process because it can either support or hinder the ability of the client to optimally perform essential work functions. Results of the assessment also inform treatment planning; once environmental factors affecting cognitive performance are identified, compensatory adaptations can be applied to either the entire employment environment (macrosystem adjustment) or the individual worker's environment (microsystem adjustment) to maximize productivity. Often, a combination of these two approaches is used, such as when the printers for an entire office floor are placed in one isolated room to cut down on ambient noise (macrosystem), while the employee with a selective attention disability is given noise-cancelling ear phones to reduce the distracting sounds of the office (microsystem adjustment).

A variety of adjustments can be made to the physical environment of a workplace to address the effect of biomechanical, ergonomic, or musculoskeletal impairment on work performance (see Chapter 15 for a more detailed description of the physical assessment and adaptation of a work environment). Some of these adaptations can also have an ancillary beneficial effect on cognitive performance; for example, when fluorescent lighting is replaced by natural alternatives to improve environmental light levels and reduce physical eye strain, an indirect benefit is that individuals with brain injuries, who can be especially susceptible to irritation from fluorescent lighting systems, may be able to concentrate for longer periods of time.

When addressing cognitive deficits, social environment constructs should be assessed in addition to evaluating the physical environment. It is important to be aware that the social environment of a workplace is multidimensional and includes management and coworker culture. If the management culture is not receptive to making reasonable accommodations to enable an individual with a cognitive disability to perform essential job functions, it can invalidate therapist recommendations (even though the employer may be legally responsible to provide those accommodations). On the same token, if the coworkers of an individual with a disability are at best unsupportive—or at worst antagonistic—the social environment can significantly affect an individual's ability to effectively perform essential job tasks.

The academic and clinical preparation of occupational therapy practitioners enables them to appreciate the impact of social support and social capital on occupational performance, and client-centered assessments such as the Moos Work Environment Scale (WES) provide objective data to support those subjective social environment observations. The WES is a yes-or-no survey that evaluates both physical and social constructs of work environments, such as coworker cohesion, supervisory support, and work pressure. Three forms of the WES are available to assess the work environment as the worker experiences it, the worker's ideal workplace environment, and what an employee may expect out of a work environment (Moos, 1994). When dealing with an individual with a cognitive or perceptual disability, the WES should be completed in conjunction with a jobsite visit whenever possible to provide the best overall picture of the work environment.

Importance of Interdisciplinary Assessment

It is not uncommon for occupational therapy practitioners, speech-language pathologists, and neuropsychologists to address functional cognitive and perceptual deficits in their respective courses of treatment as part of an overall team effort. At any stage of the work-specific CFE, deficits or functional limitations may present that fall outside the scope of occupational therapy practice or a clinician's own skill set. In these cases, it is important for the occupational therapy practitioner to look to other members of the health community to assist in providing best practice.

Speech-Language Pathology Assessment

The ability to express and receive meaningful communication is potentially the most complex cognitive process that a worker must perform during a return-to-work attempt. If breakdowns in an individual's fundamental ability to communicate are identified via the interviews, screens, or measures administered in any stage of the assessment, it is important to refer to a speech-language pathologist for a thorough evaluation of the client's communication needs. After assessing the client, the speech-language therapist can then inform the treatment team of communication strategies to ensure the therapeutic intervention is most effective.

Neuropsychological Assessment

If cognitive difficulties are reported in the stage 1 interview or are displayed in stages 2, 3, and 4, a full cognitive assessment may be appropriate to inform evaluation and treatment of the worker. Neuropsychological evaluation includes the use of an individually designed battery of well-standardized objective tests to evaluate the client's cognitive domains. This form of assessment is accomplished independently of the effects of the environment, the demands of the occupation, or other competing cognitive processes. Establishing a baseline of cognitive domain performance can be useful in identifying foci of treatment, but utilizing the results of a neuropsychological evaluation without the information from the other stages of the assessment to predict how a worker may perform complex essential job functions is inappropriate because of ecological validity concerns. Using the results of the neuropsychological evaluation in conjunction with performance on the various stages of the assessment presents a more effective and theoretically sound approach when dovetailing the professions of occupational therapy and neuropsychology.

Disability Case Management

Because of the challenges facing occupational therapy practice in this day and age, executing and coordinating the wide variety of services that can inform work assessment is often beyond the finite time resources of the practicing clinician. The role of case management is traditionally filled by social work or nursing, but occupational therapy practitioners are also becoming case managers more frequently in a variety of settings. Although not technically involved in the assessment process, a case manager can ensure that all of the necessary services identified through all stages of the assessment can be coordinated and funded in the most effective manner.

Case Resolution

Stage 1: Interview and Background Information Including an Occupational History

The JPM was completed with Stan. To accurately assess the essential functions of Stan's job, the occupational therapist contacted Stan's employer and obtained a job description for his position. Given the complex nature of his work, an appropriate O*NET description was not available. Using the job description as the basis for the interview, the occupational therapist and Stan selected the 10 most important essential job functions of his job. Stan then rated each one on a 1 to 10 scale for his ability to perform the function and his satisfaction with his performance. From his responses on the JPM, three essential job functions were targeted as a priority for treatment. Stan's wife was then asked to rate how she felt Stan would be able to do these three job functions given what she has seen at home since his injury. She indicated that she did not have the expertise to respond to the technological issues raised in the JPM, but she was able to rate his ability to manage multiple task demands and interact with others. The first- and third-person ratings on these three essential job functions are listed in Table 13.5.

While Stan did not identify other essential job tasks noted on the JPM to be of particular concern, these should be revisited at the end of the entire assessment; the cognitive and perceptual deficits identified during the assessment can then be used to confirm whether or not the other JPM job functions should be included as a focus of treatment. The third-party JPM from Stan's wife indicates that a close family member is rating Stan's performance at a similar level, and therefore an awareness deficit is not suspected. These assumptions should be confirmed during the performance-based assessment activities in stage 3.

Stage 2: Cognitive Screening and Baseline Status Tests

The results of the stage 2 assessment (Table 13.6) found that Stan's general cognitive status and perception are intact; however, the TMT score indicates impairment in Stan's cognitive flexibility. Impairment scores on the TMT can reveal a cognitive impairment in one or more of the cognitive domains. Given the highly cognitive nature of

Table 13.5 Stan's Results on the Job Performance Measure (First and Third Person)

Essential Job Function	First-Person Rating		Third-Person Rating
	Performance	Satisfaction	Performance
1. Keep up with and integrate technology advancements with the products he markets and sells, including needs assessment of his clients	3	1	N/A
2. Manage multiple, ongoing task demands related to training, sales, customer relations	1	1	2
3. Meet performance-incentive goals, which require an increased workload (majority of his salary)	2	1	1

Table 13.6 Stan's Results on Stage 2: Cognitive Screening and Baseline Status Tests

Domain	Assessment	Results
General cognitive status	Short Blessed Test (SBT)	Within normal limits
Neglect, visual field loss, aphasia	National Institutes of Health Stroke Scale (NIHSS)	0–No impairment
Perceptual screen	Occupational Therapy–Adult Perceptual Screening Test (OT-APST)	Within normal limits
Cognitive flexibility	Trail Making Test (TMT)	Deficient

Stan's job and his work-related goals, the occupational therapist referred Stan to neuropsychology for a full cognitive assessment.

Stage 3: General Measures of Cognition in Occupations

For stage 3, Stan completed the CTPA. After receiving the directions but before completing the assessment, Stan was asked to self-rate how he felt he would perform on the assessment. Quantitatively, Stan did not complete any of the tasks, made four out of six executive decisions to complete the tasks, and completed 20 percent of the inventory control task. Stan reached the cutoff for the assessment at 30 minutes, and therefore his performance efficiency was calculated by the sum of tasks completed added to the number of executive decisions made divided by total time in minutes $(0 + 4)/30 = 13$ percent. Qualitatively, Stan had difficulty organizing the tasks in order to effectively complete the work, he had difficulty alternating between tasks and frequently forgot what he was doing, had difficulty remembering the directions, and forgot both of the prospective memory tasks. Stan's performance was significantly lower than that of controls, and his performance indicated difficulty with the essential job functions identified in stage 1. In addition, Stan's self-rating of his ability to perform the CTPA

(case study continues on page 300)

before the assessment was consistent with his actual performance, and therefore he was determined to have intact awareness related to his ability to work.

Stage 4: Cognitive Tests for Specific Domains

In lieu of formal assessment in stage 4, Stan had a full cognitive profile completed by a neuropsychologist. The results of the assessment found (1) mild deficits in higher-level cognitive abilities, (2) deficits in word retrieval, and (3) short-term memory deficits. More specifically, within higher-level cognitive abilities, Stan had difficulties with rule-governed behavior and with tasks that required set-shifting, planning, and hypothesis testing. Using the models discussed earlier, the occupational therapist concluded that Stan's higher-level cognitive function deficits would impact his supervisory attentional system, which is necessary to accomplish novel/nonroutine tasks. This conclusion is consistent with the difficulty Stan reported with managing multiple tasks at one time and organizing and integrating all of the information about his products on the JPM during stage 1 of the assessment. Short-term memory is memory that is held online for a short period of time and not consolidated through rehearsal; however, given that the model for memory indicates that information passes through the short-term store to the long-term store, it is plausible to conclude that Stan's ability to form new long-term memories may also be impacted. This is consistent with his difficulty with learning about the new technologies at his office.

The pattern of deficits documented by the neuropsychologist indicate difficulty with the essential job functions identified by the JPM; however, Stan's difficulty with word retrieval and short-term memory had not been identified to date, and therefore these findings should be compared with the JPM to identify other essential job functions this could impact. Comparison to Stan's JPM revealed one other essential job function that could be impacted by his deficits: *lead team meetings and respond to concerns from team members and customers*. This job function should be included as a priority in treatment as well.

Stage 5: Environmental Assessment

The environmental assessment of Stan's worksite reinforced concerns raised by the subjective interview data gathered in stage 1 of the assessment as well as his performance difficulties on the CTPA in stage 3. Stan's office layout is a typical cubical labyrinth surrounded by offices on the periphery. Stan's peripheral office has no door and no privacy blinds. Environmental distractions include noise from phones, faxes, computers, radios, and coworkers measured at 70 decibels; two large copiers located near his office; an active overhead paging system; and an overall hectic pace exhibited by the workers. On the WES, Stan's ratings indicated that there was a considerable difference between his ideal levels of "coworker cohesion" and "managerial control" and the levels of the environment in which he worked before his injury.

Chapter Summary

Using the CFE as a framework for a cognitive-perceptual work assessment, information gathered through the five stages of the assessment can be integrated to examine the relationship between the person factors (cognition and perception), the environment (workplace), and the occupations (essential job functions) to determine Stan's capabilities and limitations related to work (Table 13.7). From this analysis, the occupational therapist can develop with the client the necessary goals for treatment and select the appropriate interventions to address these goals.

The OTPF identifies work as an area of occupation and also identifies cognitive and perceptual constructs under body structures/body functions: mental functions (AOTA, 2008). Traditionally, little focus has been placed on work rehabilitation compared to the other occupation domains, particularly the cognitive and perceptual

Table 13.7 Analysis of the Results of Stan's Work-Focused Cognitive Functional Evaluation

Essential Job Function Deficit	Domain Effected	Assessment to Support Findings
Keep up with and integrate technology advancements with the products he markets and sells, including needs assessment of his clients	Higher-level cognitive functions, short-term/long-term memory	JPM, neuropsychological evaluation, CTPA
Manage multiple, ongoing task demands related to training, sales, customer relations	Higher-level cognitive functions, short-term/long-term memory	JPM, neuropsychological evaluation, CTPA
Meet performance-incentive goals, which require an increased workload (majority of his salary)	Higher-level cognitive functions, short-term/long-term memory	JPM, neuropsychological evaluation, CTPA
Lead team meetings and respond to concerns from team members and customers	Higher-level cognitive functions, word-retrieval, short-term memory	Neuropsychological evaluation

CTPA, Complex Task Performance Assessment; JPM, Job Performance Measure

deficits that impact the ability to return to work. This is a crucial area for occupational therapy practitioners to be involved with given our unique skill set and our focus on occupational performance. The work-focused CFE can be used to establish the occupational therapy practitioner's role in this area and support new populations in returning to work that have largely gone underserved when the focus has been primarily on musculoskeletal injuries.

References

Adams, R. L., Parsons, O. A., Culbertson, J. L., & Nixon, S. J. (eds.). (1996). *Neuropsychology for Clinical Practice: Etiology, Assessment, and Treatment of Common Neurological Disorders*. Washington, DC: American Psychological Association.

American Occupational Therapy Association (AOTA). (2008). Occupational therapy practice framework: Domain and process, 2nd ed. *American Journal of Occupational Therapy, 62*, 625–683.

Atkinson, R. C., & Shiffrin, R. M. (1968). Human memory: A proposed system and its control processes. In K. W. Spence & J. T. Spence (eds.), *The Psychology of Learning and Motivation*, Vol. 8 (pp. 742–775). London: Academic Press.

Baum, C. M., Connor, L. T., Morrison, T., Hahn, M., Dromerick, A. W., & Edwards, D. F. (2008). Reliability, validity, and clinical utility of the Executive Function Performance Test: A measure of executive function in a sample of people with stroke. *American Journal of Occupational Therapy, 62*(4), 446–455.

Brott, T., Adams, H. P., Jr., Olinger, C. P., Marler, J. R., Barsan, W. G., Biller, J., et al. (1989). Measurements of acute cerebral infarction: A clinical examination scale. *Stroke, 20*(7), 864–870.

Burgess, P. W. (2000). Strategy application disorder: The role of the frontal lobes in human multitasking. *Psychological Research, 63*(3), 279–288.

Cohen, N. J. (1984). Preserve learning capacity in amnesia: Evidence for multiple memory systems. In L. R. Squire & N. Butters (eds.), *The Neuropsychology of Memory* (pp. 88–103). New York: Guilford Press.

Cooke, D. M., McKenna, K., & Fleming, J. (2005). Development of a standardized occupational therapy screening tool for visual perception in adults. *Scandinavian Journal of Occupational Therapy, 12*(2), 59–71.

Cooke, D. M., McKenna, K., Fleming, J., & Darnell, R. (2005). The reliability of the Occupational Therapy Adult Perceptual Screening Test (OT-APST). *British Journal of Occupational Therapy, 68*(11), 509–517.

Cooke, D. M., McKenna, K., Fleming, J., & Darnell, R. (2006a). Construct validity and ecological validity of the Occupational Therapy Adult Perceptual Screening Test (OT-APST). *Scandinavian Journal of Occupational Therapy, 13*(1), 49–61.

Cooke, D. M., McKenna, K., Fleming, J., & Darnell, R. (2006b). Criterion validity of the Occupational Therapy Adult Perceptual Screening Test (OT-APST). *Scandinavian Journal of Occupational Therapy, 13*(1), 38–48.

Fleming, J. M., Strong, J., & Ashton, R. (1996). Self-awareness of deficits in adults with traumatic brain injury: How best to measure? *Brain Injury, 10*(1), 1–15.

Graf, P., & Schacter, D. L. (1985). Implicit and explicit memory for new associations in normal and amnesic subjects. *Journal of Experimental Psychology, Learning, Memory, and Cognition, 11*(3), 501–518.

Hartman-Maeir, A., Katz, N., & Baum, C. M. (2009). Cognitive functional evaluation (CFE) process for individuals with suspected cognitive disabilities. *Occupational Therapy In Health Care, 23*(1), 1–23.

Kaskutas, V., & Seaton, M. (2008). *The Job Performance Measure: A job analysis tool and assessment of perceived work task performance*. Paper presented at the 2008 American Occupational Therapy Association Conference and Expo, Long Beach, CA.

Katz, N., & Hartman-Maeir, A. (2005). Higher-level cognitive functions: Awareness and executive functions enabling engagement in occupation. In N. Katz (ed.), *Cognition & Occupation Across the Lifespan* (pp. 3, 12, 13). Besthesda, MD: AOTA Press.

Katzman, R., Brown, T., Fuld, P., Peck, A., Schechter, R., & Schimmel, H. (1983). Validation of a short orientation-memory concentration test of cognitive impairment. *American Journal of Psychiatry, 140*(6), 734–739.

Law, M., Baptiste, S., Carswell, A., McColl, M. A., Polatajko, H., & Pollock, N. (1998). *The Canadian Occupational Performance Measure*, 3rd ed. Toronto: Canadian Association of Occupational Therapy.

Lezak, M., Howieson, D. B., & Loring, D. W. (2004). *Neuropsychological Assessment*, 4th ed. New York: Oxford University Press.

Matheson, L., Kaskutas, V., & Seaton, M. (2003). Work rehabilitation for occupational therapists. Paper presented at the Part 2, Advanced Assessment and Intervention, WebEx Distance-Based Educational Programming.

Moos, R. H. (1994). *A Social Climate Scale: Work Environment Scale Manual*, 3rd ed. Palo Alto, CA: Consulting Psychologists Press

Norman, D. A., & Shallice, T. (1986). Attention to action: Willed and automatic control of behavior. In R. J. Davidson, G. E. Schwart & D. Shapiro (eds.), *Consciousness and Self-Regulation: Advances in Research and Theory* (3–18). New York: Plenum Press.

North Carolina Employment Security Commission. (2009). O*NET Online. Retrieved from http://online.onetcenter.org.

Prigatano, G. P. (2005). Disturbance of self-awareness and rehabilitation of patients with traumatic brain injury: A 20-year perspective. *Journal of Head Trauma Rehabilitation, 20*, 19–29.

Robertson, I. H., Ward, T., Ridgeway, V., & Nimmo-Smith, I. (1994). *The Test of Everyday Attention Manual*. Reading, England: Tames Valley Test Company.

Shallice, T., & Burgess, P. W. (1991). Deficits in strategy application following frontal lobe damage in man. *Brain and Cognition, 114*(Pt. 2), 727–741.

Sohlberg, M. M., & Mateer, C. (2001). *Cognitive Rehabilitation: An Integrative Neuropsychological Approach*. New York: Guilford Press.

Tulving, E. (1991). Concepts of human memory. In L. Squire, N. Weinberger, G. Lynch, & J. McGaugh (eds.), *Memory: Organization and Locus of Change* (pp. 3–34). New York: Oxford University Press.

Wilson, B., Cockburn, J., & Baddeley, A. (1985). *The Rivermead Behavioral Memory Test*. Reading, England: Thames Valley Test Company.

Wilson, B. A., Evans, J. J., Emslie, H., Alderman, N., & Burgess, P. (1998). The development of an ecologically valid test for assessing patients with a dysexecutive syndrome. *Neuropsychological Rehabilitation, 8*(3), 213–228.

Wolf, T., Morrison, T., & Matheson, L. (2008). Initial development of a work-related assessment of dysexecutive syndrome. *Work, 31*(2), 221–228.

World Health Organization. (2001). *International Classification of Functioning, Disability and Health*. Geneva: World Health Organization.

Glossary

Alternating attention is the ability to shift focus of attention and move between multiple tasks.

Attention is the ability to selectively focus on stimuli.

Declarative memory is long-term memory that can consciously be recalled.

Divided attention is the ability to focus attention on multiple tasks simultaneously; it is the highest level of attention.

Ecologically valid means representative of the real world.

Episodic memory is long-term declarative memory of past events.

Focused attention is the ability to respond to stimulus; it is the lowest level of attention.

Habituation is diminution of behavioral response to repeated stimulus.

Higher-level cognitive functions are cognitive functions responsible for planning and organizing behavior; also called executive functions.

Long-term memory is memory that, through rehearsal, has been consolidated and stored and can be recalled for an extended period of time.

Memory is the ability to encode, store, and recall information.

Memory consolidation is the process of how short-term memories are rehearsed and then stored as long-term memories.

Nondeclarative memory is long-term memory that cannot consciously be recalled.

Perceptual priming is long-term, nondeclarative memory for shapes and objects.

Procedural memory is long-term, nondeclarative memory for skills.

Prospective memory is long-term, declarative memory for future events and intentions.

Selective attention is the ability to maintain focus in the face of competing stimulus.

Semantic memory is long-term, declarative memory for general world knowledge.

Sensitization is amplification of behavioral response to repeated stimulus.

Short-term memory is memory of information that can be recalled only for a short period of time while the information is used; also called working memory.

Sustained attention is the ability to maintain attention during activity.

Resources

O*NET(Occupational Information Network)

http://online.onetcenter.org

Short Blessed Test

http://alzheimer.wustl.edu/About_Us/PDFs/Short%20Blessed%20Test%20-%20Washington%20University%20Version.pdf

National Institutes of Health Stroke Scale (NIHSS)

www.strokecenter.org/trials/scales/nihss.html

Trail Making Test

www.healthcare.uiowa.edu/igec/tools/cognitive/trailMaking.pdf

Executive Functions Performance Test (EFPT)

http://crrg.wustl.edu/outcome_assessment.html

Occupational Therapy–Adult Perceptual Screening Test (OT-APST)

www.functionforlife.com.au?

14 Preventing Injuries in the Workplace
Ergonomics

Kathryn Maltchev

Key Concepts

The following are key concepts addressed in this chapter:

- Ergonomics is an interdisciplinary field focused on the interactions of the person and the environment.
- Ergonomic considerations include assessment of body mechanics and posture, material handling, repetition, static positions, anthropometrics, and environmental elements.
- Traditional ergonomics is the middle layer, in terms of detail, of a comprehensive approach to reducing injury risk. Macroergonomics is a larger organizational process, while ergokinesis focuses on the specific contributions and limitations of the worker.

Case Introduction

Carolyn was a nursing supervisor at a large nursing facility. Multiple nurses and nursing assistants had obtained back, neck, and shoulder injuries from lifting and handling the residents. Two nursing assistants were unable to return to work due to the severity of their injuries. Carolyn was frustrated and upset every time an injury occurred, because she knew these injuries were putting a hardship on her employees, not only on the ones who were injured but also on staff who were required to work extra hours with higher case loads. She also noticed the facility was spending tens of thousands of dollars per year on claims, and good people were losing their livelihoods. Carolyn felt if she could address the problems up front, she could make a big impact on the work lives of her employees and save the company money over time.

Before moving to the facility, Carolyn had worked with an occupational therapist who specialized in ergonomics, so she called to see what she could do. Carolyn initially contracted with the occupational therapist to perform an assessment of the physical job requirements for nurses and nursing assistants, review injury data to identify trends and primary risk factors, and conduct several specialized ergonomic evaluations. Once the evaluation was completed, the occupational therapist provided a detailed report outlining findings, conclusions, and recommendations to Carolyn and several other decision-makers. The group agreed they needed to make some changes. They devised a plan and budget based on the occupational therapist's evaluation.

Ergonomics Defined

Ergonomics is the study of humans, objects, or machines, and the interactions among them. The term ergonomics is of Greek origin based on *ergos,* meaning "work" and *nomos,* meaning "law." The International Ergonomics Association (2000), which represents active ergonomics societies in more than 40 countries, defines ergonomics as "the scientific discipline concerned with understanding the interactions among humans and other elements of a system, and the profession that applies theory, principles, data and methods to design, in order to optimize human well-being and overall system performance." The term *human factors* is used interchangeably with ergonomics in some countries.

Ergonomics is a unique field of study that embodies a true interdisciplinary approach to improving the work–worker interaction. It draws from the fields of engineering, medicine, technology, toxicology, psychology, industrial design, kinesiology, occupational safety, and a host of others. While ergonomics can become very complex in certain focus areas, such as engineering and industrial design, the focus for this chapter is on basic concepts and how they relate to occupational therapy. It is important to understand how occupational therapy practitioners are uniquely equipped and qualified to function in the realm of ergonomics.

Systems

The underlying objective in ergonomics is to obtain safe, comfortable, and efficient work environments. It seeks to match the cognitive and physical requirements of the job to the capabilities of the worker. The person is seen as an extension of the work-related system. Senge (1990) described systems by stating, "Business and other human endeavors are systems bound by invisible fabrics of interrelated actions. When we tend to focus on snapshots of isolated parts of the system, our deepest problems never seem to get solved (p. 7)." In general, *systems* are any object, machine, or activity in which the worker must engage and the context in which they function. To fully understand ergonomics, it is important to understand the concept of systems and how they are used.

To better illustrate this, occupational therapy terminology can be used to define systems in the area of activities of daily living (ADL). In occupational therapy, the person's environment, including the contexts, activity demands, and their effect on occupational performance, drives goals and outcomes (AOTA, 2008). For example, a poor layout of a bathroom can decrease safety or increase fall risks and decrease performance. A client may be fully independent bathing in the rehabilitation clinic that has bathroom doors wide enough for the use of a walker and a walk-in shower. This is a good system match between the client or user and the environment. However, at home, the client has a narrow door she must sidestep through with her walker, thus increasing risk of tripping and time required to access the bathroom. She must also navigate a bath tub with sliding glass doors, which further increases risk and may ensure the client is no longer able to perform bathing independently. This is a poor system match between the user and the environment. Use of the walker, the sink, the towel racks, the commode, and anything else she must interact with in that bathroom contributes to increasing the activity demands within the context of bathing and toileting. In ergonomics, the patient, the environment, and how they interact encompass the system.

A more traditional ergonomic example can be found in a manufacturing plant. The plant is having production issues related to multiple people being off work due to musculoskeletal sprain and strains. There is also a need to improve the quality of the final product and the efficiency at which it is produced. Jackson, the plant manager, pulls his top people together to look at the problem and suggest solutions. Steve is an engineer and recommends a new piece of equipment that promises better output and would reduce worker interaction with the machinery. Susan is a safety manager and recommends better employee training and incentives for higher productivity and injury reduction. Rob, the occupational therapy practitioner and ergonomic consultant, recommends a better task design that will optimize the user–machine interaction while decreasing the physical requirements of the workers. This may be accomplished by better equipping the new machine suggested by Steve with spring-loaded levers that reduce the amount of force required to operate them and lowering the panel of buttons to make them easier to reach, thereby decreasing strain on the shoulders, increasing efficiency, and increasing accessibility of maintenance panels so that workers need not get into awkward positions to perform daily checks and repairs (which also ensures these tasks are done and not avoided). They may also institute a rotational schedule and break-compliance program to reduce muscle fatigue and energy expenditure. Neither Susan's nor Steve's suggestions are wrong, but only the ergonomic example maximizes both the machine operations and the user capabilities.

Ergonomics considers the person as a full member of the system. In alignment with traditional understanding of occupational performance, the performance skills, the context, the activity demands, and the client factors cannot be separated when applying ergonomics. The overall objective in ergonomics is to externally maximize the performance skills of the worker by modifying the context and activity demands. A machine may be highly reliable and efficient in and of itself, but if the user must work in awkward positions or with forces exceeding a person's safe capabilities, performance skills diminish and can result in potential injury (see Box 14.1).

In alignment with traditional understanding of occupational performance, the performance skills, the context, the activity demands, and the client factors cannot be separated when applying ergonomics.

Ergonomic Considerations

Body Mechanics and Posture

For the body to maximize strength, mobility, and stability, alignment to the center of gravity is important. The *center of gravity* is determined by maximizing use of the skeletal system, minimizing joint and muscular stress, so that the lines of action flow through noncompressible structures. These lines then flow directly to the base of support, which is typically the feet when standing and the feet and buttocks when sitting. For example, when lowering to sit, the upper body automatically moves forward as the buttocks move back toward the seat. This helps redistribute weight to maintain stability over the base of support. If the upper body was restricted and not allowed to move forward, such as in a confined workspace, sitting would still be possible but would require significant increased lower extremity strength and stabilization to safely perform the task. Without the alignment over the center of gravity and along the base of support, the muscles become fatigued, increasing risk of injury to the muscle and supported joints (Champagne, Descarreaux, and Lafond, 2008; Kankaanpaa, Taimela, Laaksonen, Hanninen, and Airaksinen, 1998; Pscione and Gamet, 2006). Figure 14.1 shows good alignment to the center of gravity with neutral postures during different types of tasks, and Figure 14.2 shows poor alignment that would result in increased risk of injury.

Box 14.1 Ergonomic Considerations

1. Body mechanics and posture	**4.** Anthropometrics
2. Manual handling	**5.** Environmental considerations
3. Repetitive and static tasks	

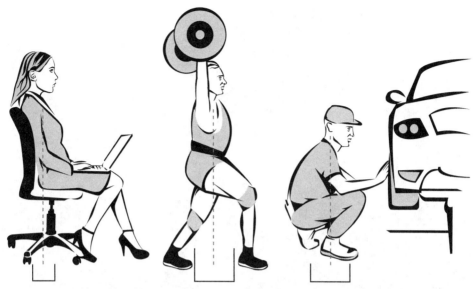

Figure 14.1 Center of gravity and good posture. The dotted line represents an approximate axis of gravitational pull, and the open box represents the base of support. Notice that with good posture, the lines of gravitational pull are lined up directly over the base of support.

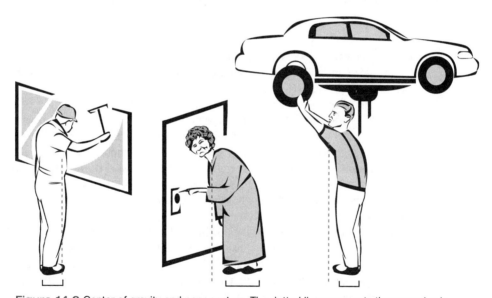

Figure 14.2 Center of gravity and poor posture. The dotted line represents the general axis of gravitational pull, and the open box represents the base of support. The axis of gravitational pull can be moved away from the base of support due to reaching, added weight, poor posture, and other factors.

Many studies indicate increased musculoskeletal injury rates when forces are applied outside a joint's center of gravity. Hoogendoorn and colleagues (2000) described postural positioning that contributes to low back pain. They found that trunk flexion of at least 60 degrees for as little as 5 percent of the day, trunk rotation of at least 30 degrees for as little as 10 percent of the day, and lifting at least 25 kilograms (about 55 pounds) more than 15 times per day are moderate risk factors for low back pain (Fig. 14.3). Another study by Sengupta and Das (2004) found that oxygen uptake (VO_2), heart rate, and myoelectric activity (measured by electromyography [EMG]) in the anterior deltoid, erector spinae,

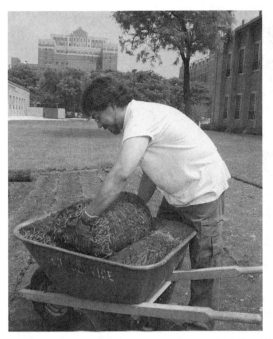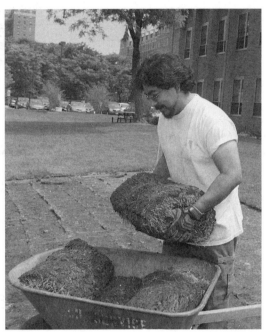

Figure 14.3 Trunk flexion and rotation, particularly while lifting or lowering, can put a person at significant risk for back pain.

and upper trapezius increased significantly when performing a repetitive upper extremity task in maximum and extreme reaching levels as compared to keeping the arms close to the body during task performance.

Higher muscular tension and tissue stress occur when an extremity is moved away from its base of support. For example, one might correlate the head sitting on the spine to a bowling ball attached to the top of a long spring. If the bowling ball is moved off the top of the spring but remains attached, it is no longer being supported through gravity and the spring's compression. Increased stress is placed on the side of the spring opposite to the bowling ball as the spring stretches or opens to counteract the weight of the ball. If fluid existed in the middle of the spring, the fluid would be pushed away from the bowling ball and toward the open side of the spring. Over time, the spring's original shape would be altered even with removal of the bowling ball. Similarly, when the head and shoulders are brought in front of the body, as with slumped or forward-bending postures, they are no longer fully supported by the spine through gravity. The head must now rely on the ligaments in the cervical and upper thoracic spine and muscles along the back of the neck and upper shoulders to hold its weight. The nucleus pulposi in the disks are also pushed toward the posterior spine, placing significant stress to these structures.

Joints should be kept as close as possible to a neutral position, which maximizes use of the center of gravity. In neutral positioning, the muscles, tendons, and ligaments are minimally stretched, resulting in less stress to these structures and the joints they support. *Neutral positioning* also reduces compression and stretch of nerves and blood vessels. This posture includes keeping elbows at the sides to reduce reaching, wrists straight (not bent or deviated), head or ears in line with the shoulders, shoulders in line with the hips, and hips in line with the feet without rotation of the spine. The elbows, hips, and knees are slightly flexed while keeping the lumbar curve. This position is considered a resting or relaxed position. Many ergonomic principles are based on maintaining a body position as close as possible to neutral.

It is important to keep in mind that neutral positioning is not always equivalent to comfort. Over time, the body adjusts to positions it is put in for prolonged periods by shortening and tightening some ligaments and muscles and stretching others. Changing postural habits takes time and many reminders. The person who typically reclines to the point where shoulder reaching is required or sits on the edge of the seat without use of the backrest may find it challenging to sit back in the seat without leaning or slumping. Others who keep their head far forward, such that the ears are several inches in front of the shoulders, often find it very uncomfortable to move the head back into alignment and may have difficulty maintaining the position. Visual cues and verbal acknowledgments can go a long way in changing longstanding patterns.

Manual Handling

Lifting, lowering, carrying, pushing, and pulling are common examples used in describing maintenance of neutral postures and keeping the force or object as close as possible to the center of gravity and base of support. The object being handled, often called the *load,* should be situated as close to waist height as possible. When multiple levels are necessary, such as on a shelving unit, the heaviest objects should be placed at waist height or below to maximize use of the stronger muscles in the lower extremities. Lighter objects should be placed on the higher shelves. The load should be held as close to the body as possible with no trunk rotation during the lift or carry (Fig. 14.4). The type of load, including the size, shape, and availability of handles, also contributes to the difficulty of the lift. Several lifting standards have been written to provide guidance on maximum load or weight allowances based on body position and load qualities. Descriptions of a few standards, including the most commonly used National Institute of Occupational Safety and Health (NIOSH) equation, are found in Chapter 15.

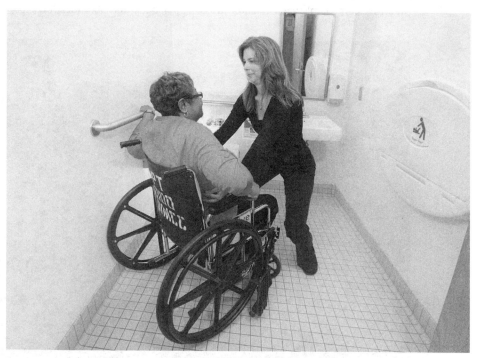

Figure 14.4 Using proper body mechanics and managing a load can be difficult during job tasks that combine lifting and turning, especially in small work spaces.

Repetitive and Static Tasks

Repetitive motions and static positioning outside neutral postures can result in muscle fatigue, joint stress, and increase injury risk (Le, et al., 2009; Navar, Zhou, Lu, and Solomonow, 2006; Sbriccoli, et al., 2004). Repetitive tasks and the conditions or problems they create vary widely but are almost always characterized by neurologic and musculoskeletal disorders. As nerves and tendons are repeatedly pulled through their protected structures, an inflammatory response can occur. Often, this repetition is accompanied by an associated force, increasing pressure and friction. For example, meatpackers have shown a higher incidence of stenosing flexor tenosynovitis (trigger finger) due to holding powered knives and using the index finger to activate a trigger repeatedly throughout the day (Gorsche, et al., 1998). With prolonged repetitive activities, nerves are often affected in general, nonspecific patterns, presenting as diffuse arm pain. Neural tension places the nerve at risk for injury anywhere along its length, not just along the joint that is moving. They are particularly vulnerable in areas where the nerves are relatively fixed and where they pass near hard surfaces such as bone (Butler, 1991). It is important when evaluating arm pain to include a full evaluation of the entire upper extremity. Workers often present with hand-based symptoms, such as numbness and tingling in the hand and fingers or aching in the wrist, that is actually being caused by compression in the cervical spine or muscular compression of the nerve(s) anywhere along its path.

Static positioning can also result in musculoskeletal injuries as well as vascular compromise. When muscles are contracted for prolonged periods of time, oxygenation reduces and the muscles tighten. It is thought that because the nervous system consumes a high percentage of oxygen in the blood, reduction or constriction of blood supply to the muscles further hinders neural uptake of oxygen, thereby causing discomfort and pain (Pritchard, Pugh, Wright, and Brownless, 1999). Static muscle contractions can occur both with whole-body positions, such as crouching or forward bending, or with sustained individual joint position, such as shoulder flexion or wrist extension (see Fig. 14.5). People often carry significant tension in the upper back and shoulder muscles, keeping the

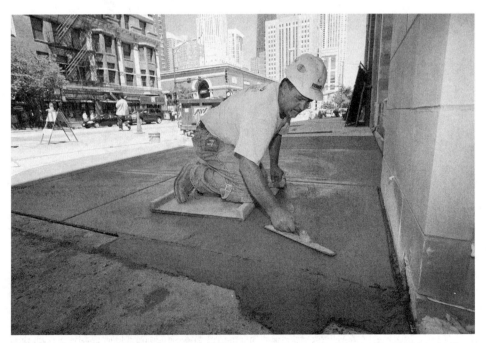

Figure 14.5 Prolonged postures and repetitive movements can result in significant stress on the body and create varied problems for workers.

shoulders elevated even though they believe they are at rest. This is another type of positioning with static muscle contraction, even though the person may not be fully aware of the posture.

Another important consideration with certain static postures is vascular compromise. Prolonged standing or crouching can create vascular challenges such as varicose veins. Veins are designed to use surrounding musculature to help pump returning blood flow back into the body. When the muscles are not activating on a regular basis, blood can pool and create painful swelling of the lower extremities.

Rest is important to muscle and cardiovascular recovery and increasing blood flow to surrounding tissues. Breaks, stretching, and alternating physically demanding tasks with nonphysically demanding tasks are good techniques to help reduce energy expenditure and decrease the effects of nonneutral positions, repetitive activities, and static postures. Generally, more frequent short-duration rest or stretching breaks are recommended for static activities, while repetitive or cyclic activities generate increased energy demand and therefore require additional or longer periods of rest (Hoops, Zhou, Lu, Solomonow, and Patel, 2007). Rest breaks should be used prior to muscle exhaustion due to the significant increased recovery time needed to avoid injury.

Anthropometrics

Anthropometrics is the measurements, sizes, and proportions of the human body. These measurements are commonly used by designers and engineers to standardize equipment and furniture to maximize use and safety. The height of fixed shower heads, sinks, and kitchen cabinets; the width of doors; the depth of car seats; the height of stairs; and the height and depth of chairs in classrooms and offices most likely were all designed with anthropometrics in mind.

Anthropometric data is used routinely in ergonomics to "specify the physical dimensions of workspaces, equipment, vehicles, and clothing to ensure that these products physically fit their users" (Bridger, 2009, p. 75). Because physical characteristics vary widely, information collected in anthropometric tables almost always refer to a particular population. Typically, designers of workstations and materials identify the potential users for their product. They then design to maximize usability for as much of the identified population as possible. For example, when designing a new school desk for seventh graders in Canada, anthropometric data for measurements such as leg length, sitting height, reach distances, torso length, and seat width for Canadian seventh graders would be collected. When possible, a goal of accommodating 90 percent of the potential users guides the design. Adjustability is highly valued as a means to reach this objective (Bridger, 2009). However, there are also occasions when only a small percentage of the user population must be considered. For example, shower height primarily affects tall users, whereas placement of switches mainly affects shorter users or those in wheelchairs.

A user–design mismatch can increase risk of injury, decrease efficiency and usability, alter postures, and deter use. Any tall, broad-shouldered individual sitting in the middle seat of a standard airplane can report on the challenges and discomfort of a design–user mismatch. Evidence of poor design is common. Car cup holders that require reaching behind the body to use, keypads so small that wrong or multiple buttons are hit, and medicine bottles that are difficult for the older population to open are examples of designs that did not account for the standard user. Anthropometrics are an important component to ergonomics and should always be taken into account when adjusting workstations or equipment.

Environmental Considerations

Many physical factors in a worker's environment can affect performance, safety, health, and general well-being. Noise, vibration, lighting, and contact stress are examples of such issues (see Box 14.2). Guidelines have been established by various organizations to help maintain safe levels of external factors and reduce the user's exposure. While this list is far from complete, it provides an overview of some of the most common issues found in working environments.

Noise can be a sound of any kind but is often considered a loud or unexpected sound that is unpleasant to the ears. While sound can be measured objectively, noise tends to be more subjective and is typically linked with excessive sound. When in excess, sound can result in hearing loss, associated speech impairment, psychological stress, sleep disturbances, and other health issues. To avoid these problems, noise should not exceed 85 decibels (OSHA, 2002). Hearing protection should be worn when noise cannot be lowered. In contrast, when ambient noise reaches below 30 decibels, intermittent sounds can cause significant distraction. Many offices that use cubicles add low-frequency static so that conversations, typing, and other activities in adjacent cubicles are not as distracting.

Whole-body and hand/arm *vibration* are two issues that should be considered when assessing potential injury risk. Vibration can produce several bodily responses, including motion sickness; resonance in the head, spine, and gastrointestinal system; blurred vision; and postural and upper body destabilization (Griffin, 1990). Although there is some evidence of general health issues related to vibration (Wikstrom, Kjellberg, and Landstrom, 1994), this chapter focuses on two of the more common complaints: low back pain and Raynaud's disease.

A few studies have linked whole-body vibration and back injuries. Bovenzi and Hulshof (1999) completed a review of epidemiologic studies on the effects of whole-body vibration on the spine. They found several studies linking whole-body vibration with low back pain, sciatic pain, and degenerative changes. However, they caution that supportive evidence overall is weak. Lings and Leboeuf-Yde (2000) found similar results in their review but further described a link between duration of exposure and frequency of low back pain. More recent studies are helping build stronger support for keeping whole-body vibration as low as possible and continuing to address it as an ergonomic concern (Bovenzi, 2009; Palmer, et al., 2008; Tiemessen, Hulshof, and Frings-Dresen, 2008). Maintaining machinery, improving vehicle suspension, using seat isolation or dampening, and using pneumatic springs or hydraulic lifts can help decrease vibration or its conduction.

Raynaud's disease is a vascular condition in which the arteries supplying extremities (such as the fingers, toes, and nose) narrow, limiting blood flow to those areas. They become cold, numb, and often painful. The symptoms usually increase with a cold environment or during times of stress (MayoClinic.com, 2009). When Raynaud's disease is associated with vibrating hand tools, it is often called "white finger." Raynaud's disease has been strongly linked to use of vibrating hand tools, even in short duration cycles (Barregard, Ehrestrom, and Marcus, 2003; Griffin, Bovenzi, and Nelson, 2003). It is important to reduce hand-tool vibration either by modifying the task to reduce use of power tools or by reducing transmission of vibration. Vibration can be reduced in a number of ways: using low-vibration equipment, adding antivibration materials to tool handles, installing antivibration mounts to support tools and reduce handling, and using of antivibration gloves. These solutions have varied effectiveness and should be evaluated and reviewed closely.

Box 14.2 Environmental Considerations

1. Noise	**3.** Lighting
2. Vibration	**4.** Contact stress

Lighting is important to occupational performance. The amount of light in an area or on a work surface must be sufficient for the task being performed, maximizing safety and efficiency while reducing eyestrain. Tasks that require more detail or focus require more light. For example, the standard light intensity for normal activities is 200 to 750 lux. More detailed tasks, such as studying or small parts repair, may require additional task lighting over 1000 lux. Light intensity can be measured using special devices called photometers if light is identified as a concern (Dul and Weerdmeester, 2008).

Reflections and flicker both contribute to discomfort related to lighting. Workstations should be arranged such that reflections and shadows are avoided. For example, if an office worker is sitting next to a sunny window, which direction should he face? If he faces the window, the light will reflect off his desk and papers, causing eyestrain. If he faces away from the window, the light will reflect off his computer monitor, again causing discomfort. His best position would be to sit at a 90-degree angle away from the window and add curtains or tint to reduce the amount of light coming through.

Flicker is caused by changes in power or voltage supplying the light source. In a work environment, most complaints related to flicker are from computer monitors and fluorescent lighting. Although most of the flickering that occurs is not noticeable, people report increased headaches and eyestrain with high flickering monitors and lights. Replacing bulbs, switching to incandescent lights and flat panel monitors, and using energy-efficient fluorescent bulbs can all assist in reducing flicker.

Contact stress occurs when occasional or constant contact occurs between a hard surface and a part of the human body, such as the wrists, elbows, fingers, thighs, or feet. The resultant localized pressure can restrict blood flow; hinder nerve, tendon, or muscle function; and break down soft tissue over long periods of time. Contact stress can occur from a variety of actions: using scissors or pliers, standing at conveyer belts that rub or press on the thighs, leaning on the arm rests of chairs, kneeling, and resting the wrists on a desk while typing or mousing (see Fig. 14.6). Recommendations for contact stress are related to avoidance when possible and softening or cushioning a surface when contact is unavoidable. For example, using spring-loaded and automatic tools to reduce handling or force, instruction in reduction of leaning or resting on hard surfaces, and distributing contact to larger surface areas can help reduce and prevent injuries.

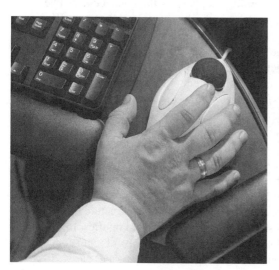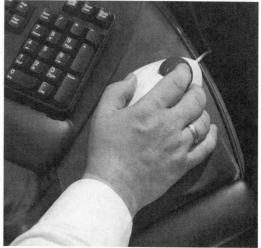

Figure 14.6 Use of a mouse can result in repetitive motions and contact stress that can become problematic.

Occupational Therapy in Ergonomics: Defining Value

Ergonomics means different things to different people and has been defined in a multitude of ways. Almost any health-, engineering-, or safety-related field has a specialty group working in an ergonomics arena, and they all have something to contribute. However, if occupational therapy practitioners believe that the skills provided through the profession offer something unique to the field, the benefit of using an occupational therapy practitioner over or in conjunction with other professionals should be clearly described. How is that value defined? The Occupational Therapy Practice Framework states: "Engagement in occupation includes both the subjective (emotional or psychological) aspects of performance and the objective (physically observable) aspects of performance. Occupational therapists and occupational therapy assistants understand engagement from this dual and holistic perspective and address all aspects of performance" (AOTA, 2008, p. 628). No truer words could be written about the role of occupational therapy in ergonomics.

The concept of systems was introduced at the beginning of this chapter with a basic description of the interaction between the person and the immediate environment. But that is just a middle layer of a complex approach that requires a holistic view of the work, the worker, and the environment. The larger organizational picture provided through macroergonomics and the more detailed individual picture provided through ergokinesis give occupational therapy practitioners the full view. It is like an onion: separate individual layers work together to create the whole.

Macroergonomics

In the systems approach, the additional outer layer of physical, cultural, social, and temporal contexts casts a wider web around the client and provides further insight into the bigger picture of occupational performance. Additional factors—such as available support systems of coworkers, family, and friends; feeling rushed due to external pressures; or a physician's perception of a client's abilities—can all affect the client's independence, safety, and efficiency with a task.

Macroergonomics is an organizational design structure that allows flexibility in the physical work environment. This flexibility emphasizes the connection between the individual and the interrelationship of social, physical, and technical factors (Hendrick and Kleiner, 2002). The objective of macroergonomics is to implement management and organizational factors that promote healthy, safe work practices and performance. A primary goal is establishing these practices within the work culture so that harmony is achieved to the point that workers are efficient, content, and successful. While *microergonomics* (or traditional ergonomics) focuses more on the physical environment, macroergonomics focuses on the overall structure and the interconnectedness of psychosocial, technologic, environmental, and individual or client factors. There has been some discussion related to the need for better integration between macroergonomics and microergonomics (Genaidy, Sequeira, Rinder, and A-Rehim, 2009). This integration is where occupational therapy can thrive.

Often, observations of how workers engage with each other and management can provide great insight into the work culture and organizational structure. Fick (2008) describes how work culture and policies can influence work-related injuries. In her example, a company is supportive of early discomfort reporting to help avoid more complicated injuries. The employees feel empowered and encouraged to resolve issues early. However, the company also begins to incentivize managers to limit the number of work-related injuries reported. Employees may perceive that any report of discomfort would result in retaliation from management. Occupational therapy practitioners can use the information to inform management of potential unintended consequences of established policies and resolve employee concerns.

Worker motivation can also affect performance and be guided by organizational structure. Chebykin, Bedny, and Karwowski (2008) describe a challenge vocational schools faced in the old Soviet Union. The job task students learned was highly repetitive, and the only required measurement was the quality of the completed product. Students described the tasks as monotonous and often had difficulty transitioning into the increased productivity demands of a work environment. Researchers found that by the end of the training program, students had developed their own production standards. The attempt to implement new requirements was ineffective. However, in a similar training group, time standards were introduced at the beginning. By adding a challenging component before students set their own standards, not only did motivation and job satisfaction increase, but the students voluntarily increased their performance standards each day of the training. A work culture that valued productivity and efficiency was created. Further, the increased productivity did not decrease quality, as feared initially. Determining the appropriate standard was important. If the production standard was too high, students would not have been able to meet the goal. The lack of success could have resulted in the new time standard being disregarded. However, if the standard was too low, sufficient challenge and resulting feeling of accomplishment would be diminished. The self-generated increase in production standards may not have occurred. Organizational structure, such as the time standard, can be used to provide strong motivational components to enhance job satisfaction and efficiency.

Occupational therapy practitioners need additional training to be fully effective in addressing macroergonomics, organizational structure, and complex behaviors. Rice (2008) emphasizes the importance of understanding limitations faced by therapists in this field and referring to appropriate additional resources when needed. In this vein, Fick (2008) described where occupational therapy practitioners can excel. She reported that groups such as "purchasing, human resources, sales, and even the safety department often work as separate and isolated parts of the same system, leaving the consulting therapist to put the pieces together so that crucial alignments can be gained between the therapist's recommendations and other parts of the system." Often, the occupational therapy practitioner's role is to identify the root issues and facilitate communication among all involved parties. This may also include identifying gaps and adding outside resources when necessary. By identifying the root issues and addressing them along all levels, occupational therapy practitioners can greatly impact injury prevention and resolution.

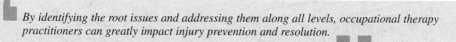

By identifying the root issues and addressing them along all levels, occupational therapy practitioners can greatly impact injury prevention and resolution.

Ergokinesis

On the opposite end of the larger systems approach of macroergonomics, *ergokinesis* is a detailed approach to the application of human anatomy and physiology, body mechanics, disease management, and psychosocial factors as they interact in an occupational environment (Maltchev, 2008). It is the study of how the worker connects with his or her occupational context and activity demands. The term ergokinesis is derived from *ergo,* meaning work, and *kinesis,* meaning movement. It is a highly specialized subset of existing practice in behavioral ergonomics, building on traditional biomechanical approaches, health promotion, and individual disease management. It places the focus on the individual and how he or she physically and psychologically adjusts to the physical, social, and organizational environment. Ergokinesis is not a substitute for traditional ergonomics, which should always be addressed. But it is an enhancement of resources to address specific worker behavior and adaptation in both individual and group contexts. Figures 14.7 and 14.8 compare the traditional engineering-based ergonomic approach to the worker-based approach of ergokinesis.

Case Example

Several years ago, Tim was referred for occupational therapy services due to complaints of general right arm pain and fatigue with symptoms of thoracic outlet syndrome. He worked as a station operator who packaged light bulk goods for a major food manufacturer. His job was to take four or five items at a time off the conveyer belt and place them in boxes for shipping. He was covered under work-related benefits and continued working his regular job while seeing the occupational therapy practitioner at the beginning of his shift.

A thorough clinical evaluation indicated significant tension and slight overdevelopment of the right scalenus, levator scapulae, and the upper trapezius muscles. Tim had rounded, protracted shoulders with a moderate forward head posture. His right shoulder remained slightly elevated even at rest. All his findings were consistent with his symptoms, and it was theorized that due to his posture, positioning, and muscular overdevelopment,

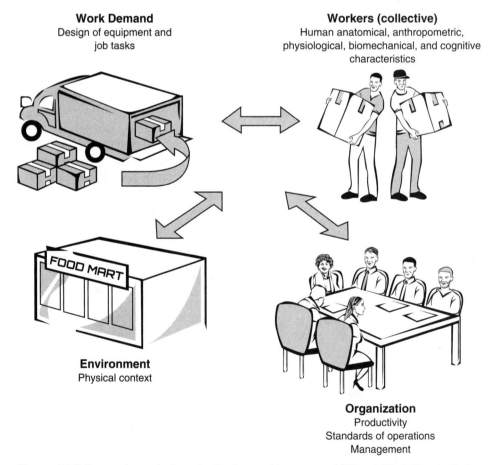

Figure 14.7 Ergonomics seeks to understand general human capabilities and limitations to design equipment, job tasks, environments, and systems to maximize safe human performance.

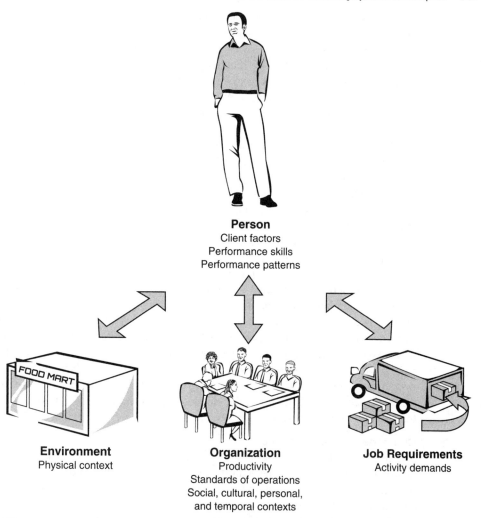

Person
Client factors
Performance skills
Performance patterns

Environment
Physical context

Organization
Productivity
Standards of operations
Social, cultural, personal,
and temporal contexts

Job Requirements
Activity demands

Figure 14.8 Ergokinesis places an emphasis on how individual workers interact with occupational contexts and activity demands through client factors and performance skills and patterns.

the scaleni were compressing the brachial plexus with additional symptom magnification through tightness in the levator and upper trapezius.

It was recognized that something Tim was doing, either at home or at work, was contributing to the muscle imbalance in his neck and shoulder. Because he was under work-related benefits and because he reported that most of his symptoms improved when off work but increased throughout his shift, the focus began with his job. Multiple conversations were initiated with his case manager, safety officer, and an onsite ergonomist. They had done several adjustments to the workstations the year before, and it was felt they were now ergonomically sound. The employees had gone through training and were heavily engaged in the ergonomics process through buddy ergo evaluations and self-reporting opportunities.

Tim improved significantly with therapy through increased awareness of his posture and correction of the muscle imbalances. However, he continued to express an increase in symptoms at the end of a long workday. Finally, after working with Tim for several weeks and receiving an invitation from the food manufacturer, the occupational therapy practitioner was able to visit Tim at work and watch him as he performed his job duties. His workstation was, in fact, set up very well, and Tim was very efficient while performing the task. The conveyer and the boxes were set slightly below elbow height and required minimal turning or reaching. However, after a while of observation, the therapist noticed that Tim became tense when the product was not spaced evenly, and every time he picked up the packages from the conveyer belt, he slightly elevated and protracted his right shoulder while laterally flexing his neck. While the movements were small and probably would not have otherwise been noticed or generated concern, they occurred 6 to 8 times per minute for 8 hours per day.

Kinesio taping was used for sensory feedback, and Tim's safety team was recruited to encourage Tim to keep his neck and shoulders level and relaxed. Tim was also instructed in stretches and exercises specifically addressing the physical requirements of his job and to counteract job-related movement patterns. Stress reduction techniques were used to facilitate proper breathing and general muscle tension reduction. These changes resulted in full resolution of Tim's symptoms.

Two very important lessons came out of this case. First, practitioners should always strive for observation and instruction in a person's natural environment, at home, work, school, or play. Tim quickly adjusted to physical and verbal cues and rarely lost muscular control with activity performed in the clinic. Even with the best physical recreation of tasks, the natural environment offers different demands and may bring out learned behavior that is an associated response of the task and the environment. The second lesson learned was that injury can occur even with ergonomically designed workstations and with proactive employers who strongly support work-injury prevention measures. Tim's company had obviously placed ergonomics as a priority, and while they had reduced injuries overall, they continued to have challenging cases. There was a need to better understand the employees as individuals and the unique physical, cognitive, and psychosocial aspects they brought to work performance (see Fig. 14.9).

Components of Ergokinesis

The first component of ergokinesis is *client factors* such as cardiovascular, sensory, and neuromuscular functions. These are large contributors to musculoskeletal pain and work dysfunction and often need individualized attention. In the preceding example, Tim demonstrated an abnormal movement pattern that created pain and injury. Addressing the general ergonomic issues of workstation design did not resolve his discomfort. Special observation skills, knowledge of normal muscle tone functions and kinesthetics, and an understanding of how stress can present itself physically all contributed to the successful resolution of the case. A good foundation in anatomy, physiology, and disease processes can significantly assist in identifying client factors affecting performance. Whether a client is facing age-related changes, is very tall or very short, has a disability, or just has a muscle or posture imbalance, addressing specific client factors can enhance occupational performance in the workplace.

For example, a worker who is obese may begin to report some knee and ankle discomfort yet have no detectable injury. Studies have indicated that obesity is associated with degenerative and inflammatory processes. Although not yet fully defined, the additional loading of joints and muscles seems to negatively affect the mechanics related to ambulation (Wearing, Henning, Byrne, Steele, and Hills, 2006). By understanding the disease processes related to obesity and the particular factors affecting the client, the occupational therapy practitioner can address the contributing issues before a true injury occurs. Depending on the job and observed biomechanics, additional support such as leaning opportunities and level walking surfaces may be needed to reduce stress on tendons and ligaments. He or she may benefit from instruction in dynamic standing activities to help support the joints. Strengthening of weakened muscles and stretching of overly tight muscles and joints could also improve occupational performance. And, depending on the

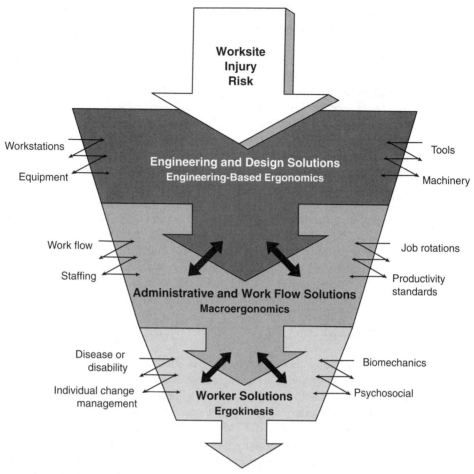

Figure 14.9 The general flow of ergonomic assessment and intervention from a systems approach. Work-related injuries and illnesses are reduced by a holistic approach to addressing multiple levels of the system.

work culture and acceptability, additional resources related to a healthy diet and exercise program can be provided.

Companies are emphasizing earlier reporting of potential work-related injuries and illnesses. This is providing a greater opportunity for occupational therapy practitioners to identify and resolve issues very early in the disease process. Most contributing factors can be identified and addressed through simple worksite observation. However, significant or unresolved pain, restricted movement, numbness or tingling, or other concerning reports or observations warrant additional evaluation. It is important to be familiar with potential limitations or restrictions on occupational therapy licensure and governmental regulations for injury reporting and medical referral.

The second component of ergokinesis is modification and accommodation. Layla was a 62-year-old woman who contacted her work-based ergonomics program, which was headed by an occupational therapist. She reported wrist and hand pain that increased while working on her computer. During the initial workstation evaluation, it was noted her metacarpal phalangeal (MCP) and interphalangeal (IP) joints were red and swollen. She reported a rheumatoid arthritis flare and needed recommendations. In addition to standard ergonomic instructions, the occupational therapist provided information about joint protection and pain reduction strategies related to her job tasks. Voice recognition software and workload sharing were used as a means to reduce hand use during periods of inflammation. After obtaining a prescription from her rheumatologist, special joint splints were fitted for her wrist and fingers to decrease development of joint deformity while minimizing interference with her work. To maintain joint mobility and decrease stiffness, she was also encouraged to slightly increase her activity level when the inflammation resolved per regulations by her personal physician.

Layla reported that she had never been referred for occupational therapy before and had only requested the ergonomic evaluation because it was offered through her employer. Because the employer contracted with an occupational therapist for this service, additional measures were identified and taken to help Layla remain in her job long term. Five years later, Layla continues to successfully manage her arthritis at work through occasional adjustments and recommendations by her occupational therapist and physician.

It is no revelation that occupational therapy practitioners are specialists in modifying activities or demands to meet the needs of people with physical, cognitive, or emotional challenges. While traditional ergonomics focuses on changing the work environment to meet the needs of the average user, it is within the realm of ergokinesis where individual needs are met (see Box 14.3). With aging workforces, returning veterans, and improved technologies to assist people with disabilities and chronic illnesses, the need for qualified clinicians to help merge the ability of specialty populations and work capabilities is great. Occupational therapy practitioners can be great advocates and facilitators in this process. Refer to Chapter 16 for more information related to the ADA and its implications in work and industry.

The final component of ergokinesis is effecting individual behavior and motivational change. Psychosocial issues such as worker identity and job stress can affect occupational performance and individual health. Studies have also indicated that a worker's perception of control over his or her environment directly relates to improved physical performance and overall health (Karasek and Theorell, 1990). It is important to recognize the worker as both a role and identity. A lack of perceived control affects the worker's perception not only of the work but of his or her role in it. People desire to be perceived as unique and valuable contributors. Chapter 2 discusses the importance of the worker role and considerations in addressing identity-related issues in a work environment.

Job stress is a well-known predictor of work-related pain and injury. Bongers, Kremer, and ter Laak (2002), in their review of psychosocial risk factors associated with upper extremity problems, found upper extremity pain and injury were consistently correlated with work- and non-work-related stress. In addition, Nakata and colleagues (2006) reported a greater risk of occupational injury among manufacturing employees who have high quantitative workloads, high cognitive demands, and low job satisfaction. Interestingly, they also described gender differences where low social supports from colleagues and family correlated with work-related injuries in women, while future job ambiguity correlated with injuries among men. Review Chapter 11 for additional information on how psychosocial factors impact the worker.

In a traditional work environment, addressing these issues can be challenging. Effecting change in either an organization or an individual takes time. However, simple solutions can often make big impacts. Education is an important place to start. Workers are more

---

Box 14.3 Components of Ergokinesis

1. Client factors
2. Modification and accommodation
3. Motivational change

likely to adopt a desired behavior if they understand how it will affect them (Nieuwenhuijsen, 2004). Occupational therapy practitioners should have a firm understanding of the methods and supportive evidence used in practice so they can relay appropriate information to their clients. Workers must buy into not only the program but also the professional who is leading it.

Task analysis can be used to determine simple and complex factors influencing behaviors. The question should be asked: What can be done to encourage a desired behavior? Solutions might include involving the worker in a decision-making process, keeping items such as mechanical lifts near high-usage areas, and integrating ergonomics programs with other available resources such as employee assistance and wellness programs. Establishing relationships on multiple levels, with employees and upper management, is important in gaining trust and creating a work culture that encourages open discussion.

Moving Forward

Ergonomics is a varied specialty that can be complex in nature. It interweaves and becomes a part of most considerations discussed in this book. Additional study is highly recommended to learn more about detailed ergonomic concepts and application of ergonomic theory. Specialty certification is available through national organizations, and more information can be found in the resources listed at the end of this chapter.

Occupational therapy practitioners are already equipped with many of the primary skills that differentiate the profession in ergonomics. As mentioned previously, a good understanding of anatomy, physiology, biomechanics, disease processes, psychosocial factors, task analysis, and other standard occupational therapy curriculum provides important foundational concepts that are pivotal in both general ergonomics and ergokinesis. Every location, company, person, and work group will present with unique challenges. Although the setting is different from traditional practice areas, many identified goals and outcomes are the same. Develop an understanding of the unique skills occupational therapy practitioners offer and define the value moving forward.

Chapter Summary

Ergonomics is a multifaceted science focusing on the interaction of the person and the environment. Through a systems approach, ergonomics seeks to ensure that the cognitive and physical aspects of the job match the capabilities of the worker. Occupational therapy practitioners uniquely understand how occupational performance can be influenced by the interrelationship of performance skills, context, activity demands, and client factors. In ergonomics, similar elements encompass the system.

Assessment of ergonomic factors include many considerations. Body mechanics and posture can effect muscle fatigue and tissue stress when force is applied outside the base of support. Material handling is important to evaluate because excessive force not handled properly can increase risk of injury. Attention should also be given to repetitive movements and static positions, which can cause inflammation, reduce blood flow, and reduce neural uptake of oxygen. Anthropometrics and several environmental considerations are also important components of ergonomics.

A comprehensive approach to addressing work-injury prevention involves multiple layers. While microergonomics, or traditional ergonomics, focuses primarily on the physical environment, macroergonomics is an organizational structure that addresses the interaction of psychosocial, cognitive, and work structure factors. Work culture, productivity demands, organizational policies, and others encompass macroergonomics. On the opposite side of the spectrum, ergokinesis is a more detailed process focusing on the individual and his or her interaction with the physical, psychosocial, and organizational components of the job. Although additional study is needed in many aspects of a comprehensive ergonomic approach, occupational therapy practitioners have a unique foundation for addressing injury prevention on multiple levels.

Case Resolution

 Based on the recommendations presented by the occupational therapist, Carolyn and the other nursing home decision-makers decided on the following ergonomic and injury prevention measures:

- Three mechanical lifts were immediately purchased, and they set a 5-year plan to fit each patient room with a mechanical lift. The goal at the end of 5 years was to create a no-lift environment to protect both residents and staff.
- A new management system was created to assess resident needs and abilities. This information was used to arrange caseloads for nursing assistants, ensuring a more even distribution of residents according to level of assistance required, cognitive ability, and weight.
- Two initial training sessions for staff and supervisors were scheduled to educate them on biomechanics, injury prevention, early reporting and identification of symptoms, and equipment use. Supervisors were trained to learn how to motivate employees to use the new techniques and mechanical lifts consistently.
- All new hires were required to go through the initial training.
- Before all lifts were purchased, a priority system for using existing lifts was put into place. Available lifts were to be used for high-injury-risk populations (such as maximum transfer assistance and obesity) and kept in a centralized area for easy access.
- For nontransfer patient handling (positioning, turning, dressing, etc.), therapeutic transfers (bearing weight for patients in rehabilitation), and for transfers not considered high risk, staff was required to go through additional training once per year to ensure carryover of learned biomechanics and safety techniques.
- The occupational therapist contacted a colleague at a local gym and coordinated a discount in membership and personal training fees to assist employees in increasing strength and cardiovascular fitness.
- Policies and procedures were put into place on how to handle new injuries and return-to-work issues through injury investigations and root cause analysis.
- The occupational therapist was asked to screen anyone reporting minor discomfort related to their job to assist with early identification and resolution of injuries.
- Light-duty and alternative-duty placements were provided to employees to allow for earlier return to work and graduated work reentry.

The occupational therapist continued to work with Carolyn for continuous improvement. After 5 years, Carolyn reported to her management team that no injuries had occurred over the previous 3 years. Associated cost savings, including cost per claim, overtime, absenteeism, and staff turnover, was in the hundreds of thousands. Employee morale had improved significantly, which resulted in overall improved resident care.

References

American Occupational Therapy Association (AOTA). (2008). Occupational therapy practice framework: Domain and process, 2nd ed. *American Journal of Occupational Therapy, 62,* 625–683.

Barregard, L., Ehrenström, L., & Marcus, K. (2003). Hand-arm vibration syndrome in Swedish car mechanics. *Occupational and Environmental Medicine, 60*(4), 287–294.

Bongers, P. M., Kremer, A. M., & ter Laak, J. (2002). Are psychosocial factors, risk factors for symptoms and signs of the shoulder, elbow, or hand/wrist? A review of the epidemiological literature. *American Journal of Industrial Medicine, 41*(5), 315–342.

Bovenzi, M. (2009). Metrics of whole-body vibration and exposure-response relationship for low back pain in professional drivers: A prospective cohort study. *International Archives of Occupational and Environmental Health, 82*(7), 893–917.

Bovenzi, M., & Hulshof, C. (1999). An updated review of epidemiologic studies on the relationship between exposure to whole-body vibration and low back pain (1986–1997). *International Archives of Occupational and Environmental Health, 72*(6), 351–365.

Bridger, R. S. (2009). *Introduction to Ergonomics.* London: Taylor & Francis.

Butler, D., & Jones, M. A. (1991). *Mobilisation of the Nervous System.* Melbourne, Australia: Churchill Livingstone.

Chebykin, O. Y., Bedny, G. Z., & Karwowski, W. (2008). *Ergonomics and Psychology: Developments in Theory and Practice.* Boca Raton, FL: CRC Press/Taylor and Francis.

Champagne, A., Descarreaux, M., & Lafond, D. (2008). Back and hip extensor muscles fatigue in healthy subjects: Task-dependency effect of two variants of the Sorensen test. *European Spine Journal, 17*(12), 1721–1726.

Dul, J., & Weerdmeester, B. (2008) *Ergonomics for Beginners: A Quick Reference Guide.* Boca Raton, FL: CRC Press.

Fick, F. (2008). Ergonomic assessment and solutions: More than musculoskeletal risk factors. *Work Programs Special Interest Section Quarterly* / American Occupational Therapy Association 22, 1–4.

Genaidy, A. M., Sequeira, R., Rinder, M. M., & A-Rehim, A. D. (2009). Determinants of business sustainability: An ergonomics perspective. *Ergonomics, 52*(3), 273–301.

Gorsche, R., Wiley, J. P., Renger, R., Brant, R., Gemer, T. Y., & Sasyniuk, T. M. (1998). Prevalence and incidence of stenosing flexor tenosynovitis (trigger finger) in a meat-packing plant. *Journal of Occupational and Environmental Medicine, 40*(6), 556–560.

Griffin, M. J. (1990). *Handbook of Human Vibration.* London: Academic Press.

Griffin, M. J., Bovenzi, M., & Nelson, C. M. (2003). Dose-response patterns for vibration-induced white finger. *Occupational and Environmental Medicine, 60*(1), 16–26.

Hendrick, H. W., & Kleiner, B. M. (2002). In H. W. Hendrick and B. M. Kleiner (eds.), *Macroergonomics: Theory, Methods, and Applications.* Mahwah, NJ: Earlbaum.

Hoogendoorn, W. E., Bongers, P. M., de Vet, H. C., Douwes, M., Koes, B. W., Miedema, M. C., et. al. (2000). Flexion and rotation of the trunk and lifting at work are risk factors for low back pain. *Spine, 25*(23), 3087–3092.

Hoops, H., Zhou, B. H., Lu, Y., Solomonow, M., & Patel, V. (2007). Short rest between cyclic flexion periods is a risk factor for a lumbar disorder. *Clinical Biomechanics, 22*(7), 745–757.

International Ergonomics Association. (2000). What is ergonomics? Retrieved from http://www.iea.cc/browse.php?contID=what_is_ergonomics.

Kankaanpää, M., Taimela, S., Laaksonen, D., Hänninen, O., & Airaksinen, O. (1998). Back and hip extensor fatigability in chronic low back pain patients and controls. *Archives of Physical Medicine and Rehabilitation, 79*(4), 412–417.

Karasek, R., & Theorell, T. (1990). *Healthy Work: Stress, Productivity, and the Reconstruction of Working Life.* New York: Basic Books.

Le, B., Davidson, B., Solomonow, D., Zhou, B. H., Lu, Y., Patel, V., & Solomonow, M. (2009). Neuromuscular control of lumbar instability following static work of various loads. *Muscle and Nerve, 39*(1), 71–82.

Lings, S., & Leboeuf-Yde, C. (2000) Whole-body vibration and low back pain: A systematic, critical review of the epidemiological literature 1992–1999. *International Archives of Occupational and Environmental Health, 73*(5), 290–297.

Maltchev, K. (2008). Ergokinesis: A new person-centered approach to ergonomics. Short course presented at AOTA Annual Conference in Long Beach, CA.

MayoClinic.com. (2009). Reynaud's disease. Retrieved from www.mayoclinic.com/health/raynauds-disease/DS00433.

Nakata, A., Ikeda, T., Takahashi, M., Haratani, T., Hojou, M., Fujioka, Y., et. al. (2006). Impact of psychosocial job stress on non-fatal occupational injuries in small and medium-sized enterprises. *American Journal of Industrial Medicine, 49*(8), 658–669.

Navar, D., Zhou, B. H., Lu, Y., & Solomonow, M. (2006). High-repetition cyclic loading is a risk factor for a lumbar disorder. *Muscle and Nerve, 34*(5), 614–622.

Nieuwenhuijsen, E. (2004). Health behavior change among office workers: An exploratory study to prevent repetitive strain injuries. *Work, 23*(3), 215–224.

Occupational Safety and Health Administration (OSHA). (2002). *Hearing Conservation.* Washington, DC: U.S. Department of Labor.

Palmer, K. T., Harris, C. E., Griffin, M. J., Bennett, J., Reading, I., Sampson, M., & Coggon, D. (2008). Case-control study of low-back pain referred for magnetic resonance imaging, with special focus on whole-body vibration. *Scandinavian Journal of Work and Environmental Health. 34*(5), 364–373.

Piscione, J., & Gamet, D. (2006). Effect of mechanical compression due to load carrying on shoulder muscle fatigue during sustained isometric arm abduction: An electromyographic study. *European Journal of Applied Physiology 97*(5), 573–581.

Prichard, M. H., Pugh, N., Wright, I., & Brownless, M. (1999). A vascular basis for repetitive strain injury. *Rheumatology, 38*(7), 636–639.

Rice, V. J. B. (2008). Macroergonomics. In K. Jacobs (ed.), *Ergonomics for Therapists* (pp. 37–45). St. Louis, MO: Mosby.

Sbriccoli, P., Yousuf, K., Kupershtein, I., Solomonow, M., Zhou, B. H., Zhu, M. P., & Lu, Y. (2004). Static load repetition is a risk factor in the development of lumbar cumulative musculoskeletal disorder. *Spine, 29*(23), 2643–2653.

Senge, P. (1990). *The Fifth Discipline.* New York: Doubleday/Currency.

Sengupta, A. K., & Das, B. (2004). Determination of worker physiological cost in workspace reach envelopes. *Ergonomics, 47*(3), 330–342.

Tiemessen, I. J., Hulshof, C. T., & Frings-Dresen, M. H. (2008). Low back pain in drivers exposed to whole-body vibration: Analysis of a dose-response pattern. *Occupational and Environmental Medicine, 65*(10), 667–675.

Wearing, S. C., Hennig, E. M., Byrne, N. M., Steele, J. R., & Hills, A. P. (2006) Musculoskeletal disorders associated with obesity: A biomechanical perspective. *Obesity Reviews, 7*(3), 239–250.

Wikstrom, B. O., Kjellberg, A., & Landstrom, U. (1994). Health effects of long-term occupational exposure to vibration: A review. *International Journal of Industrial Ergonomics, 14*(4), 273–292.

Glossary

Ergonomics is the study of matching work and work tasks to the worker.

Systems are any object, machine, or activity in which the worker must engage and the context in which they function.

Center of gravity is the point at which weight or mass of the body or objects is evenly distributed and balanced.

Neutral posture is a stance that maintains body position over the center of gravity while optimizing muscle and joint functions and keeping the natural curves of the spine without twisting.

Manual handling is any activity involving pushing, pulling, lifting, lowering, or carrying an object or person.

Load is an object or person being lifted, carried, pushed, or pulled.

Anthropometrics is the measurements, sizes, and proportions of the human body.

Noise is a loud or unexpected sound that is unpleasant to the ears.

Flicker is fluctuating light.

Contact stress is pressure where there is occasional or constant contact between a hard surface and a part of the human body, such as the wrists, elbows, fingers, thighs, or feet.

Microergonomics is interaction of humans, objects, and machines; traditional ergonomics.

Macroergonomics is a larger organizational view of ergonomics that allows flexibility in the physical work environment to implement management and organizational factors that promote healthy, safe work practices and performance.

Ergokinesis is application of human anatomy and physiology, body mechanics, disease management, and psychosocial factors as they interact in an occupational environment.

Resources

Occupational Health and Safety Administration (OSHA) Ergonomics

www.osha.gov/SLTC/ergonomics/index.html

Board of Certification in Professional Ergonomics

www.bcpe.org

Ergonomics for Therapists, 3rd ed., by Karen Jacobs (Boston: Butterworth-Heinemann, 2008).

15 Assessing and Modifying the Workplace

Ev Innes

Key Concepts

The following are key concepts addressed in this chapter:

- Two approaches to *work-related assessments* to determine potential risks to workers and intervene to prevent injuries are reviewed: the person-centered approach and the systems approach.
- Ergonomic assessments encompassing a wide range of work analyses that define work demands and identify risks and approaches to ergonomic assessment are described.

Case Introduction

Sharon is an occupational therapist employed by a company that provides injury prevention and ergonomic assessment services to industry to identify existing and potential risks to workers and makes recommendations to address these risks. Sharon has received a number of new referrals that include the following:

- A manufacturing company that has several areas reporting much higher numbers of workers' compensation claims than others. The claims relate to musculoskeletal disorders affecting workers' upper limbs, necks, and backs. The company has requested an assessment of these areas to identify risks and advice on how to control them.
- An aged-care facility that wishes to implement a minimal-manual-handling/no-lift policy and introduce equipment that will assist staff to safely transfer residents. The facility wants to know how much this measure will reduce the risk of injuries associated with manual handling.

Sharon's responsibility is to determine the appropriate assessments that must be conducted in order to assess risks and make appropriate recommendations.

Introduction

Occupational therapy practitioners conduct a range of work-related assessments (WRAs), including workplace assessments (WPAs) and job analyses. WPAs focus on "the interaction between the worker, the job and the work environment . . . in order to identify suitable duties, including an overview of the physical environment, job demands and working conditions" (Innes and Straker, 2002, p. 55). Job analyses are often conducted in conjunction with, or as part of, a WPA and include "analysis of the work demands (intellectual, physical, sensory and perceptual), workstation design, equipment used and the work environment" (p. 56). The need to conduct assessments at the worksite is seen as crucial by occupational therapy practitioners internationally (e.g., Canelón, 1995; Innes, 1997; Joss, 2007; Lysaght, 1997). In New South Wales (NSW), Australia, for example, a return-to-work (RTW) plan for an injured worker cannot be approved unless a WPA has been conducted to ensure that the proposed duties are suitable and the work environment is safe (WorkCover NSW, 2000).

These definitions of WPAs tend to focus on the match between an injured worker, the specific job performed, and the work environment. Occupational therapy practitioners also conduct WPAs to determine potential risks to workers and intervene to prevent injuries. These two approaches have been described by Bohr (1998, p. 230) as either a *person-centered approach* "when the objective is the early identification of the signs and symptoms of a problem or returning the injured worker to the job," or a *systems approach* "if the objective of the analysis is primary prevention . . . [which] affords the opportunity to design or alter work systems to maximize the match between the worker and the system."

Ergonomic assessment "is a more generic term used . . . to describe a wide range of work analyses that define work demands and identify risks. [The term] *ergonomic assessment* implies a process of evaluation without specifying the tools to be used to collect and analyze data" (p. 231).

The focus of this chapter is on ergonomic assessments that may be used by occupational therapy practitioners when conducting WPAs with either a person-centered or systems approach. A range of specific ergonomic assessment tools are described as part of a comprehensive approach to environmental assessment.

Workplace-Based Assessments

From a person-centered approach, a thorough analysis of the client's job, work environment, and skills is necessary to accurately pinpoint areas of match or mismatch, which benefits employers and others (e.g., referring doctor, rehabilitation counselor, insurer, rehabilitation coordinator). Such an analysis and matching reveals areas for the individual client that may require remediation or upgrading. It also assists with the development of appropriate workplace-based rehabilitation programs; selection of suitable duties; and modification of workplace tools/equipment, techniques, and/or environment (Fig. 15.1).

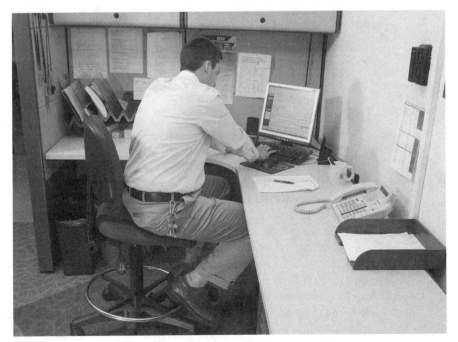

Figure 15.1 WPAs can help determine discrepancies among a worker's abilities, work setting, and tasks to assist in finding the best fit for the worker.

A WPA is a specific occupational rehabilitation service and is defined by WorkCover NSW (2000, p. 3) as:

A specialized on-site assessment of the worker's pre-injury duties and/or potential suitable duties with the same or different employer [in order] to:

- Identify the critical demands of all work tasks (physical, psychological, social, and environmental),
- Establish the work-related performance criteria against which the worker's functional capacity is to be evaluated,
- Identify methods of temporarily or permanently modifying/mitigating the work demands to facilitate a safe return to work, and
- Identify workplace-based strategies, which will assist the worker with restoring his/her tolerance to the available duties.

Both occupational therapy practitioners and physical therapy practitioners have the appropriate competencies for performing WPAs (WorkCover NSW, 2000). The competencies required to perform a WPA include:

- Possessing qualifications and training in relevant health sciences.
- Preparing for the assessment.
- Identifying and assessing duties and tasks that are suitable for the worker:
  - Critical work demands of the preinjury and/or available work tasks are analyzed in terms of:
    - Physical demands.
    - Psychological and cognitive demands.
    - Social demands.
    - Environmental demands.
  - Work-related performance criteria are established from the analyzed duties and tasks.
- Using multiple data sources and data-collection methods to identify and assess duties and tasks (at least three data sources and three data-collection methods must be used).
- Identifying and negotiating methods of temporarily or permanently modifying the demands of the work tasks to address the worker's needs.
- Identifying and negotiating workplace-based strategies to promote functional restoration of the worker.
- Documenting and communicating assessment decisions.

When using a *systems approach* to determine the potential for injury at a workplace and implement a preventive strategy, similar competencies are required. The difference, however, is the ability to identify risks before people have been injured and to recommend strategies and interventions that are appropriate for a wider range of people rather than for just the injured worker.

Workplace-Based Assessment Process

When assessing the workplace, it is essential to gain the confidence and cooperation of all concerned by:

- Informing those persons whose jobs are under analysis why it is being done and what is hoped will be achieved.
- Stating how the information will be collated and used.
- Asking for their contributions—the workers will probably know more about their jobs than you can observe.
- Ensuring good communication at all times among the occupational therapy practitioner, the client, the employer representative(s), rehabilitation coordinators, and union representative(s).

In this way, uncertainties can be answered and the likelihood of better and more accurate information to analyze is increased.

The amount of detail included in the assessment, the presentation of information, and the critical items of information about a job or workplace will vary depending on the purpose for which the results of the assessment/analysis are to be used. Variation must always be considered when data are being assembled, recorded, and reported.

Data-Collection Methods Used in WPAs

A range of methods can be used to conduct WPAs. Any of the methods may be used, but each has advantages and disadvantages that must be considered. Therefore, common practice is to use more than one data-collection method. For example, WorkCover NSW (2000) stipulates that *three or more data-collection methods* must be used when conducting WPAs.

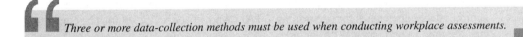

Three or more data-collection methods must be used when conducting workplace assessments.

Using multiple data-collection methods allows occupational therapy practitioners to obtain an overall picture of the situation under evaluation and is consistent with the approach used by ergonomists (Stanton and Young, 2001). Consideration must be given to whether *qualitative* and/or *quantitative* information is required on the basis of the questions that need to be addressed. Quantitative information is produced by "formal measurement processes that rely on technical skill in using the tools available to record measurements and analyzing those measurements mathematically and scientifically" (Bohr, 1998, p. 234). Qualitative information relies "on the synthesis of technical data, descriptive information, research results, and professional judgment to describe parameters that cannot be easily quantified, such as job processes and work flow, work stress, or motivation" (p. 234). Both methods are required for a comprehensive and thorough analysis of a workplace environment and the jobs performed there.

The methods most commonly used are:

- *Observation* (of the job duties, tasks, task elements, work environment).
- *Interview* (with the workers, employer representatives, coworkers).
- *Measurement* (of the job duties, tasks, task elements, work environment).
- *Checklists* and general ergonomic assessments.

Observation

Observation is a method commonly used by occupational therapy practitioners. Observations can provide valuable information on how jobs are performed, including work flow and pace (Bohr, 1998), as well as unique or idiosyncratic aspects that apply only to the particular workplace or job. This method is often used in workplaces where jobs have a high degree of manual or physical input.

Observations should be repeated several times and backed up by interviews to clarify any points as necessary. Occupational therapy practitioners often use digital cameras or camcorders to record job performance and work environments to review information and identify issues that may have been missed during the onsite visit. A wide range of standardized observational tools can be used to provide more detailed information; however, most practitioners do not use these tools when conducting assessments at the worksite. The reasons for limited use of these tools are thought to be due to (1) the time required to apply them and then analyze the data obtained, (2) lack of training and experience using them, and (3) failure of the tools to provide the information required. Some of the most common observation-based tools are described later in this chapter.

When observing at the workplace, practitioners must be aware that their presence may interfere with workers' activities, or the workers' techniques may change as a result of being observed. Observations can be a time-consuming and costly method to obtain data, but it provides more detail about work environments and the jobs performed there.

> *When observing at the workplace, practitioners must be aware that their presence may interfere with workers' activities, or the workers' techniques may change as a result of being observed. Observations can be a time-consuming and costly method to obtain data, but it provides more detail about work environments and the jobs performed there.*

Interviews

As part of a WPA, interviews are usually conducted with individual workers and/or employer representatives (such as the supervisor), then followed up with observation at the workplace. To be effective, the occupational therapy practitioner must understand the job and the workers performing it (Bohr, 1998). Interviews are considered a subjective method of data collection, but they "provide an opportunity to verify job data regarding routine and infrequent job tasks, to gain an understanding of work flow patterns and sequences, and to obtain worker perspectives of physical and mental work stresses" (p. 237).

When using interviews as part of a wider ergonomic analysis, slightly different procedures are used to assess the workplace than when assessing an individual worker. A representative sample of workers and supervisors are interviewed away from the job to gain maximum work activity information. The results of the interviews are recorded in a standardized format. The responses of several interviews are usually combined into a simple job description. Questionnaires may also be used to obtain information from a larger number of people in a consistent manner.

Measurement

Specific tasks, task elements, or functional requirements are measured with a focus on the physical demands of the job. This may include the number of repetitions that occur; heights, weights, dimensions of equipment or the environment; vibration; and specific body postures and movements. Also, the time taken to perform tasks or tolerances required (e.g., sitting, standing) and the distances covered are measured. Environmental measurements may also include measures of lighting, noise, and temperature (Bohr, 1998).

Formal measurements are usually considered to be more objective than observations alone or than information gained via interviews. Formal measurements are strongest when combined with information obtained through observations and interview to reinforce the data obtained. Measurements also provide information that can be compared with regulations and standards. Specific recommendations for change or modification based on accurate measurements can be made rather than "guesstimated." It should be acknowledged that taking formal measurements can interfere with workers' activities, and measurement is a time-consuming and costly method, but the process provides more accurate and detailed data.

> *Formal measurements are strongest when combined with information obtained through observations and interview to reinforce the data obtained.*

Checklists and General Ergonomic Assessment

There are almost as many ergonomic and job analysis checklists as there are practitioners who conduct assessments of work. Checklists have been described as "the ubiquitous method" (Stanton and Young, 2001, p. 1903) and are the most commonly used ergonomic method of analysis (Dempsey, McGorry, and Maynard, 2005; Stanton and Young, 2001). Each occupational therapy practitioner has his or her preferred checklist or has developed a custom-made list based on components from others (Dempsey, et al., 2005). Two main types of checklists have been identified: (1) analysis checklists and (2) action checklists. *Analysis checklists* present a list of items that are analyzed and evaluated by the user. They are useful for inventory purposes to ensure that important aspects of a job or workplace are considered, to identify problem areas, and to compare different jobs or workplaces. *Action checklists* present a list of actions that can be taken to improve the existing designs or conditions and are useful for prioritizing improvement options and training needs (Kogi, 2001).

Checklists rely on the observation skills of the people using them and are often based on subjective assessment that may lack precision. The role of checklists in WPA is "as one of a range of practical evaluation tools for conducting social dialogue between employers, workers, users, and others concerned" (Kogi, 2001, p. 1750). Many occupational health and safety authorities in various countries have a range of checklists available. Many are also published in various ergonomics texts, such as *Kodak's Ergonomic Design for People at Work* (Chengalur, Rodgers, and Bernard, 2004). Examples of two analysis checklists used for job analyses are shown in Figures 15.2 and 15.3.

Other WPA Methods

Other, less common data-collection methods can also be used. These include *activity sampling* and *work participation.*

Activity sampling involves taking a large number of observations made at random intervals during a complete working cycle and provides a snapshot of what the worker is actually doing and how often a task is performed or repeated (see Fig. 15.4). It is considered an accurate method, as the information is obtained over a period of time, however, it is time-consuming and it is still necessary to conduct interviews with workers in order to interpret results.

The work participation method requires the occupational therapy practitioner to perform the work. It is only possible to use this method where the tasks are simple operations requiring little or no instruction, as in the case of some manual or technical tasks (e.g., simple process work, such as assembling two or three components, or packing products). The therapist must learn the job and then work alongside the regular worker. There are obvious safety and training concerns related to this form of assessment, so extreme caution must be used when choosing this method of data collection. While work participation can provide firsthand accurate information, it requires time to learn the job, and the practitioner is unlikely to have the same level of skill and expertise as an experienced worker performing the job.

Assessment of Physical Demands of Jobs

Several surveys have been conducted to identify the ergonomic assessment tools most commonly used by certified professional ergonomists in the United States (Dempsey, et al., 2005) and Canada (Pascual and Naqvi, 2008). Similar surveys have not been conducted with occupational therapists in work-related practice; therefore, the results for ergonomists provide a guide to the types of tools that are commonly used.

Job Task Analysis—Completed for *each* job task in whole work position

Business Division	Site Name	Job Title	Task
	Retail Store	Shelf Packer	Check & Repack Shelves

Task Descripton: Push loaded cages from stock reserve to shop floor, open boxes with box cutter, and remove items to place on shelves. May require help with large items. Shelf height ranges from 15 cm to 180 cm. Weights up to 15 kg for a single person lift.

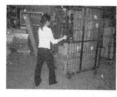 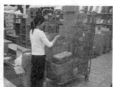 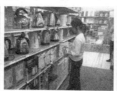 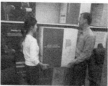

Key Physical Demands

Physical Demands of Task and % of Work Time Allocated	Never 0%	Occasional 1%–33%	Frequent 34%–66%	Constant 67%–100%	Occasional High Frequency	Comments
Sitting	✓					• Note if sustained posture • Opportunity to change postures • Total time in position • Max time before break • Type of seating
Standing			✓			• Not if sustained posture • Opportunity to change postures • Total time in position • Max time before break • Type of floor surface
Walking			✓			• Indicate distance • Max distance • Type of surfaces
Steps/stairs		✓				• Indicate number of steps/stairs • Frequency of climbing
Squatting		✓				• Sustained or repetitive • Associated with which aspects of task?
Kneeling, crawling		✓				• Sustained or repetitive • Distance crawled • Associated with which aspects of task?
Looking up		✓				• Associated with which aspects of task?
Looking down		✓				• Associated with which aspects of task?
Bending spine forward		✓				• Associated with which aspects of task?
Twisting spine to side		✓				• Associated with which aspects of task?
Bending backward	✓					• Associated with which aspects of task?
Working with hands above shoulder height		✓				• Associated with which aspects of task?

Figure 15.2 Example analysis checklist—Retail store shelf packer.

Job Task Analysis—continued

Key Physical Demands

Physical Demands of Task and % of Work Time Allocated	Never 0%	Occasional 1%–33%	Frequent 34%–66%	Constant 67%–100%	Occasional High Frequency	Comments
Reaching forward or sideways >30 cm		✓				• Associated with which aspects of task?
Gripping or grabbing			✓			• Associated with which aspects of task? • Objects gripped/grasped
Fine hand coordination		✓				• Associated with which aspects of task?
Lifting floor to waist		✓				• Indicate weight range (see MH freq chart)
Lifting at waist height		✓				• Indicate weight range (see MH freq chart)
Lifting waist to overhead		✓				• Indicate weight range (see MH freq chart)
Carrying			✓			• Indicate weight range & distance (see MH freq chart)
Pushing		✓				• Indicate weight range & type of floor surface
Pulling		✓				• Indicate weight range & type of floor surface (if appropriate)
Dragging	✓					• Object/time dragged • Distance
Forceful push or pull	✓					• Associated with which aspects of task?
Force using one hand or one side of body		✓				• Associated with which aspects of task?
Exerting force in an awkward posture	✓					• Associated with which aspects of task?
Holding, supporting, or straining	✓					• Associated with which aspects of task?
Exposure to heat	✓					• Describe circumstances • Comment on temperature range • Opportunity for temp control
Exposure to cold	✓					• Describe circumstances • Comment on temperature range • Opportunity for temp control
Other (e.g., exposure to dust, noise)						• Describe circumstances

Figure 15.2—cont'd

Job Task Analysis—continued

Adaptive Devices Available	Brief Description of Use
e.g., carton cutter	e.g., used to cut cardboard boxes open to access goods
e.g., step ladder	e.g., used to place or retrieve goods on high shelves
e.g., wheeled cages	e.g., used to transport multiple boxes of goods up to truck in loading dock

Frequency is defined as follows:
- **Continuous** or **constant**—activity or condition exists 2/3 or more (>67%) of the time (i.e., approximately 5 hours or more of an 8-hour day).
- **Occasional high frequency**—activity or condition exists at a frequent or constant rate (see below), but for short periods of time (indicate length of time this occurs).
- **Frequent**—activity or condition exists from 1/3 to 2/3 (33%–66%) of the time (i.e., approximately 2.5 to 5 hours of an 8-hour day).
- **Infrequent**—activity or condition exists up to 1/3 (<33%) of the time (i.e., less than 2.5 hours of an 8-hour day).

For some tasks it may be more appropriate to consider the number of repetitions performed. **Materials-handling** tasks are those that involve lifting, lowering, carrying, pushing, and pulling. **Nonmaterials-handling** tasks are those that involve repetitive movements not associated with materials handling (e.g., repetitive hand movements, reaching, bending/stooping, squatting/crouching).

Frequency	Materials Handling	Nonmaterials Handling
Infrequent	1–2 repetitions/day	
Occasional	2–32 repetitions/day OR 1–5x/hr OR <1x/10 min	1–100 repetitions/day OR ≤15x/hr OR ≤1x/4 min
Frequent	33–200 repetitions/day OR 6–30x/hr OR 1x/10 min to 1x/2 min	101–800 repetitions/day OR 15–120x/hr OR 1x/4 min to 1x/30 sec
Constant	>200 repetitions/day OR >30x/hr OR >1x/2 min	>800 repetitions/day OR 120x/hr OR ≥1x/30 sec

Based on Blankenship (1994).

Figure 15.2—cont'd

The most common direct measurement techniques were use of grip-and-pinch dynamometers and push/pull force sensors (Dempsey, et al., 2005). The most popular observational techniques included the psychophysical material handling data (also known as Snook/Mital tables, or Liberty Mutual manual materials handling tables), National Institute of Occupational Safety and Health (NIOSH) lifting equation, body discomfort maps, Rapid Upper Limb Assessment (RULA), and Rapid Entire Body Assessment (REBA) (Dempsey, et al., 2005; Pascual and Naqvi, 2008). In the United States, more than 70 percent also used ergonomic checklists (Dempsey, et al., 2005).

The following sections discuss several observational techniques frequently referred to in the literature addressing whole-body postural assessments, manual handling risk assessments, and upper limb posture and hand-use assessments.

Whole-Body Postural Assessment

Manual Tasks Risk Assessment
The Manual Tasks Risk Assessment (ManTRA) was developed to assist health and safety inspectors audit workplaces for compliance with the Queensland Manual Tasks Advisory

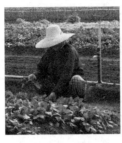 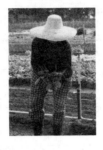 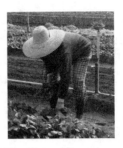

Description:
1. Stand over radish plant and squat or bend at waist while bilaterally reaching forward.
2. With two hands, grasp the plant by its leaves just above the soil.
3. Pull radish from soil.
4. Shake to loosen and remove soil from roots.
5. Secure with a rubber band or plastic tie.
6. Place to the side.

Environment: Outdoors, during daylight hours

Duration: Task performed for up to 2 hours at a time

Equipment: Gloves, hat, sunglasses, boots, and sleeve protectors

Frequency
1. Never 0%
2. Infrequent 1%–25%
3. Occasional 26%–50%
4. Frequent 51%–75%
5. Constant 76%–100%

Physical Demand	Frequency	Comments
Standing	5	Sustained
Reaching: Forward	5	Sustained, also involves twisting and bending at waist
Neck postures: Flexion	5	Sustained
Extension	2	
Rotation	2	
Shoulder postures: Abduction	2	
Flexion	5	Sustained up to 100º through whole task, bilateral
Shoulder postures: Flexion	3	Repetitive, bilateral
Extension	2	
Pronation	3	Repetitive, bilateral
Supination	2	
Fine hand coordination	2	
Gripping/grasping	5	Repetitive
Lifting: Floor-to-knee transfer	2	
Pulling	5	Repetitive, while bent at waist
Forceful push or pull	5	Repetitive, light load
Exposure to extreme temps	5	Work outdoors
Exposure to chemicals	5	Fertilizer and pesticides Low level exposure
Bending	5	Bend at waist with knees slightly bent Lumbar spine: ++flexion Thoracic spine: flexion

Figure 15.3 Example analysis checklist—Pulling and bunching red radish.

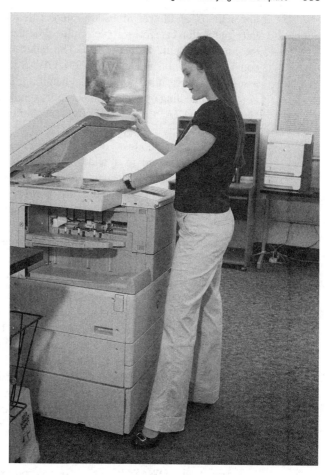

Figure 15.4 Activity sampling can provide a snapshot of the task and the frequency with which it is performed.

Standard and to assess exposure to musculoskeletal risk factors. When used in the workplace, ManTRA is used by a team, including workers who perform the tasks assessed and staff responsible for manual task risk management (Burgess-Limerick, et al., 2004). ManTRA has been used in a variety of workplaces, such as mining, food production, construction, and health (Burgess-Limerick, et al., 2005; Burgess-Limerick, Joy, Straker, Pollock, and Cliff, 2006; Chim, 2006; Straker, Burgess-Limerick, Pollock, and Egeskov, 2004; Torma-Krajewski, Hipes, Steiner, and Burgess-Limerick, 2007).

A task is assessed as a whole rather than as task elements and is based on a specific person's performance of the task, not on people in general. The tool "combines information about the total time for which a person performs the task in a typical day (exposure) and the typical time for which the task is performed without break (duration)" (Burgess-Limerick, et al., 2004, p. 2). Four body regions (lower limbs, back, neck/shoulder, and arm/wrist/hand) are each considered for five characteristics of the task (cycle time, force, speed, awkwardness, and vibration) (Burgess-Limerick et al., 2004). Scores are calculated, and intervention may be indicated if certain critical values are exceeded.

Ovako Working Posture Analyzing System

The Ovako Working Posture Analyzing System (OWAS) was developed as a "practical method for identifying and evaluating poor working postures" (Karhu, et al., 1977, p. 199). It requires observation of work tasks every 30 or 60 seconds, and the postures of the back, upper limbs, and lower limbs are rated. The various posture combinations are classified into four action categories to determine whether intervention is required and how quickly the problem should be addressed. The length of time spent in various postures is also considered (Mattila and Vilkki, 1999). OWAS is considered easy to use and is focused on assessing posture, not risk of manual handling. Therefore, if you wish to determine the risk of manual handling operations, other tools should be used (Pinder and Monnington, 2002), such as ManTRA, the NIOSH lifting equation, or manual handling assessment charts (Health and Safety Executive, 2003).

The OWAS method was originally developed for use in the Finnish steel industry, but it has also been used in a wide range of other areas, including the mining industry (Heinsalmi, 1986); with cleaners, mechanics, construction workers, dairy farmers, nurses (Mattila and Vilkki, 1999); and in the building industry (Monk, 1998), fishing industry (Scott and Lambe, 1996), and seafood retail industry (Weigall and Simpson, 2002). OWAS has also been suggested for use in occupational rehabilitation (Pratt, 1993). Interrater and test–retest (intrarater) reliability of OWAS is considered good (de Bruijn, Engels, and van der Gulden, 1998).

Rapid Entire Body Assessment

The Rapid Entire Body Assessment (REBA) was developed as a postural analysis tool sensitive to the type of unpredictable working postures found in health-care and other service industries (Hignett and McAtamney, 2000). It has been used to assess jobs in health care and hospitals (Hignett and McAtamney, 2000; Janowitz, et al., 2006), supermarkets (Coyle, 2005), and dental professions (Nasl, Hossenini, Shahtaheri, Golbabaei, and Ghasemkhani, 2005). REBA's approach and scoring system are based on the Rapid Upper Limb Assessment (RULA; McAtamney and Corlett, 1993). Scoring is based on trunk, neck and leg postures and load or force (combined score), upper and lower arms, wrist and coupling (combined score), and an activity rating (Hignett and McAtamney, 2000). The assessment results are then converted into recommendations for action (Hignett and McAtamney, 2000; Pinder and Monnington, 2002).

As with the OWAS, REBA is focused on assessment of posture rather than manual handling risk (Pinder and Monnington, 2002). It is sensitive to detecting changes or improvements following ergonomic intervention. However, its focus is biomechanical and workplace changes based on task repetition, length of shifts, and other factors that affect worker performance are not reflected in REBA scores (Coyle, 2005). Initial studies indicate that REBA has acceptable interrater reliability; however, more detailed examination of reliability and validity is recommended by REBA's developers (Hignett and McAtamney, 2000).

Manual Handling Risk Assessment

Manual handling is a common feature of many jobs, so determining the risk associated with this task is usually an essential component of WPAs, both from person-centered and systems perspectives. An extensive and thorough review of the literature on manual handling risk assessment was conducted by Straker (1997), in which he examined the various approaches to manual handling tasks. He differentiated between single and combination manual handling tasks. Single manual handling tasks are lifting, lowering, pushing, pulling, or carrying; combination manual handling tasks "involve a sequence of single tasks such as pulling a box to the edge of a shelf, lifting the box, carrying it to a new shelf, lowering it and pushing it into place" (p. 3).

Straker concluded that a range of approaches and methods are available "to assess the risk in single manual handling tasks. Although there is often consistency between approaches and methods, there are important differences. It therefore appears likely that a range of approaches and methods are needed to adequately capture the risk in any single task manual handling situation" (p. 82).

The approaches used to assess the risks of manual handling tasks include psychophysical (e.g., maximum acceptable weight [MAW]), physiological (e.g., heart rate, energy expenditure/oxygen consumption), biomechanical, and other approaches that include psychological methods (e.g., discomfort, exertion) (Straker, 1997). These psychological methods are often included as psychophysical approaches.

For example, for low- to moderate-frequency lifts (≤ 6/min), the psychophysical method of determining MAW set over a 20- to 40-minute period appears to reflect reasonable physiological loads for most manual handling tasks. Methods to determine MAW include the psychophysical tables developed by Snook and Ciriello (1991), and the combined approach tables by Mital, Nicholson, and Ayoub (1997). These are also called the Snook/Mital tables or Liberty Mutual manual materials handling tables.

Higher lifting frequencies, however, result in physiological loads exceeding recommended limits. Physiological methods using heart rate and energy expenditure are useful only for repetitive tasks of moderate to high frequency (Straker, 1997). Discomfort ratings (visual analogue scale [VAS]), and exertion scales (Borg's Rate of Perceived Exertion [RPE] scale) are useful measures to evaluate tasks performed for short periods of time and require no sophisticated equipment. However, these methods are "potentially affected to some extent by wider factors such as motivation and social situation" (p. 65), as is MAW.

Where resources are plentiful and the task is very important, Straker recommends "direct measurement using psychophysical, physiological and psychological measures in combination with biomechanical modeling" (p. 111). In reality, it is extremely unlikely that practitioners have the luxury of the time and cost involved in applying these approaches, as well as the skill and expertise to use all these methods. It is therefore suggested that where resources are limited or the single manual handling task is uncommon (Fig. 15.5), the tables by Snook and Ciriello (1991) or Mital and colleagues (1997)—that is, the Liberty Mutual manual materials handling tables—are used together with biomechanical modeling (Straker, 1997).

For combination manual handling tasks, the methods available are "direct measurement, estimation from single task assessment by direct substitution, estimation from modeling using single task values, or estimation from modeling using combination task worker and work situation characteristics" (Straker, 1997, p. 108). There are limitations with each of these approaches for combination manual handling tasks, and Straker considers that where there are limited resources there is "little option but to accept a much less accurate method" (p. 113). The options suggested are substitution estimates based on single task methods, but the probable large margin of error must be acknowledged.

Manual Handling Regulations and Codes of Practice

Most developed countries have manual handling regulations or codes of practice endorsed by national occupational health and safety authorities. In the United Kingdom, for example, the Health and Safety Executive provide guidance material on the *Manual Handling Operations Regulations 1992 (as amended)* and have developed Manual Handling Assessment Charts (MAC) to assist employers in assessing the manual handling risk of lifting, carrying, and team handling operations. The MAC is designed to be used by health and safety inspectors to identify the most common risk factors in manual handling tasks and can also be used by others, such as employers, safety officers, and clinicians. It considers load weight and frequency, hand distance from the lower back, trunk twisting and sideways bending, postural constraints, grip on the load, floor surface, and other environmental factors for lifting and carrying. Additional items for carrying are carry distance and obstacles

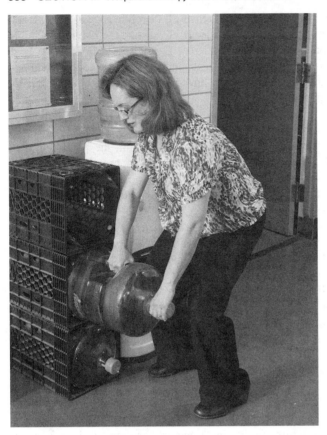

Figure 15.5 Manual handling demands are present in many jobs.

en route; and for team operations, communication, coordination, and control is included (Health and Safety Executive, 2009). A risk score is provided for each item and overall, enabling prioritization of risk control measures.

In Australia, the National Standard and Code of Practice for manual tasks (Australian Safety and Compensation Council, 2007a, 2007b) includes a manual handling risk assessment covering postures and movements, forces, duration, vibration, thermal environment, and work organization and work practices. Where a factor is identified, control options are provided to assist with managing the risk.

Some Australian states also provide additional information on risk assessments regarding manual tasks, including manual handling of people, which has specific risk factors inherent in the tasks performed (Workplace Health and Safety Queensland, 2001; WorkSafe Victoria, 2006).

New Zealand also has a manual handling code of practice (New Zealand Department of Labour, 2001), while the European Agency for Safety and Health at Work (2007) has a checklist for identifying manual handling risks and uses the MAC and Key Indicator Method for more in-depth risk assessment of manual tasks.

All these organizations provide detailed information on how to conduct risk assessments associated with manual tasks, and most also provide suggestions for control measures when risks are identified.

Revised NIOSH Lifting Equation

The United States' revised NIOSH lifting equation is used to calculate a recommended weight limit (RWL) for bilateral lifts in occupational settings. A lifting index (LI) is calculated to determine the physical strain of a specific lifting task: the higher the LI, the greater the risk for low back injury. A number of factors are considered when calculating the equation: horizontal distance of the worker from the load at the start and end of the lift, vertical distance of the load from the floor, vertical displacement of the load, frequency of the lift, duration of the task, degree of trunk rotation, and quality of the handles/coupling available (Waters and Putz-Anderson, 1999). A recent development provides a method for determining a *sequential lifting index* for situations in which "workers rotate between a series of manual lifting rotation slots or elements at specified time intervals during the course of a work shift" (Waters, Lu, and Occhipinti, 2007, p. 1761).

As a tool for practitioners, however, the revised NIOSH lifting equation "far exceeds what most would consider practical in the quick but discerning evaluation of workplace risk factors" (Focht, 2008, p. 184). Therefore, while occupational therapy practitioners need to be aware of the revised NIOSH lifting equation, it is unlikely that many will use it in practice, preferring instead to use faster and simpler tools that nonetheless provide information on manual handling risks.

Seated Tasks

Many jobs now require extended periods of work in seated positions, often at a workstation that involves computer use or interacting in some way with an input device, screen, or other technical device. Adopting a sedentary posture and using computers or other input devices for prolonged periods of time have been associated with a range of musculoskeletal disorders, including back and neck pain and cumulative trauma disorders. With the increased use of technology across the age range, young children at school are also developing musculoskeletal problems associated with computer use, including laptops. It is therefore essential that occupational therapy practitioners are aware of the risks associated with sedentary postures and the seating and equipment requirements for these tasks for people of all ages.

Many tools, usually in the form of checklists, are available for assessing the suitability of the workstation and the postures adopted when using the equipment. Some focus on the suitability of the equipment; others address how the equipment is set up. There was no literature located that recommends one checklist or assessment over another. It is therefore left to practitioners to determine which tool best suits their needs. Many have been developed and/or made available through the national occupational health and safety organizations.

Upper Limb Postural Assessment

Quick Exposure Check

The Quick Exposure Check (QEC) is designed to assess workers' exposure to risks for work-related musculoskeletal disorders of four body areas (back, shoulders and arms, hands and wrists, and neck) before and after an ergonomic intervention (David, et al., 2005; David, et al., 2008; Li and Buckle, 1999). A 3-point scale is used to rate posture, movement frequency, weight, duration, exertion, vibration, and stress (David, et al., 2005; David, et al., 2008). It involves both the practitioner/observer and the workers who have direct experience in performing the job in conducting the assessment and identifying possible areas for change (David, et al., 2005; David, et al., 2008; Li and Buckle, 1999). The QEC "encourages consideration of changes to workstations, tools, equipment and working methods to eliminate, or at least minimize, levels of exposure. This should be done in discussion with the workers(s). Those who have regular involvement in performing the task may have good suggestions for improvement" (David, et al., 2005). The tool focuses primarily on physical workplace factors but also includes the evaluation of psychosocial factors (David et al., 2008).

The QEC has acceptable intraobserver and interobserver reliability and test–retest reliability (David, et al., 2008; Ozcan, Kesiktas, Alptekin, and Ozcan, 2008). Studies of usability and validity show it is applicable and valid for application to a wide range of work activities. The developers report that with practice, tasks can normally be assessed within 10 minutes. While a scoring system is used, further work is required to determine how various scores are interpreted. However, exposure levels have been proposed to guide priorities for intervention, and the developers recommend that practitioners use the scoring system for "before and after" comparisons of exposure to the main risk factors (David, et al., 2008).

Rapid Upper Limb Assessment

The Rapid Upper Limb Assessment (RULA) was developed "to investigate the exposure of individual workers to risk factors associated with work-related upper limb disorders" (McAtamney and Corlett, 1993, p. 91). It is intended for use as a screening tool and as part of a broader ergonomic survey covering epidemiological, physical, mental, environmental, and organizational factors (McAtamney and Corlett, 1993, 1994). RULA assesses biomechanical and postural loading of the whole body, with particular focus on the neck, trunk, and upper limbs.

Deciding at what point of the work cycle to perform a RULA assessment is important. It can be based on the posture held for the longest time, the "worst" posture adopted, or taken at regular intervals over the working period (McAtamney and Corlett, 1994). The postures for the upper arm, lower arm, and wrist and forearm ("wrist twist") are scored. Static loading or repetition and force/load scores are then estimated. This is repeated for the neck, trunk, and legs. Combining these scores produces a grand score used to determine an action level indicating whether the posture is acceptable or requires investigation and change (Corlett, 2001; McAtamney and Corlett, 1993). Right and left upper limbs can be scored separately if necessary. See Figure 15.6 for a RULA score sheet.

RULA was originally developed using workers in the garment-making industry, computer operators, and workers performing a variety of manufacturing tasks (McAtamney and Corlett, 1993, 1994). It has also been used with formwork carpenters (Lee, Chan, and Hui-Chan, 2001), truck drivers (Massaccesi, et al., 2003), in the retail seafood industry (Weigall and Simpson, 2002), in automotive assembly plants (Drinkaus, et al., 2003), and to assess the impact of different mouse positions when doing a computer task (Cook and Kothiyal, 1998).

Construct validity of the RULA method has been established with significant associations between RULA scores and reported pain (Massaccesi, et al., 2003; McAtamney and Corlett, 1993). Interrater reliability indicated "high consistency of scoring" (McAtamney and Corlett, 1993, p. 98).

Strain Index

The Strain Index is a semiquantitative job analysis method used to identify jobs that expose workers to increased risk of developing distal upper extremity (elbow, forearm, wrist, hand) disorders. The Strain Index produces a score representing the product of six task variables: (1) intensity of exertion, (2) duration of exertion, (3) exertions per minute, (4) hand/wrist posture, (5) speed of work, and (6) duration of task per day (Moore and Garg, 1995, 2001). It was originally developed for use in a pork-processing plant and has also been used in turkey processing (Knox and Moore, 2001) and automotive assembly (Drinkaus, et al., 2003).

The Strain Index has good test–retest and interrater reliability (Stephens, Vos, Stevens, and Moore, 2006; Stevens, Vos, Stephens, and Moore, 2004), and has demonstrated predictive validity (Knox and Moore, 2001; Moore and Garg, 1995). When compared to RULA, however, results had very little correlation, indicating that results were not interchangeable and the instruments measured different constructs. It was recommended that if

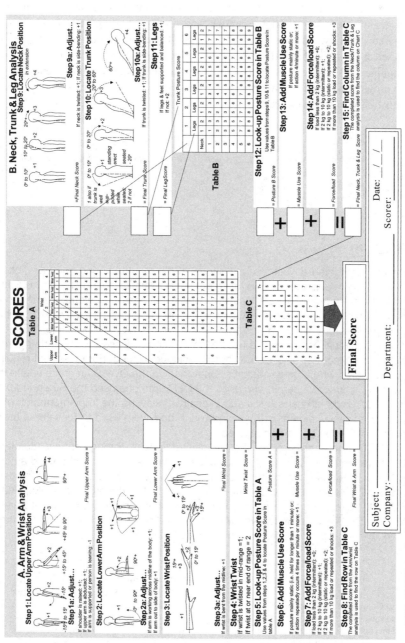

Figure 15.6 RULA score sheet.

the job involved high hand intensity, the Strain Index could be used, while if it involved awkward upper limb postures, the RULA could be used (Drinkaus, et al., 2003).

Chapter Summary

There are many tools available to assess the physical work demands of jobs. Those presented in this chapter include a range of assessment approaches from simple checklists that guide observation to more complex and time-consuming tools with acceptable reliability and validity. Occupational therapy practitioners must consider the referral question and select the tools that will enable them to best answer it. As with any new or different technique or assessment, these tools require practice to develop proficiency; however, they also provide the occupational therapy practitioner with an expanded repertoire of assessments to use in the workplace.

Occupational therapy practitioners must consider the referral question and select the tools that will enable them to best answer it.

Case Resolution

Sharon conducted a walk-through survey of the manufacturing company, observing tasks in the relevant areas and using a checklist (similar to Fig. 15.2) to quickly identify aspects that required a more detailed analysis, interviewing workers and supervisors, and examining injury records. She identified the tasks associated with high incidences of upper limb and back injuries and also those with higher risk of injury. For tasks that required manual handling, she used ManTRA and assessed each worker in the area to determine his or her level of risk for the tasks performed. For tasks that required several static whole body postures, Sharon used the OWAS. In areas where there were upper limb concerns, she used the QEC, and she used the Strain Index when tasks required high hand force and intensity. Following the implementation of recommendations to reduce risk, the assessment tools were used to reevaluate the tasks to determine if the risk had decreased.

In the aged-care facility, Sharon again did a walk-through survey, identifying high-risk tasks and interviewing workers and supervisors. This time she used a checklist specifically focused on manual handling of people, such as the one developed by Workplace Health and Safety Queensland (2001). For the high-risk tasks, Sharon used REBA to assess the postures associated with transferring residents, before and after the introduction of assistive lifting/transferring devices, which were part of the minimal-manual-handling/no-lift program that was introduced.

References

Australian Safety and Compensation Council. (2007a). National code of practice for the prevention of musculoskeletal disorders from performing manual tasks at work. Retrieved from www.safeworkaustralia .gov.au/ NR/rdonlyres/65298783-6262-4D0D-A41D-13296040703D/0/ASCC_ManualTasks_COP.pdf.

Australian Safety and Compensation Council. (2007b). National standard for manual tasks. Retrieved from www.safeworkaustralia.gov.au/NR/rdonlyres/ 514BC761-49D7-4127-A4AD-315735101F3D/0/ 2239DEWRNationalStandards_FINAL.pdf.

Blankenship, K. L. (1994). *The Blankenship System Functional Capacity Evaluation: The Procedure Manual,* 2nd ed. Macon, GA: Blankenship Corporation.

Bohr, P. C. (1998). Work analysis. In P. M. King (ed.), *Sourcebook of Occupational Rehabilitation* (pp. 229–245). New York: Plenum Press.

Burgess-Limerick, R., Dennis, G., Straker, L., Pollock, C., Leveritt, S., & Johnson, S. (2005). Participative ergonomics for manual tasks in coal mining. In *Conference*

Proceedings of the Queensland Mining Industry Health & Safety Conference 2005 (pp. 73–79). Townsville, Qld: Queensland Mining Industry.

Burgess-Limerick, R., Joy, J., Straker, L., Pollock, C., & Cliff, D. (2006). *Implementation of an ergonomics program intervention to prevent musculoskeletal injuries caused by manual tasks* (Coal Services Health & Safety Trust Research Grant Final Report). Brisbane, Qld: University of Queensland.

Burgess-Limerick, R., Straker, L., Pollock, C., & Egeskov, R. (2004). Manual Tasks Risk Assessment Tool (ManTRA) V 2.0. Retrieved from http://ergonomics.uq.edu.au/download/mantra2.pdf.

Canelón, M. F. (1995). Job site analysis facilitates work reintegration. *American Journal of Occupational Therapy, 49*(5), 461–467.

Chengalur, S. N., Rodgers, S. H., & Bernard, T. E. (2004). *Kodak's Ergonomic Design for People at Work,* 2nd ed. Hoboken, NJ: Wiley.

Chim, J. (2006). Ergonomics workload analysis for the prevention of musculoskeletal disorders in food services in the health sector. In HFESA (ed.), *Human Factors & Ergonomics Society of Australia 42nd Annual Conference Proceedings,* University of Technology, UTS, Sydney, November 20–22.

Cook, C. J., & Kothiyal, K. (1998). Influence of mouse position on muscular activity in the neck, shoulder and arm in computer users. *Applied Ergonomics, 29*(6), 439–443.

Corlett, E. N. (2001). Assessing the risk of upper limb disorders. In W. Karwowski (ed.), *International encyclopedia of ergonomics and human factors,* Vol. 3 (pp. 1461–1465). London: Taylor & Francis.

Coyle, A. (2005). Comparison of the Rapid Entire Body Assessment and the New Zealand Manual Handling "Hazard Control Record" for assessment of manual handling hazards in the supermarket industry. *Work, 24*(2), 111–116.

David, G., Woods, V., & Buckle, P. (2005). Further development of the usability and validity of the Quick Exposure Check (QEC). Retrieved from www.hse.gov.uk/research/rrpdf/rr211.pdf.

David, G., Woods, V., Li, G., & Buckle, P. (2008). The development of the Quick Exposure Check (QEC) for assessing exposure to risk factors for work-related musculoskeletal disorders. *Applied Ergonomics, 39*(1), 57–69.

de Bruijn, I., Engels, J. A., & van der Gulden, J. W. J. (1998). A simple method to evaluate the reliability of OWAS observations. *Applied Ergonomics, 29*(4), 281–283.

Dempsey, P. G., McGorry, R. W., & Maynard, W. S. (2005). A survey of tools and methods used by certified professional ergonomists. *Applied Ergonomics, 36*(4), 489–503.

Drinkaus, P., Sesek, R., Bloswick, D. S., Bernard, T., Walton, B., Joseph, B., et al. (2003). Comparison of ergonomic risk assessment outputs from Rapid Upper Limb Assessment and the Strain Index for tasks in automotive assembly plants. *Work, 21*(2), 165–172.

European Agency for Safety and Health at Work. (2007). SLIC risk assessment and training tools on manual handling. Retrieved from http://osha.europa.eu/en/topics/msds/slic/.

Focht, D. (2008). Lifting analysis. In K. Jacobs (ed.), *Ergonomics for Therapists,* 3rd ed. (pp. 173–190). St Louis, MO: Mosby Elsevier.

Health and Safety Executive. (2009). Manual handling assessment chart (MAC) tool. Retrieved from www.hse.gov.uk/msd/mac/.

Health and Safety Executive (Health and Safety Laboratory). (2003). Manual handling assessment charts. Retrieved from www.hse.gov.uk/pubns/indg383.pdf.

Heinsalmi, P. (1986). Method to measure working posture loads at working sites (OWAS). In N. Corlett, J. Wilson, & I. Manenica (eds.), *The Ergonomics of Working Postures* (pp. 100–104). London: Taylor & Francis.

Hignett, S., & McAtamney, L. (2000). Rapid entire body assessment (REBA). *Applied Ergonomics, 31*(2), 201–205.

Innes, E. (1997). Work assessment options and the selection of suitable duties: An Australian perspective. *New Zealand Journal of Occupational Therapy, 48*(1), 14–20.

Innes, E., & Straker, L. (2002). Workplace assessments and functional capacity evaluations: Current practices of therapists in Australia. *Work, 18*(1), 51–66.

Janowitz, I. L., Gillen, M., Ryan, G., Rempel, D., Trupin, L., Swig, L., et al. (2006). Measuring the physical demands of work in hospital settings: Design and implementation of an ergonomics assessment. *Applied Ergonomics, 37*(5), 641–658.

Joss, M. (2007). The importance of job analysis in occupational therapy. *British Journal of Occupational Therapy, 70*(7), 301–303.

Karhu, O., Harkonen, R., Sorvali, P., & Vepsalainen, P. (1981). Observing working postures in industry: Examples of OWAS application. *Applied Ergonomics, 12*(1), 13–17.

Karhu, O., Kansi, P., & Kuorinka, I. (1977). Correcting working postures in industry: A practical method for analysis. *Applied Ergonomics, 8*(4), 199–201.

Knox, K., & Moore, J. S. (2001). Predictive validity of the Strain Index in turkey processing. *Journal of Occupational & Environmental Medicine, 43*(5), 451–462.

Kogi, K. (2001). Basic ergonomics checklists. In W. Karwowski (ed.), *International Encyclopedia of Ergonomics and Human Factors,* Vol. 3 (pp. 1747–1750). London: Taylor & Francis.

Lee, G. K. L., Chan, C. C. H., & Hui-Chan, C. W. Y. (2001). Work profile and functional capacity of formwork carpenters at construction sites. *Disability & Rehabilitation, 23*(1), 9–14.

Li, G., & Buckle, P. (1999). Current techniques for assessing physical exposure to work-related musculoskeletal risks, with emphasis on posture-based methods. *Ergonomics, 42*(5), 674–695.

Lysaght, R. (1997). Job analysis in occupational therapy: Stepping into the complex world of business and industry. *American Journal of Occupational Therapy, 51*(7), 569–575.

Massaccesi, M., Pagnotta, A., Soccetti, A., Masali, M., Masiero, C., & Greco, F. (2003). Investigation of work-related disorders in truck drivers using RULA method. *Applied Ergonomics, 34*(4), 303–307.

Mattila, M., & Vilkki, M. (1999). OWAS methods. In W. Karwowski & W. S. Marras (eds.), *Occupational Ergonomics Handbook* (pp. 447–459). Boca Raton, FL: CRC Press.

McAtamney, L., & Corlett, E. N. (1993). RULA: A survey method for the investigation of work-related upper limb disorders. *Applied Ergonomics, 24*(2), 91–99.

McAtamney, L., & Corlett, N. (1994). R.U.L.A.—A rapid upper limb assessment tool. In S. A. Robertson (ed.), *Contemporary Ergonomics 1994* (pp. 286–291). London: Taylor & Francis.

Mital, A., Nicholson, A. S., & Ayoub, M. M. (1997). *A Guide to Manual Materials Handling,* 2nd ed. London: Taylor & Francis.

Monk, V. (1998). Postural assessment of building industry tasks using the Ovako Working Posture Analysing System. *Journal of Occupational Health & Safety – Australia & New Zealand, 14*(2), 149–155.

Moore, J. S., & Garg, A. (1995). The Strain Index: A proposed method to analyze jobs for risk of distal upper extremity disorders. *American Industrial Hygiene Association Journal, 56*(5), 443–458.

Moore, J. S., & Garg, A. (2001). The Strain Index. In W. Karwowski (ed.), *International Encyclopedia of Ergonomics and Human Factors,* Vol. 3 (pp. 1598–1600). London: Taylor & Francis.

Nasl, S. J., Hossenini, M. H., Shahtaheri, S. J., Golbabaei, F., & Ghasemkhani, M. (2005). Evaluation of ergonomic postures of dental professions by Rapid Entire Body Assessment (REBA), in Birjand, Iran [Farsi]. *Journal of Dentistry, 18*(1), 61.

New Zealand Department of Labour. (2001). Code of practice for manual handling. Retrieved from www.osh.dol.govt.nz/order/catalogue/pdf/manualcode.pdf.

Ozcan, E., Kesiktas, N., Alptekin, K., & Ozcan, E. E. (2008). The reliability of Turkish translation of quick exposure check (QEC) for risk assessment of work related musculoskeletal disorders. *Journal of Back & Musculoskeletal Rehabilitation, 21*(1), 51–56.

Pascual, S. A., & Naqvi, S. (2008). An investigation of ergonomics analysis tools used in industry in the identification of work-related musculoskeletal disorders. *International Journal of Occupational Safety & Ergonomics, 14*(2), 237–245.

Pinder, A. D. J., & Monnington, S. C. (2002). Benchmarking of the manual handling assessment charts (MAC). Retrieved from www.hse.gov.uk/research/hsl_pdf/2002/hsl02-31.pdf.

Pratt, L. (1993). *The modification of OWAS and RULA for use in occupational rehabilitation.* Paper presented at the 29th Annual Conference of the Ergonomics Society of Australia, December 1–3, Perth, WA.

Scott, G. B., & Lambe, N. R. (1996). Working practices in a perchery system, using the OVAKO Working Posture Analyzing System (OWAS). *Applied Ergonomics, 27*(4), 281–284.

Snook, S. H., & Ciriello, V. M. (1991). The design of manual handling tasks: Revised tables of maximum acceptable weights and forces. *Ergonomics, 34*(9), 1197–1213.

Stanton, N. A., & Young, M. S. (2001). A survey of ergonomics methods. In W. Karwowski (ed.), *International Encyclopedia of Ergonomics and Human Factors,* Vol. 3 (pp. 1903–1907). London: Taylor & Francis.

Stephens, J.-P., Vos, G. A., Stevens, E. M. J., & Moore, J. S. (2006). Test–retest repeatability of the Strain Index. *Applied Ergonomics, 37*(3), 275–281.

Stevens, E. M. J., Vos, G. A., Stephens, J.-P., & Moore, J. S. (2004). Inter-rater reliability of the Strain Index. *Journal of Occupational & Environmental Hygiene, 1*(11), 745–751.

Straker, L. (1997). *A Critical Appraisal of Manual Handling Risk Assessment Literature.* Louisville, KY: International Ergonomic Association Press.

Straker, L., Burgess-Limerick, R., Pollock, C., & Egeskov, R. (2004). A randomized and controlled trial of a participative ergonomics intervention to reduce injuries associated with manual tasks: Physical risk and legislative compliance. *Ergonomics, 47*(2), 166–188.

Torma-Krajewski, J., Hipes, C., Steiner, L., & Burgess-Limerick, R. (2007). Ergonomic interventions at Vulcan Materials Company. *Mining Engineering, 59*(11), 54–58.

Waters, T. R., Lu, M. L., & Occhipinti, E. (2007). New procedure for assessing sequential manual lifting jobs using the revised NIOSH lifting equation. *Ergonomics, 50*(11), 1761–1770.

Waters, T. R., & Putz-Anderson, V. (1999). Revised NIOSH lifting equation. In W. Karwowski & W. S. Marras (eds.), *The Occupational Ergonomics Handbook* (pp. 1037–1061). Boca Raton, FL: CRC Press.

Weigall, F., & Simpson, K. (2002). Manual handling methods in the retail seafood industry: Final report. Retrieved from www.workcover.nsw.gov.au/Publications/OHS/ManualHandling/manualhandlingretailseafoodindustry.htm.

WorkCover NSW. (2000). Workplace assessment OR 03 manual for assessors. Retrieved from www.workcover.nsw.gov.au/Publications/WorkersComp/InjuryManagement/Pages/wkplassess.aspx.

Workplace Health and Safety Queensland. (2001). Manual tasks involving the handling of people: Code of practice 2001. Retrieved from www.deir.qld.gov.au/workplace/pdfs/handlingpeople_code2001.pdf.

WorkSafe Victoria. (2006). Transferring people safely. Retrieved from www.worksafe.vic.gov.au/wps/wcm/resources/file/eba01b0b3051426/transferring_people_safely.pdf.

Glossary

Ergonomic assessment is "a more generic term used . . . to describe a wide range of work analyses that define work demands and identify risks. Ergonomic assessment implies a process of evaluation without specifying the tools to be used to collect and analyze data" (Bohr, 1998, p. 231).

Job analysis is "analysis of the work demands (intellectual, physical, sensory, and perceptual), workstation design, equipment used and the work environment" (Innes and Straker, 2002, p. 56).

Workplace assessment (WPA) is "the interaction between the worker, the job, and the work environment . . . in order to identify suitable duties, including an overview of the physical environment, job demands and working conditions" (Innes and Straker, 2002, p. 55).

Resources

National Agencies

Canadian Centre for Occupational Health and Safety (CCOHS)

www.ccohs.ca

European Agency for Safety and Health at Work (EU-OSHA)

osha.europa.eu/en

Health and Safety Executive (HSE) (United Kingdom)

www.hse.gov.uk/index.htm

National Institute of Occupational Safety and Health (NIOSH) (U.S. Centers for Disease Control & Prevention)

www.cdc.gov/NIOSH/

New Zealand Department of Labour—Health and Safety Site

www.osh.dol.govt.nz/index.html

Occupational Safety and Health Administration (OSHA) (U.S. Department of Labor)

www.osha.gov

Safework Australia (Australian Safety and Compensation Council)

http://safeworkaustralia.gov.au

Tools

Liberty Mutual Manual Materials Handling Tables

http://libertymmhtables.libertymutual.com/CM_LMTablesWeb/taskSelection.do?action=initTaskSelection

Rapid Upper Limb Assessment (RULA) (online version)

www.rula.co.uk

WinOWAS (A Computerized System for the Analysis of Work Postures)

http://turva1.me.tut.fi/owas/

Ergonomic Resources and Tools

CUErgo (Cornell University Ergonomics Web)

http://ergo.human.cornell.edu

Humanics Ergonomics—Ergonomics Resources

www.humanics-es.com/recc-ergonomics.htm#tools

Thomas E. Bernard—Analysis Tools for Ergonomists

http://personal.health.usf.edu/tbernard/ergotools/index.html

Kodak's Ergonomic Design for People at Work, 2nd ed. by S. N. Chengalur, S. H. Rodgers, and T. E. Bernard (Hoboken, NJ: Wiley, 2004).

Occupational Therapy Work-Related Policy and Programming

Section IV focuses on key incentives to work and work-related legislation and policy. While much of the focus of these chapters is on policy in the United States, information from countries worldwide is also included. Chapter 16 explains the ADA and provides examples of how occupational therapy practitioners are involved in its application. Chapter 17 reviews key policies and legislation in the United States, Canada, Israel, and the United Kingdom, and discusses how occupational therapy is involved in work-related services in each of these countries. Finally, Chapter 18 describes how work-related program development and marketing can be combined with occupational therapy conceptual practice models and knowledge to develop evidence-based work-related services.

16 The Americans With Disabilities Act (ADA)

Shoshana Shamberg

Key Concepts

The following are key concepts addressed in this chapter:

- The United States has a long history of legislation that has progressively provided increased protection and rights for accessibility for Americans.
- The Americans With Disabilities Act (ADA) consists of five titles addressing different areas of compliance required to eliminate discriminating practices toward persons with disabilities: (1) employment practices, (2) state and local transportation, (3) public accommodations, (4) telecommunications, and (5) miscellaneous provisions.
- A reasonable accommodation is any modification or adjustment to a work environment that enables a qualified applicant or employee with a disability to perform essential job functions.
- Consultation related to the ADA is an expanding area of practice for occupational therapy practitioners.

Case Introduction

Janis Moore is a software engineer and employee of Sonar Tel, a large corporate telephone company. Ms. Moore has worked for Sonar Tel for approximately 8 years. Because of paraplegia resulting from a spinal cord injury sustained 13 years ago, she uses a power wheelchair for mobility inside the building and a manual wheelchair to go to and from work and home. Ms. Moore also has a medical diagnosis of fibromyalgia, which, during acute episodes, impacts her ability to use her hands for tasks such as maneuvering her manual wheelchair, computer keyboarding, holding a telephone, and opening doors. She also has some memory deficits, exacerbated by stress and fatigue, which require her to use compensation techniques.

Helen Smith is a personnel manager for Sonar Tel who previously has worked with multiple employees who had a range of impairments and disabilities that impacted their ability to perform the essential functions of their jobs. Ms. Smith is aware that many accommodations are simple and relatively inexpensive. The costs of accommodations most often are far less than the costs associated with decreased performance and/or the cost of turnover and training of new employees.

Ms. Smith has requested consultation with an occupational therapy practitioner with whom she has worked in the past to address accessibility issues impacting Ms. Moore's ability to perform her job and access her worksite. Sonar Tel is a large company and so has resources to provide accommodations that might not be considered "reasonable" for smaller employers. In consultation with Sonar Tel management, Ms. Smith has asked that accommodations and changes to the environment be identified that might benefit all employees and make it easier to hire and employ persons with disabilities in the future.

Introduction

This chapter introduces occupational therapy practitioners to the Americans With Disability Act (ADA) adopted in the United States in 1990. The chapter also overviews the specialty practice area of accessibility consultation. A historical overview of the ADA provides the framework for examining the potential to expand occupational therapy services in this area. Occupational therapy practitioners have historically advocated for and provided training to assist individuals with disabilities to live independently and to pursue occupational performance in the worker role. Therefore, ADA consulting is a perfect fit with practitioners' existing knowledge and skills base bolstered by additional training in how federal guidelines and legislation guide services and supports. With firm knowledge of the civil rights guaranteed to Americans with disabilities, practitioners can ensure their clients the greatest level of civil rights protection in all aspects of service.

ADA consultation is an expanding area of practice. It can be provided by professionals with various educational and training backgrounds, but the focus on function and performance of occupations in the environment make occupational therapy practitioners particularly well suited for ADA consultation. Some occupational therapy practitioners offer ADA consultation as a major component of their work-related practice, offering service, for example, to companies regarding provision of reasonable accommodations. Other occupational therapy practitioners, such as those who see clients in supported living or vocational preparation or rehabilitation programs, also benefit from understanding the ADA as they help prepare their clients for work settings in which they may request reasonable accommodation.

> *ADA consultation is an expanding area of practice. It can be provided by professionals with various educational and training backgrounds, but the focus on function and performance of occupations in the environment make occupational therapy practitioners particularly well suited for ADA consultation.*

Independent living is defined as control over one's life based on the choice of acceptable options that minimize reliance on others. This includes making decisions about performing everyday activities, such as managing personal and financial affairs, participating in day-to-day life in the community, fulfilling a range of social roles, and making decisions that lead to self-determination and the minimization of physical and psychological dependence on others (Frieden and Cole, 1985).

Occupational therapy practitioners are trained to understand the dynamic interplay between the individual and the environment (see Fig. 16.1). They recommend modifications to facilitate a person's ability to function with the maximum independence in a particular environment, whether work, home, school, or community. The practitioner evaluates the unique requirements of the individual through a comprehensive assessment process, which includes observation of the client's ability to perform daily activities while considering the demands of the environment, need for modification and adaptation, and application of appropriate legislative guidelines to ensure compliance. Each federal law has different applications, and knowledge is crucial to ensure that appropriate recommendations are provided to clients and their support services, including employers, landlords, and social service networks. Making recommendations may involve determining the physical and cognitive skills required for self-care, communication, accessibility, adaptive equipment, and occupational performance. The occupational therapy practitioner's

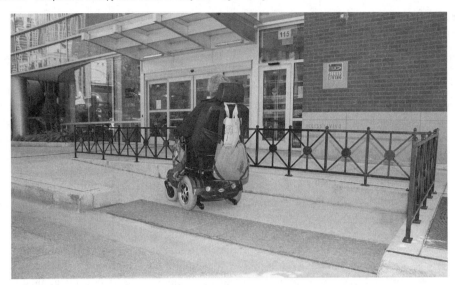

Figure 16.1 Occupational therapy practitioners specially trained in accessibility have knowledge of architectural barriers and environmental design and construction; they can assist organizations in designing accessible entrances and environments.

knowledge of disease, trauma, neurology, movement (kinesiology), psychological function, ergonomics, sociocultural issues, support services, task analysis, and interdisciplinary consultation are crucial to effective provision of ADA consultation services to clients, employers, medical professionals, architects, contractors, designers, and human resource personnel.

Occupational therapy intervention programs in proper body mechanics, injury prevention, work simplification, activities of daily living (ADL), organizational skills, and pain and stress management can also help maximize the client's success at living independently in the community. Removal of physical barriers to ensure accessibility from the home en route to the jobsite or school is crucial.

Jobsite analysis combined with the practitioner's familiarity of environmental barriers and human performance can be used to determine specific accessibility problems and formulate solutions to modify homes, public areas, or workstations to maximize function and safety. Injured workers are guaranteed their right to return to their jobs if they are able to perform their duties. Occupational therapy practitioners employed in work hardening programs have maintained a significant role in assisting employees, employers, and human resource personnel in determining *reasonable accommodations* to enable qualified employees with a physical or mental disability to work. As described by the U.S. Equal Employment Opportunity Commission (EEOC, 2005), reasonable accommodation is "any change or adjustment to a job or work environment that permits a qualified applicant or employee with a disability to participate in the job application process, to perform the essential functions of a job, or to enjoy benefits and privileges of employment equal to those enjoyed by employees without disabilities." Occupational therapy practitioners specially trained in accessibility have knowledge of architectural barriers, environmental design and construction, architectural equipment and installation, accessibility standards, government regulations, and funding sources—and they know when and where to apply this knowledge.

Reasonable accommodations must be identified and considered in context because the resources available to an employer are considered in determining what is reasonable. For example, changes to a work schedule for an employee working for a large company

Table 16.1 Three Examples of Reasonable Accommodations

Problem	Cost	Accommodation Example
Water fountain too high to access from wheelchair	Low	Install paper cup dispenser at accessible height on the side or front of the water fountain.
Door width too narrow for walker or wheelchair to move through comfortably	Medium	Widen doorway to minimum of 36-inch clearance or more. Install electronic door opener.
Entrance is accessed by two landings with 12 steps each. The three-story building has stairways connected at each level	High	Install wheelchair lift on stairs leading to main door and an elevator to access each floor level.

with many workers to support the change is considered reasonable, but it may be considered unreasonable for a small company where the schedule changes require hiring additional employees. A reasonable accommodation is not necessarily the "best," the most expensive solution. For example, if an employee's wheelchair prevents him or her from getting close enough to the desk, a new workstation might be purchased; this might be the accommodation most preferred by the employee, but it would also be expensive. A reasonable and less expensive option would be putting risers on the existing desk to raise its height.

A few additional examples of reasonable accommodations are provided in Table 16.1. In each example, the problem and an accommodation are identified. The first example is low cost, the second is medium cost, and the third is high cost. As mentioned previously, even the high-cost accommodation may be considered reasonable depending on the resources of the employer. The process of identifying, negotiating, and providing reasonable accommodations can be complicated, and practitioners should pursue additional training and education to develop competencies in this area of consultation and practice.

Another critical concept related to determining whether accommodations are reasonable is that of undue hardship. According to the EEOC (2002), a determination of undue hardship should be made on the basis of the following factors:

- The nature and cost of the accommodation needed.
- The overall financial resources of the facility making the reasonable accommodation; the number of persons employed at this facility; the effect on expenses and resources of the facility.
- The overall financial resources, size, number of employees, and type and location of facilities of the employer (if the facility involved in the reasonable accommodation is part of a larger entity).
- The type of operation of the employer, including the structure and functions of the workforce, the geographic separateness, and the administrative or fiscal relationship of the facility involved in making the accommodation to the employer;
- The impact of the accommodation on the operation of the facility

History of Accessibility Legislation

With congressional approval of the ADA in 1990, 43 million Americans with disabilities were awarded civil rights protection through extension of equal rights protection established by the Civil Rights Act of 1964. The ADA is an attempt to correct the many pitfalls of earlier legislation aimed at providing services and rights for people with disabilities and a method of enforcement of specialized regulations through the courts.

Vocational rehabilitation- and disability-related legislation dates back to 1916 when disabled soldiers were awarded rehabilitation services and vocational retraining. In 1920, the Vocational Rehabilitation Act led the way for future legislation in this area. Federal legislation addressing accessibility began in 1954 with the Hospital Survey and Construction Act (or the Hill-Burton Act; Pub.L. 83-565) designed to correct construction and design problems in federally funded hospitals. The Architectural Barriers Act of 1968 (Pub.L. 90-480) created the U.S. Architectural and Transportation Barriers Compliance Board (ATBCB), now known as the Access Board, which was authorized to study architectural design and develop standards for the construction of accessible buildings. Their findings are called the *Minimum Guidelines for Accessible Design (MGRAD)*. The Rehabilitation Act of 1973 (Pub.L. 93-112) expounded the powers of the ATBCB, which was authorized to enforce federal accessibility requirements in federally funded buildings and programs as well as in transportation facilities. These standards, created by representatives from Housing and Urban Development (HUD), General Services Administration (GSA), Department of Defense (DOD), and the U.S. Postal Service, are called the Uniform Federal Access Standards (UFAS). The UFAS is based on MGRAD and guidelines of the American National Standards Institute (ANSI), a private organization. The Fair Housing Act of 1988 established the Fair Housing Act Accessibility Guidelines (FHAAG) for multifamily housing of four units or more and civil rights housing protection for persons with disabilities. The ADA mandates enforcement of accessibility rights in both the public and private sectors. The UFAS and FHAAG were incorporated in establishing the Americans with Disabilities Act Accessibility Guidelines (ADAAG). Title III of the ADA, which covers accessibility of public accommodations, requires the use of ADAAG; however, state and local accessibility regulations must be considered in the design or modification process. The most restrictive regulations are the ones that govern new construction.

The ADA promotes the integration of individuals with disabilities into the mainstream of American society. It seeks to prevent discrimination against persons with disabilities by extending to them the same civil rights protection guaranteed under the law to individuals on the basis of race, creed, sex, national origin, and religion. The ADA extends this protection to employment, public accommodations, state and local government services, transportation, and telecommunications. Employment rights are enforced through the EEOC on a complaint-by-complaint basis. For facilities open to the public, accessibility guidelines created by the ATBCB and accessibility-related complaints are enforced by the U.S. Department of Justice (DOJ).

> *The ADA promotes the integration of individuals with disabilities into the mainstream of American society. It seeks to prevent discrimination against persons with disabilities by extending to them the same civil rights protection guaranteed under the law to individuals on the basis of race, creed, sex, national origin, and religion.*

In the United States, 14 million disabled people are willing and able to work but remain unemployed largely due to environmental barriers limiting their access to the workplace and ability to function at their potential for the job they are qualified to perform (Rehabilitation Research and Training Center, 2009). Four million Americans have mobility problems, 9 million Americans have hearing loss, and 9 million Americans have visual impairments. This population represents a vast reservoir of manpower and consumerism if given equal opportunities to participate in the mainstream of society (i.e., housing, leisure, community services, purchasing products, and employment). Dependence on government assistance can be minimized and quality of life can be maximized by providing equal opportunities for independent living. The removal of environmental and social barriers is the initial step. Access to technology enables a qualified worker with a disability to compete for jobs on an equivalent level as those without disabilities.

ADA Consultation Services

The ADA consists of five titles addressing different areas of compliance required to eliminate discriminating practices toward persons with disabilities: (1) employment practices, (2) state and local transportation, (3) public accommodations, (4) telecommunications, and (5) miscellaneous. Occupational therapy practitioners can provide consultation and intervention in each of these areas. As outlined in the Occupational Therapy Practice Framework: Domain and Process, occupational therapy clients include persons, organizations, and populations (AOTA, 2008). Occupational therapy ADA consultation and intervention is provided with each of these client groups. The following section describes areas of occupational therapy practice consultation and intervention to assist with ADA compliance. Examples of consultation for each of the five titles of the ADA are provided in Table 16.2.

Title I: Employment

Job site analysis is used in the development of job descriptions to identify the following: (1) the essential and marginal functions of a job; (2) environmental, cognitive, and psychological

Table 16.2 Titles of the ADA and Occupational Therapy Consultation

Title of the ADA	Example of Occupational Therapy Consultation
Title I: Employment Practices	Consultation for an adaptable workstation for a computer and other office equipment. Hands-free equipment like phones and intercom systems for communication. Voice-activated environmental control units for lights, doors, and electronic devices.
Title II: Public Accommodations (State and Local Transportation)	Ensure that the local library and courthouse accommodate people with disabilities, especially in providing accessible parking, entry, bathrooms, and computer stations.
Title III: Public Accommodations (and Commercial Facilities)	Ensure all doctor's offices, shopping centers, theaters, and other private businesses open to the public have accessible parking, entry, maneuverability, bathrooms, and so on. See ADAAG for design requirements.
Title IV: Telecommunications	Ensure communications systems (TDD/TTY, fax machine, and relay systems) are accessible to people with impaired hearing. Accessible websites that interface with accessible software and electronic features of computer systems and Internet are required.
Title V: Miscellaneous Provisions	Title V includes technical provisions that guide implications of the other acts, such as anticoercion and antiretaliation provisions for pursuing rights under the ADA.

demands; (3) worksite modifications; and (4) recommendations for assistive devices, adaptive equipment, and auxiliary aids.

Using jobsite analysis data, a written document can be formulated to provide employers with accurate, job-specific information for job applicants and human resource staff. Occupational therapy practitioners consult to human resource personnel on how to use the functional job description as a tool during the interview process. Practitioners can promote sensitivity training to coworkers and supervisors to promote positive interaction and effective working environments with persons with or without disabilities. This can be critical in promoting a smooth entry or return of a person with a disability to the workplace.

Occupational therapy practitioners provide consultation to employers on assessing the occupational performance of individuals to determine their ability to perform essential functions of the job. If accommodations are needed, the practitioner can recommend tasks and worksite modifications and adaptations, specialized equipment, auxiliary aids, job restructuring, and flexible scheduling. Workstations must be safe, organized, efficient, and usable to minimize adverse or excessive movement according to the specific requirements of the worker to prevent injury and to maximize function and independence (see Fig. 16.2). Common elements include location and physical design of the workstation, mobility (steps, ramps, etc.), restroom facilities, hazards, atmospheric conditions, common areas (water fountains, telephones, food services), and emergency services (first aid, fire escape, extinguishers, and alarms).

Occupational therapy practitioners can assist employers in determining whether an individual poses a direct threat to himself or herself and can suggest methods to minimize risks. Injury prevention programs may be implemented through therapy practitioner consultation. This can include developing postoffer, job-related employee screenings and evaluations for high-risk injury positions.

Consultation to rehabilitation counselors and employees can assist in modifying work environments according to the specific functional requirements of an injured worker who is returning to the work place (see James Mueller's *The Workplace Workbook: An Illustrated Guide to Job Accommodation and Assistive Technology* for the design of workstations for specific disabilities). Box 16.1 presents case example of consultation related to Title I.

Title II: State and Local Governments and Transportation

Occupational therapy practitioners can apply their knowledge of accessibility requirements, adaptive equipment, mobility limitations, and communication requirements to create accessible bus, railway, airplane, and subway systems. Because occupational therapy consumers can be individuals, organizations, and/or communities, consultants may also assist libraries, government agencies, and publically funded programs to provide universal

---

Box 16.1   Case Example of ADA Title I, Employment

Michael is a 40-year-old business owner with amyotrophic lateral sclerosis (ALS) who uses a power wheelchair independently but is dependent on transfers, toileting, and feeding. He uses a computer with a mouth stick and trackball. Michael created an office space at home that is visually and electronically networked with his office manager at his business office. They communicate and meet regularly with staff via Skype (remote voice and video communication software) and conference calling. Michael's home office computer is networked to his business office system. He has a flexible schedule to accommodate his ALS needs and caregiving. He can use e-books, scan most documents into the computer, and sign legal papers with an electronic signature.

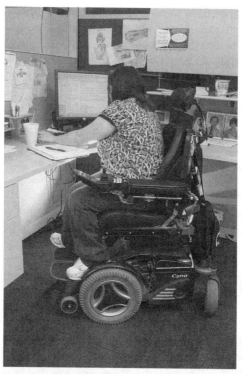

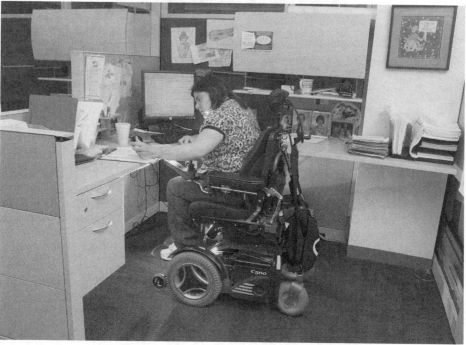

Figure 16.2 Accommodations to workstations, such as raising the height of the desktop, allow an employee who uses a motorized wheelchair to access her desk and computer.

access for people with a wide range of disabilities. Consultants can help consumers identify accommodations to existing systems as well as help to apply principles of universal design to develop accessible systems that support function among persons both with and without disabilities. Principles of universal design are discussed later in this chapter. Box 16.2 presents a case example of consultation related to Title II.

Title III: Public Accommodations

Occupational therapy practitioners can facilitate compliance with ADA's Title III by consulting architects, engineers, contractors, businesses, professional organizations, disability groups, and the consumer to determine how to create accessible environments within the parameters of government guidelines. These places, as specified in the ADA, include settings such as movie theaters, health clubs, restaurants, hotels, office buildings, malls, grocery stores, libraries, physicians' offices, and hospitals. Accessibility of programs, goods, and services means that these places must be able to be approached, entered, and used by all people, including individuals with disabilities. Therapy practitioners can recommend adaptive equipment, auxiliary aids, policy changes, reasonable accommodations (alternative methods of providing equivalent services), and environmental adaptations to remove barriers. Accessibility is crucial to a person's ability to live independently in the community. The application of universal design principles to the construction of homes and public spaces can make those environments safer, more comfortable, and more usable for all persons (see Fig. 16.3). An environment should be adaptable to the changing needs of populations. Box 16.3 presents a case example of consultation related to Title III.

Box 16.2 Case Example of ADA Title II, State and Local Governments

Maxine is a 40-year-old woman with cerebral palsy who uses a power wheelchair for mobility, is employed by the federal government, and uses accessible public transportation to get to and from work. She requires no accommodations other than wheelchair accessibility at work, which has been provided. She lives independently in her own home.

While Maxine was traveling from work to home one day, the bus driver stopped suddenly. Maxine's wheelchair was thrown sideways because the wheelchair tie down was not functioning properly. Maxine's leg was severely bruised. When she told the driver she was in severe pain and needed medical care, he told her he did not have a cell phone and could not help her to access medical care. He left her at the bus stop and told her to obtain help at a fire station a block away.

Maxine's doctor was located nearby, so she went directly to his office for an assessment of her injury. He suggested she go to the emergency room if her leg felt hot or started swelling. She went home and the next morning went to the emergency room in horrible pain. She was diagnosed with cellulitis due to her injury combined with poor circulation, and she was admitted to the hospital—the beginning of months of treatments for continuous infections. Maxine lost her job because of her multiple hospitalizations and inability to work. Her ability to transfer to and from her wheelchair independently was impacted, she never recovered her strength, and she developed shoulder problems due to the physical stress.

The services of an accessibility consultant were obtained by Maxine's personal injury lawyer to determine if there was evidence of negligence by the bus driver, county bus services, and their maintenance of safety procedures and bus equipment. It was determined that the safety equipment on the bus was malfunctioning, and the driver, who should have had a working cell phone, was negligent and inappropriately left the injured customer without assistance for medical care. The Department of Transportation (DOT) provided assistance to the accessibility consultant in determining ADA compliance issues and policies and procedures for dealing with customers with disabilities and emergencies that may arise during transit. Maxine's medical charts were reviewed for preexisting conditions and to determine actual injury due to negligence of the county transit system. Due to the consultation services provided to her lawyer, Maxine obtained a financial settlement for her medical care, loss of employment, and personal injury. The consultation services included a complete analysis of relevant ADA issues and a written report, deposition, and expert witness testimony.

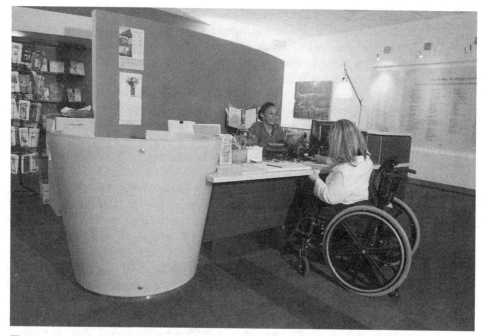

Figure 16.3 This reception desk in an office building is designed to allow a person using a wheelchair to pull up to the desk to complete forms and use the desktop.

Box 16.3   Case Example ADA Title III, Public Accommodations

The services of an accessibility consultant were requested by a local children's museum and its architectural team to determine if accessibility guidelines had been properly applied in the design and construction of the exhibits. The museum was concerned about ADA Title III compliance (regarding architectural design related to a privately funded project) for both children with disabilities and adults who may be accompanying the children in the museum. Title II also was applicable because of state- and local-government funding. In addition, a $5 million grant from the Department of Education placed this project under Section 504 of the Rehabilitation Act for program accessibility. Architectural plans as well as a script describing how to participate in each exhibit was provided, and a small tabletop model of each exhibit was viewed.

The accessibility consultant simulated various disabilities to find any spaces that presented barriers for visitors in relation to ADAAG and UFAS recommendations for ADA and Section 504 compliance. The consultant also reviewed children's accessible design guidelines because the facility was to be used by this population. Program accessibility included the need for alternative formats for written information, sign language interpreters, tactile cues and wayfinding for persons with reading and cognitive disabilities, and additional safety and design considerations for children. Architectural problem areas included lack of a continuous accessible route wide enough for wheelchair and walker access throughout each exhibit; variation of grasping sizes and strength requirements for manipulating exhibit materials; and varying heights of work surfaces, electronic controls, and equipment used in museum activities for different age levels and wheelchair access. The need for equal access to play areas for both able-bodied visitors and wheelchair users and the need for spaces for transfers and maneuvering, adequate lighting to address low vision, and sound absorption for high levels of sounds in open spaces were identified. Services included a written report of the compliance issues, relevant legislation, and ideas to address the needs for specialized populations and situations beyond basic legal compliance guidelines.

Title IV: Telecommunications

The ADA requires that individuals with hearing and speech impairments must be provided the ability to communicate via relay systems and assistive technology (telecommunication devices for the deaf [TDDs], text telephones [TTYs], Braille keyboards, etc.). Occupational therapy practitioners can offer consultation to telecommunications companies on providing the most appropriate devices and training related to visual and auditory impairments. Title IV of the ADA requires telephone companies to provide continued voice transmission relay services that allow people with hearing and speech impairments to communicate over the telephone through a teletypewriter. Telecommunications relay services, or TRS, enables telephone conversations between people with and without hearing or speech disabilities (see Fig. 16.4). TRS relies on communications assistants (CAs) to relay the content of calls between TTY users and traditional handset users (voice users). For example, a TTY user may telephone a voice user by calling a TRS provider (or relay center), where a CA will place the call to the voice user and relay the conversation by transcribing spoken content for the TTY user and reading text aloud for the voice user.

Reasonable accommodations for the hearing impaired might include amplified telephones and other assistive listening devices; visible accommodations to communicate audible alarms and messages; alarms that are both audible and visual; and, for deaf employees who rely on sign language, provision of qualified sign language interpreter services. Further, the ADA requires employers to ensure employees or job applicants with hearing impairment can communicate effectively when necessary (see Fig. 16.5). The key words *when necessary* extend this requirement to include accommodations not only for job tasks but also for special occasions and meetings, training, job evaluations, and communication concerning work, discipline, or job benefits. It also includes regular work-related communication and employee-sponsored benefits and programs. Box 16.4 presents a case example of consultation related to Title IV.

Title V: Miscellaneous Provisions

Title V of the ADA relates to miscellaneous provisions and clarifies application of Titles I through IV. Title V states that both the States and Congress are covered by the ADA. It provides for recovery of legal fees for successful proceedings pursuant to the ADA and establishes a mechanism for technical assistance along with specific instructions to many

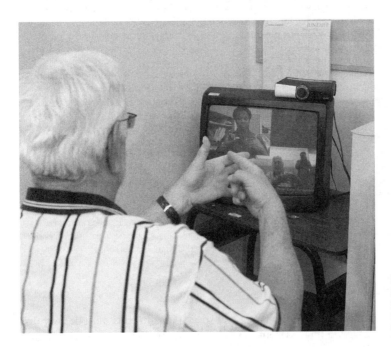

Figure 16.4 Various communication devices allow a person with speech or hearing difficulties to communicate with others in the workplace.

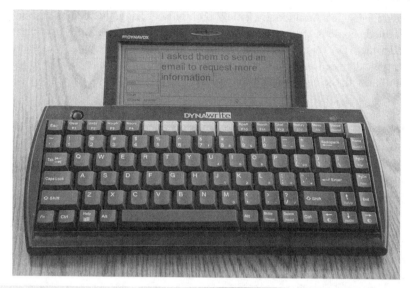

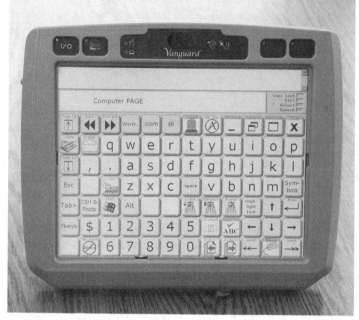

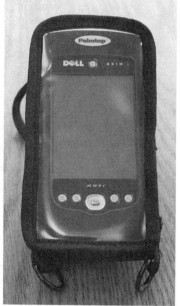

Figure 16.5 Telecommunication relay services or the use of video services allow a person who is deaf or who has a hearing limitation to communicate with others.

Box 16.4 Case Example ADA Title IV, Telecommunications

Dave, a worker with deafness and low vision, was hired by a local furniture company to manage office telemarketing and plan events for customer appreciation days. Dave can provide all communication using an adapted computer and e-mail communication with tracking software with both visual and auditory output. Tactile cues were provided on his keyboard and in the office for labeling drawers and cabinets. Special lighting was installed with adjustable intensity and nonglare bulbs and fixtures. Alternative formats and access for written materials were provided as needed, as were TDD/TTY for communication and a sign language interpreter.

federal agencies. Additionally, Title V prohibits coercing, threatening, or retaliating against disabled people or those attempting to aid people with disabilities in asserting their rights under the ADA (North Carolina State University, 2010). Occupational therapy practitioners typically need not focus on Title V in their consultation service, but they should still be familiar with the civil rights it represents.

Universal Design Applications for Increasing Accessibility

Environments created using the elements of universal design are accessible, adaptable, aesthetic, and affordable; they are barrier-free and provide features that can be used by people with a wide range of abilities and needs across the life span. A universal design approach facilitates occupational performance not only for persons with disabilities but for all persons. An *accessible* environment may be used, approached, and entered easily, especially by persons with disabilities. An *adaptable* environment is one that is built or modified so that adaptation to individual and changing needs can be accomplished without structural change using universal design features. *Life-span design* incorporates accessible and adaptable features for use as occupants grow older to accommodate changes in functional ability. A *barrier-free* environment is built or altered to remove obstacles and maximize accessibility. By modifying the home, workplace, tasks, and behavior, a person can compensate for age-related changes or disability and maximize comfort, safety, and independence.

> *A universal design approach facilitates occupational performance not only for persons with disabilities but for all persons. An* accessible *environment may be used, approached, and entered easily, especially by persons with disabilities. An* adaptable *environment is one that is built or modified so that adaptation to individual and changing needs can be accomplished without structural change using universal design features.*

A public accommodation is considered if all people, including those with disabilities, can approach, enter, and use all points of contact. A partial list of the critical points and requirements set forth in the ADAAG is presented in Box 16.5 and briefly described here (U.S. Access Board, 2002):

- *Accessible route:* An accessible site must have a continuous, unobstructed path connecting all elements and spaces of a building or facility (e.g., route from parking space to the entrance).
- *Signage:* The ADAAG specifies the proportion, size, location, symbol usage, and level of contrast for character signage. Letters must contrast with background and must be raised. Raised letters or numbers used to mark buildings, rooms, or offices must be placed on the right or left of the door between 54 and 66 inches from ground/floor level.
- *Parking spaces:* Accessible parking spaces are required in every parking lot that services employees or visitors according to the number of total spaces for nondisabled. The formula is specified in the ADAAG. The parking spaces must be conveniently located and marked for use by people with disabilities. Accessible spaces must have a minimum width of 12 feet, 5 feet of which serve as a drop-off zone, with a side aisle for wheelchair lift access and side entry to vehicles. The accessible parking area must be connected by an accessible route to an accessible entrance.

> ### Box 16.5   ADA Guideline Points of Contacts
>
> - Accessible ramp/lifts
> - Controls
> - Signage
> - Warning signals
> - Parking spaces
> - Lighting
> - Approaches
> - Public telephone/water fountains
> - Doors/doorways
> - Bathrooms
> - Stairs
> - Automatic teller machines
> - Elevators
> - Floor surfaces, pattern and color contrast, and minimization of perceptual distortions

- *Approaches:* Paths must be a minimum of 36 inches wide. Pathways should be constructed of firm, smooth, nonslip continuous surfaces. Any surface greater in slope than 1 inch within 20 inches in length (1:20, or 5%) is defined as a ramp. Exterior, uncovered ramps should have a maximum slope of 1:20 or 5%. Covered and interior ramps may have a maximum slope of 1:12, or 8%. Ramps must have handrails and curb guards as well as nonslip surfaces. Landings must be provided at the base and top of each ramped area. These landings must be no further than 30 feet apart.
- *Doors and doorways:* A doorway must have a clear opening of 36 inches (32 inches with door open) and must be operable by a single effort. Doorway entrances must be level at grade (1/2 inch or lower threshold) and have an accessible swing clearance. Fire doors are exempt from accessibility guidelines. Turnstile or revolving entrances are not accessible, and an alternative must be provided. Electronically controlled door openers, intercom systems, and other entry devices will provide increased access where needed (see Fig. 16.6).

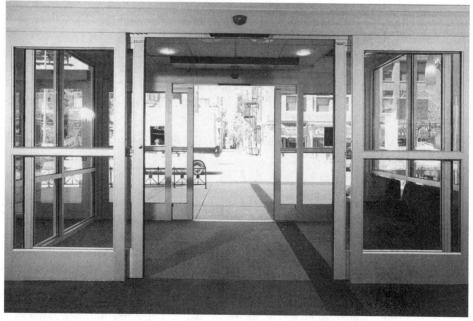

Figure 16.6 Sliding glass doors that operate on sensors and are timed to allow persons who ambulate slowly or who use wheelchairs are one example of universal design.

- *Stairs:* Stairs must have consistent tread and riser dimensions, be equipped with handrails, drain properly, have adequate lighting, and have nonslip surfaces.
- *Elevators:* Elevators should be automatically operated, have a cab door width of at least 32 inches, have protective door and reopening devices, have door and signal timing for hall calls, have a door delay for cab calls, have auditory cues, and have a minimum area required for wheelchair accessibility.
- *Controls:* Switches and controls for light, heat, ventilation, windows, draperies, fire alarms, and all similar controls must be placed within reach of people in wheelchairs, preferably around 42 inches from the floor. Controls on such items as water faucets and door handles must be able to be manipulated using the "closed fist test" (operating a control or handle with only one hand closed in a fist). Levered handles, Good Grips knob adapters, and automatic controls are acceptable under this test for use by people with manipulation and hand impairments.
- *Warning signals:* Warning signals must be both visual and audible and located at appropriate accessible points, as designated by ADAAG. Fire or exit signage must be at least 7 feet from the floor.
- *Lighting:* Adequate, nonglare lighting should be provided with electrical outlets and rocker style or pressure-sensitive switches located at accessible heights.
- *Public telephones/water fountains:* A public telephone must be placed so that the coin slot, dial, and headset can be reached by someone in a wheelchair. Phones for people with hearing impairments should be labeled as such with clear visual operating instructions. Coin slots should not be more than 54 inches off the floor. Similarly, water fountains should be fully accessible. The fountain should not be recessed in a wall, if possible. Its controls should be located at the front of the unit. A wall-mounted unit should not be located more than 36 inches off the floor. An accessible cup dispenser and a telephone amplification device are examples of reasonable accommodations.
- *Bathrooms:* Bathrooms are more susceptible to accidents than are most other environments. The following modifications reduce the likelihood of accidents and increase accessibility: installing grab bars in toilet stalls; rearranging and widening toilet partitions to increase maneuverability; opening clearance under sinks and counters; insulating hot water pipes under sinks; lowering paper dispensers; raising toilet seats and installing accessible flushing levers; lowering mirrors or providing full-length mirrors; installing automatic controls on toilet, sinks, and doors.
- *Automated teller machines:* ATMs must be usable for people with disabilities. Accommodations may be as simple as installing an angled mirror to enable a person in a wheelchair to see the ATM screen, or they may require major redesign and retrofitting of the unit. Tactile cues, Braille, and/or voice prompts must be provided for people with visual impairments.

The U.S. Access Board (2002) provides in-depth specifications (www.access-board.gov/ada).

Therapy Practice Assessment and Application for Specific Disabilities

The most common disabling illnesses that may require accommodation in the workplace include stroke, arthritis, multiple sclerosis, neurological illness, cancer, amputation due to diabetes or injury, respiratory disease, AIDS, and lifelong illness from birth, such as mental retardation, cerebral palsy, spina bifida, and muscular dystrophy. Traumatic injuries include spinal cord injury, brain trauma, hip and limb fractures, back injuries, and hand injuries. Age-related changes also can place a person at risk for accidents and falls because of slower reactions to danger, cognitive difficulties related to memory and problem-solving, limited movement, decreased agility and muscle strength, and visual and hearing deficits.

The occupational therapy practitioner assesses the strengths and weaknesses of a person in the following areas:

- Mobility, balance, body mechanics, strength, and range of motion when reaching, pushing, pulling, bending, lifting, stooping, and turning with or without assistive devices.
- Activity tolerance and endurance.
- Safety and security.
- Environmental obstacles/barriers and their removal.
- Sensory processing including visual perception and acuity, motor skills, hearing and auditory processing, and so on.
- Level of independence in self-care, community living, and occupational tasks.
- Cognitive skills such as memory, impulsivity, perception, problem-solving, concentration, attention span, and comprehension.
- Psychological considerations, including stress management, coping mechanisms, emotional stability, and communication skills related to job tasks.
- Sociocultural issues, including support systems (both those in place and those needed), such as family support, job coaching, community support services, and disability advocacy.
- Installation and use of specialized adaptive equipment and assistive technology.
- Hand function and ability to access and manipulate machinery, equipment, furniture, and so on.
- Employee and employer concerns and medical precautions.

Chapter Summary

The ADA does not require businesses to provide accommodations that impose "undue hardship" on business operations. Designing and implementing accommodations may be simple or complex depending on the limitations of the environment and the abilities of the individual. According to research findings by the Job Accommodations Network, of 890 employers who, over an 18-month period, supplied cost information related to accommodations they had provided, almost half (49.4%) reported that there was no direct cost for the accommodation. Many employers gave changing a work schedule as an example of a no-cost accommodation. The remaining 50.6% said the accommodation they had made resulted in a typical cost of $600. The majority of accommodations that had a cost (84.7%) entailed a one-time only expense. The remaining (15.3%) included either an annual cost or a combination of one-time and annual costs for the accommodation (Schartz, Hendricks, and Blanck, 2006). Thorough assessment by a trained therapy practitioner accessibility consultant of the environment and the person who will function in that environment is crucial to formulating accurate recommendations, installing adaptive equipment, and removing environmental barriers.

Collaboration among occupational therapy practitioners, interior designers, architects, contractors, employers, and employees with disabilities is necessary to create the most functional design solutions in the most cost-effective manner. Collaboration among occupational therapy practitioners and employers, their resource personnel, and employees can help maximize the work environments, increase productivity, reduce hazards and discriminatory practices, and promote positive attitudes concerning disabilities and ADA implementation. Everyone benefits from environments, products, services, and technologies designed for persons with disabilities.

If a task is made easier or an environment accessible, those without disabilities often find the same task or environment more accommodating. Everyone has benefited from the establishment of elevators, curb cuts in sidewalks, and telephone amplification devices, to mention just a few. Advocacy for the removal of social, physical, and psychological barriers in our communities and in our workplaces is an important role for therapy practitioners. Educating the public concerning ADA and its benefit to society is crucial to its success. Occupational therapy practitioners have the knowledge, training, and experience to be excellent resources.

Case Resolution

After Ms. Smith, the personnel manager, requested consultation with an occupational therapy practitioner, the following services related to providing accommodations under the ADA were provided: (1) review of the employee job description to determine functional problems and spaces to be analyzed, including job-related and self-care tasks, architectural elements, office equipment, and environmental barriers impacting access, productivity, and safety; (2) observation of Ms. Moore performing the identified essential functions of her job while accessing parking, ramps, entrances, her workstation, bathrooms, cafeteria, and the copy center; (3) recommendations to the client and employer concerning reasonable accommodations and appropriate assistive technology to eliminate barriers, (4) a written report that included specific ideas for job task and environmental modifications and specialized equipment; and (5) technical assistance resources.

Problem areas identified that influenced performance of essential job requirements included (1) use of a standard computer keyboard, (2) grasping and manipulating the telephone, (3) getting in and out of the office building, and (4) and accessing some office spaces safely and efficiently. Working together, the occupational therapy practitioner, Ms. Smith, and Ms. Moore identified a number of accommodations to be implemented: (1) remodeling a bathroom to improve accessibility for Ms. Moore and all employees, (2) providing a storage area for her supplies and wheelchairs, (3) moving Ms. Smith to a larger workstation cubicle, (4) negotiating a flexible schedule with the ability to work at home, (5) assigning a permanent accessible parking spot, (6) making simple adjustments to her computer workstation, and (7) sharing tasks that involved difficult-to-access locations, such as mailroom and copy center tasks, with other employees.

The recommended solutions included many changes that would benefit users both with and without disabilities and would enable Ms. Moore to perform her job to the best of her ability. These included adapting the ramp slope (20 inches of length for every 1 inch of height) to decrease steepness and installing supports with graspable handrails on both sides of stairs and ramps to improve mobility using her manual wheelchair. Signage on ramps for direction of traffic would enable her to control and minimize the stress of using her manual wheelchair up and down the ramp. Installation of an automatic door opener, as well as an intercom system to call for help if needed, was suggested. In the bathroom, adaptations for safe maneuvering and transfer and for improved hygiene were suggested. Increased space and ergonomic design of her workspace cubicle were suggested to improve efficiency, energy conservation, and body mechanics to prevent further stress and injury. Hands-free equipment was also suggested to minimize stress on her joints and stressful positions. Suggestions for accessing the cafeteria services, vending machines, pay phones, water fountains, elevator controls, and so on, were provided, including a means of calling for assistance and adapting the heights of controls. A flexible work schedule, which included time for her to rest in the middle of the day on a couch located in a quiet, unused storage room, was easily provided. She could easily extend her workday to make up for time needed to rest.

References

American Occupational Therapy Association (AOTA). (2008). Occupational therapy practice framework: Domain and process, 2nd ed. *American Journal of Occupational Therapy, 62,* 625–683.

Americans With Disabilities Act of 1990 (ADA), Pub.L. No. 101-336, §2, 104 Stat. 328 (1991), pp. 101–336.

Freiden, L., & Cole, J. A. (1985). Independence: The ultimate goal of rehabilitation for spinal cord-injured persons. *American Journal of Occupational Therapy, 39*(11), 734–739.

Mueller, J. (1990). *The Workplace Workbook 2.0: An illustrated Guide to Job Accommodations and Assistive Technology.* Washington, DC: Dole Foundation.

North Carolina State University. (2010). Online Americans with Disabilities Act (ADA) Training presented by the Office for Equal Opportunity. Retrieved from www.ncsu .edu/project/oeo-training/ada/title_5.htm.

Rehabilitation Research and Training Center on Disability Statistics and Demographics. (2009). *Annual Disability Statistics Compendium: 2009.* New York: Hunter College. Retrieved from www.disabilitycompendium.org.

Schartz, H. A., Hendricks, D. J., & Blanck, P. (2006). Workplace accommodations: Evidence based outcomes. *Work, 27*(4), 345–354.

U.S. Access Board. (2002). ADA accessibility guidelines for buildings and facilities. Retrieved from www.accessboard.gov/adaag/html/adaag.htm.

U.S. Equal Employment Opportunity Commission (EEOC). (2002). Undue hardship issues. Retrieved from www.eeoc.gov/policy/docs/accommodation.html#undue.

U.S. Equal Employment Opportunity Commission (EEOC). (2005). The ADA: Your employment rights as an individual with a disability. Retrieved from www.eeoc.gov/facts/ada18.html.

Glossary

An **accessible environment** may be used, approached, and entered easily, especially by persons with disabilities.

An **adaptable environment** is one that is built or modified so that adaptation to individual and changing needs can be accomplished without structural change using universal design features.

A **barrier-free** environment is built or altered to remove obstacles and maximize accessibility.

Life-span design incorporates accessible and adaptable features for use as occupants grow older to accommodate changes in functional ability.

Reasonable accommodation is any modification or adjustment to a work environment that enables a qualified applicant or employee with a disability to perform essential job functions.

Resources

ABLEDATA

www.abledata.com

Phone: (800)227-0216
ABLEDATA is a database of information on assistive technology and rehabilitation equipment designed to serve persons with disabilities and rehabilitation professionals.

Abilities OT Services and Seminars

www.aotss.com

Phone: (410)358-7269; e-mail: info@aotss.com
At this site, you can find technical assistance, publications, and Internet and onsite training programs for medical and design/build professionals on home modifications, jobsite modifications, disability legislation compliance, and assistive technology.

Access Board

www.access-board.gov\ada-aba\guidenprm.html

The Access Board has extensive information, publications, and technical assistance services to address the government regulations for compliance with such laws as ADA, the Rehabilitation Act, and the Architectural Barriers Act. A hard copy of accessibility guidelines can be obtained by calling (202)272-5434.

Adaptive Environments Center

www.adaptenv.org

347 Congress Street, Suite 301
Boston, MA 02210
Phone: (617)695-1225; fax: (617)482-8099

American Occupational Therapy Association (AOTA)

www.aota.org

Phone: (800)729-2682
The AOTA site lists of environmental access specialists in occupational therapy by region and sources for technical assistance information on home modifications and assistive technology.

American Society of Interior Designers (ASID)

www.asid.org

608 Massachusetts Avenue, N.E.
Washington, DC 20002-6006
Phone: (202)546-3480; fax: (202)546-3240

American Institute of Architects (AIA)

www.aia.org

1735 New York Avenue, NW
Washington, DC 20006
Phone: (800)AIA-3837; fax: (202)626-7547; e-mail: infocentral@aia.org

Center for Universal Design

www.design.ncsu.edu/cud

The Center for Universal Design is one of the major national resource and educational centers for environmental design for people with disabilities and universal access. The center offers extensive publications and conducts trainings nationwide.

Concrete Change/Visitability Resources

www.concretechange.org

600 Dancing Fox Road
Decatur, GA 30032
Phone: (404)378-7455

Easter Seals

www.easter-seals.org/resources/easy.asp

230 West Monroe Street, Suite 1800
Chicago, IL 60606
Phone: (800)221-6827; (312)726-6200; (312)726-4258 (TTY)

Future Home Foundation

www.thefuturehome.net

12900 Jarrettsville Pike
Phoenix, MD 21131
Phone: (410)666-0086; e-mail: cdavidward@aol.com

HUD USER

www.huduser.org

Publications by HUD focused on housing issues. Most are free or minimal shipping costs.
Phone: (800)245-2691; TDD: (800)483-2209; e-mail: huduser@aspensys.com

IDEA: Center for Inclusive Design & Environmental Access

www.ap.buffalo.edu/~idea/index.html

School of Architecture and Planning
State University of New York at Buffalo
Buffalo, NY 14214-3087
Phone: (716)829-3485; fax: (716)829-3256
This site also hosts the Home Modification list information.

National Association of Home Builders Research Center

www.nahb.com or www.nahbre.org

400 Prince George's Center Boulevard
Upper Marlboro, MD 20774-8731
Phone: (301)249-4000; fax: (301)249-0305

National Resource Center on Supportive Housing & Home Modification

www.homemods.org

University of Southern California
Andrus Gerontology Center
3715 McClintock Avenue
Los Angeles, CA 90089-0191
Phone: (213)740-1364; fax: (213)740-7069

Trace Research and Development Center

www.trace.wisc.edu

This site offers technical assistance, ABLEDATA, product information, publications, and assistive technology resources.

Volunteers for Medical Engineering

www.vme.org

2301 Argonne Dr.
Baltimore, MD 21218(410)243-7495

Government Agencies

Access Board

www.access-board.gov

ADA Barrier Removal Checklist

www.usdoj.gov/crt/ada/racheck.pdf

Equal Employment Opportunity Commission (EEOC)

www.EEOC.gov

Federal Communication Commission (FCC)

(202)632-7260; TDD: (202)632-6999

Department of Transportation (DOT)

www.DOT.gov

U.S. Department of Justice (DOJ)

www.DOJ.gov

National Council on Disability (NCD)

www.ncd.gov

Additional Resources

ADAPT (Advocacy for Independent Living)

www.adapt.org

Adaptive Environments Center

www.adaptenv.org

Association of TECH ACT Programs

www.ataporg.org

DATI Fair Housing and AT Resources

www.dati.org/newsletter/issues/2002n3/MultifamilyConstruction.html

Designing a More Usable World

www.trace.wisc.edu/world

Ramp Building Design Guide

www.design.ncsu.edu/cud/pdf_files/rampbooklet296final.pdf

Rebuilding Together (formerly Christmas in April Program)

www.rebuildingtogether.org

Trace Research and Development Center for Assistive Technology

www.trace.wisc.edu

Volunteers for Medical Engineering

www.vme.org

AARP: Home Modifications Guide

www.aarp.org/families/home_design/

Accessible Home Tour: Assistive Technology Partners

www.uchsc.edu/atp/adapted_home/adapthome.htm

Adaptable Bathrooms Manual

www.abilitycenter.org/webtools/links/adaresources/AdaptableBath.pdf

17 Work Incentives and Policies in the United States and Around the World

Vicki Kaskutas

Contributors: Navah Ratzon and Tal Zimanboda (Israel), Annick Thibodeau (Canada), and Susan Prior (United Kingdom)

Key Concepts

The following are key concepts addressed in this chapter:

- Occupational therapy practitioners must always consider the policy environment when providing work performance assessment, intervention, and prevention services to individuals and populations.
- Workers' compensation benefits vary by state and occupational therapy practitioners must be aware of the variations in coverage.
- Work incentives and public policies that can help individuals with work interruptions in the United States, Canada, Israel, and the United Kingdom.

Case Introduction

The client Rena is a 50-year-old female electrician who has a long history of spinal stenosis with resultant lower extremity numbness while standing. Two months ago, she fell from a ladder while working, sustaining a fracture to her right calcaneus. The fracture has healed, but scar tissue has led to tarsal tunnel syndrome. She is referred to the outpatient work rehabilitation center by an orthopedic surgeon, who has placed no medical restrictions on Rena's return-to-work preparations. The workers' compensation insurance company approves 3 weeks of therapy. Rena takes medication for hypertension, hypothyroidism, and depression. She receives total temporary disability pay from workers' compensation but is worried that her employer will fire her because she has been off work for 2 months. You tell Rena about the Family and Medical Leave Act, which provides for up to 12 weeks of medical leave and protects her from being fired. Because Rena will be returning to work in 3 weeks, the FMLA will protect her position and allow her to take days off work for follow-up medical treatment or to manage symptom fluctuations.

For Rena to tolerate prolonged standing on concrete floors required by her job, a custom foot orthotic is recommended. Referral for orthotic fabrication is requested from the physician, and the workers' compensation case manager is informed. It is close to her return-to-work date, but Rena still cannot tolerate squatting to wire electrical outlets for more than 5 minutes at a time. Using a stool, however, Rena can perform this essential job function without pain, so you recommend that she request a stool from her employer as a reasonable accommodation under the Americans with Disabilities Act.

Rena returns to work as scheduled. Six weeks later, she comes to the clinic for modifications to her foot orthosis by physical therapy. She reports that the stool successfully resolved her problem with low-height work, but the lower extremity numbness and pain from spinal stenosis limits her ability to stand for long periods and to climb ladders and stairs. The occupational therapist suggests that Rena ask for additional accommodations that will help her perform the essential functions of the job but remind her that climbing ladders is a critical job function. She is provided with suggestions for managing her symptoms and advised to consider vocational rehabilitation to train for a less physically demanding job. In the state where Rena was injured, workers' compensation is required to pay for vocational rehabilitation services if the individual is unable to work. Rena states she had hoped to work 4 more years as an electrician so she would be eligible for a full pension; she therefore must consider her options carefully.

Introduction

Individuals with disabling conditions interface with many public policies that can impact their recovery, ranging from provision of medical care to returning to employment. These federal, state, and local policies, laws, and standards also affect the delivery of occupational therapy; therefore, practitioners must be familiar with them and know how to navigate the policy environment. Occupational therapy practitioners must always consider the policy environment when providing work performance assessment, intervention, and prevention services to individuals and populations. This chapter explores the policy environment and discusses the impact that policy may have on day-to-day practice. It presents various categories of policy, including workers' compensation, employment of protected individuals (preventing discrimination in employment), employee leave, disability insurance, workplace safety, and policies the employer must abide by. A discussion of work-related incentives and policies in the United States, Canada, Israel, and the United Kingdom provides a broad view of how various countries manage issues affecting practitioners delivering work-related services. This chapter is a guide to the current policies that affect delivery of services to address work performance, but it must be recognized that policy changes occur over time. Occupational therapy practitioners must stay up to date with the current policy environment in their country, region, and community to best meet the needs of the individual client.

Incentives to Companies That Employ Individuals With Disabilities

The number of individuals with a disability in the workforce remains disproportionately low in the United States. In December 2009, only 36.4 percent of individuals with a disability were in the labor force (U.S. Bureau of Labor Statistics).

Despite many programs and resources for employers and individuals with disabilities, the number of individuals with a disability in the workforce remains disproportionately low in the United States (Fig. 17.1). For example, according to the U.S. Bureau of Labor Statistics (2010), in December 2009, only 36.4 percent of individuals with a disability were in the labor force, versus 82.5 percent for individuals without disability. The unemployment rate (not seasonally adjusted) for individuals with disabilities was 13.8 percent for individuals with a disability compared with 9.5 percent for those with no disability. The U.S. Department of Labor's *Office of Disability Employment Policy* (ODEP) provides leadership on disability employment policies and practices through research yielding authoritative and credible data on employment of people with disabilities. There are several programs to increase employment rates among individuals with disabilities and many resources to assist with hiring individuals with disabilities. The *U.S. Office of Personnel Management* streamlines the hiring process for federal agencies and departments, and ensures U.S. laws protecting the rights of individuals with disabilities, veterans, and others are protected in this process. The *Workforce Recruitment Program for College Students with Disabilities* (WRP) is a resource for federal agencies and private businesses nationwide to identify qualified temporary and permanent employees from a variety of fields. Applicants are highly motivated postsecondary students and recent graduates eager to

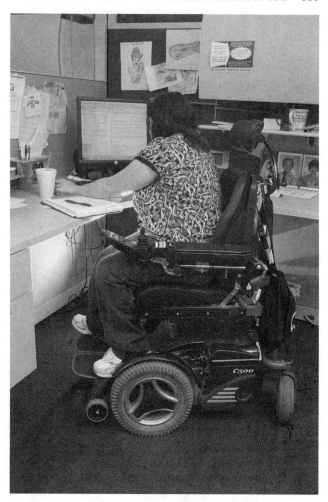

Figure 17.1 Despite laws against discrimination and the existence of incentives for employers, the percentage of persons with disabilities who wish to work who are in the workforce remains much lower than that of persons without disabilities.

prove their abilities in the workforce. The *Employer Assistance and Resource Network* (EARN) provides employers with free consulting services and resources to support the recruitment and hiring of people with disabilities. The Resources section at the end of this chapter lists the website addresses of these and other agencies.

Employers who hire an individual with a disability may be eligible for $2,400 to $15,000 in tax credits to cover the cost of accommodations and to make workplaces accessible. These are described in the IRS Code Section 44. The Disabled Access Credit provides a nonrefundable credit for small businesses (businesses that had $1 million or less in earnings or had no more than 30 full-time employees in the previous year) that incur expenses for the purpose of providing access to persons with disabilities. The Architectural Barrier Removal Tax Deduction encourages businesses of any size to remove architectural and transportation barriers to the mobility of persons with disabilities and the elderly. Businesses may claim a deduction of up to $15,000 a year for qualified expenses for items that normally must be capitalized. The Work Opportunity Credit provides eligible employers with a tax credit up to 40 percent of the first $6,000 of first-year wages of a new employee if the employee is part of a "targeted group" (Internal Revenue Service, 2011).

Individuals With Work-Related Injuries or Illnesses

Many clients referred to occupational therapy for work-related services are eligible for workers' compensation. Workers' compensation provides medical services, temporary wage replacement (TTD), and permanent partial disability (PPD) for individuals who sustained their work injuries or illnesses on the job (Box 17.1). Federal law requires that employers with more than six employees provide services under workers' compensation. Workers' compensation laws are administered at the state level except for federal government employees (covered by the Federal Employees' Compensation Act) and certain other groups, such as employees who work on the navigable waterways (covered by the Longshore and Harbor Workers' Compensation Act).

Workers' compensation laws vary among states; therefore, occupational therapy practitioners must become familiar with the laws in the state(s) where their patients work. Workers' compensation is usually provided by an insurance company, but many large employers are self-insured, which means that the employer, rather than an insurance company, pays the benefits and administers the program. Workers' compensation costs depend on many factors, such as the type of business and previous rate of work injuries. Medical benefits include physician services, diagnostic tests, hospitalization, surgery, and rehabilitation. Workers' compensation costs are managed similarly to health insurance. Choice of medical providers is granted to the individual with the work injury or illness in some states; in other states, the employer makes these choices. The workers' compensation provider may use a third-party administrator to oversee the day-to-day management of the case; this service is often performed with more complicated cases. Case managers may serve as an advocate for the individual with a work injury or illness, explaining the job duties or environment to the physician, explaining the medical condition or plan of care to the employer, or explaining the plan of care or rehabilitation regime to the individual.

In addition to providing the diagnosis, prescribing tests and medications, and deciding the course of treatment, the treating physician is responsible for deciding whether time off of work is necessary. If the physician certifies that the individual is unable to perform his or her work duties because of job-related illness or injury, the employer must provide partial income to help replace lost wages; this is called temporary total disability (TTD). The amount of the income varies among states; 66 percent of customary pay is common. These wages are usually not subject to federal or state income taxes. Most states cap the weekly pay, yet there is a wide range among states. The physician is a critical factor in workers' compensation cases not only for provision of medical care but also for certification of temporary disability. Therefore, the state's workers' compensation law regarding choice of medical providers can impact the overall cost of the claim.

After individuals recover from their work injury or illness, they may still have some long-term functional impairment or disability. Individuals who suffer a permanent loss of function due to the work injury or illness are financially reimbursed for this permanent loss

---

Box 17.1 Workers' Compensation Benefits

Benefits mandated by workers' compensation in all states include:

- Total temporary disability (TTD)
- Fees for medical and rehabilitation services and prescription medications
- Partial permanent disability (PPD)

Some states require additional benefits:

- Vocational rehabilitation

whether they can return to work or not. This is referred to as permanent partial disability (PPD). The method for computing the amount of permanent functional loss and the financial implications varies by state. Traditionally, PPD settlements have been decided by the degree of impairment of the injured body part/system. In some cases, this determination is based on joint range of motion measurements. A more functionally based system is evolving in some regions, with settlement amounts depending on functional abilities and degree of disability, rather than impairment level measures like range of motion. Some states provide vocational rehabilitation for individuals who cannot perform their previous job on a permanent basis. Vocational rehabilitation provides assessment and rehabilitation for a new vocation, including job training, adaptive equipment purchase, modification of job tools and environment, and even college education. It is important for the occupational therapy practitioner to know if vocational rehabilitation is provided under the workers' compensation law, as this may affect the long-term employment plans for the client.

Workers' compensation is a *no-fault law*, meaning that no fault is assumed by either the employer or the injured individual. Individuals cannot sue their employer; however, they can seek legal representation at any point to assist with their claim. Employers may not dismiss individuals because they experienced a workplace injury or illness. However, if the employee was not following workplace safety procedures, disciplinary action may be taken in accordance with the employer's policies. The employer would still be required to provide medical care, TTD, and PPD if indicated. Employees receiving benefits are susceptible to other workplace policies or events, such as dismissal due to prolonged work absence and layoff due to downsizing or closure. It is important for occupational therapy practitioners to encourage clients to explore workplace policies that can impact long-term employment. For example, an individual may be able to prevent job loss due to prolonged work absence by filing for a leave of absence under the Family and Medical Leave Act (FMLA) or taking advantage of a short-term disability policy he or she may have at work or through private insurance.

> *Workers' compensation is a* no-fault law, *meaning that no fault is assumed by either the employer or the injured individual. Individuals cannot sue their employer; however, they can seek legal representation at any point to assist with their claim.*

Occupational therapy practitioners must understand the workers' compensation laws that apply to their patients and become skilled in the nuances of working with these cases. Referral generation may be driven by the case manager, insurance company, or employer in workers' compensation cases; however, the individual with the work injury is always the client. It is important to collaborate with these workers' compensation professionals to provide a customized treatment program to meet the needs of the individual with the work injury or illness. The physician ensures that the client's structural impairments are adequately healed and provides expert opinion as to whether or not performance of on-the-job material handling, work positions, or exposures is contraindicated. Because occupational therapy practitioners are experts in measuring functional abilities and addressing occupational performance, our opinions are often the best predictors of return-to-work capacity. Therefore, practitioners who address work performance issues must have excellent clinical reasoning. Occupational therapy practitioners combine the use of standardized assessments, client performance during work simulations, observations, and information regarding the ability of the workplace to support the client's needs when making return-to-work recommendations. The needs of the employer, insurance company, case manager, and physician are considered, but the primary focus is on the well-being of the individual with the work injury or illness. Because the client sustained his or her injury or illness while performing work duties, it is critical to ensure that return to these customary work tasks will not be harmful to the client. The client should demonstrate that he or she can safely and reliably perform activities at levels of demand that closely match the work duties prior to being returned to work. It is important for occupational therapy practitioners to balance the need to increase the client's capacity to levels competitive at work with ensuring that he or she is not exposed to factors that could prevent healing or be potentially harmful. Individuals may not always be able to use proper body mechanics or work methods while performing job duties due to longstanding habits, structural changes, muscle fatigue, job demands, or workplace factors; therefore, the therapist helps the client identify practical solutions that promote both productivity and safety.

Because occupational therapists are experts in measuring functional abilities and addressing occupational performance, our opinions are often the best predictors of return-to-work capacity.

Individuals dealing with work injuries or illnesses often face many stressors in addition to the structural and functional impairments due to their diagnoses. These stressors include the inability to work or perform other required roles in the home and community, interruption of habits and routines, loss of social support systems that existed at the workplace, decreased income and the negative consequences of financial limitations, potential long-term disability, and the emotional consequences and strain that revolve around all of these life changes. It is important for the occupational therapy practitioner to identify issues that are critical to each client and address all of these issues that are within the scope of practice as described by the Occupational Therapy Practice Framework: Domain and Process (AOTA, 2008). Occupational therapy practitioners are uniquely qualified and well prepared to address the broad range of issues that must be managed in workers' compensation cases. To optimize clients' occupational performance at work, practitioners may need to draw on multiple approaches and frames of references or conceptual practice models, such as cognitive-behavioral, empowerment, social learning, environmental, and biomechanical approaches. Practitioners may need to advocate to the insurance company or employer to get payment and resources to address the wide range of problems that prevent the client from returning to work, be they physical, emotional, health-maintenance related, environmental, or job specific. This may include advocating for additional therapy visits, coverage of a broader range of procedural codes, use of workplace tools during rehabilitation, negotiated work schedules, environmental modifications at the workplace, or changes in work duties or methods.

Individuals dealing with work injuries or illnesses often face many stressors in addition to the structural and functional impairments due to their diagnoses. These stressors include the inability to work or perform other required roles in the home and community, interruption of habits and routines, loss of social support systems that existed at the workplace, decreased income and the negative consequences of financial limitations, potential long-term disability, and the emotional consequences and strain that revolve around all of these life changes.

In some cases, adversarial relationships can develop during a workers' compensation case. Since the employer's cost for workers' compensation insurance depends on the number and severity of workers' compensation claims, many employers prefer injured workers return to work quickly to prevent prolonged temporary total disability, and insurance companies closely manage the medical and rehabilitation expenses. In an effort to keep staffing levels optimal and prevent loss of full wages, employers may modify the work duties or schedule to accommodate decreased work capacities of the individual; however, they are not required to make accommodations for individuals with temporary disabilities. For example, an employer may assign an injured worker to alternative work duties that are within the individual's limited physical capacities. The employee may perceive this as not allowing adequate time to recover, but there are many negative consequences of prolonged work disability. An employer who does not maintain contact with the individual may be perceived as neglecting him or her; however, the employer may not want the individual to feel forced to share medical information or to feel pressured to return to work. On the other hand, an employee may be anxious to return to work in a limited capacity, but the employer may not allow this.

Medical care is another area that can lead to misunderstandings. The injured individual may prefer his or her family physician to provide care, whereas the employer may use a specific occupational medicine physician due to the physician's expertise in treating work injuries or a keen knowledge of the work demands. However, the individual may have a therapeutic relationship with his or her family physician that may prove to be beneficial in managing the widespread effects of some work injuries and illnesses. Occupational therapy practitioners need to maintain neutrality and objectivity with all parties involved in a workers' compensation claim, yet always be an advocate for the client. Often, advice the client receives from his or her attorney, friends, or family members facilitates inactivity, negative feelings, and depression; therefore, the therapist may be the only individual in the client's life to promote well-being. By helping the individual maintain a positive attitude and by avoiding entanglement in adversarial relationships, the therapist can promote proactive problem-solving, occupational performance, and overall well-being.

Occupational therapy practitioners must be detail oriented and vigilant in documentation of workers' compensation cases. Occasionally, occupational therapy records are deposed or the practitioner must testify in workers' compensation cases. Practitioners must comply with any subpoenas and may require legal advice. Many of the policies discussed in this chapter may also affect a client with a work injury or illness, such as the Americans with Disability Act (ADA), FMLA, and Social Security Disability Insurance (SSDI). It is of utmost importance that occupational therapy practitioners working with individuals with work injuries or illnesses are well versed in these policies and learn how to help their clients navigate through the often confusing policy environment.

Employment of Protected Populations

The United States has in place many policies to prevent employment discrimination of specific categories of individuals, including age, race, sex, disability, and religion (Box 17.2). These laws affect employers with 15 or more employees and are governed by the Equal Employment Opportunity Commission (EEOC). These policies are important for new employees, individuals returning to work after work-related injury or illness, individuals with health conditions or disabilities, and individuals participating in rehabilitation services.

> **Box 17.2 Select U.S. Employment Policies Relevant to Occupational Therapy Practitioners**
>
> - Title VII of the Civil Rights Act of 1964
> - Civil Service Reform Act of 1978
> - Pregnancy Discrimination Act of 1978
> - Age Discrimination in Employment Act of 1967
> - Americans with Disabilities Act of 1990
> - Americans with Disabilities Amendments Act of 2008
> - Rehabilitation Act of 1973
> - Genetic Information Nondiscrimination Act of 2008
> - Vietnam Era Veterans' Readjustment Assistance Act of 1972
> - Uniformed Services Employment and Reemployment Rights Act of 1994
> - Education and Employment Program Amendments of 1991
> - Fair Labor Standards Act of 1938

Title VII of the *Civil Rights Act of 1964* states that employers are not allowed to make employment decisions based on sex, race, or religion. The *Civil Service Reform Act of 1978* requires fair and equitable treatment in all aspects of personnel management without regard to political affiliation, race, color, religion, national origin, sex, marital status, age, or disabling condition. The *Pregnancy Discrimination Act of 1978* prohibits sex discrimination on the basis of pregnancy, childbirth, or related medical conditions. It is important for occupational therapy practitioners to understand these employment laws and their impact on work services. For employment testing, this means that testing protocols cannot be gender biased; therefore, material-handling tests of strength must treat males and females the same. If a job requires individuals to be able to perform tasks on high surfaces or to lift heavy weights, males may perform more successfully than females because of their body size, which is not discriminatory if the test is based on actual job demands. However, assessments that advance the amount of weight lifted for males and females at different rates based on gender are discriminatory. Assessments that use gender-driven norms may also be considered discriminatory; therefore, it is more appropriate to use criterion-referenced assessments for employment decisions. The occupational therapy practitioner must always ensure the safety of individuals participating in return-to-work or preemployment testing. These decisions must be performance driven and not gender based.

The *Age Discrimination in Employment Act of 1967* protects individuals 40 years of age and older from employment discrimination. Assessments and rehabilitation programs must be delivered consistently to individuals of all ages (Fig. 17.2). Occupational therapy practitioners must carefully interpret assessment results that use age-referenced norms; criterion-referenced tests based on actual job requirements are preferred. For example, some cognitive assessments adjust for age by awarding extra points to individuals over a certain age, and some physical assessments use age-referenced norms. Physiological changes do occur as a result of the maturation process. With age, bone, muscle, and tendons heal at different rates; muscle fiber content changes; the nervous system becomes less plastic; the brain changes; and agility, balance, and coordination may decrease. Many individuals develop age-related health conditions, such as osteoarthritis, cardiovascular disease, or Alzheimer's disease, that can complicate recovery from illness or injury and interfere with ability to work. Although occupational therapy practitioners cannot assume these age-related conditions and changes are present or the same among individuals, it is their responsibility to ensure the safety of clients at all times during assessment and rehabilitation. As it is for all individuals, it is important to screen aging clients to identify structural and functional impairments before subjecting them to work performance testing. However, this screening cannot discriminate against older individuals in any way.

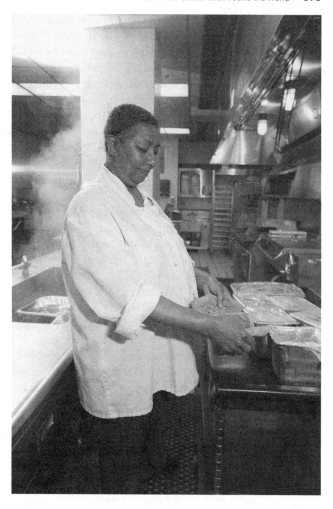

Figure 17.2 The Age Discrimination in Employment Act of 1967 protects the rights of older workers in the workplace.

The *Americans with Disabilities Act of 1990* is addressed in detail in Chapter 16. It is essential for the occupational therapy practitioner to understand the effects of the ADA on day-to-day work practice. Section 501 of the *Rehabilitation Act of 1973*, a precursor to the ADA, prevents employment discrimination of individuals with disabilities by federal agencies and programs receiving federal funding. All benefits under this act are similar to the ADA, but they apply to private employers; therefore, occupational therapy practitioners can defer to the ADA. It is the occupational therapy practitioner's responsibility to provide reasonable accommodations during testing and rehabilitation with individuals with qualified disabilities who can perform the essential functions of the job. Whether writing job descriptions, designing or performing postoffer preemployment screens, administering functional capacity evaluations, or delivering rehabilitation programs, practitioners must ensure that protocols, equipment, environments, and facilities do not discriminate against individuals with disabilities in any manner. Individuals with qualified disabilities who can perform the essential functions of the job must be provided with reasonable accommodations both in the occupational therapy clinic and the workplace. It is the occupational therapy practitioner's responsibility to help individuals identify the accommodations that are needed and to help the client advocate for these accommodations. Please refer to Chapter 16 for further details about the Americans with Disabilities Act.

The *Genetic Information Nondiscrimination Act of 2008* (GINA) is a new law that prohibits discrimination by health insurers and employers based on individuals' genetic information. Genetic information includes the results of genetic tests to determine whether someone is at increased risk of acquiring a condition (such as some forms of breast cancer) in the future as well as an individual's family medical history. The law prohibits the use of genetic information in making employment decisions, restricts the acquisition of genetic information by employers and others, imposes strict confidentiality requirements, and prohibits retaliation against individuals who oppose actions made unlawful by GINA or who participate in proceedings to vindicate rights under the law or aid others in doing so. The same remedies available under Title VII of the Civil Rights Act and the ADA, including compensatory and punitive damages, are also available under Title II of GINA. Although the effects of this law on provision of occupational therapy may be limited, it is important for practitioners to realize the existence of this new law.

Several laws promote employment and job advancement of veterans, including employment within the federal government of disabled veterans expanded job opportunities for veterans and disabled veterans, and veterans with service-connected disabilities. The *Vietnam Era Veterans' Readjustment Assistance Act* (VEVRAA) requires employers that have federal contracts or subcontracts entered into before December 1, 2003, of $25,000 or more and/or federal contracts or subcontracts entered into on or after December 1, 2003, of $100,000 or more to provide equal employment opportunities for certain veterans with disabilities. VEVRAA specifically prohibits discrimination against covered veterans with disabilities in the full range of employment activities. The *Uniformed Services Employment and Reemployment Rights Act of 1994* (USERRA) prohibits employment discrimination against a person on the basis of past military service, current military obligations, or intent to serve (www.dol.gov/vets/programs/userra/main.htm). The *Veterans Education and Employment Program Amendments of 1991* require expanded job opportunities for veterans and disabled veterans. Occupational therapy practitioners working with veterans should explore these laws in more detail and consider their possible effect on preemployment services, return-to-work programs, and rehabilitation. Given the recent influx in young veterans of employment age, excellent opportunities for occupational therapy practitioners to provide work services with this population exist.

The *Fair Labor Standards Act of 1938* (FLSA) and its subsequent amendments establish minimum wage, youth employment standards, and wages for workers with disabilities. The FLSA establishes 18 years as the minimum age for employment based upon job and hours. Minors ages 16 to 17 years may work an unrestricted number of hours in nonhazardous jobs (FLSA defines specific dangerous occupations). Minors ages 14 to 15 years may work outside of school hours in nonhazardous jobs in retail, food service, and gasoline service establishments. Work hours are limited to no more than 3 hours on a school day, 18 hours in a school week (23 hours for those enrolled in approved work experience and career exploration programs), 8 hours on a non–school day, or 40 hours in a non–school week. Minors of any age may deliver newspapers; perform in radio, television, movies, or theatrical productions; work for their parents in their solely owned nonfarm businesses (except at jobs deemed hazardous); or gather evergreens and make evergreen wreaths. The FLSA also authorizes employers who receive a certificate from the U.S. Department of Labor's Wage and Hour Division to pay wages less than the federal minimum wage to workers who have disabilities. The special minimum wage is based on the productivity of the individual worker as compared to experienced workers who do not have disabilities who perform essentially the same type, quality, and quantity of work in the same geographic area. Occupational therapy practitioners working with youth and individuals with disabilities must be familiar with details of the FLSA and understand its effects on provision of work programming.

Policies for Medical Leave

The *Family and Medical Leave Act* provides individuals with up to 12 weeks of medical leave in a 12-month period for serious health conditions of the employee or a member of his or her immediate family (child, spouse, or parent). The leave may be taken intermittently or on a reduced leave schedule when medically necessary. Employers must continue employee health insurance benefits during the leave and restore employees to the same or equivalent position upon completion of the leave. The individual does not receive pay for the medical leave, but he or she may use accrued sick or vacation pay. It is important for individuals dealing with medical conditions to abide by their employer's absentee policies to prevent job loss during recuperation. Private employers with 50 or more employees working within 75 miles of the employee's worksite must provide leave under the FMLA, as must all public agencies and private and public elementary and secondary schools, regardless of the number of employees. Employees are eligible to take FMLA leave if they have worked for their employer at least 12 months and have worked for at least 1,250 hours over the 12 months immediately prior to the leave. The U.S. Department of Labor enforces the FMLA.

In addition to the federal law requiring FMLA, several states have enacted their own family and medical leave laws. The amount of leave and benefits and the criteria for eligibility varies for many of these state-enacted medical leave laws; therefore, practitioners must research these laws in their state. Because employers are not required to hold employment for individuals who are dealing with health conditions who do not file for leave under the FMLA, it is important for occupational therapy practitioners to ensure that clients understand the FMLA and file for it in a timely manner.

Disability Payment Programs

Individuals with disabilities who are unable to work may qualify for disability pay under federally mandated programs, such as *Supplemental Security Income (SSI)* and *Social Security Disability Insurance (SSDI),* or under private insurance programs such as employer-provided or privately purchased short- or long-term disability policies. These programs provide limited income to qualified individuals for either a specified or an undefined time period. The SSDI and SSI programs share many concepts and terms, but there are also many important differences in the rules affecting eligibility and benefit payments. Many individuals are eligible for benefits under both programs. Occupational therapy practitioners in many areas of practice should become familiar with SSI and SSDI to ensure that eligible clients are aware of benefits of these programs. Income and medical care are basic needs that must be met in order for clients to maximize their occupational performance.

SSDI and SSI define disability for individuals 18 years and older as "the inability to engage in any substantial gainful activity because of a medically determinable physical or mental impairment(s) that is expected to result in death, or has lasted or is expected to last for a continuous period of not less than 12 months." Substantial gainful activity (SGA) describes a level of work activity and earnings. Work is "substantial" if it involves doing significant physical or mental activities, or a combination of both. For work activity to be substantial, it can be performed on a part-time or full-time basis. "Gainful" work activity is work performed for pay or profit, work of a nature generally performed for pay or profit, or work intended for profit, whether or not a profit is realized. SGA is used to determine initial eligibility and to decide if disability continues after return to work; however, SGA is not a factor in determining initial eligibility for SSI benefits in individuals with blindness. The monthly SGA level for 2011 is $1,640 for statutorily blind individuals and $1,000 for nonblind recipients (Social Security Administration [SSA], 2010).

SSI is a federal income supplement program that provides monthly benefits to individuals who have limited income and resources and who are disabled, blind, or age 65 or older. Benefits are available to adults and children. SSI is funded by general tax revenues of the U.S. Treasury and administered by the Social Security Administration (SSA). Benefits are not based on prior work. In most states, SSI beneficiaries also get Medicaid to pay for hospital stays, doctor bills, prescription drugs, and other health costs. Recipients are eligible for food stamps in most states.

SSDI provides monthly cash benefits to individuals who are unable to work for a year or more because of a disability (SSA, 2011b). To qualify for benefits, the individual must have worked long enough and recently enough in positions that paid into Social Security. The individual must have accrued 40 credits of employment, 20 of which were earned in the last 10 years. The number of work credits needed to qualify for benefits depends on age. Work credits are based on total yearly income; four credits are the maximum that can be earned in 1 year. The income amount required for a credit changes from year to year. In 2009, one credit was earned for each $1,120 of wages or self-employment income; $4,480 is required to earn four credits for the year.

Individuals must meet strict guidelines in order to receive SSDI. The individual must have earned less than $1,000 per month in wages over the past year, and the condition must interfere with basic work-related activities, be severe enough to be on the SSA medical list for the major body systems (SSA, 2011a), or be of equal severity to medical conditions on this list. Claimants must provide medical evidence of the impairment(s) and the severity of the impairment(s) from their licensed physician or other acceptable professional; evidence includes medical reports, hospital records, and reports from public and private agencies and from non-medical sources such as schools, social workers and employers, and other practitioners. If the individual's condition is at the same level of severity as a medical condition on the list, the condition must interfere with the individual's ability to perform his or her previous work. The final step is to determine if the individual can adjust to other work, considering the medical conditions and age, education, past work experience, and any transferable skills. If the individual meets all of the criteria, the claim is approved.

Individuals initially denied the benefit may reapply. An individual may seek the assistance of a disability specialist or attorney to secure benefits. The monthly disability benefit is based on the individual's lifetime average earnings covered by Social Security. This amount appears on the yearly statement sent by the SSA or can be determined using the SSA benefit calculator. Payments from workers' compensation or other disability programs may affect the amount of the disability benefit. SSDI income is not taxable at the federal or state levels. After an individual has been receiving SSDI for 2 years, he or she becomes eligible for Medicare, which provides partial payment for medical and surgical services, hospital expenses, health screenings, diagnostic tests, and medication. Benefits continue until the individual is able to work on a regular basis or reaches full retirement age, at which time the benefits automatically convert to retirement benefits.

Employment Programs

The *Ticket to Work Program* provides SSI and SSDI beneficiaries with employment services, vocational rehabilitation services, or other support services necessary to find, enter, and retain employment (SSA, 2011d). The goal of the program is to assist beneficiaries in obtaining employment and working toward financial independence (see Table 17.1). After receiving a ticket for services from the SSA, the individual chooses an employment network to coordinate and provide vocational rehabilitation services or other support services to help him or her find and maintain employment. As of 2010, there were 103 Work Incentives Planning and Assistance projects across the United States to work with SSA beneficiaries with disabilities on job placement, benefits planning, and career development. Individuals participating in the Ticket to Work Program may be eligible for work incentives, which allow for cash payments and/or health care to continue until

Table 17.1 Comparison of the SSDI and SSI Disability Programs

	SSDI	SSI
Source of payments	Disability trust fund.	General tax revenues.
Minimum initial qualification requirements	Must meet SSA's disability criteria. Must be "insured" due to contributions made to FICA based on own payroll earnings or those of spouse or parents.	Must meet SSA's disability criteria. Must have limited income and resources.
Health insurance coverage provided	Medicare. Consists of hospital insurance (Part A), supplementary medical insurance (Part B), and Medicare Advantage (Part C). Voluntary prescription drug benefits (Part D) are also included. Title XVIII of the Social Security Act authorizes Medicare.	Medicaid. Medicaid is a jointly funded, federal-state health insurance program for low-income and needy individuals. It covers certain children, some or all of the aged, blind, and/or disabled who are eligible to receive federally assisted income maintenance payments. Title XIX of the Social Security Act authorizes Medicaid. The law gives the states options regarding eligibility under Medicaid.
How monthly benefits are computed	Payment is based on average earnings covered by Social Security over the individual's lifetime. The amount may be reduced if also receiving workers' compensation payments (including Black Lung payments) and/or public disability benefits, such as certain state and civil service disability benefits. Other income or resources do not affect the payment amount. Monthly payment amount is adjusted each year to account for cost-of-living changes.	Beginning with the federal benefit rate ($674 for a qualified individual and $1,011 for a qualified couple in 2009), countable income is subtracted, and any state supplement added. All income is not factored in. The income amount left after making all allowable deductions is *countable income.* There are several ways to exclude income. Federal benefit rate is adjusted each year to account for cost-of-living changes.
Is a state supplemental payment provided?	There is no state supplemental payment with the SSDI program.	Many states pay some individuals who receive SSI an additional amount called a *state supplement.* The amounts and qualifications for state supplements vary by state.

Adapted from SSA (2011c).

the individual achieves his or her work goal and financial independence. The amount of income allowed under these work incentives varies between SSI and SSDI.

Employment support is provided under SSI and SSDI to assist individuals in becoming as self-sufficient as possible through work. Employment supports can help individuals find a job or start a business, protect cash and medical benefits while working, save money to go to school, or make it easy to begin receiving benefits after returning to work. SSDI employment supports provide long-term help to allow individuals to test their ability to work, or to continue working, and gradually become self-supporting and independent. In general, individuals have at least 9 years to test their ability to work. This includes full cash payments during the first 12 months of work activity, a 36-month extended eligibility period, and a 5-year period in which cash benefits again can resume without a new application. Individuals may continue to have Medicare coverage during this time or even longer. SSI employment supports offer ways to continue receiving SSI checks and/or Medicaid coverage while working. Some of these provisions can increase the individual's net income to help cover special expenses. If the individual cannot receive SSI checks because his or her earnings are too high, eligibility for Medicaid may still continue. In most cases, if the individual loses his or her job or cannot continue working, benefit checks can be resumed without filing a new application.

The *Workforce Investment Act of 1998* (WIA) consolidates federal job training and employment programs into a nationwide system of One-Stop Career Centers, which offer a wide range of employment services, vocational rehabilitation, adult education, welfare-to-work, and vocational education activities. WIA also prohibits discrimination against individuals with disabilities who apply for, participate in, or are employees of any program or organization that receives federal financial assistance under WIA or that provides programs/activities as part of the One-Stop system.

Vocational Rehabilitation

Since the early 1900s, numerous federal laws have been enacted to establish vocational rehabilitation services for individuals with disabilities. The *Smith-Fess Act of 1920*, also known as the Vocational Rehabilitation Act, authorized the establishment of a state-federal vocational rehabilitation program for civilians with physical disabilities. These services included vocational guidance, training, occupational adjustment, prostheses, and placement services, all of which had to be specifically linked to a vocational objective and could not include physical restoration or "socially-oriented" rehabilitation. The *Barden-LaFollette Act of 1943* (Vocational Rehabilitation Act Amendments) expanded public rehabilitation eligibility to include the emotionally disturbed and mentally retarded, increased service to include physical restoration, and removed the ceiling on appropriation. The *Vocational Rehabilitation Act Amendments of 1954* provided the basis for future expansion through greater financial support, research and demonstration grants, professional preparation grants, state agency expansion and improvement grants, and grants to expand rehabilitation facilities. The *Vocational Rehabilitation Act Amendments of 1965* accelerated the expansion and improvement of services by allotting federal funds to state agencies, funding statewide planning for growth, and providing grants to expand rehabilitation facilities. The *Rehabilitation Act Amendments of 1974* assists states in operating statewide comprehensive, coordinated, effective, efficient, and accountable programs of vocational rehabilitation to assess, plan, develop, and provide vocational rehabilitation services for individuals with disabilities, consistent with their strengths, resources, priorities, concerns, abilities, capabilities, interests, and informed choice, so that such individuals may prepare for and engage in gainful employment. The *American Recovery and Reinvestment Act of 2009*

(ARRA) appropriates \$540 million in new funding for the Vocational Rehabilitation State Grants program to help individuals with disabilities, especially those with the most significant disabilities, prepare for, obtain, and maintain employment.

Vocational rehabilitation counselors serve as gatekeepers to finance rehabilitation services, education, training, and equipment to support return to work. Occupational therapy practitioners collaborate with vocational rehabilitation counselors in many ways. Vocational rehabilitation may contract with occupational therapy and rehabilitation agencies to enhance work capacities and identify accommodations needed to return to work. Occupational therapy practitioners may direct clients to funding for vocational exploration and training, transportation, and equipment to support return to work. Because vocational rehabilitation is provided at the state level, practitioners should contact their state agency for referral information and resources (see Vocational Rehabilitation under Resources at the end of this chapter).

Retirement Income

Social Security benefits replace a portion of earnings upon retirement, death, or disability. Individuals who pay Social Security taxes can earn up to four credits per year, and 40 credits are needed to qualify for benefits. Individuals who retire after reaching full retirement age receive full retirement benefits, whereas those who retire before reaching full retirement age receive reduced benefits for life. Full retirement age is 65 years for those born before 1937; it increases gradually for those born after that time. For example, 66 years is the full retirement age for individuals born between 1943 and 1954, and 67 years for those born after 1960. Individuals delaying benefits beyond full retirement age, or age 70 years, receive increased benefits depending on birth year. Individuals may take early retirement, as early as age 62; however, their benefits are reduced permanently. Individuals can continue to work and still receive retirement benefits. Earnings in (or after) the month full retirement age is achieved will not reduce benefits; however, benefits are reduced if earnings exceed certain limits for the months before full retirement age.

Medical Insurance Programs

It is important for all individuals to receive medical services, so medical insurance is essential. Individuals may qualify for Medicare or Medicaid, and some may qualify for both Medicare and Medicaid. *Medicare* is the United States' basic health insurance program for people age 65 or older and many people with disabilities. Although the full retirement age is rising, individuals should still apply for Medicare benefits within 3 months of their 65th birthday, as Medicare medical insurance (Part B) may cost more money if individuals wait to apply. Medicare provides hospital insurance (Part A), which helps pay for inpatient hospital care and certain follow-up services; medical insurance (Part B), which helps pay for doctors' services, outpatient hospital care, and other medical services; Medicare Advantage plans (Part C), which are available to some individuals; and prescription drug coverage (Part D). New SSDI recipients are not eligible for Medicare until they have been on SSDI for 2 years; it is important for individuals to secure alternative health insurance during this time.

Medicaid is a health-care program for people with low income and limited resources. Individuals receiving benefits may have to pay a small part of the cost for some medical services. Medicaid is a state-administered program. Each state sets its own guidelines regarding eligibility and services. Factors considered in determining eligibility include age, pregnancy, disability, and blindness; income and resources; and citizenship status. Individuals receiving SSI are usually eligible for Medicaid. Special rules apply to those who live in nursing homes and to disabled children living at home. Eligibility for children is based on the child's status. Information is available from the Centers for Medicare and Medicaid Service (see Resources at the end of this chapter).

The *Consolidated Omnibus Budget Reconciliation Act of 1985* (COBRA) entitles individuals who lose their health benefits to choose to continue group health benefits provided by their group health plan for limited periods of time under certain circumstances; such as voluntary or involuntary job loss, reduction in the hours worked, transition between jobs, death, divorce, and other life events. Qualified individuals may be required to pay the entire premium for coverage up to 102 percent of the cost to the plan. The *American Recovery and Reinvestment Act of 2009* provides for premium reductions of 65 percent for COBRA health premiums.

Occupational therapy practitioners should be aware of eligibility requirements for Medicare and Medicaid so they can assist clients in obtaining these resources. Medicare or Medicaid reimburses for many occupational therapy services that are needed to enhance work performance services; therefore, therapists should be aware of how to bill appropriately to ensure that necessary work assessment and rehabilitation services are covered for clients. It is also important to ensure that clients consider applying for COBRA benefits to extend medical insurance after termination or layoff.

Job Accommodation Network

The Job Accommodation Network (JAN) is not a policy or law but a resource provided by the federal government through ODEP to facilitate employment and retention of workers with disabilities. JAN provides employers, employment providers, individuals with disabilities and their family members, and other interested parties with information on job accommodations, entrepreneurship, and related subjects. JAN provides free, one-on-one consulting services for both private and government employers, including consultation about all aspects of job accommodations, information about federal initiatives and hiring programs, and referral to other resources. Through JAN, employers can learn about hiring and retaining qualified employees with disabilities, accommodation options and practical solutions, their responsibilities under the ADA and Vocational Rehabilitation Act and amendments, how to reduce workers' compensation and other insurance costs, accessibility requirements, and more. Individuals with disabilities can learn about their rights under U.S. law; their accommodation options; and organizations, resources, support groups, and government and placement agencies. Services for rehabilitation professionals include facilitating placement of clients through accommodation assistance, brainstorming accommodation options, finding local resources for workplace assessment, and providing information about and resources for device fabrication and modification. Occupational therapy practitioners can benefit from using JAN, referring their patients to JAN, and encouraging employers to consult with JAN experts.

Occupational Information Network

The Occupational Information Network (O*NET) is the nation's primary source of occupational information. The O*NET database contains information on hundreds of standardized

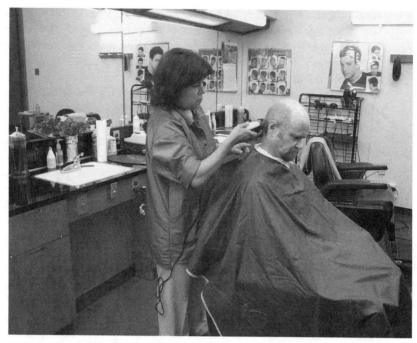

Figure 17.3 The work tasks, knowledge, skills, abilities, activities, tools and technology, work context, job zone, interests, work styles, work values, and wages and employment trends for trades such as barbers can be found in the O*net database.

and occupation-specific descriptors. The database, which is available to the public at no cost, is continually updated through surveys of a broad range of workers from every occupation. O*NET defines work tasks, knowledge, skills, abilities, activities, tools and technology, work context, job zones, interests, work styles, work values, and wages and employment trends (Fig. 17.3). Constructs on O*NET can be sorted by importance or level of performance for the job. O*NET can help occupational therapy practitioners understand their clients' job in order to help prepare them for return to work. O*NET allows for cross-walking among various occupations with common characteristics, so it is useful for occupational therapy practitioners performing vocational exploration.

Standards and Guidelines for Workplace Safety

The *Occupational Safety and Health Act of 1970* (OSH Act) created the Occupational Safety and Health Administration (OSHA) and the *National Institute of Occupational Safety and Health* (NIOSH). OSHA, under the U.S. Department of Labor, is responsible for developing and enforcing workplace safety and health regulations. NIOSH is the federal agency responsible for conducting research and making recommendations for the prevention of work-related injury and illness; it is part of the Centers for Disease Control and Prevention.

The OSH Act covers all employers and their employees in the United States except for self-employed persons, farms that employ only immediate family members, employers monitored by other federal agencies (mining, nuclear energy and weapons, some transportation industries), and employees of state and local governments in states operating without an OSHA-approved state plan. The OSH Act encourages states to develop and operate their own job safety and health programs; however, OSHA must approve and monitor them. Most states adopt standards identical to the federal ones, but others vary somewhat. See the Resources at the end of the chapter for OSHA-related websites.

Federal OSHA standards are grouped into four major categories: general industry, construction, maritime (shipyards, marine terminals, longshoring), and agriculture. Employers must be familiar with the standards applicable to their businesses and must eliminate hazards. The best method to comply with standards is to implement engineering controls to remove exposure to the physical hazard or toxic substance; however, if the exposure cannot be removed, administrative controls and personal protective equipment are appropriate to describe the procedures and equipment required when exposed to the hazard. Employees must comply with all rules and regulations that apply to their own actions and conduct. Even in areas where OSHA has not set forth a standard addressing a specific hazard, employers are responsible for complying with the OSH Act's "general duty" clause, which states that each employer shall furnish a place of employment free from recognized hazards that are causing or are likely to cause death or serious physical harm to his employees.

Requirements for all industry sectors allow employees, designated representatives, and OSHA access to relevant medical records, including records related to employees' exposure to toxic substances. Employers are required to provide employees with personal equipment designed to protect them against certain hazards and to ensure that employees have been effectively trained on the use of the equipment. Equipment can include protective helmets, eye protection, hearing protection, hard-toed shoes, and equipment for special operations. Manufacturers and importers of hazardous materials are required to conduct hazard evaluations of their products; products found to be hazardous under terms of the standard must be labeled hazardous on their containers, and the first shipment of the material to a new customer must include a Material Safety Data Sheet (MSDS). Employers must use these MSDSs to train their employees to recognize and avoid the hazards presented by the materials. The OSH Act grants employees the right to file a complaint with OSHA about safety and health conditions in their workplaces without their identity being revealed to their employers, to contest the amount of time OSHA allows for correcting violations of standards, and to participate in OSHA workplace inspections.

All covered employers must complete an Injury and Illness Incident Report (Form 301) when a recordable work-related injury or illness occurs that results in either death, days away from work, restricted work activity or job transfer, medical treatment beyond first aid, or loss of consciousness. Employers must also log work-related injuries and illnesses on the Summary of Work-Related Injuries and Illnesses form (Form 300a), including the extent and severity of each case and specific details about what happened and how it happened. This form must be posted in a visible location so employees are aware of the injuries and illnesses that occur in their workplace.

It is important for occupational therapy practitioners addressing work performance with individuals or populations to be familiar with OSHA regulations. Practitioners providing treatment to workers with acute injuries should know what makes a work injury recordable. An employer seeking to keep an injury from being recordable may discourage ongoing medical treatment, restricted work, or time off of work. Practitioners providing services at the worksite can review Form 301 to gain information about causation and identify ways to assist the injured worker to prevent future incidences. The Form 300a log can provide a snapshot of the types of injuries occurring at a worksite, which can be useful to practitioners designing preventive interventions. Methods of meeting OSHA compliance standards can be useful in these interventions (engineering controls, administrative controls, and personal protective equipment). Practitioners must ensure that workers can perform their work duties while abiding by safety standards required at their workplace. For example, it is more difficult (albeit safer) for a worker wearing steel-toe work boots, protective clothing, and a full-body harness to walk and climb than if wearing a t-shirt and loose-fitting pants. Therefore, equipment that restricts or hinders movement in any way must be considered in assessment and rehabilitation, and personal protective equipment and methods required on the job must be tested or simulated during assessment and/or intervention. Practitioners who provide services at the worksite *must maintain personal safety* as they assist employers and employees in promoting workplace safety. For example, practitioners who borrow equipment and supplies from the employer must maintain and use such equipment safely at the worksite as well as in the clinical environment, which includes following MSDS guidelines where applicable. Also, practitioners must collaborate with the employer to ensure that all adaptive equipment or accommodations meet OSHA industry-specific and general safety standards. Practitioners providing services at the worksite should inquire about safety training and safety equipment that are required for entry into the workplace.

OSHA provides Ergonomics Program Management Guidelines for various industries, including meatpacking plants, nursing homes, shipyards, and grocery stores. Practitioners working with these industries should consult these guidelines. OSHA also offers many electronic tools and resources to assist occupational therapists and others working with industry. Although the Ergonomics Standard of 1999 was rescinded, it contains many useful resources for identifying and abating musculoskeletal risks. NIOSH also has many resources—checklists, assessments, workplace solutions, interventions, research grants, and videotapes, to name a few—that can assist occupational therapists addressing work performance. See Resources at the end of the chapter.

The *American National Standards Institute* (ANSI) oversees the creation and use of thousands of voluntary consensus standards to assure the safety and health of consumers, employers, and the environment, and it oversees accreditation programs that assess conformance to standards. ANSI standards are voluntary, not required like OSHA standards. Although occupational therapy practitioners' involvement with ANSI is generally limited, those in industry rehabilitation and consulting should know that ANSI exists.

Legal System

Occupational therapy practitioners working with individuals with interruptions in their ability to work may interact with the legal system. Since occupational therapy practitioners are experts at assessing work abilities, they may be required to testify in a deposition or court hearing about an individual's abilities to perform his or her previous job or any competitive employment. They may be asked to explain results of testing or details of the rehabilitation program in workers' compensation cases and sometimes to provide an opinion regarding an individual's sincerity of effort. They may also be asked to serve as an expert witness. No matter what the reason, the practitioner should be well informed of the policies involved in the case.

Work Incentives and Policies in Canada, Israel, and the United Kingdom

This chapter so far has provided an overview of work incentives and work-related policies and legislation in the United States. The next section of provides brief overviews of work incentives and related policy in three foreign countries: Canada, Israel, and the United Kingdom. As we become more *globally connected,* we share information and learn from our colleagues around the world. As we do so, we must keep in mind the variations in how different countries provide support to persons with injuries or disabilities who want to work.

Work Incentives and Policies in Canada

Referrals to Occupational Therapy in Canada

The Canadian health-care system consists of a public sector in which services are covered by public funds and a private sector in which services are covered by various sources. Canada provides universal, comprehensive coverage for medically necessary hospital and physician services on the basis of need rather than the ability to pay. The severity of the condition and the urgency of the treatment required must be considered while providing services in the public sector. Because the public sector often has insufficient resources to assess and treat injured workers without delay, occupational therapists in the private sector see a significant portion of this population.

In Canada, as in the United States, a master's degree is required to become an occupational therapist. Support personnel, sometimes called occupational therapy assistants, provide client care and treatment under the supervision of an occupational therapist and may have a college diploma or have on-the-job training. As support personnel, they are knowledgeable in the field of occupational therapy and are involved in the provision of occupational therapy services in self-care, work, and leisure occupations. Canada does not require certification for occupational therapy assistants.

Occupational therapy services are widely used in both the public and private sectors for the following:

- Assessment of work capacity after an injury or illness to assist with return to work, including assignment of work tasks, ability to tolerate environmental demands, timing of return to work, identification of necessary accommodations, and/or prevention of future injury or illness.
- Assessment of ability to perform job requirements, such as return-to-work testing or reassignment testing, although occupational therapy services seem underused for preemployment/post–job offer testing.
- Analysis of jobs to quantify exposure, identify essential functions, identify risks, and make ergonomic recommendations.
- Intervention for individuals to prepare them for return to work through work hardening programs and during progressive return to work.
- Prevention of work injuries and maintaining physical and mental health, including group educational sessions and one-on-one coaching.
- Assessment of work capacity to identify if a person meets the definition for work disability pay according to the definition of partial and/or total disability stated at the provincial level, federal level, or by private disability insurers.
- Support to the employee, the employer, and the payer during the return-to-work process through efficient communication, seeing the "big picture," and using problem-solving skills.

How Widely Is Occupational Therapy Used for Work-Related Service Provision?

Although other health-care professionals offer similar services, occupational therapists in Canada are often considered experts in the areas of functional ability assessments, work hardening programs, jobsite assessments, ergonomic recommendations, and return-to-work support. An occupational therapist's thoroughness with task analysis, knowledge of the work market and the workforce, and ability to support work capacity with both standardized testing and extensive work simulation may be partly responsible for their consideration as experts in Canada. Also, the ability to address multiple aspects of a situation by considering the physical, psychological, and social aspects of the worker in his or her environment makes the occupational therapist a key player to assist in the return-to-work process.

Critical Laws and Policies Guiding Work-Related Services
Disability Determination Laws

The Canadian Human Rights Act prohibits all discrimination on the grounds of disability (Canadian Human Rights Commission, 2007). The prohibition is also found in the Canadian *Charter of Rights and Freedoms,* which made Canada the first country in the world to include the protection of persons with disabilities in its Constitution. Therefore, the Canadian Human Rights Act prevails over all other laws described in this section. The Canadian Human Rights Act mandates that an employer shall not discriminate against a person who displays or is afflicted by a disability as long as that person can perform the essential functions of the job. Employees or potential employees have the right to request reasonable accommodations to allow them to perform these essential functions unless they create undue hardship for the employer in terms of health, safety, or cost. In this area, occupational therapy can aid both employees and employers. While considering strategies to accommodate a worker, the occupational therapist must keep in mind that an employer must consider moving the employee to other positions or changing duties, but the employer does not have to create an entirely new position. Also, the employer is not required to maintain a disabled employee in a position that is not useful or productive in the context of its operations.

Employment Laws: Labour Standards Act

Labor standards fall under the federal or the provincial authority depending on the worker's job sector. Canada has 10 provinces: Alberta, British Columbia, Manitoba, New Brunswick, Newfoundland and Labrador, Nova Scotia, Ontario, Prince Edward Island, Quebec, and Saskatchewan. The federal Canada Labour Code (R.S.C., 1985) applies to:

- Works or undertakings connecting a province with another province or country, such as railways, bus operations, trucking, pipelines, ferries, tunnels, bridges, canals, telephone and cable systems.
- All extra-provincial shipping and services connected with such shipping, such as longshoring.
- Air transport, aircraft, and airports.
- Radio and television broadcasting.
- Banks.
- Defined operations of specific works declared by Parliament to be for the general advantage of Canada or of two or more provinces, such as flour, feed and seed cleaning mills, feed warehouses, grain elevators, and uranium mining and processing.
- Federal Crown corporations engaged in works or undertakings that fall within section 91 of the Constitution Act, 1867, or that are an agency of the Crown (e.g., the Canadian Broadcasting Corporation and the St. Lawrence Seaway Authority).

Under federal jurisdiction, employees with 3 months of continuous employment have up to 12 weeks of employment protection for absences due to illness. Otherwise, the labor law falls under provincial jurisdiction where the details and application differ among provinces.

Provincial authority is derived from the "property and civil rights" subsection of the Constitution Act of 1867. The right to enter into contracts is a civil right, and because labor laws impose certain restrictions on contracts between employers and employees, they fall within provincial authority as property and civil rights legislation. Provinces also have the right to legislate on local works and undertakings.

In general, each province's labor laws are similar because one of their main goals is to protect the worker's employment for a certain period of time during a leave of absence. The coverage period varies from 12 to 26 weeks per year depending on the province and is available only to employees who worked a minimum specified time (usually 3 or 6 months). The eligibility period also varies among provinces. An extension to this leave may be granted in certain circumstances. For example, in Quebec province, the leave may be up to 104 weeks if the person is unable to work as a result of being a victim of a criminal act.

In case of disability, employees having worked a minimum number of hours at the current job may benefit from unemployment insurance for up to 15 weeks. Both federal and provincial labor laws create opportunities for occupational therapy practitioners to help workers return to their occupation within the period of time the job is protected in order to prevent loss of employment.

Systems to Compensate Workers With Disability (Canada Pension Plan, Quebec Pension Plan, Private Disability Insurers, Workmen's Compensation Board)

The Workmen's Compensation Act varies among provinces. If the duty to provide accommodations is not fully explicit in a province's workmen's compensation act, the act usually makes reference to the Canadian Human Rights Act. As noted earlier, the duty to accommodate has created opportunities for occupational therapy to work with both employees and employers to identify accommodations. Further, the disability system has created multiple opportunities for occupational therapists to assist in the determination of fitness for duty by performing functional ability evaluations.

Canada provides financial incentives for the disability system to help workers who are receiving wage replacement benefits to return to work, and this has created significant opportunities for work hardening programs.

As employers see value in workers being fully ready to resume their work safely, they are more open to having a portion or the totality of the work hardening program performed at the worksite. Performing a work hardening program within the natural work environment makes it more relevant when determining workers' ability to resume performing the essential functions of their job. Employers have a financial incentive to return workers to the worksite as soon as possible, even if it is not to their original occupation. That financial incentive is even more direct in the cases of workers receiving workmen's compensation benefits. Light duties are often used in that context, and the assistance of occupational therapy practitioners is often sought to help determine possible tasks to fit the worker's current level of function. Practitioners can also help workers ease back into their regular job by gradually increasing the complexity of the tasks being performed under light duty.

Medical Leave Laws

As previously indicated, disabled employees having worked a minimum number of hours at the current job may benefit from unemployment insurance for up to 15 weeks. Sick leave in Canada is covered in six jurisdictions. A seventh jurisdiction, Ontario, provides emergency leave to certain employees in cases of illness, injury, or medical emergency. All such leave is unpaid. The implementation of these laws varies greatly from one jurisdiction to the next. Here are a few examples:

- In Quebec, employees with 3 months of uninterrupted service are allowed up to 26 weeks of employment protection against dismissal, suspension, or transfer because of an absence due to illness or accident. A similar provision exists under federal jurisdiction: employees with 3 months of continuous employment are allowed up to 12 weeks of employment protection for leaves due to illness. Also in Quebec, an extension of up to 52 weeks may be granted if the worker's child or spouse is considered missing or committed suicide. Also in Quebec, an extension of up to 104 weeks may be granted if the worker must care for a minor child who was a victim of a criminal act or if the worker's child or spouse was the victim of a criminal act that resulted in death.

- Newfoundland and New Brunswick provide employees 5 days of leave per year if they have been employed with the same employer for a continuous period of 6 months and 90 days respectively.
- In Saskatchewan, provisions regarding sick leave are more family-centric. In fact, an employer may not dismiss, suspend, lay off, demote, or discipline an employee with at least 13 weeks of service because of absence due to a personal illness or injury or, interestingly, due to the illness or injury of a dependant who is a member of the employee's immediate family. An employee's job is protected for absences not exceeding 12 weeks per year in case of serious injury or illness, or 12 days in a calendar year for illnesses or injuries that are not serious. In addition, the period of job protection is extended to 26 weeks for employees on workers' compensation. There is nevertheless an exception in the latter case. Employees with a demonstrated record of chronic absenteeism that is unlikely to improve are not entitled to this leave. An employer may require that an employee provide a medical certificate in such instances.
- Employees in the Yukon are entitled to one day without pay per month of employment, up to a maximum of 12 days.

Under federal jurisdiction, an employee may be assigned to a different job if he or she is unable to perform his or her previous work. In Quebec, an employee may be assigned to comparable employment after an absence of 4 weeks.

No matter which jurisdiction they fall under, employers are prohibited from dismissing, suspending, demoting, disciplining, or laying off an employee because of absence (except for just cause) during the period of medical leave.

These provisions give occupational therapy practitioners the opportunity to help workers return to their occupation within the period of time the job is protected, thereby preventing loss of employment.

Compassionate Care Leave
The duration of compassionate care leave usually varies from 8 to 12 weeks depending on the province. An employee can also take this leave due to his or her own serious illness or injury. In addition, an employee with at least 13 weeks' service is entitled to up to 12 unpaid days' leave per year for nonserious illness or injury (of the employee and/or an immediate family member), unless it can be demonstrated that the employee has a record of chronic absenteeism and there is no reasonable expectation of improved attendance. An employer is prohibited from dismissing, suspending, laying off, demoting, or disciplining an employee because of absence (except for just cause) during the period of absence compassionate care leave.

These provisions provide an opportunity for occupational therapy practitioners to help workers return to their occupation within the period of time the job is protected, thereby preventing loss of employment. They also create an opportunity for occupational therapists to provide preventative services by giving the worker under compassionate care leave the tools to better manage the additional workload (combining personal and professional responsibilities), the stress caused by the uncertainty of the situation, and similar concerns that may persist when the person returns to work.

Health and Safety Laws
Each province has its own occupational health and safety act and regulations. Federal health and safety regulations fall under Part II of the Canada Labour Code (R.S.C., 1985).

Canadian occupational health and safety legislation is primarily based on three fundamental rights of workers:

- The right to be informed of known or foreseeable safety or health hazards in the workplace.

- The right to participate in the prevention of occupational accidents and diseases either as members of joint health and safety committees or as health and safety representatives.
- The right to refuse dangerous work and be protected against dismissal or disciplinary action following a legitimate refusal.

Employers are responsible for providing a safe workplace environment. In 2004, Quebec province added a provision to the Labour Standards Act that forces employers to address any workplace psychological harassment. This opens up the definition of workplace safety to consider both the physical and psychological well-being of workers. A similar initiative was introduced for employees working under federal jurisdiction. Such initiatives create a unique opportunity for occupational therapists to actively participate in making workplaces safer for all workers and to help with the prevention of illness and injuries both physical and psychological.

Evidence-Based Practice in Canada
Licensing entities emphasize the need for occupational therapists to keep their professional knowledge up to date through continuing education and to apply evidence-based practice. The Canadian Association of Occupational Therapy (CAOT) requires applicants in all provinces to have successfully completed a master's degree in order to obtain an occupational therapy license. According to the COTA, education in a professional master's program provides the necessary opportunity and environment to support development of competencies for evidence-based and occupation-based intervention.

At this point, reimbursement practices do not explicitly require an occupational therapist to use evidence-based practices, but it is indirectly required because the payer expects a quick and efficient resolution of the work disability. Therefore, the occupational therapist must follow an evidence-based practice to be able to respect cost and duration constraints imposed by payers.

Work-Related Services Reimbursement and Referral Sources
The main referral sources for work-related occupational therapy include physicians, workmen's compensation boards, motor vehicle insurance providers (public or private depending on the province), private disability insurance providers, employers, unions, lawyers, and private individuals. In the private sector, the referral source is usually the payer except when the referral is made by the physician. The services are sometimes reimbursed by private health insurance plans, although occupational therapy services are often not covered. There are also private-pay clients who pay out of pocket. For services rendered to a population level, occupational therapy services are sometimes paid by employers for educational sessions offered to their employees.

A physician's referral is required for any assessment and treatment under workmen's compensation and public motor vehicle insurance. Some private health insurance may require a physician's referral for assessment and treatment. In the context of disability insurance, no physician's referral is required for assessment-only services (e.g., functional ability assessment, jobsite assessment, ergonomic assessment). Even though private disability insurance policies do not require a physician's referral to initiate treatment, tight collaboration with the treating physician is often sought before treatment begins because the payer wants the occupational therapy treatment to be part of the physician's global treatment plan, and it is usually the treating physician who must preapprove any return-to-work activities.

What Are the Biggest Challenges to Providing Work-Related Services in Canada?
The role of occupational therapists when treating workers with physical dysfunction is now well established. Unfortunately, payers, employers, workers, and the general population still need to be educated as to how occupational therapists can help workers with

mental health conditions. Mental health conditions, including depression and anxiety, will soon be the number one reason for worker absences, and occupational therapists can play a key role to treat and prevent these conditions. Occupational therapists may require assistance in creating educational tools to inform people of their abilities to address mental health conditions. They may also require assistance to better market their services.

Since many health insurance policies do not cover occupational therapy, patients tend to visit other health-care providers whose services are covered. Because of a payer's financial constraints, treatment is sometimes terminated before achieving a maximum level of function. This may sometimes lead to suboptimal care for the patient's condition when occupational therapy services are required. More needs to be done to bring awareness to insurance companies, employers, employee groups, and unions to address this issue and get occupational therapy included in the list of services covered by health insurance policies.

What Are the Biggest Benefits to Providing Work-Related Services in Canada?

Referrals are being made much earlier in the disability process, thereby making it easier for occupational therapy services to have a greater impact sooner, which also helps in cost containment. Occupational therapy services are increasingly being used for the prevention of work injuries and disabilities instead of just for treatment, which helps in the ultimate goal: keeping people healthy!

Work Incentives and Policies in Israel

Referrals to Occupational Therapy in Israel

Work rehabilitation and prevention services in Israel are provided by occupational therapists in a variety of settings. As in Canada, occupational therapy assistants are not certified, although persons in therapy-support roles may hold this title in some settings. Those services are provided either through health services or through the Ministry of Industry, Trade and Labor (n.d.) and the National Insurance Institute of Israel.

Assessment, intervention, and recommendations for work rehabilitation are done sometimes during hospitalization in rehabilitation centers. Work rehabilitation services are more commonly provided in the community where prevocational rehabilitation, vocational rehabilitation, and job placement is done by occupational therapists. At the first stage, the process includes evaluation of work capacity and the ability to return to work using interviews, questionnaires, onsite analysis (rarely done), different kinds of functional capacity evaluations, and simulators (e.g., VALPAR work samples). In the next stage, the work rehabilitation process is implied in vocational rehabilitations centers, supported occupation setups, protected occupation centers, and the free market. In all these different organizations, occupational therapists are part of a team that evaluates, trains, and mediates clients' return to work. All services are provided to a variety of people with different disabilities, such as physical disabilities, mental illness disabilities, and mental retardation.

In addition, a few Israeli companies have occupational therapists present at the workplace. Most of these companies are high-tech companies that use ergonomic services in particular. Occupational therapists providing ergonomic job redesign services generally are hired for independent projects by employers who wish to resolve specific issues or promote goodwill, or an occupational therapist who wishes to market this type of service may offer it as an independent initiative.

Postoffer screening in Israel is virtually nonexistent except in the armed forces, fire brigade, and police departments where occupational therapists are usually not involved.

Some unique vocational rehabilitation services are provided mainly by occupational therapists in Israel. For example, the Karten CTEC (Computer-aided Training Education and Communication) Centres offer information technology training and experience for people with a wide range of disabilities and mental health problems not only to develop skills needed for employment but also to encourage a growth in personal confidence and self-esteem. The information technology program can form part of a more comprehensive work preparation program. The centers provide assistive technology assessment, training program, workstation evaluation, and consulting services; if accessibility modifications are needed, it is part of the treatment given (Karten Network, 2011).

Another special and unique service provided by occupational therapists is the use of *virtual reality* as an assessment and treatment tool in work rehabilitation. Applications have been directed at a variety of clinical populations, including those with cognitive and metacognitive deficits. In this context, the most common use is in driving rehabilitation. Virtual environments provide the opportunity for repeated learning trials and offer the capacity to gradually increase the complexity of tasks while decreasing therapist support and feedback.

Other special techniques include integrating 3-D motion analysis into clinics and ergonomic interventions. Computerized 3-D analysis is used for diagnostic workup and therapeutic interventions in, for example, the office workplace.

Occupational therapists in Israel provide work-related services:

- Assessment, evaluation, work rehabilitation services, modification of the work environment, and assistive technology in relationship to the work demands.
- Ergonomic assessment and modifications in the work environment.
- Assessment of and training for people with disabilities to promote work skills to be used in the free or protected market according to the findings of each client.

How Widely Is Occupational Therapy Used for work-Related Service Provision?

Occupational therapists are part of a team of social workers, psychologists, and other professionals. In some cases, occupational therapists are an integral part of the team, and in others they provide consultation services.

Critical Laws and Policies Guiding Work-Related Services

Israel Health Law

In January 1995, a new national health insurance law was enacted in Israel, which allowed registration of every resident to one of four public health funds. These funds provide, among other medical services, rehabilitation services to their insured members. When necessary, the members may, through their insurance provider, purchase services from public or private hospitals or other health-service providers. Through this law, a package of elementary medical services was defined to guarantee all citizens readily available comprehensive rehabilitation.

The government-set health-service package encompasses a broad range of medical treatments in the fields of rehabilitation, including occupational therapy services.

Equality of Rights Law

In 1998, legislation was proposed to give equal rights to people with disability in Israel. In order to implement the law, new regulations were initiated, and today most of these regulations are still in draft state. Although these regulations are still being reviewed before enactment, the Israeli Ministry of Industry, Trade and Labor has begun a process of incentives to help people with disability be included in employment in the open market. This process includes the following steps:

- Incentives for the employer:
  - *Accommodations*—The Ministry of Industry, Trade and Labor helps in funding accommodations needed to employ a specific person with disability.
  - *Support*—Employers receive assistance in employing people with disability.

- Incentives for the person with disability:
  - ○ *Encouragement*—The Ministry of Industry, Trade and Labor developed an assistance plan to encourage people with disability to become employed and start businesses. This encouragement includes training, counseling, support groups, education, assistance in developing employment plans, and more.
  - ○ *Positions*—Government offices are encouraged, when appropriate, to open positions for people with disabilities and to do business with companies that employ or are owned by people with disability.
  - ○ *Evaluation of employability*—Employability of people with disability is assessed. On the basis of the evaluation, they receive recommendations for training or workplace adaptations and, when required, future reevaluation.
- Incentives for the employer and person with disability:
  - ○ *Adapted minimum wage*—The employability of the person with disability is evaluated and his or her performance is compared to that of an average worker to calculate an adapted minimum. If the percentage of employability of a person with a disability as compared to an average worker is found to be between 25 and 50 percent, the percentage paid from minimum wage is 75 percent; if it is between 50 and 75 percent, the percentage paid is 50 percent; if it is 75 percent and over, the percentage paid is one third of minimum wage
  - ○ *Surveillance*—Accommodations and incentives in the workplace is a new procedure under new regulations in Israel; therefore, surveillance is carried out in order to examine, evaluate, and understand the needs in the field.
  - ○ *Mental health law*—In 2000, a law was enacted concerning rehabilitation for people with mental illness in the community. The object of this law is to help people with mental illness rehabilitate and to integrate with the community, enabling them to obtain the highest possible degree of functional independence and quality of life. To help promote and implement the rights of people with mental illness and to further these objectives, special rehabilitation services were established. Occupational therapists were recognized, among other occupations, to help in this process, which includes evaluation, employment training, and employment mediation to enable people with mental illness to work according to their ability, skills, and preferences in the open market, in supported work (a rehabilitation program enabling protected work experience in the open market), or in sheltered work.

Evidence-Based Practice in Israel

Occupational therapists in Israel are obligated to evidence-based practice, and the various employers of occupational therapists in Israel (health services; the Ministry of Industry, Trade and Labor; and the National Insurance Institute of Israel) require evidence-based practice. Nevertheless, the areas of ergonomics and work rehabilitation often benefit from pioneering approaches, and in these cases, occupational therapists choose the best practice on the basis of their experience, or they initiate research to explore new ideas.

Work-Related Services Reimbursement and Referral Sources

Services are covered according to the place the service is given; health services are covered by health insurance; services provided by the Ministry of Industry, Trade and Labor are covered by the state; and the National Insurance Institute of Israel absorbs the costs of its own services.

Occupational therapists are involved in many employment services; each service has a unique procedure of referral and function. Occupational therapists are on staff in most health services and are generally paid by their employer. In health services, referral to occupational therapy services is most commonly made by physicians. In return-to-work rehabilitation for people with mental health illnesses, the client is referred to a multidiscipline committee, which reviews the matter and advises the client regarding rehabilitation. The client can apply for services by himself or herself or can be referred by his or her therapist, psychiatrist, or a family member. In supported and protected employment services, occupational therapists are part of staff and provide service upon need. In services given by the Ministry of Industry, Trade and Labor and the National Insurance Institute of Israel, consultation of occupational therapists is supplied by individual case or for a specific project. It is important to mention that occupational therapy services do not yet exist in all areas concerning employability; there are still areas where physicians, psychologists, and social workers are more commonly part of staff.

What Is the Biggest Challenge to Providing Work-Related Services in Israel?

Involvement of occupational therapists in prevention programs in Israel is limited at this point. It seems appropriate that one challenge in Israel should deal with marketing and implementing the knowledge and abilities of occupational therapists to contribute to workplace injury prevention programs.

Additionally, occupational therapists in Israel should attempt to be more involved with rehabilitation in the workplace. Active rehabilitation in the actual working environment may contribute to earlier return to work. In addition, this type of rehabilitation may help clients return to their initial workplace or to an alternative workplace more successfully. When possible, helping clients return to their job prior to finishing rehabilitation is ideal because treatment can continue in the actual work position.

What Are the Biggest Benefits to Providing Work-Related Services in Israel?

Occupational therapists in Israel are usually part of a rehabilitation team that follows the client-centered model, focusing not on the injury alone but also on the client's needs, abilities, personal will and choices, and so on. The uniqueness of occupational therapists in this team is the ability to consider the person, the environment, and the task as one unit.

Employers benefit from the occupational therapist's approach to safety, ergonomics, work environment, and productivity. Addressing such issues reduces the number of days lost to sick leave, consequently improving productivity.

Team members such as physicians, social workers, and other professionals working in employment rehabilitation benefit from the occupational therapists' knowledge and perspective, improving their ability to make return-to-work decisions.

The Israeli system benefits when people are rehabilitated after occupational therapy intervention and can return to work, no longer needing compensation or unemployment allowance.

Work Incentives and Policies in the United Kingdom

Referrals to Occupational Therapy in the United Kingdom

The majority of occupational therapists in the United Kingdom practice in either the publically funded National Health Service or the Social Care Sector. A smaller proportion are employed by "third-sector" organizations (charities and not-for-profit agencies) or are in private practice. In relation to employment, some are employed to provide condition-management programs through Department of Work and Pension services or in occupational health services of public- and private-sector employers.

In response to the growing awareness of the health and economic benefits of employment, many governmental policies regarding vocational rehabilitation have been adopted. The College of Occupational Therapists (2011), the United Kingdom's professional body, aims to ensure access to occupational therapy within all vocational rehabilitation services in the United Kingdom and to ensure that occupational therapists working across all sectors consider the employment needs of service users (Barnes, Holmes, and College Of Occupational Therapists, 2009; College of Occupational Therapists, 2007).

An occupational therapist's role in vocational rehabilitation could include:

* Asking service users about their work aspirations.
* Vocational assessments.
* Worksite assessments.
* Job analysis.
* Work hardening/conditioning.
* Condition management.
* Case management.
* Recommendations and negotiations for reasonable adjustments to work tasks or environment.
* Advising employers.

How Widely Is Occupational Therapy Used for Work-Related Service Provision?

There is concern that due to the increasing demand for vocational rehabilitation, the United Kingdom faces a shortfall in workforce capacity in this specialism. Professionals who currently contribute to vocational rehabilitation include occupational therapists, case managers, physiotherapists, psychologists, Jobcentre Plus personal advisers, disability employment advisers, and employment support workers. Occupational therapists have been identified as having the capacity and skills to make a significant contribution to this agenda (Sainsbury Centre for Mental Health and College of Occupational Therapists, 2008), highlighting the profession's understanding of the significant impact occupation and employment have on a person's health and well-being. A recent high-profile review of health and employment led by Dame Carol Black (2008) identified occupational therapy as one of several health professions with a role in vocational rehabilitation. Currently, provision varies widely across the United Kingdom.

Critical Laws and Policies Guiding Work-Related Services

The policy context for vocational rehabilitation services in the United Kingdom is complex, in part due to devolution. Vocational rehabilitation is influenced by policy related to health, employment, and welfare. This is a period of significant change in each of these policy areas. Responsibility for health policies is devolved to each of the four UK nations: Scotland, England, Northern Ireland, and Wales, while responsibility for employment and welfare policies is held by the UK Judiciary. Recent policy initiatives have highlighted the need for integrated services that support unemployed people in finding employment, help people at risk of losing work due to health issues to retain employment, and help to maintain the health and well-being of employees (Black, 2008; Great Britain Department of Work and Pensions & Department of Health [GBDWP/DH], 2008, HM Government, 2009; National Social Inclusion Programme, et al., 2006; Scottish Executive 2005, 2006; Scottish Executive and National Health Service in Scotland, 2007). There is a "moral, social and economic case" for supporting people with health conditions to work (GBDWP/DH, 2008, p. 5). In 2006, a government-commissioned review established the positive relationship between employment and improved health (Waddell and Burton, 2006). Government departments have since acknowledged that such a wide agenda cannot be achieved by health alone and "requires integrated responses and integrated solutions" (Future Vision Coalition, 2009, p. 7).

Mental health conditions are now the most common reason for claiming health-related benefits in the United Kingdom and are therefore the focus of many initiatives. Most recently, policies have focused on supporting people experiencing mental health conditions to retain or gain employment (GBDWP/DH, 2009; HM Government, 2009).

It is recognized that the UK welfare system is unsustainable. During the last UK recession, many people who were unemployed were placed on incapacity benefits, resulting in "a lost generation of workers" (Sainsbury Centre for Mental Health and the College of Occupational Therapists, 2008, p. 6). It is vital at times of economic uncertainty that every effort is made to support people's aspirations to work (GBDWP/DH, 2008).

Sickness Absence and Welfare

Beginning in April 2010, procedures for sickness absence changed. Certification of illness remains the responsibility of general practitioners, but "sick note" was replaced by a statement of fitness to work. These notes may recommend a period of absence but can now make recommendations to employers for circumstances under which the person could work, which may be altered hours or amended duties, for example. The aim is to reduce periods of absence and avoid alienation from the workplace because it is known that the longer a person is off work, the less likely he or she is to return to employment. This new procedure is supported by recently established "fit for work services," which aim to help people stay in work or return to work more quickly. Several pilot sites have been created throughout the United Kingdom and will be robustly evaluated.

For people who are workless, there have also been recent changes in the welfare system. *Dame Carol Black's Review of the Health of Britain's Working Age Population* (2008, p. 13) highlighted "historical failures" of health-care and employment support evidenced by the rates of incapacity benefits. The Welfare Reform Act (2009) tackled this issue. Previously, people not in employment due to health problems claimed incapacity benefit; this has now been replaced for new claimants by the Employment and Support Allowance. To receive this benefit, a claimant must take part in one or more work-focused health-related assessments to identify

(a) the extent to which a person still has capability for work, (b) the extent to which his capability for work may be improved by the taking of steps in relation to his physical or mental condition, and (c) such other matters relating to his physical or mental condition and the likelihood of his obtaining or remaining in work or being able to do so, as may be prescribed. (Welfare Reform Bill, 2009, p. 9)

The outcome of this assessment may be that the person has limited capacity for work and is therefore assigned to a support group that offers a higher level of benefit. Others must engage in a work-related activity with the aim of obtaining work.

Legislation

Legislation that protects the rights of individuals with health problems to work and while at work includes the following:

Disability Discrimination Act 2005, which requires employers to make reasonable adjustments to accommodate employees who are or have become disabled.
Human Rights Act 1998, which outlines individuals' rights, including the right to work.
Health and Safety at Work Act 1974, which ensures that the health and safety of everyone at work is protected.
Employment Rights Act 1996 and Employment Act 2002 (Dispute Regulations) 2004, which ensures fair procedures in relation to dismissal, disciplinary, and grievance actions.

Evidence-Based Practice in the United Kingdom

Practicing occupational therapists in the United Kingdom must be registered with the Health Professions Council (HPC) and are bound by its standards; these include a requirement to maintain fitness to practice (HPC, 2007).

The Sainsbury Centre for Mental Health (2007) recommends that the United Kingdom develop a vocational rehabilitation workforce capable of providing evidence-based services. A recent high-profile review focused on supporting people with mental health conditions who are workless into paid employment (Perkins, Farmer, and Litchfield, 2009), concluding with a recommendation to provide greater access to the individual placement and support model of vocational rehabilitation. This report has informed subsequent policy development. Several centers of excellence have been developed in England with the support of the Sainsbury Centre for Mental Health. Recent cross-governmental policies indicate an intention to provide access to individual placement and support services throughout the United Kingdom.

Vocational rehabilitation services may also work to standards laid down by the Vocational Rehabilitation Association (VRA; 2008) or the UK Rehabilitation Council (UKRC; 2009). Both sets of standards identify good practice but are not mandatory. Those of the UKRC were commissioned by the Department for Work and Pensions to enable commissioners and purchasers to be better informed about what they are buying.

How Are Work-Related Services Reimbursed?

Most UK vocational rehabilitation services are funded through taxes in public-funded national health services or Department for Work and Pensions services. Taxes may also fund social services commissioned by third-sector organizations.

Recent policy documents suggest large employers should shoulder some of the responsibility for funding vocational rehabilitation services, citing the strong economic case for intervening early and supporting people to keep them in work.

Private-practice occupational therapists may be funded through private health-care insurance, employers, or self-funding individuals.

What Are the Biggest Challenges to Providing Work-Related Services in the United Kingdom?

Recent policy initiatives have highlighted the need to dispel myths that people with mental health problems are unable to work and to raise awareness among health professionals, employment services, employers, and service users that securing and maintaining work is a realistic goal. Antistigma campaigns in the United Kingdom play a positive role in breaking down barriers to achieving vocational goals that people may experience.

The United Kingdom is currently experiencing increasing unemployment, so securing paid work is becoming more challenging. However, several policy developments are based on the fact that the costs of the country's long-term failure to manage ill health and return people to work are no longer sustainable. There is also concern that positive developments in vocational rehabilitation led by recent policy may be hampered by a shortfall in workforce capacity.

What Are the Biggest Benefits to Providing Work-Related Services in the United Kingdom?

There are clear imperatives for provision of effective vocational rehabilitation services:

- Supporting people with health problems back into employment improves their health.
- Healthier people at work can contribute to the economy.
- Improving employment rates and health of people at work reduces health-related costs.

Chapter Summary

As in every other area of practice, occupational therapy practitioners must be aware of the policies and legislation that affect clients and their circumstances. Such awareness enables the clinician to provide the best care and advocate for the client.

Employment is guided by many laws and policies, including workers' compensation, disability legislation and regulation, antidiscrimination legislation for protected populations, and a variety of work incentives and policies to promote employment. Being aware of federal- and state-based regulatory bodies and resources is critical for the occupational therapy practitioner in the provision of work-related care.

Case Resolution

You see Rena in your clinic about 2 years after she was discharged from occupational therapy. She is getting physical therapy for lower extremity symptoms associated with spinal stenosis. She states that she has been off work for 10 months and has been terminated at work. Rena notes that she cannot perform the standing, walking, climbing, and material handling required of an electrician. She states that her depression has worsened, and she was not determined to be a good candidate for vocational rehabilitation due to problems with concentration and anxiety. Because Rena's problems are not work-related, she is not receiving workers' compensation, and because she has not accrued adequate work credits at the unions, she does not qualify for retirement at this time. She states that short-term disability through her union is nearing the end of the policy period and that her health insurance will run out soon. Rena appears distraught and hopeless.

You ask Rena if she has long-term disability through her union. She does not know but states that she will find out. You also suggest that if she has not made over $1,000 per month, she may qualify for Social Security Disability Income after she has been off of work for 1 year. Her long work history and spinal stenosis may qualify her for SSDI, and you explain that if she is denied, she should reapply. You tell Rena that she should consider using COBRA to continue health-care benefits because she will not be eligible for Medicare until she has been on SSDI for 2 years. You give Rena written information about these benefits and tell her to call you if she needs help. She is very appreciative of your suggestions.

This case demonstrates how occupational therapy practitioners can assist clients with work interruptions by understanding federal, state, and local policies and work incentives.

References

American Occupational Therapy Association (AOTA). (2008). Occupational therapy practice and framework: Domain and process. *American Journal of Occupational Therapy, 62,* 625–683.

Barnes, T., Holmes, J., & College of Occupational Therapists. (2009). *Occupational Therapy in Vocational Rehabilitation: A Brief Guide to Current Practice in the UK.* London: College of Occupational Therapists.

Black, C. (2008). *Dame Carol Black's Review of the Health of Britain's Working Age Population: Working for a Healthier Tomorrow.* London: Stationery Office.

Canada Labour Code. (R.S.C., 1985, c. L-2). Retrieved from www.hrsdc.gc.ca/eng/labour/labour_law/index.shtml.

Canadian Charter of Rights and Freedoms. Part I of the Constitution Act, 1982, Schedule B to the Canada Act 1982 (UK), 1982, c 11. Retrieved from www.efc.ca/pages/law/charter/charter.text.html.

Canadian Human Rights Commission. (2007). Canadian Human Rights Act: Overview. Retrieved from www.chrc-ccdp.ca/about/human_rights_act-eng.aspx.

Civil Rights Act of 1964. Pub.L. 88-352, 78 Stat. 241 (1964).

College of Occupational Therapists. (2007). *Recovering Ordinary Lives: The Strategy for Occupational Therapy in Mental Health Services 2007–2017.* London: The College.

College of Occupational Therapists. (2008). *The College of Occupational Therapists' Vocational Rehabilitation Strategy.* London: The College.

College of Occupational Therapists. (2011). Home page. Retrieved from www.cot.co.uk/Homepage/.

Disability Discrimination Act 2005. UK Public General Acts, 2005 c. 13. Retrieved from www.legislation.gov.uk/ukpga/2005/13/contents.

Employment Act 2002. UK Public General Acts, 2002 c. 22. Retrieved from www.legislation.gov.uk/ukpga/2002/22/contents.

Employment Rights Act 1996. UK Public General Acts, 1996 c. 18. Retrieved from www.legislation.gov.uk/ukpga/1996/18/contents.

Future Vision Coalition. (2008). A new vision for mental health: Discussion paper. Retrieved from www.cpft.nhs.uk/LinkClick.aspx?fileticket=xdbP4HigeHo%3D&tabid=646&mid=1360&language=en-GB.

Great Britain Department for Work and Pensions & Department of Health (GBDWP/DH). (2008). *Improving Health and Work: Changing Lives. The Government's Response to Dame Carol Black's Review of the Health of Britain's Working-Age Population.* Norwich, England: Stationery Office.

Great Britain Department for Work and Pensions & Department of Health (GBDWP/DH). (2009). *Working Our Way to Better Mental Health: A Framework for Action.* London: Stationery Office.

Health and Safety at Work Act 1974. UK Public General Acts, 1974 c. 37. Retrieved from www.legislation.gov.uk/ukpga/1974/37/contents.http://www.hse.gov.uk/legislation/hswa.htm

Health Professions Council. (2007). Standards of proficiency—Occupational therapists. Retrieved from www.hpc-uk.org/publications/standards/index.asp?id=45.

HM Government. (2009). *Work, Recovery and Inclusion: Employment Support for People in Contact with Secondary Mental Services.* London: National Mental Health Development Unit.

Human Rights Act 1998. UK Public General Acts, 1998 c. 42. Retrieved from www.legislation.gov.uk/ukpga/1998/42/contents.

Israel Government Portal Labor Laws. (n.d.). Ministry of Industry, Trade and Labor information. Retrieved from www.gov.il/FirstGov/TopNavEng/Engoffices/ EngMinistries/EngIndustry/EngIndustryLaws/.

Karten Network. (2011). Karten CTEC Centres.[Information regarding Computer-aided Training Education and Communication Centres]. Retrieved from http://karten .djmsandpit.info/?p=650.

National Social Inclusion Programme, National Institute for Mental Health in England (NIMHE), & Care Services Improvement Partnership (CSIP). (2006). Vocational services for people with severe mental health problems: Commissioning guidance. Retrieved from http://www .dh.gov.uk/en/Publicationsandstatistics/Publications/ PublicationsPolicyAndGuidance/DH_4131059.

Perkins, R., Farmer, P., & Litchfield, P. (2009). *Realising Ambitions: Better Employment Support for People with a Mental Health Condition.* Norwich, England: Stationery Office.

Sainsbury Centre for Mental Health. (2007). *Mental Health at Work: Developing the Business Case.* London: Sainsbury Centre for Mental Health.

Sainsbury Centre for Mental Health & College of Occupational Therapists. (2008). Vocational rehabilitation: What is it, who can deliver it, and who pays? Retrieved from www.centreformentalhealth.org.uk/pdfs/vocational_ rehab_what_who_paper.pdf.

Scottish Executive. (2005). *Healthy Working Lives: A Plan for Action.* Edinburgh: Scottish Executive.

Scottish Executive. (2006). *Workforce Plus: An Employability Framework.* Edinburgh: Scottish Executive.

Scottish Executive & National Health Service in Scotland. (2007). *Co-ordinated, Integrated and Fit for Purpose; A Delivery Framework for Adult Rehabilitation in Scotland.* Edinburgh: Scottish Executive.

Scottish Government. (2009). *Towards a Mentally Flourishing Scotland: Policy and Action Plan.* Edinburgh: Scottish Government.

Social Security Administration (SSA). (2010). Substantial gainful activity. Retrieved from www.socialsecurity.gov/ OACT/COLA/sga.html.

Social Security Administration (SSA). (2011a). Disability evaluation under Social Security. Retrieved from www.ssa.gov/disability/professionals/bluebook/ AdultListings.htm.

Social Security Administration (SSA). (2011b). Disability planner: Social Security protection if you become disabled. Retrieved from www.ssa.gov/dibplan/index.htm.

Social Security Administration (SSA). (2011c). The Red Book: Overview of our disability programs. Retrieved from www.ssa.gov/redbook/eng/overview-disability.htm.

Social Security Administration (SSA). (2011d). Ticket to Work. Retrieved from www.ssa.gov/work/aboutticket .html.

U.S. Bureau of Labor Statistics. (2010). Labor force statistics from the current population survey. Retrieved from www.bls.gov/cps/cpsdisability.htm.

U.S. Internal Revenue Service. (2011). Tax benefits for businesses who have employees with disabilities. Retrieved from www.irs.gov/businesses/small/article/0,,id= 185704,00.html.

United Kingdom Rehabilitation Council. (2009). Rehabilitation standards version 1.0. Retrieved from www.rehab-council.org.uk/UKRC/pages/DownloadForm.aspx? Type=Standards.

Vocational Rehabilitation Association–UK. (2008). VRA Standards of Practice. Retrieved from www.vra-uk .org/civicrm/contribute/transact?reset=1&id=10.

Wadell, G., & Burton, A. K. (2008). *Is Work Good for Your Health and Well-being?* London: Stationery Office.

Welfare Reform Act 2009. UK Public General Acts, 2009 c. 24. Retrieved from http://www.legislation.gov.uk/ukpga/ 2009/24/contents.

Workforce Recruitment Program. (2011). Welcome to the 2011 Workforce Recruitment Program for College Students with Disabilities (WRP). Retrieved from https://wrp.gov/LoginPre.do?method=login.

U.S. Acts

ADA Amendments Act of 2008, Pub.L. 110-325, 2008, 122 Stat. 3553, 3553-54 (codified as amended at 42 U.S.C. § 12101 Note).

Age Discrimination in Employment Act of 1967, Pub.L. 90-202, Dec. 15, 1967, 81 Stat. 602 (29 U.S.C. 621 et seq.).

American Recovery and Reinvestment Act of 2009, (ARRA), Pub.L. 111_5, Feb. 17, 2009, 123 Stat. 115, H.R. 1.

Americans with Disabilities Act of 1990, Pub.L. 101-336, July 26, 1990, 104 Stat. 327 (42 U.S.C. 12101 et seq.).

Civil Rights Act of 1964, Pub.L. 88-352, July 2, 1964, 78 Stat. 241.

Civil Service Reform Act of 1978, Pub.L. 95-454, Oct. 13, 1978, 92 Stat. 1111.

Consolidated Omnibus Budget Reconciliation Act of 1985, Pub.L. 99-272, Apr. 7, 1986, 100 Stat. 82.

Fair Labor Standards Act of 1938, ch. 676, 52 Stat. 1060 (29 U.S.C. 201 et seq.).

Family and Medical Leave Act of 1993, Pub.L. 103-3, Feb. 5, 1993, 107 Stat. 6 (5 U.S.C. 6381 et seq.; 29 U.S.C. 2601 et seq.).

Federal Employees' Compensation Act of 1916, Sept. 7, 1916, ch. 458, 39 Stat. 742.

Genetic Information Nondiscrimination Act of 2008, Pub.L. 110-233, 122 Stat. 881.

Longshore and Harbor Workers' Compensation Act, Mar. 4, 1927, ch. 509, 44 Stat. 1424 (33 U.S.C. 901 et seq.).

Occupational Safety and Health Act of 1970, Pub.L. 91-596, Dec. 29, 1970, 84 Stat. 1590 (29 U.S.C. 651 et seq.).

Pregnancy Discrimination Act of 1978, Pub.L. 95-555, Oct. 31, 1978, 92 Stat. 2076 (42 U.S.C. 2000e(k)).

Rehabilitation Act Amendments of 1974, Pub.L. 93-516, title I, Dec. 7, 1974, 88 Stat. 1617.

Rehabilitation Act of 1973, Pub.L. 93-112, Sept. 26, 1973, 87 Stat. 355 (29 U.S.C. 701 et seq.).

Uniformed Services Employment and Reemployment Rights Act of 1994 (USERRA), Pub.L. 103-353, codified as amended at 38 U.S.C. §§ 4301–4335.

Uniformed Services Employment and Reemployment Rights Act of 1994, Pub.L. 103-353, Oct. 13, 1994, 108 Stat. 3149.

Veterans Education and Employment Program Amendments of 1991, Pub.L. 101-237, title IV, Dec. 18, 1989, 103 Stat. 2078.

Vietnam Era Veterans' Readjustment Assistance Act of 1972, Pub.L. 92-540, Oct. 24, 1972, 86 Stat. 1074.

Vietnam Era Veterans' Readjustment Assistance Act of 1974, Pub.L. No. 93-508, § 404(a), 88 Stat. 1578, 1594 (codified as amended at 38 U.S.C. §§ 2021-2026).

Vocational Rehabilitation Act (Smith-Fess Act of 1920), June 2, 1920, ch. 219, as added July 6, 1943, ch. 190, §1, 57 Stat. 374 (29 U.S.C. 31 et seq.).

Vocational Rehabilitation Act Amendments of 1943 (Barden-LaFollette Act), July 6, 1943, ch. 190, 57 Stat. 374.

Vocational Rehabilitation Act Amendments of 1954, Aug. 3, 1954, ch. 655, 68 Stat. 652.

Vocational Rehabilitation Act Amendments of 1965, Pub.L. 89-333, Nov. 8, 1965, 79 Stat. 1282.

Workforce Investment Act of 1998, Pub.L. 105-220, Aug. 7, 1998, 112 Stat. 936.

Glossary

Consolidated Omnibus Budget Reconciliation Act of 1985 (COBRA) allows individuals in the United States who lose their health benefits the right to continue group health benefits provided by their group health plan for limited periods of time under certain circumstances.

Medicaid is a U.S. health-care program for people with low income and limited resources.

Medicare is a U.S. health insurance program for people age 65 or older and many people with disabilities.

Material Safety Data Sheet (MSDS) is a document with information regarding the properties of hazardous items and their safe use.

Permanent partial disability (PPD) is financial reimbursement for individuals who suffer a permanent loss of function due to work injury or illness regardless of whether they can return to work.

Social Security Disability Insurance (SSDI) is a U.S. federal program that provides monthly cash benefits to individuals who are unable to work for a year or more because of a disability.

Supplemental Security Income (SSI) is a U.S. federal income supplement program that provides monthly benefits to individuals who are disabled, blind, or age 65 or older and have limited income and resources.

Substantial gainful activity (SGA) is a level of work activity and earnings.

Temporary total disability (TTD) is partial income paid by employees to help replace lost wages of individuals who cannot perform their work duties due to job-related illness or injury.

Resources

America's Career Resource Network
www.acrnetwork.org

American National Standards Institute (ANSI)
www.ansi.org

Centers for Medicare and Medicaid Service
www.cms.hhs.gov/home/medicaid.asp
www.cms.hhs.gov/home/medicare.asp

Federal Workers' Compensation
www.dol.gov/dol/topic/workcomp/index.htm

Job Accommodation Network
www.jan.wvu.edu

National Human Genome Research Institute
www.genome.gov/24519851

National Institute of Occupational Health and Safety
www.cdc.gov/niosh/about.html

Occupational Information Network
http://online.onetcenter.org

U.S. Office of Personnel Management
www.opm.gov/index.asp

Vocational Rehabilitation (State Rehabilitation Agencies)
www.rehabnetwork.org/directors_contact.htm

Workers' Compensation Resource
http://topics.law.cornell.edu/wex/Workers_compensation

Workforce Recruitment Program for College Students with Disabilities (WRP)
https://wrp.gov/LoginPre.do?method=login

Equal Employment Opportunity Commission

Age Discrimination in Employment Act of 1967
www.eeoc.gov/laws/statutes/adea.cfm

Civil Rights Act of 1964
www.eeoc.gov/laws/statutes/titlevii.cfm

Pregnancy Discrimination Act of 1978
www.eeoc.gov/laws/types/pregnancy.cfm

Occupational Safety and Health Administration

Ergonomics Program Management Guidelines
www.osha.gov/dts/osta/oshasoft/index.html

Ergonomics Standard of 1999
www.osha.gov/pls/oshaweb/owadisp.show_document?p_table=FEDERAL_REGISTER&p_id=16305

OSH Act
www.osha.gov/pls/oshaweb/owasrch.search_form?p_doc_type=OSHACT&p_toc_level=0&p_keyvalue=OshAct_toc_by_sect.html

OSHA eTools and Electronic Products for Compliance Assistance
www.osha.gov/dts/osta/oshasoft/index.html

Social Security

Social Security Disability Insurance Program
www.socialsecurity.gov/pgm/links_disability.htm

Social Security Retirement
www.socialsecurity.gov/retirement/

Supplemental Security Income
www.socialsecurity.gov/pgm/links_ssi.htm

Ticket to Work
www.socialsecurity.gov/work/

U.S. Department of Labor

U.S. Office of Disability Employment Policy (ODEP)
www.dol.gov/odep/

Consolidated Omnibus Budget Reconciliation Act of 1985 (COBRA)
www.dol.gov/ebsa/faqs/faq_compliance_cobra.html

Employer Assistance and Resource Network (EARN)
www.dol.gov/odep/programs/earn.htm

Employment Laws: Department of Labor
www.dol.gov/compliance/guide/index.htm

Fair Labor Standards Act (FLSA)
www.dol.gov/whd/flsa/index.htm

Family and Medical Leave Act
www.dol.gov/compliance/laws/comp-fmla.htm

Safety and Health Standards: Occupational Safety and Health
www.dol.gov/compliance/guide/osha.htm

Uniformed Services Employment and Reemployment Rights Act of 1994 (USERRA)
www.dol.gov/vets/programs/userra/main.htm

Vietnam Era Veterans' Readjustment Assistance Act (VEVRAA)
www.dol.gov/compliance/laws/comp-vevraa.htm

Workforce Investment Act of 1998 (WIA)
www.dol.gov/odep/pubs/ek01/act.htm

18 Developing and Marketing Work-Related Services

Brent Braveman

Key Concepts

The following are key concepts addressed in this chapter:

- The health-care system in the United States is a large, complex, dualistic system complicated by involvement of both the government and private industry.
- Marketing is a complex, multistep process that includes assessment of the internal and external environments of your organization and development of programming and marketing communications.
- Program development shares some steps with the marketing process, and marketing and program development are often completed in sync with each other.
- Just as occupational therapy practitioners combine multiple practice models to design intervention for clients, program developers combine multiple program development and practice models to design programs of service delivery.

Case Introduction

Alicia is an occupational therapist with 4 years of experience in traditional hospital-based settings. Before becoming an occupational therapist, Alicia spent 2 years in the Peace Corps and has a strong interest in working with underserved and disadvantaged populations. The values of volunteerism and social justice were instilled in Alicia by her parents at an early age, and she pictures herself working in the community in a non-profit service organization. She is working part time on a clinical occupational therapy doctorate (OTD) with a focus on professional leadership and advanced clinical practice. Her doctoral program requires that she complete a 20-credit applied project. Alicia explored options for her project and decided to complete a project that involved working with an underserved population and would help her transition her career into less traditional practice focused more on community-based intervention.

By networking with her peers, school faculty, and other occupational therapy practitioners on social media sites such as Facebook and OT Connections (the social media site of the American Occupational Therapy Association [AOTA]), Alicia found other occupational therapy practitioners with similar interests. Based on the recommendation of a new colleague, Alicia contacted her local AIDS service organization (ASO) that provides case management and transitional living services for persons living with HIV/AIDS to explore unmet needs of the residents. She learned that the most pressing unmet need for most of the residents is assistance in finding and sustaining employment. Because most of the residents also have histories of mental illness and/or substance abuse and many grew up in poorer neighborhoods with limited educational and training backgrounds, they face significant barriers to employment.

As part of her OTD project, Alicia decided to enroll in a course on developing theory-based and evidence-based occupational therapy programming. The primary assignment for this course is to develop a framework for a new program. Alicia approached the ASO and suggested that she would like to use the organization and the development of prevocational and vocational services using a supported employment approach as the focus for her class project. She also suggested that she could continue working with the organization and complete her 20-credit OTD project at the organization and work to put the new program in place. The program director of the ASO saw this as a unique opportunity to take advantage of knowledge and skills that were not currently in place at the organization and agreed to develop a learning and volunteer contract with Alicia to carry out her class assignment and her OTD project.

Introduction

As described throughout this text, occupational therapy practitioners provide work-related interventions in a wide range of settings, including hospitals and medical clinics, school systems, communities, nonprofit agencies, standalone vocational rehabilitation programs, and the workplace itself. Clients include injured workers, organizations, employers, and communities. Occupational therapists and occupational therapy assistants assume a wide variety of roles within these programs and have moved beyond providing direct intervention to administrative roles, consultative roles, case management, and developing and marketing programs within organizations and as private entrepreneurs.

Marketing and program development are topics often included in entry-level occupational therapy texts and educational programs, and they are critical functions completed by managers and entrepreneurs in the area of work-related intervention (Braveman, 2006b; Braveman, 2009; Richmond, 2003). Marketing and program development are closely related, and both are complicated processes that typically require much time, effort, advanced skills, and in-depth knowledge. The complexity of marketing and program development should not be underestimated. Full discussions of either process are beyond the scope of this book, and readers are highly encouraged to use materials and resources specific to the marketing process or developing a program of service if involved in significant efforts. However, because they are so important to successfully establishing and implementing effective work-related programming, they are overviewed in this chapter. More in-depth resources are suggested at the end of the chapter. Before moving into these reviews, a brief overview of the scope of work-related services is provided. Most of these areas of service are also addressed in more depth in other chapters of this book.

The Scope of Occupational Therapy Work-Related Services

Rising health-care costs and difficult economic times continue to draw attention and debate to our complex dualistic health-care system. *Dualistic* means that both the government (federal, state, and local) and private business and industry are involved in the delivery of health care in the United States. In regard to work-related practice, dualism is illustrated through policies, laws, and systems such as the Americans with Disabilities Act (ADA) and the workers' compensation system. Our federal and state governments are involved in providing vocational preparation and rehabilitation services. At the same time, many private businesses and nonprofit private agencies are also involved in providing vocational rehabilitation, injury prevention, return-to-work services, and other work-related services. An increasing number of occupational therapy practitioners have become successful entrepreneurs and business owners. Additionally, a growing number of occupational therapy practitioners function as consultants to promote full participation of persons with disabilities and challenges of all types in our workforce.

An increasing number of occupational therapy practitioners have become successful entrepreneurs and business owners. Additionally, a growing number of occupational therapy practitioners function as consultants to promote full participation of persons with disabilities and challenges of all types in our workforce.

Occupational therapy practitioners provide assessment, consultation, and intervention in wide range of work-related practice settings and programs. Some of the most common are listed in Table 18.1 along with brief descriptions. Many of these settings are discussed in depth throughout this book.

Marketing and Program Development

The Marketing Process

Many people think *marketing* refers to advertising or promoting a product or service. Although product promotion is one element of marketing, the full marketing process includes many other aspects and can be extraordinarily complex. Occupational therapy practitioners who want or need to assess the needs of the target populations they serve and

Table 18.1 Types of Work-Related Services Provided by Occupational Therapy Practitioners

Setting	Description
Vocational preparation and habilitation	Focuses on the development and improvement of basic work skills to facilitate supported or competitive employment. Assists in integrating the role of worker with other life roles and developing identity and competence as a worker.
Vocational rehabilitation	Assists persons with a work history who have left the workplace due to an injury or onset of an impairment or disability to return to a specific workplace or to work in general.
Supported employment • Developmental disabilities • Mental health	Focuses on meeting the needs of individuals with disabilities assuming that all individuals, regardless of the nature or extent of their disabilities, should have the opportunity and support to work in the community. Practitioners work to locate and/or modify meaningful jobs in the community and provide training and supports at the job site.
Injury prevention and ergonomics • Functional capacity evaluation • Workplace consultation	Intervenes with individuals and/or a workplace to prevent injury and maximize health and function through assessment of the fit between a worker and the environment.
Preemployment/postoffer screening • Job Analysis	Screens potential employees to establish their ability to perform the essential elements of a job after a job offer is extended but before the employee begins. Often combined with analysis of jobs at a workplace to identify the essential functions of a particular job.
Onsite work programs	Delivers work-related services, including prevention, consultation, and postinjury rehabilitation at the work site. Intervention with injured workers often focuses on returning the worker to the job as soon as possible, which may involve negotiating light-duty alterations to a job.

Table 18.1   Types of Work-Related Services Provided by Occupational Therapy Practitioners—cont'd

Setting	Description
School-based transition services	Services provided under the Individuals with Disabilities Education Act (IDEA) focus on assisting adolescents and young adults with disabilities to make the transition from school- and education-based settings to work.
Community-based programs • Homelessness programming	A wide range of community-based and nonprofit agencies provide services to populations such as the homeless, persons fleeing domestic violence, and persons living with HIV/AIDS, mental illness, and addiction to substances. Services range from teaching basic skills such as computer skills to supported employment and training programs for specific trades, such as working in restaurants or hotels.
Employer consultation • Job and ergonomic analysis • ADA consultation	Services provided directly to employers and organizations can include job and ergonomic analysis, injury prevention programs, and consultation on implementation of the ADA, such as identifying reasonable accommodations for employees with disabilities.
Case management	Case managers help clients secure services and coordinate their delivery to be as comprehensive and effective as possible. Assessment of clients' long-term needs, evaluation of resources, locating and accessing additional resources, and guiding clients and providers through the interaction of complex systems is often a role of the case manager.

design, develop, and promote new products and services to meet those needs will likely need some education or training beyond their entry-level education. Many persons pursue advanced education and graduate degrees and spend their entire careers developing skills in marketing and program development. Luckily, many larger organizations have on staff marketing professionals who can guide and aid you in the process.

Components of the Marketing Process

Braveman (2006c) described the marketing process as comprising four major components or steps. These steps are often combined with efforts such as program development, program evaluation, and outcomes assessment. Each of the four components of the marketing process is briefly described in Box 18.1 and is outlined in the next section of this chapter. The involvement of occupational therapy practitioners in each step can vary widely: for example, small business owners or entrepreneurs may be integrally involved in all the steps, direct service practitioners may only assist with data collection or another piece of the process, and occupational therapy managers may spend most of their time consulting and collaborating with a marketing professional.

Organizational Assessment

The first step of the marketing process involves collecting data and information to examine the internal influences that will impact the development of your product or service. Organizational assessments examine factors such as your organization's reputation in the community, the staff's qualifications, type and quality of equipment, available space, geographic location, and level of administrative support for new programs (Braveman, 2006c). Organizational assessments are conducted to establish a comprehensive understanding of the resources available to develop and promote your product. The organizational assessment also identifies potential obstacles and constraints. This is also the time to network with key stakeholders within your organization or business to make sure you

---

Box 18.1 Components of the Marketing Process

- *Organizational Assessment:* Examination of the factors within an organization that influence the development and promotion of a new product or service.
- *Environmental Assessment:* Examination of the data, information, and other forms of evidence, including the needs of target populations, that will guide the development and promotion of a new product or service.
- *Market Analysis:* Use of the information gained during organizational and environmental assessments to validate perceptions of the wants and needs of the target populations that will receive a new product or service.
- *Marketing Communications:* Packaging and promoting a product so the target populations and other key stakeholders in the new product or service have a clear understanding of what the product or service is and how it may be accessed.

(Braveman, 2006c; reprinted with permission)

---

all share the same goals and vision of your organization's future. A common first step is to review the mission statement of your business or department and consider your new product in light of your mission. Coordinating organizational assessment activities with others in the organization is also an effective way to establish new working relationships with experts who can help you with later steps of the marketing process.

A common and useful tool for assessing both the organization and the environment is *SWOT (strengths, weaknesses, opportunities, and threats) analyses.* SWOT analyses can be conducted by combining a review of key documents or reports (financial reports, outcome statistics, program evaluation, or accreditation reports) with staff interviews, discussions, or structured brainstorming exercises. SWOT analyses may also be completed with a focus on developing a particular product or service.

Large organizations routinely collect various types of data and information such as referral rates, payer mix, and geographic location of target populations. Occupational therapy practitioners planning new services and products will find this information helpful. In smaller organizations, this information may not be as readily available, and the practitioner may need to be more resourceful to find the information needed for the marketing and development of new products. Braveman (2006c) suggested some simple strategies to aid with data collection during the organizational assessment. These strategies are presented in Box 18.2.

Box 18.2 Simple Strategies for Organizational Assessment

- Conduct informational interviews with other department directors over coffee or a meal to learn more about the skills, resources, and needs of other disciplines.
- Obtain your boss's permission to announce a potential product or service you are considering in a meeting, in a newsletter, or on a Listserv, and ask for input or concerns from your peers.
- Ask your boss and representatives from departments such as planning, marketing, publications, or business affairs if there are routine reports produced that might be helpful to you that you are not currently receiving.
- To obtain information from physicians, nurses, or other internal customers, conduct a short survey of needs, resources, or limitations by visiting other departments' staff meetings.
- Complete a SWOT analysis with your department; enlist other department directors to do the same and share the results.
- Spend an hour reviewing your organization's website and note the relevant services offered by other departments that might have some synergy with one of your existing or future products or services.

(Braveman, 2006c; reprinted with permission)

Environmental Assessment

An environmental assessment helps determine needs and existing resources by examining data and information such as demographics, cultural trends, health-care utilization patterns, political and regulatory issues, new technologies, and socioeconomic status of the target populations served by your organization. Learning about your competitors and the products and services currently offered as well as gaps in offered services in the existing marketplace is also completed as part of the environmental assessment. The extent to which this type of data and information is available in your organization will vary a great deal. Some organizations may aggressively collect data such as reimbursement patterns or discounts to payers, but other organizations are surprisingly unsophisticated in their monitoring of the external environment. Some of the types of data and information you might use to evaluate the needs and resources of your target populations include population demographics (age, marital status, socioeconomic data, insurance status, etc.), payer mix for particular catchment areas, and organizational plans for future space and resource allocation.

Collecting data and information about target populations, payers, and competitors can be tremendously complex, particularly in areas with large populations and multiple providers, but some simple strategies, presented in Box 18.3, can be used in almost any setting.

Market Analysis

A market analysis uses the data and information collected in your organizational and environmental assessments to validate your perceptions of the wants and needs of your target population(s). The desired outcome of your market analysis is a *marketing plan* that coordinates and applies information about your organization or business, your current and planned products and services, the objectives, and the strategies to guide your marketing activities and communication with your target populations about your occupational therapy products and services (Richmond, 2003).

Market analyses for services that will require a large investment of capital are often quite complex and comprehensive. Few occupational therapy departments have the resources to complete complex analyses, and this may be true for many small businesses. However, some of the same strategies that can be used to collect primary data and information from your target populations as part of your environmental analysis can be used in the market analysis to validate your perceptions of the needs, resources, and limitations of the same target populations.

Box 18.3 Simple Strategies for Environmental Assessment

- Use the Internet, phonebook, and professional association directories to identify competitors in the area who are already serving your target population and review their websites and brochures to learn about their products and services.
- Conduct informational interviews with leaders of community-based organizations or public health officials concerned with the health and wellness of your target population.
- Conduct informal or formal focus groups with members of your target population.
- Have a booth or table at a health fair, community festival, street fair or collaborate with others in your organization to offer free screenings during which you can also collect information about your target population.
- Identify the physicians providing services to your target population, and collect information by visiting their offices, conducting mail or telephone surveys, or offering a continuing education event or meeting where you might be able to collect information on their perceptions of your target population's needs, resources, and limitations.

Marketing Communications

Marketing communications is the step in the marketing process during which you package and promote your product or service. Marketing communications involves devising methods of communicating with your target populations (customers), including potential clients, payers, and referral sources. Distinguishing between your various types of customers helps to guide promotional efforts. Sometimes the client is also the payer, but when the client and payer are different, as in the case of a client who has insurance, it can be much more effective to identify the specific concerns of each customer and devise related but separate communications.

Marketing communications also involves determining who must be educated about products and services you provide as well as the most successful medium to deliver your message. Braveman (2006c) described a simple and helpful set of concepts called the *Four P's of Marketing:* (1) product, (2) price, (3) place, and (4) promotion.

> *It can be tempting to agree to provide a service assuming you will be able to learn what you need to know in time, but the fastest way to lose potential customers is to promise more than you can deliver.*

Identifying your *product* means clearly defining the scope and boundaries of what you are and are not prepared to deliver. It can be tempting to agree to provide a service assuming you will be able to learn what you need to know in time, but the fastest way to lose potential customers is to promise more than you can deliver. For example, consider the case of Frank, who opened his own consulting business after working for a local rehabilitation system for several years. Frank was skilled at conducting job analyses, preemployment screenings, workstation evaluations, and ergonomic assessments to prevent injury in common office settings. While he had some exposure to the ADA and in the past had made simple recommendations for reasonable accommodations, he had no formal training in ADA consulting and was unfamiliar with the complexities of the regulation. After a few months of working on his own, Frank completed some preemployment screens for a large employer who was very happy with his work. The director of human resources asked Frank about the other services he offered and specifically about consultation on employment policies and the ADA. Worried that he might lose a potentially big customer, Frank assured the HR director that he could provide anything the company needed. However, Frank delivered his reports and documentation. They were vague and in places contradictory. When questioned, he was unable to clearly and confidently provide answers. The HR director lost confidence in Frank's abilities and stopped using him not only for ADA consultation but altogether. In situations like Frank's, it is tempting to try to accommodate such requests to grow your business faster. But it is important to avoid promising an enthusiastic customer a service that you are not prepared to deliver. Failing to deliver on such promises is the fastest way to squelch a program's potential. By defining your product carefully in advance and being honest about what you can and cannot deliver, you will develop trust with your current customers and a positive business reputation for potential customers, and you will grow your business faster.

Purchasing a product or service incurs a number of different costs. One type of cost, of course, is the financial cost or *price* of your product. In addition to financial costs are other, less obvious types of cost to a consumer that will influence the success of a new product or service. These can be related to convenience or time, such as whether your customer needs to travel to you and if doing so is easy or difficult. Other costs may be more psychological or emotional, such as whether clients may experience physical or psychological discomfort by using your services. Some of these other types of costs are described in Box 18.4. While you may not be able to avoid these costs, you may be able to identify ways to minimize them.

Place is where your service is delivered or where your product is available to your customers. While this may seem straightforward, when it comes to most occupational therapy services, providers have become more flexible as competition for limited reimbursement has increased. Entrepreneurs and business owners find that flexibility in schedules and providing services on days and at times when customers are available, such as evenings and weekends, may provide an edge over your competitors. Consider providing work-related consultative services to an employer that has workers on shifts 24 hours a day, 7 days a week. Will you make your services available at 3 a.m.? The rise of *onsite work programs* that provide rehabilitative services at the workplace of injured workers is a great example of using the concept of *place* not only to provide convenience to customers but also to provide services in an *evidence-based* manner. When you provide work-related services in the client's real-world setting, the client misses less time from work and costs may be saved for both the payer and the employer because the injured worker can return to light duty more quickly. The occupational therapy practitioner may also more effectively influence the social factors that can affect return to work, such as the injured worker's relationship with his or her boss and coworkers.

Promotion of your services may include internal promotion if you are introducing a new product or service and want your coworkers' support in establishing the new offering as well as promoting the product or service to potential customers. Identifying everyone in your organization who will benefit from your new venture or will want to understand it can be critical to success. Keeping others informed allows them to support you and to identify any challenges you may not have considered. For example, will increased volume of visits have an impact on the workload of another department? Will billing or collection forms and services need to be updated? Sharing your plans with all potential internal stakeholders and identifying their potential concerns can help avoid some uncomfortable and unnecessary circumstances.

External promotion calls for a carefully coordinated effort by all stakeholders who are interested in providing services or products to the same target population. By collaborating with coworkers, you can develop an action plan for promoting your products and services to various target populations. Braveman (2006c) suggested that answering the following questions can help you begin to develop an action plan for external promotion:

1. Who is the target population of your product or service (i.e., the consumers)?
2. Besides the consumer or direct beneficiary of your product or service, who else is either an internal or external customer (e.g., nurses, physicians, payers)?
3. What are the primary goals of your consumers and customers?
4. Who will be involved in deciding where to go for services?
5. What is the most efficient and effective way to reach your consumers and customers?

Box 18.4 Nonmonetary Costs Associated With Product or Service Use

- Time costs such as the time involved in getting to or using your service, including the time away from paid employment or family.
- Emotional or psychological costs associated with admitting the need for your service.
- Physical costs such as pain associated with a treatment.
- Monetary costs beyond direct charges for services, such as costs for parking or travel to and from your service location.

Selecting Promotional Media

Strategies and methods to communicate with potential customers about your product or service are called promotional media, which are varied and can be used in many different combinations. Choosing the most effective promotional media may be straightforward or complex depending on whether you will be promoting your product or service internally, externally, or both. The available time and financial resources may limit your choice of promotional strategies. This may be especially true for the new consultant, small business owner, or budding entrepreneur. Recognizing the advantages and disadvantages of each form of promotional media will also help you narrow your options and make a selection. The advantages and disadvantages of some of the most common forms of promotional media are presented in Table 18.2. In addition to the strategies listed in Table 18.2, other methods of promoting a new product or service to a target population might include exhibiting at a continuing education conference; developing a free speakers' bureau; offering an inservice education program to physicians, nurses, or other target populations; or holding an open house in your department or program (Braveman, 2006c).

This section introduced you to the marketing process and its four steps: (1) organizational assessment, (2) environmental assessment, (3) market analysis, and (4) marketing communications. Hopefully, you now recognize that the process of identifying the needs, resources, and limitations of your organization and of various target markets can be

Table 18.2 Advantages and Disadvantages of Common Forms of Promotional Media

Communication Method	Advantages	Disadvantages
Face-to-face meetings	• Lower cost depending on number • Can customize message and alter based on response • Can evaluate customer reaction more easily	• Time intensive, can reach fewer contacts • May be perceived as an interruption
Brochures and direct mail	• Can reach larger number of contacts with one effort • Provides contact information in sustainable form for future • Time investment in development only	• Higher cost depending on number and quality • Fixed message • Difficult to evaluate customer reaction and effectiveness of effort • May be difficult to reach the decision-maker
Telephone solicitations	• Lower cost • Can customize message and alter based on response • Can reach larger number of contacts	• May be perceived as an interruption • May be difficult to reach the decision-maker
Seminars	• Can customize message and alter based on response • Can evaluate customer reaction more easily • Establishes a relationship with attendees that can be developed	• Higher cost • Time intensive, can reach fewer contacts • Difficult to evaluate customer reaction and effectiveness of effort
Television, radio, and print advertising	• Can reach larger number of contacts with one effort • Provides contact information in sustainable form for future • Time investment in development only	• Higher cost • Fixed message

extraordinarily complex. The value of developing collaborative relationships with others in your organization, community, and profession who can help you with marketing functions was stressed. By developing effective collaborations with key individuals in your organization or the community (including other business owners, *even* your competitors), you can more easily identify resources to find information that will help you justify the need for a new work-related product or service and to promote it when developed.

Marketing can be complex, and the novice occupational therapy practitioner, business owner, or entrepreneur may feel overwhelmed when first learning about the diverse range of activities that must be completed when exploring the development of a new work-related product or service. For more complex situations, it may be wise to consider hiring a marketing consultant, but even the novice can use related skill sets, such as those involved in developing new programs. The program development process is discussed next.

The Program Development Process

Directors and managers of work-related services may often be responsible for developing, planning, implementing, and evaluating programming. Like the marketing process, program development can vary in complexity from developing new or updated clinical protocols within existing programs to developing whole new lines of services. More complicated program development may call for the use of multiple theories and new approaches to organizing interventions. In-depth exploration of the various theories, conceptual practice models, and knowledge that might be used in the development of work-related services is beyond the scope of this chapter. Braveman (2006b) provided a more in-depth discussion in a chapter on program development in *Leading and Managing Occupational Therapy Services: An Evidence-Based Approach.* Table 18.3 summarizes some key terms related to the types of knowledge used in the development of occupational therapy work-related services.

Most work-related services rely on a combination of concepts from the occupational therapy paradigm to guide thinking about what the service should be and on occupational therapy conceptual practice models and related knowledge from other disciplines to define more specifically what problems are addressed, what services are provided, what outcomes are expected, and how outcomes will be achieved.

Most work-related services rely on a combination of concepts from the occupational therapy paradigm to guide thinking about what the service should be and on occupational therapy conceptual practice models and related knowledge from other disciplines to define more specifically what problems are addressed, what services are provided, what outcomes are expected, and how outcomes will be achieved. Consider, for example, providing onsite work rehabilitation to a worker returning to light duty after a shoulder injury. When developing the overall program approach, an occupational therapy practitioner might design a program by relying on multiple theories and models from occupational therapy and related disciplines, such as the biomechanical frame of reference, the model of human occupation (MOHO), the cognitive model, motor control, disability studies, social cognitive theory, the transtheoretical model of change, and the health belief model (Kielhofner, 2008; McLeroy, Bibeau, Steckler, and Glanz, 1988; Prochaska, DiClemente, and Norcross, 1992; Strecher, DeVillis, Becker, and Rosenstock, 1986).

Table 18.3 Key Terms

Theory	A theory provides an explanation of how or why a particular phenomenon occurs and how that phenomenon might be influenced. Theories are often composed of both general concepts that refer to larger chunks of reality and specific concepts that refer to the elements of which they are organized.
Frame of reference	A frame of reference is a structure for guiding practice by delineating the beliefs, assumptions, definitions, and concepts within a specific area of practice. Frames of reference employ existing theory and focus on developing methods of applying that theory in occupational therapy.
Conceptual practice model	A conceptual practice model generates theory and the methods (e.g., assessments and intervention strategies) used by therapists in their everyday work to apply that theory. Each model addresses some phenomena related to occupational functioning (e.g., motivation, perception, movement) and specifies theory and tools for application pertaining to particular kinds of problems in that area.
Paradigm	A paradigm is knowledge that specifically addresses the identity and perspective of the occupational therapy profession. The paradigm articulates a shared vision of members of the field that defines the nature and purpose of the discipline.

In addition to using models that guide what services to provide, a model that guides how to organize service (e.g., program development models) is needed. The literature is full of discussions of approaches to program development, and case examples of programs can be found in the occupational therapy literature (Braveman, 2006a; Braveman, Goldbaum, Goldstein, Karlic, and Kielhofner, 2001; Braveman, Kielhofner, Belanger, Llerena, and de las Heras, 2002; Braveman, Sen, and Kielhofner, 2001; Brownson, 2001; Grossman and Bortone, 1986; Scaffa, 2001).

Just as the focus varies among theories, conceptual practice models, and frames of reference that guide clinical decision-making with individual clients, the focus varies among different program development models. Some program development models are more focused on systematic levels and help us decide where and with whom to intervene to address a particular challenge or health problem. Other models are more useful in guiding decision-making once a setting and population for an intervention is known (Braveman, 2006c).

For example, the ecological model of health promotion describes five societal levels at which intervention could be planned: (1) the intrapersonal level, (2) the interpersonal level, (3) the organizational level, (4) the community level, and (5) the public policy level (McLeroy, et al., 1988). See Figure 18.1.

While the ecological model is very helpful in deciding *where* one might intervene once a particular challenge or health problem is identified, it is not useful in deciding *how* to intervene or what the major intervention elements of a program involve. A simple model used numerous times in the occupational therapy literature includes four processes (see Fig. 18.2):

- *Needs Assessment:* Describing the target population, naming perceived and felt needs, and analyzing available resources and constraints both internal and external to the organization or context in which the program is being planned.

Public Policy: Policies, program, and regulations of local, state, and federal bodies are examined for opportunities to influence or regulate behavior.

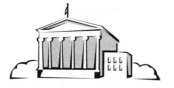

Organizational: Interrelationships among organizations or within existing social networks are examined for opportunities to influence behavior.

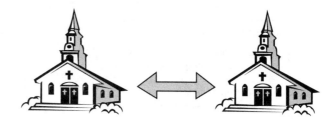

Institutional: Structures within organizations and their programs, policies, and procedures are examined for opportunities to influence behavior.

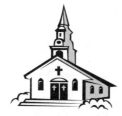

Interpersonal: Relationships and interactions with persons such as friends, family, and peer groups are examined for opportunities to influence behavior.

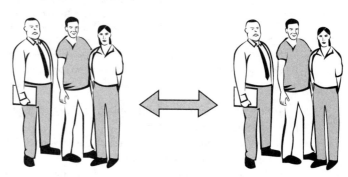

Intrapersonal: Individual factors and characteristics such as knowledge, beliefs, and values that may influence behavior.

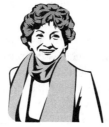

Figure 18.1 The ecological model of health promotion.

Needs Assessment

- Describe the needs of the target population and the community in which population resides
- Identify resources and constraints
- Choose conceptual practice models to address the underlying mechanism of action related to desired change

Program Evaluation

- Measure the effects of the program against the goals of the program
- Start program evaluation at the beginning (needs assessment) by identifying desirable outcomes

Program Planning

- Define a focus
- Plan to plan by identifying who must be involved in planning to assure success
- Establish goals and objectives
- Establish methods to integrate the program into the existing system
- Develop referral systems

Program Implementation

- Implement plans according to pre-established goals, objectives, and action plan
- Document actions taken and results
- Communicate results, concerns, and actions taken to key stakeholders
- Coordinate and solve problems with the team and consumers

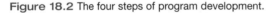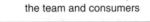

Figure 18.2 The four steps of program development.

- *Program Planning:* Identifying the steps and sequence of actions to be taken to plan for initiation of the program.
- *Program Implementation:* Initiating intervention first in trial format and then in a more formal and sustained manner.
- *Program Evaluation:* Assessing the impact and quality of program processes and outcomes and making continuous improvements in efficiency and effectiveness—an ongoing process.

It is rare that we begin the process of developing work-related services without knowing most of the critical variables, such as the setting in which the program will be delivered and who will receive the services. Because this is true and most intervention calls for a combination of theories or practice models, it is most useful to begin by identifying a program development model that will help guide you. To explain further, here is an example of how several models might be used in combination. Imagine that you are concerned with how clinical depression affects retention rates in the workplace and are interested in developing preventative services to decrease the negative effects of depression on employment. The ecological model of health promotion may help you to decide *where* to intervene and to do so at the intrapersonal, interpersonal, organizational, and community levels. To plan the steps of developing your program, you use the four-step program development model presented in Figure 18.2. As you plan your program, you know that you need a model that helps you understand motivation and why older adults may choose to become involved in various occupations, so you select the model of human occupation. As you develop specific intervention components, you find a need to address psychological aspects and cognitive of function such as social interaction, attention, memory, and problem-solving. To address these problems, you rely on related knowledge such as the cognitive model and the psychiatric rehabilitation model in combination with MOHO. Chapter 4 presents several occupational therapy conceptual practice models, including the Canadian model of occupational performance and engagement (CMOP-E), MOHO, and the biomechanical model. The transtheoretical stages of change model, the psychiatric rehabilitation model, and the social model of disability are also presented. The next section looks at a few other models that are useful in understanding work-related problems and in developing work-related services.

The Health Belief Model

The health belief model (HBM) was originally developed in the 1950s through an initiative by the U.S. Public Health Service. The HBM describes the influence of individuals' beliefs on specific health behaviors. The model suggests that choices about health behaviors are influenced by four sets of perceived beliefs:

- Perceived susceptibility such that the more a person believes he or she is susceptible to a health problem, the more likely he or she is to take action.
- Perceived seriousness such that the more serious a person believes a health problem to be, the more he or she is likely to take action.
- Perceived benefits such that the more beneficial a person believes a health behavior to be, the more likely he or she will take action.
- Perceived barriers such that the more difficult a person believes it to be to overcome the barriers to acting, the less likely he or she will take action.

In addition, the model includes a *cue to action,* which is thought to act as a trigger for making a decision about a particular health behavior (acting or not acting). Cues to action may be internal (such as pain or discomfort) or external (such as the presence of others involved in the behavior). An internal cue such as tingling in the wrist might cue a person with carpal tunnel syndrome to take a break from typing. An external cue such as seeing a safety sign reminding workers to ask for assistance when lifting heavy items might cue a worker to ask for help. The HBM can be utilized in a program to consider how to influence individual behaviors and design multiple interventions such as the various sorts of behaviors associated with injury prevention (see Fig. 18.3).

Social Cognitive Theory

Social cognitive theory (SCT) suggests that behavior is influenced by expectancies and incentives. There are three types of identified expectancies: (1) Expectancies about environmental cues or about what leads to actions are called environmental expectancies. (2) Expectancies about the consequences of one's own behavior are called outcome expectancies. (3) Expectancies about one's competence to perform a behavior necessary to achieve a particular outcome are called efficacy expectations. Incentives (or reinforcements) are the value that an individual places on particular outcomes. Examples of incentives that may influence the value of an outcome could include the praise or criticism of peers, improved perceived health, or financial impact (Bandura, 2000).

Expectancies and incentives together influence behavior. For example, a person who values the effects of frequent breaks from a computer workstation—reduced neck discomfort (incentive)—is more likely to take breaks and stretch if he or she believes that (1) working continuously without breaks poses significant health threats (environmental

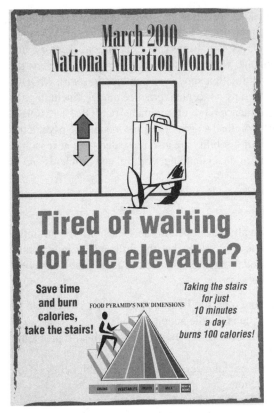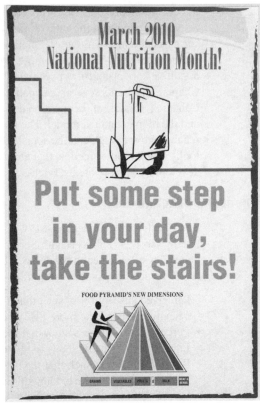

Figure 18.3 Cues to action can be delivered in simple ways in the environment, such as by posting signs as part of a health promotion effort related to nutrition, exercise, and health.

cues), (2) taking breaks and stretching will likely decrease the threats and lead to improved health and comfort (outcome expectations), and (3) he or she is capable of adopting a new work routine incorporating breaks (efficacy expectations).

While all elements of SCT are important and helpful to the occupational therapy manager who is planning a health-related program, the concept of how to impact clients' perceived self-efficacy is of particular importance. *Self-efficacy* relates to beliefs about capabilities of performing *specific* behaviors in *particular situations;* it does not refer to a personality characteristic or a global trait that operates independently of contextual factors (Strecher, et al., 1986).

In designing occupational therapy programming intended to foster changes in occupational behavior, it is important to consider that efficacy expectations (the belief that one is capable of performing a certain behavior) are learned from primary sources; but these sources are not of equal influence. These influences are described here and summarized in Box 18.5.

The first and most influential source is learning through experience or through *performance accomplishments*. Performance accomplishments are situations in which clients have the opportunity to achieve a sense of mastery through doing. An example of a performance accomplishment is when a client uses an assistive device such as an ergonomic keyboard and discovers that he or she can be successful in using the equipment.

The second source is through observation of others involved in the behavior in question, or through *vicarious experiences*. A typical example is when we show a client a videotape of a model using assistive equipment or techniques but don't necessarily allow

> ### Box 18.5 Four Sources of Learning for Efficacy Expectations (Perceived Self-Efficacy)
>
> • *Performance accomplishments:* Learning by doing, providing a hands-on opportunity for a master experience.
> • *Vicarious experience:* Learning by observation; best if the "model" is perceived as like the client and as achieving mastery with effort rather than ease.
> • *Verbal persuasion:* Learning by listening.
> • *Physiological state as effected by self-regulatory capabilities:* Level of arousal can affect client's readiness to attempt new occupational behavior.

the client hands-on time to practice. When using vicarious experiences, it is important to remember that the use of models has been shown to be more effective when the model is perceived to achieve mastery by overcoming difficulty rather than perceived as easily meeting the challenge. So if the model used in the videotape is a young, healthy occupational therapy fieldwork student who easily uses proper body mechanics, and the client is an older worker with multiple health problems, the client may perceive that the model is "not like me," and his or her sense of self-efficacy may not be impacted. The more closely the model resembles the client in age, level of function, and other characteristics, the more likely the vicarious experience will positively affect perceived self-efficacy.

A third source of influence on perceived self-efficacy is *verbal persuasion.* Verbal persuasion is simply trying to convince a client to adopt a behavior. Trying to verbally convince a client who is experiencing neck and upper back pain to alter his or her workstation is an example of verbal persuasion. While verbal persuasion is a common method to try to convince occupational therapy clients to adopt new behavior, it is unfortunately much less effective than combining it with opportunities for performance accomplishment or to observe appropriate models.

Finally, clients' physiological and psychological states, as influenced by their *self-regulatory capabilities,* can influence his or her readiness to attempt to change behavior and can affect their perceived self-efficacy. Clients who are overly aroused because they are nervous, are fearful of pain or failure, are under the influence of sedatives, or are highly fatigued may not be well prepared to attempt to learn a new behavior. Providing multiple opportunities for the client to learn or returning to a client when he or she is more physiologically ready for intervention may increase the likelihood of successfully influencing occupational behavior.

In providing health education or in attempting to convince clients to adopt new occupational behavior that is health promoting, we must also consider the three following concepts in regard to perceived self-efficacy. Perceived self-efficacy may vary according to the *magnitude* or difficulty of the task. A client may perceive that he or she can perform the simpler task of rising from a chair while following the recommendation not to flex the hip beyond 90 degrees but may not perceive that he or she can perform the more difficult task of getting in or out of a car while following the same recommendation. Perceived self-efficacy may also vary according to the *strength* of confidence for completing a particular task in a particular situation. Strength and magnitude may be closely related, but the strength of a person's conviction that he or she can complete a behavior may be influenced by factors beyond the magnitude of difficulty of the task, such as prior experiences with similar tasks. Finally, we must consider the *generality* or the degree to which expectations about a particular behavior in a particular situation will generalize to other situations. We often practice behaviors with clients in clinic settings, assuming that they will be able to generalize the behavior to the work setting or home in which they will need to perform a particular behavior.

Choosing Conceptual Practice Models and Related Knowledge for the Development of Occupational Therapy Programming

> *A mechanism of action specifies (1) what changes, (2) how change proceeds, (3) the conditions under which an intervention achieves beneficial results, and (4) why a change may occur for certain groups of consumers and not for others.*

A key issue in selecting the theoretical underpinning of a program is to be able to identify the theoretical explanation for why a particular change occurs as a result of a specific intervention. Central to this process is identifying and understanding *mechanisms of action* (see Box 18.6). A mechanism of action specifies (1) what changes, (2) how change proceeds, (3) the conditions under which an intervention achieves beneficial results, and (4) why a change may occur for certain groups of consumers and not for others (Gitlin, et al., 2000). Because satisfactory occupational functioning depends on a wide range of occupational behaviors and because different theories or conceptual practice models are intended to address a range of phenomena, developing programming most often requires managers to use more than one practice model in combination. For example, MOHO seeks to explain the occupational nature of human beings and how we come to choose and participate in occupational forms. While MOHO recognizes that occupational performance depends on underlying capacities, such as the ability to move one's arm or to sequence a series of actions in the appropriate order to complete daily activities, it does not address how to remediate or compensate for the decreased active range of motion or impaired cognition. Thus, when designing programming for someone likely to have both motor and cognitive deficits, such as an individual with a head injury, you must rely on multiple practice models to address all of the underlying mechanisms of action necessary to facilitate satisfactory occupational functioning.

Braveman and colleagues (2002) identified four questions that can guide the selection of model(s) for program planning. These questions may be used to evaluate the appropriateness of models in regard to the phenomena they address so that various models may be effectively combined in a program. They also guide a manager in considering the pragmatic issues that arise in trying to implement programs within varied contexts, such as limitations in space, adequately trained personnel, or reimbursement. These questions are listed in Box 18.7. They are briefly explained here and applied to the development of the occupational therapy components of a work rehabilitation program.

Question 1: Does the model specify the underlying mechanisms of action necessary to facilitate the desired type of change?

Occupational therapy practitioners may be involved in a variety of interventions with a client who, for instance, has a back injury. These interventions may include activities of daily living, including self-care or home management; stress management; negotiating and

---

Box 18.6 Mechanisms of Action

- Indicate how change proceeds.
- Designate the conditions under which an intervention achieves beneficial results.
- Suggest why change may occur for certain groups of consumers and not for others.

Box 18.7   Four Questions to Guide Selection of Conceptual Practice Models in Program Planning

---

1. Does the model specify the underlying mechanisms of action necessary to facilitate the desired type of change?
2. Is there sufficient evidence to support application of the model(s) to the consumer group and the type of change you wish to facilitate?
3. Does the model(s) fit with the social, cultural, political, professional, and financial contexts in which the program must be implemented?
4. Does implementation of the model have any special requirements for space, equipment, or personnel?

---

managing accommodations in the workplace; proper and adapted body mechanics; and environmental and job modification. The mechanisms of action that underlie return to satisfactory occupational performance in each of these areas are different, and no single conceptual practice model addresses all the necessary mechanisms. Table 18.4 gives examples of areas of intervention, hypothesized mechanisms of action, and a proposed conceptual practice model for facilitating improved occupational performance. It highlights the need to combine conceptual practice models to address all the key mechanisms of action to be addressed by a single occupational therapy program.

Question 2: Is there sufficient evidence to support application of the model(s) to the consumer group and the type of change you wish to facilitate?

The process of evaluating evidence requires developing specific clinical questions. Assuming that the most important clinical question—Is there evidence to support that work rehabilitation for persons with back injury is effective?—has been answered to the satisfaction of the program developer, a next step is to identify the key components of effective programs.

Table 18.4   Examples of Areas of Intervention, Hypothesized Mechanisms of Action, and Proposed Conceptual Practice Model

Sample Areas of Intervention for a Client with a Back Injury	Hypothetical Mechanisms of Action to Explain Occupational Performance	Related Conceptual Practice Model
Assessment of levels of occupational identity and occupational competence in relationship to the worker role	Levels of commitment to work (occupational identity) and belief that one can be successful (occupational competence) can influence the level of motivation to participate in work services in order to return to work.	Model of human occupation
Self-care activities including bathing and dressing	Involvement in everyday occupational forms such as bathing while standing can improve strength and endurance of persons who are experiencing pain and decreased mobility due to an injury.	Biomechanical
Environmental modifications and adaption of job tasks	Adaptation of the environment can compensate for decreased performance capacity and increase independence.	Canadian model of occupational performance and engagement

At this point, the question that must be answered is whether there is a match between the underlying mechanisms of action thought to affect the desired occupational behavior, the key components of effective programming found in the literature (evidence), and the conceptual practice models chosen to guide program development. This matching process is an iterative one in which multiple comparisons and revisions to one's thinking are likely to be made as you discover any type of mismatch between one component and another. Figure 18.4 represents the process of evaluating the fit between the suspected mechanisms of action, the components of effective programming supported by evidence, and the phenomena addressed by conceptual practice models.

Question 3: Does the chosen practice model(s) fit with the social, organizational, cultural, political, professional, and financial contexts in which the program must be implemented?

Many factors influence program development and implementation beyond just whether the program is theoretically sound and grounded in the most recent available evidence. Social, organizational, cultural, political, professional, and economic factors may also limit the capacity of an occupational therapy practitioner to develop and implement a program in exactly the manner he or she wishes. For example, theory drawn from an occupational therapy conceptual practice model might suggest that exploration of leisure pursuits and interests as a mechanism for promoting increased physical activity would be a valuable component of a work rehabilitation program. However, the realities of limits on the services that may be provided due to reimbursement mechanisms or expectations about the focus of services by employers and payers may force compromise or alterations in program design.

Considering the full range of factors that influence how a conceptual practice model is used to guide program development can save valuable time by preventing investment of resources in program components that will be poorly received. It may also help the program developer consider ways in which the conceptual practice model (either in its entirety or broken down into its primary tenets) might be introduced to key stakeholders in the organization or delivery context so that program elements are more likely to be accepted.

Question 4: Does implementation of the model have any special requirements for space, equipment, or personnel?

While a theory supported by evidence might suggest a range of possible interventions, some interventions may require space, equipment, or personnel beyond the scope of the organization's resources. It is the responsibility of the program developer to plan for funding of staff salaries, training, new equipment, and space within available resources.

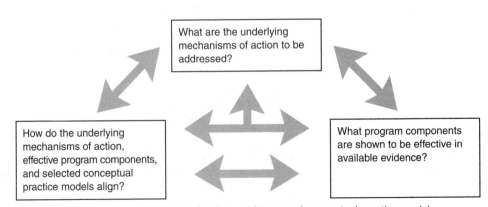

Figure 18.4 Matching mechanisms of action, evidence, and conceptual practice models.

Occupational therapy practitioners play different roles in different settings within the area of work rehabilitation, ranging from education and intervention at the worksite (which may require little equipment beyond objects used in the job) to completion of standardized functional capacity evaluations (which may require specialized equipment and have specific space demands). With the back injury client, involvement in any type of physical activity must be completed with a clear understanding of the injury and precautions to be followed, and this may require that occupational therapy practitioners have undergone training and demonstrated competencies in these areas. The resource implications of involvement in such programming must be considered early in the process of program development.

Chapter Summary

This chapter introduced and briefly reviewed the processes of marketing and program development in the context of work-related services. A primary objective of the chapter was to highlight the complexity of these processes, illustrating the wide range of information, data, methods, and theories upon which an occupational therapy practitioner must draw when involved in marketing and/or program development.

Marketing and program development are separate but related processes that require looking both within an organization and outside of it to the larger environment to identify influences and resources that might support or inhibit the development and promotion of new services. Knowledge may be drawn from the occupational therapy paradigm by using conceptual practice models such as the model of human occupation, the Canadian model of occupational performance, the biomechanical model, and others, and from related knowledge such as the ecological model of health promotion, the health belief model, or social cognitive theory. These models are often used in combination as the program developer focuses on identifying the underlying mechanisms of action that must be addressed to effectively promote change. Occupational therapy practitioners who find themselves in the position of exploring the development of new services through the marketing and program development processes are encouraged to use the many resources and descriptions found in the occupational therapy literature and to network with other professionals to assist with this complex process.

Case Resolution

As Alicia began her class assignment and her OTD project, she found that both her course instructor and her OTD advisor gave her similar advice. They both suggested she begin by reviewing the literature in occupational therapy and other fields, such as public health, to learn about the application of various models and theories related to marketing and program development. Alicia quickly learned that the marketing process is much more complex than drawing up program announcements or developing a brochure. She began to collaborate with the program director and director of development at the ASO to identify the information and data currently available that would help inform the development of the new supported employment program. While some information was readily available, they found that other information needed to be collected through assessments of the internal organization and the external environment.

Alicia quickly recognized that much of the information and data being collected and analyzed as part of the marketing process was the same information described in a simple program development model, particularly the steps of needs assessment and program planning. As she and the other staff of the ASO learned more about the perceived needs of the residents and validated these needs by continuing their organizational and environmental assessments, Alicia began to identify mechanisms of action to

(case study continues on page 422)

address in the program. She had already begun to think about which occupational therapy conceptual practice models would be appropriate to guide program and intervention planning, and she found that in real life, the processes of marketing and program development were not lockstep, with one step following the other, but were fluid, requiring her to be flexible in the collection and analysis of information.

Over the next 6 months, Alicia and the ASO staff created a plan that used what they had learned about the residents; the organization; and the local, state, and national environments and was based on sound theory and evidence from literature in occupational therapy, public health, psychology, and health promotion. As they started assessing the first residents to participate in the new supported employment program, Alicia reflected both on how much she had learned and how much more there was to know. More than anything, Alicia appreciated just how complex marketing and developing new services can be.

References

Bandura, A. (2000). Health promotion from the perspective of social cognitive theory. In P. Norman, C. Abrams, & M. Conner (eds.), *Understanding and Changing Health Behaviour from Health Beliefs to Self-Regulation* (pp. 299–342). Amsterdam: Overseas Publishers Association.

Braveman, B. (2006a). Developing evidence-based occupational therapy programming. In *Leading and Managing Occupational Therapy Services: An Evidence-Based Approach* (pp. 215–244). Philadelphia: F.A. Davis.

Braveman, B. (2006b). *Leading and Managing Occupational Therapy Services: An Evidence-Based Approach.* Philadelphia: F.A. Davis.

Braveman, B. (2006c). Marketing occupational therapy services. In *Leading & Managing Occupational Therapy Services: An Evidence-Based Approach* (pp. 333–346). Philadelphia: F.A. Davis.

Braveman, B. (2009). Management of occupational therapy services. In E. B. Crepeau, E. S. Cohn, & B. A. Boyt Schell (eds.), *Willard & Spackman's Occupational Therapy,* 11th ed. (pp. 914–928). Philadelphia: Wolters Kluwer/Lippincott Williams & Wilkins.

Braveman, B., Goldbaum, L., Goldstein, K., Karlic, L., & Kielhofner, G. (2001). *Employment Options: A Program Leading to the Employment of Persons Living with AIDS Program Manual.* Chicago: Model of Human Occupation Clearinghouse.

Braveman, B., Kielhofner, G., Belanger, R., Llerena, V., & de las Heras, C. G. (2002). Program development. In G. Kielhofner (ed.), *The Model of Human Occupation: Theory and Application,* 3rd ed. (pp. 491–519). Baltimore: Williams & Wilkins.

Braveman, B., Sen, S., & Kielhofner, G. (2001). Community-based vocational rehabilitation programs. In M. Scaffa (ed.), *Occupational Therapy in Community-based Practice Settings* (pp. 139–161). Philadelphia: F.A. Davis.

Brownson, C. (2001). Program development for community health: Planning, implementation and evaluation strategies. In M. Scaffa (ed.), *Occupational Therapy in Community-based Practice Settings* (pp. 95–116). Philadelphia: F.A. Davis.

Gitlin, L. N., Corcoran, M., Martindale-Adams, J., Malone, C., Stevens, A., & Winter, L. (2000). Identifying mechanisms of action: Why and how does intervention work? In R. Schulz (ed.), *Handbook of Dementia Caregiving: Evidence-based Interventions for Family Caregivers* (pp. 225–248). Philadelphia: Springer.

Grossman, J., & Bortone, J. (1986). Program development. In S. C. Robertson (ed.), *SCOPE: Strategies, Concepts, and Opportunities for Program Development and Evaluation* (pp. 91–99). Bethesda, MD: American Occupational Therapy Association.

Kielhofner, G. (2008). *Model of Human Occupation: Theory and Application.* Baltimore: Lippincott, Williams & Wilkins.

McLeroy, K. R., Bibeau, D., Steckler, A., & Glanz, K. (1988). An ecological perspective on health promotion programs. *Health Education Quarterly, 15*(4), 351–377.

Prochaska, J. O., DiClemente, C. C., & Norcross, J. C. (1992). In search of how people change: Applications to addictive behavior. *American Psychologist, 47*(9), 1102–1114.

Richmond, T. (2003). Marketing. In G. L. McCormack, E. G. Jaffe, & M. Goodman-Lavey (eds.), *The Occupational Therapy Manager* (pp. 177–192). Bethesda, MD: AOTA Press.

Scaffa, M. E. (2001). *Occupational Therapy in Community-based Practice Settings.* Philadelphia: F.A. Davis.

Strecher, V. J., DeVillis, B. M., Becker, M. H., & Rosenstock, I. M. (1986). The role of self-efficacy in achieving health behavior change. *Health Education Quarterly, 13*(1), 73–91.

Glossary

Dualism in health care means that both the government (federal, state, and local) and private business and industry are involved in the delivery of health care in the United States. In regard to work-related practice, dualism is illustrated through policies, laws, and systems such as the Americans with Disabilities Act (ADA) or the workers' compensations system.

Organizational assessment, the first step of the marketing process, involves collecting data and information to examine the internal influences that will impact the development of your product or service.

Environmental assessment is a step of the marketing process that examines data and information such as demographics, cultural trends, health-care utilization patterns, political and regulatory issues, new technologies, and socioeconomic status of the target populations served by your organization to help determine needs and existing resources.

Market analysis is the step in the marketing process during which you validate your perceptions of the wants and needs of your target population(s) using the data and information collected in your organizational and environmental assessments.

Marketing communications is the step in the marketing process during which you package and promote your product or service. Marketing communications involves devising methods of communicating with your target populations (customers), including potential clients, payers, and referral sources.

Mechanism of action is a condition that specifies (1) what changes, (2) how change proceeds, (3) the conditions under which an intervention achieves beneficial results, and (4) why a change may occur for certain groups of consumers and not for others

Needs assessment is the process of describing the target population, naming perceived and felt needs, and analyzing available resources and constraints both internal and external to the organization or context in which the program is being planned.

Program evaluation is the ongoing process of assessing the impact and quality of program processes and outcomes and making continuous improvements in efficiency and effectiveness.

Program implementation is the process of initiating intervention first in trial format and then in a more formal and sustained manner.

Program planning is the process of identifying the steps and sequence of actions to be taken to plan for initiation of the program.

Resources

Health Marketing Quarterly

Health Marketing Quarterly—an applied journal for marketing health and human services—is devoted to supplying how-to marketing tools for specific delivery systems. Each volume of this unique and informative journal demonstrates the applicability of marketing for specific health services. Health managers and providers will learn how to develop a thorough marketing approach and how marketing can improve awareness of opportunities, increase customer/patient satisfaction, and improve the cost-effectiveness of programs. This journal also acts as a resource manual for service managers to market current and future services. It bridges the gap between theory and application for service providers and administrators by presenting select marketing methodologies. In *Health Marketing Quarterly,* practitioners and academicians from selected delivery systems contribute valuable information targeted toward the latest growth areas in the health-care field. The journal focuses on group practice marketing, mental health marketing, long-term care marketing, marketing of ambulatory care, alternative care programs,

social services, hospitals, HMOs, health insurance, and health products.

American Marketing Association

www.marketingpower.com/

The American Marketing Association, one of the largest professional associations for marketers, has 38,000 members worldwide in every area of marketing. For over six decades, the AMA has been an essential resource providing relevant marketing information that experienced marketers turn to every day. The AMA website offers a wide array of newly expanded information, including research, case studies, and best practices in marketing. AMA's marketing journals provide access to the newest developments in marketing thought, while AMA magazines have practical applications of marketing strategies to address marketers' daily needs on the job. AMA offers specialty conferences, one-day hot topic seminars, boot camps, and workshops to help marketers build the skills that keep them ahead of emerging trends and help long-term professional development.

T & D Magazine

www.astd.org

T & D Magazine is published by the American Society of Training and Development, and its readers are degreed training and development professionals and line managers. They range from new practitioners to seasoned executives in business, government, academia, and consulting. The stated goals of *T & D Magazine* are to provide useful, how-to information on current best practices through case studies; share new technologies and their applications; report emerging trends, and address issues relevant and pivotal to the field.

American Public Health Association (APHA)

www.apha.org

APHA is the oldest and largest organization of public health professionals in the world, representing more than 50,000 members from over 50 occupations of public health. APHA is concerned with a broad set of issues affecting personal and environmental health, including federal and state funding for health programs, pollution control, programs and policies related to chronic and infectious diseases, a smoke-free society, and professional education in public health.

American Society of Training and Development (ASTD)

www.astd.org

ASTD's membership includes over 70,000 from various fields related to workplace learning and performance in over from over 100 countries. ASTD's mission is to provide leadership to individuals, organizations, and society to achieve work-related competence, performance, and fulfillment.

Index

Note: Page numbers with b indicate box; f indicate figure; t indicate table